Connections Between Diabetes Mellitus, Other Metabolic and Endocrine Dysfunctions and Cardiovascular Pathologies

Connections Between Diabetes Mellitus, Other Metabolic and Endocrine Dysfunctions and Cardiovascular Pathologies

Guest Editor

Cristina Tudoran

MDPI

Basel • Beijing • Wuhan • Barcelona • Belgrade • Novi Sad • Cluj • Manchester

Guest Editor
Cristina Tudoran
Discipline of Cardiology
University of Medicine and
Pharmacy "Victor Babes"
Timisoara
Timisoara
Romania

Editorial Office
MDPI AG
Grosspeteranlage 5
4052 Basel, Switzerland

This is a reprint of the Special Issue, published open access by the journal *Biomedicines* (ISSN 2227-9059), freely accessible at: https://www.mdpi.com/journal/biomedicines/special_issues/VLZ629F2VW.

For citation purposes, cite each article independently as indicated on the article page online and as indicated below:

Lastname, A.A.; Lastname, B.B. Article Title. *Journal Name* **Year**, *Volume Number*, Page Range.

ISBN 978-3-7258-5095-2 (Hbk)
ISBN 978-3-7258-5096-9 (PDF)
https://doi.org/10.3390/books978-3-7258-5096-9

Contents

About the Editor

Cristina Tudoran

Cristina Tudoran is a senior physician in cardiology who works at the Cardiology Clinic of the County Emergency Hospital "Pius Brinzeu" Timisoara and at the University of Medicine and Pharmacy "Victor Babes" Timisoara. She completed her PhD thesis in 2013 with "magna cum laude", and since then, she has continued her research on cardiovascular alterations in patients with various pathologies. In 2020, during the COVID-19 pandemic, her interest shifted toward investigating cardiac abnormalities in patients recovering from acute COVID-19 infection, also focusing on long-term follow-up. She published her first article on this topic in the Journal of Clinical Medicine at the beginning of 2021, shortly after the post-acute COVID-19 syndrome was first mentioned in the medical literature. Dr. Cristina Tudoran continued her research on cardiovascular abnormalities encountered in previously healthy individuals recovering from a SARS-CoV-2 infection and published over 17 articles on this topic.

Her research allowed her to fulfill the criteria for Dr. Habilitatus, obtaining her habilitation degree from the Romanian Ministry of Education in 2023. She also serves as a PhD coordinator at the University of Medicine and Pharmacy "Victor Babes" Timisoara.

She published 65 articles in Clarivate-indexed journals, has an H-index of 17, and served as Guest Editor in 11 Special Issues across various ISI-indexed journals. She is an Editorial Board Member of Frontiers for Cardiovascular Medicine and a member of the Romanian and European Society of Cardiology.

Preface

This Reprint aims to highlight new insights into significant genetic, ethnic, and socioeconomic risk factors for the diagnosis and treatment of patients with metabolic and endocrine dysfunctions and the associated cardiovascular pathology. The articles published in "Connections Between Diabetes Mellitus, Other Metabolic and Endocrine Dysfunctions, and Cardiovascular Pathologies" focus on the following three main topics: diagnostic challenges, treatment options, and uncommon associations between metabolic disorders and CVD in specific populations. The prevention and treatment of CVD during pregnancy have always posed challenges for physicians, and this Reprint provides valuable insights to enhance the management of these patients.

Cristina Tudoran
Guest Editor

biomedicines

MDPI

Editorial

Connections Between Diabetes Mellitus, Other Metabolic and Endocrine Dysfunctions, and Cardiovascular Pathologies

Cristina Tudoran [1,2,3]

[1] Department VII, Internal Medicine II, Discipline of Cardiology, University of Medicine and Pharmacy "Victor Babes" Timisoara, E. Murgu Square, Nr. 2, 300041 Timisoara, Romania; tudoran.cristina@umft.ro

[2] Centre of Molecular Research in Nephrology and Vascular Disease, University of Medicine and Pharmacy "Victor Babes" Timisoara, E. Murgu Square, Nr. 2, 300041 Timisoara, Romania

[3] County Emergency Hospital "Pius Brinzeu", L. Rebreanu, Nr. 156, 300723 Timisoara, Romania

The incidence of diabetes mellitus (DM) has progressively increased over the last decades. It still maintains its ascending trend due to the modern people's daily diet containing a large amount of glucose and lipids and the lack of physical activity, combined with the prolongation of the general population's life expectancy. According to the World Health Organization, it is estimated that around 830 million people are currently suffering from DM. MS is characterized by the coexistence of metabolic and cardiovascular (CV) risk factors in the same patient, such as dyslipidemia, elevated fasting glucose level and/or insulin resistance (IR), and increased blood pressure values or even systemic hypertension (SH). DM, metabolic syndrome (MS), and obesity are leading causes of morbidity and mortality worldwide. On the other hand, the incidence of CV disease (CVD) is also growing, especially in developing countries. This trend could at least partially explain why physicians encounter more often patients with several endocrine pathologies and/or metabolic disorders and CVD.

Physicians and researchers should not underestimate the enormous impact of DM, MS, obesity, hypothyroidism, primary aldosteronism (PA), and iron deficiency on the evolution of CVD, especially if the patient also develops heart failure (HF). Special attention should be given to pregnant women, as the onset of each of these endocrine disorders during this physiologic condition could worsen the patient's prognosis. Advances in gene regulation technology, clarification of pathophysiologic pathways in the glucose metabolism, development of new therapeutic approaches, and the use of artificial intelligence (AI) to improve diagnostic protocols open new horizons for the management of patients with various metabolic and endocrine dysfunctions, also allowing a precocious detection, even in a subclinical status, of CV alterations, thus preventing their evolution to a symptomatic disease with multiple consequences for the patient.

This Special Issue aims to highlight new insights into the significance of several risk factors (gene expression, race, ethnicity, and socioeconomic status) for the diagnosis and treatment of patients with DM and CVD and on the outcome of these individuals. The articles published in "Connections Between Diabetes Mellitus, Other Metabolic and Endocrine Dysfunctions, and Cardiovascular Pathologies" focus on three main topics: diagnostic challenges, treatment options, and uncommon associations between metabolic disorders and CVD in specific populations. The prevention and treatment of CVD during pregnancy have always raised challenges for physicians, and this Special Issue provides valuable insights for the better management of these women.

Regarding innovative diagnostic possibilities, special attention has been granted to the options offered by genetic analysis. In this regard, Stanciu et al. discuss the impact

 https://doi.org/10.3390/biomedicines13081980

of the mammalian target of rapamycin (mTOR) dysregulation on hyperglycemia and IR. MTOR is a serine/threonine protein kinase that belongs to the phosphoinositide 3-kinases (PI3K)-related protein kinase family, exerting a key role in glucose and lipid metabolism, cell growth, survival, and proliferation. mTOR hyperactivation may cause hyperglycaemia and IR, with a higher incidence in the Western population. The inhibition of mTOR, by various drugs, determines anti-inflammatory, antioxidant, and antitumoral effects, leading to decreased levels of glucose and triglycerides, and reduction of body weight. Dietary habits, proinflammatory cytokines, increased salt intake and renin–angiotensin–aldosterone system (RAAS) dysregulation induce mTOR overactivation, favoring the development of IR and AH.

Another point of interest was the early detection and effective risk assessment of DM and CVD, considering the increasing incidence of their association with impact on patients' outcomes. Advances in oculomics, exploring the relationship between retinal microvascular changes and systemic vascular health, offer a promising non-invasive approach for assessing CV risk. Retinal fundus imaging and optical coherence tomography/angiography provide critical information for precocious diagnosis of retinal vascular changes (vessel caliber, tortuosity, and branching patterns). Given the large volume of data generated during routine eye exams, there is a growing need for automated tools to facilitate diagnosis and risk prediction. Artificial intelligence (AI)-driven analysis of retinal images can accurately predict CV risk factors and events, and metabolic diseases, surpassing traditional diagnostic methods in some cases. AI-generated models achieve high sensitivity and specificity, surpassing other classical diagnostic methods. This approach highlights the potential of retinal imaging as a key component in personalized medicine, enabling more precise risk assessment and earlier intervention. It not only aids in detecting vascular abnormalities that may precede CV events, but also offers a scalable, non-invasive, and cost-effective solution for widespread screening. By integrating oculomics into routine clinical practice, healthcare providers could significantly enhance early detection and management of systemic diseases, ultimately improving patient outcomes. Fundus image analysis thus represents a valuable tool in the future of precision medicine and CV health management.

Other laboratory analyses, as the triglyceride-to-high-density lipoprotein (TG/HDL) ratio, stand out as a viable option to determine early changes in lipid metabolism associated with IR, offering a cost-effective and straightforward alternative to traditional, more complex biomarkers. This research reveals the TG/HDL ratio's predictive power across ethnicities and sexes, with specific thresholds providing greater accuracy for Caucasians, Asians, and Hispanics compared to African Americans, and for men versus women. The analysis of the TG/HDL ratio is a simple, accessible marker for IR.

The pathogenesis of diabetic kidney disease (DKD) is complex and multifactorial. It is frequently associated with different degrees of albuminuria, ranging from normoalbuminuria, microalbuminuria, to macroalbuminuria. Considering its complications and reduced number of diagnostic biomarkers, it is important to develop new biomarkers with potential roles in the early diagnosis of DKD. Glycine, tiglylglycine, kynurenic acid, and tryptophan may be considered promising biomarkers for early diagnosis of DKD and DM type 2 progression follow-up.

DM type II, along with atherosclerotic vascular disease, results in several feared complications, one of them being acute peripheral ischemia. Actual research focuses on identifying new inflammatory markers for the diagnosis, treatment of critical ischemia, and prognosis assessment. Further studies are required to define risk classes and to estimate the prognosis of critical ischemia. We also need to identify specific markers for the clinical staging of this disease in the post-revascularization phase, both in terms of surgical complications related to revascularization and of major CV events.

Another DM type 2 complication is diabetic retinopathy. The most important risk factors for the occurrence, evolution, and management of diabetic retinopathy are poor glycaemic control and longer DM duration, while the most impacting comorbidities are AH, CVD, chronic kidney disease (CKD), and dyslipidaemia. Early detection and management of systemic risk factors may avert this DM complication. However, the primary and fundamental strategy for preventing ocular complications in diabetic patients requires tight glycaemic control.

Recent data suggest that patients with DM are predisposed to develop myocardial fibrosis sooner, a contributor to adverse cardiac remodelling following acute myocardial infarction, leading to the occurrence of HF, a complex clinical syndrome caused by structural or functional dysfunction of the ventricular filling. In this regard, in the last years, new drugs have been developed, some of which are not only effective in reducing basal blood glucose levels, but they also improve the outcome of patients with HF. Other studies draw attention to the fact that most antidiabetic drugs have controversial effects on the risk of HF (thiazolidinediones, saxagliptin in the DPP-4i, and even insulin). Researchers still debate the safety of metformin in patients with HF. Emerging evidence suggests that anti-diabetic medications, such as sodium-glucose transporter 2 (SGLT2i), glucagon-like peptide-1 receptor agonists (GLP-1Ras), and dipeptidyl peptidase-4 (DPP4i), may have an important role in reducing fibrosis, improving CV outcomes, and reducing the burden of HF. SGLT2i and even GLP-1 RAs achieved positive results for HF endpoints, with SGLT2i in particular significantly reducing the composite endpoint of CV mortality and hospitalization for HF. Further understanding of the mutual pathophysiological mechanisms between HF and DM may facilitate the detection of novel therapeutic targets to improve the clinical outcome.

Another topic of this Special Issue was the diagnosis and treatment of patients with primary aldosteronism (PA) and associated comorbidities treated by general practitioners. We determined a significant association between PA and various chronic diseases, including AH, hypokalemia, hepatic steatosis, gout, CKD, obesity, and depression. Notably, PA patients exhibited a markedly higher likelihood of developing gout compared to those without PA. The findings underline the need for early detection and individualized management strategies for PA to mitigate the associated risks and improve patient outcomes.

Pregnancy is a physiologic condition that can exacerbate underlying pathologies or even cause complications endangering both mother and child. Some of these comorbidities raise diagnostic and therapeutic challenges. The pathologies debated in this Special Issue are endothelial dysfunction, SH, and hypothyroidism in pregnant women and their impact on the fetus. We also focused on methods to prevent these co-morbidities in healthy high-risk pregnant women. We demonstrated that in pregnant women with preeclampsia and pregnancy-induced hypertension, increased arterial stiffness may be involved in the pathogenesis of preterm birth, suggesting an association between fetal development and maternal endothelial dysfunction. Pulse wave analysis may be a non-invasive, reliable, clinically applicable method for assessing maternal arterial stiffness (AS). It may be more relevant to intrauterine fetal growth when associated with lower serum 25(OH)D levels. Subclinical hypothyroidism treated with levothyroxine in women with gestational DM does not increase the risk of gestational hypertensive disorders but is associated with an increased risk of prematurity. Petre et al. state that physical training, coordinated by a medical team consisting of an obstetrician, a physiotherapist, and a cardiologist, decreases systolic and diastolic blood pressure values and heart rate in healthy pregnant women. Strictly supervised physical training may reduce pregnancy-induced SH. Pulse wave velocity is also recommended for screening of elevated AS during pregnancy. Additionally, regular exercise in healthy pregnant women decreases AS, suggesting that it may help to prevent endothelial dysfunction, AS, and SH during pregnancy.

Iron deficiency (ID) is a common condition in patients with acute coronary syndrome. Although its influence on short-term follow-up appears to be uncertain, ID seems to be independently associated with a worse prognosis during the mid- to long-term follow-up of the patient. Transferrin saturation, contrary to ferritin, is not upregulated during acute conditions, which may be crucial for the non-invasive diagnosis of ID. Transferrin saturation appears to have a greater predictive value on death and other adverse events compared to ferritin or serum iron concentration, but there are new, promising, precise markers employed for non-invasive ID diagnosis in clinical practice. Iron supplementation in patients with acute coronary syndrome may have a beneficial effect on myocardial healing and left ventricular remodeling after myocardial infarction, but further research, especially on human models, is needed to support this theory.

Dumitrescu et al. point out that disadvantaged populations exhibit a significantly higher prevalence of DM, impaired glucose regulation, SH, and dyslipidemia. Another risk factor for CVD is the type of obesity, especially important in patients with DM type 1. In men, central adiposity, assessed by total, trunk, and android fat mass, is associated with higher glucose and lower glucose variability. In women, gynoid fat mass, but not other body composition parameters, is related to hyperglycemia. The observed associations of body weight and body composition with the features of daily glucose dynamics may be mediated by insulin sensitivity.

Cosoreanu et al. studied the prevalence of CV risk factors, CVD, and microvascular complications among the Roma population, underscoring the importance of considering ethnic disparities in approaching healthcare management strategies. Regarding the anthropometric and paraclinical assessments, her data evidenced different characteristics in the Roma compared to a corresponding group of non-Roma, highlighting the importance of tailoring healthcare interventions to the specific needs and cultural context of this ethnic minority.

Fukuda et al. highlight the particularities of IR in the Japanese population. In these individuals, the age-related high prevalence of DM and impaired insulin tolerance is associated with impaired insulin secretion rather than IR.

A specific situation arose at the end of 2019, when the coronavirus disease (COVID-19) resulted in a worldwide pandemic. New data regarding the multisystemic effects of the severe acute respiratory syndrome coronavirus 2 (SARS-CoV-2) emerged. Several studies determined that COVID-19 has negative effects on the glycemic control in DM and non-DM patients. Predicting post-COVID-19 diabetes is crucial for enhancing patient care and public health. Our research investigates the role of metabolic factors in predicting glycemic outcomes in patients recovering from moderate to severe COVID-19. Conventional diabetes risk factors, including body mass index and lipid profiles, showed low predictive power for post-COVID-19 glycemia. This Special Issue highlights the critical role of metabolic and inflammatory pathways in managing glycemic control in COVID-19 patients. Markers such as blood glucose, Homeostasis Model Assessment of Insulin Resistance, and high-sensitivity C-reactive protein are significant predictors of blood glucose levels, while the triglyceride/glucose index appears less helpful in this context. Early, targeted interventions based on these markers can improve patient outcomes and reduce the risk of post-COVID-19 complications, such as DM.

This compilation of articles highlights the importance of a precocious diagnosis and assessment of the risk profile in patients with metabolic diseases and CVD, especially HF, as well as in specific physiological conditions (pregnant women) and special populations (the Roma population, native Japanese, and people living in developing countries). Special interest should be given to pregnant women with subclinical hypothyroidism or with vitamin D deficiency and pre-eclampsia. Further studies are required to determine the importance of specific genetic and environmental factors and lifestyle changes on CV risk profiles in subjects with metabolic disorders for targeted interventions addressed to these high-risk populations. Continued research efforts in this area are essential for improving our understanding and refining treatment strategies to optimize patients' outcomes.

Acknowledgments: I express my gratitude to the entire editorial team of *Biomedicines*. Without their expertise and professionalism, "Connections Between Diabetes Mellitus, Other Metabolic and Endocrine Dysfunctions, and Cardiovascular Pathologies" would never have been so successful. I would also like to express my appreciation to all the contributors who chose to submit their valuable work to this Special Issue, making it possible for us to publish this pre-print.

Conflicts of Interest: The author declares no conflicts of interest.

List of Contributions:

1. Misiewicz, A.; Badura, K.; Matuszewska-Brycht, O.; Krekora, J.; Drożdż, J. Iron Deficiency as a Factor of Worse Prognosis in Patients with Acute Myocardial Infarction. *Biomedicines* **2025**, *13*, 769. https://doi.org/10.3390/biomedicines13040769.
2. Mogos, M.; Milas, O.; Socaciu, C.; Socaciu, A.I.; Vlad, A.; Gadalean, F.; Bob, F.; Cretu, O.M.; Suteanu-Simulescu, A.; Glavan, M.; et al. Urinary and Serum Amino Acids May Be Associated with Podocyte, Proximal Tubule, and Renal Endothelial Injury in Early Diabetic Kidney Disease in Type 2 Diabetes Mellitus Patients. *Biomedicines* **2025**, *13*, 675. https://doi.org/10.3390/biomedicines13030675.
3. Fukuda, K.; Haneda, M.; Kubota, N.; Araki, E.; Yamagata, K. Age-Related Glucose Intolerance Is Associated with Impaired Insulin Secretion in Community-Dwelling Japanese Adults: The Kumamoto Koshi Study. *Biomedicines* **2025**, *13*, 380. https://doi.org/10.3390/biomedicines13020380.
4. Andor, M.; Man, D.E.; Nistor, D.C.; Buda, V.; Dragan, S. The Influence of COVID-19 in Glycemic Control: Predictive Value of Inflammation and Metabolic Parameters. *Biomedicines* **2024**, *12*, 2642. https://doi.org/10.3390/biomedicines12112642.
5. Mihai, M.; Vladut, S.; Lucian, P.G.; Irina, M.E.; Victoria, N.; Claudiu, M. Subclinical Hypothyroidism and Gestational Hypertensive Disorders in a Cohort of Romanian Pregnant Women with Gestational Diabetes Mellitus: A Pilot Study. *Biomedicines* **2024**, *12*, 2587. https://doi.org/10.3390/biomedicines12112587.
6. Krieg, A.; Krieg, S.; Heuser, A.; Laverenz, U.; Istrate, V.-A.; Schott, M.; Kostev, K. Exploring the Spectrum of Comorbidities Associated with Primary Aldosteronism: Insights from a Large Real-World Case-Control Study. *Biomedicines* **2024**, *12*, 2479. https://doi.org/10.3390/biomedicines12112479.
7. Ghenciu, L.A.; Dima, M.; Stoicescu, E.R.; Iacob, R.; Boru, C.; Hațegan, O.A. Retinal Imaging-Based Oculomics: Artificial Intelligence as a Tool in the Diagnosis of Cardiovascular and Metabolic Diseases. *Biomedicines* **2024**, *12*, 2150. https://doi.org/10.3390/biomedicines12092150.
8. Dumitrescu, A.; Vitcu, G.M.; Stoica, S.; Susa, S.R.; Stoicescu, E.R. Cardiovascular Risk Factors in Socioeconomically Disadvantaged Populations in a Suburb of the Largest City in Western Romania. *Biomedicines* **2024**, *12*, 1989. https://doi.org/10.3390/biomedicines12091989.
9. Semenova, J.F.; Yushin, A.Y.; Korbut, A.I.; Klimontov, V.V. Glucose Variability in People with Type 1 Diabetes: Associations with Body Weight, Body Composition, and Insulin Sensitivity. *Biomedicines* **2024**, *12*, 2006. https://doi.org/10.3390/biomedicines12092006.
10. Ivanescu, A.; Popescu, S.; Ivanescu, R.; Potra, M.; Timar, R. Predictors of Diabetic Retinopathy in Type 2 Diabetes: A Cross-Sectional Study. *Biomedicines* **2024**, *12*, 1889. https://doi.org/10.3390/biomedicines12081889.
11. Stanciu, S.M.; Jinga, M.; Miricescu, D.; Stefani, C.; Nica, R.I.; Stanescu-Spinu, I.-I.; Vacaroiu, I.A.; Greabu, M.; Nica, S. mTOR Dysregulation, Insulin Resistance, and Hypertension. *Biomedicines* **2024**, *12*, 1802. https://doi.org/10.3390/biomedicines12081802.

12. Iurciuc, M.; Buleu, F.; Iurciuc, S.; Petre, I.; Popa, D.; Moleriu, R.D.; Bordianu, A.; Suciu, O.; Tasdemir, R.; Dragomir, R.-E.; et al. Effect of Vitamin D Deficiency on Arterial Stiffness in Pregnant Women with Preeclampsia and Pregnancy-Induced Hypertension and Implications for Fetal Development. *Biomedicines* **2024**, *12*, 1595. https://doi.org/10.3390/biomedicines12071595.
13. Li, X.; Zhou, X.; Gao, L. Diabetes and Heart Failure: A Literature Review, Reflection and Outlook. *Biomedicines* **2024**, *12*, 1572. https://doi.org/10.3390/biomedicines12071572.
14. Baneu, P.; Văcărescu, C.; Drăgan, S.-R.; Cirin, L.; Lazăr-Höcher, A.-I.; Cozgarea, A.; Faur-Grigori, A.-A.; Crișan, S.; Gaiță, D.; Luca, C.-T.; et al. The Triglyceride/HDL Ratio as a Surrogate Biomarker for Insulin Resistance. *Biomedicines* **2024**, *12*, 1493. https://doi.org/10.3390/biomedicines12071493.
15. Cosoreanu, A.; Rusu, E.; Rusu, F.; Stanciu, S.; Ungureanu, I.; Donici, M.; Visinescu, A.; Enache, G.; Radulian, G. Clinical and Metabolic Particularities of a Roma Population with Diabetes—Considering Ethnic Disparities in Approaching Healthcare Management. *Biomedicines* **2024**, *12*, 1422. https://doi.org/10.3390/biomedicines12071422.
16. Tudurachi, B.-S.; Anghel, L.; Tudurachi, A.; Sascău, R.A.; Zanfirescu, R.-L.; Stătescu, C. Unraveling the Cardiac Matrix: From Diabetes to Heart Failure, Exploring Pathways and Potential Medications. *Biomedicines* **2024**, *12*, 1314. https://doi.org/10.3390/biomedicines12061314.
17. Petre, I.; Iurciuc, S.; Buleu, F.; Petre, I.; Moleriu, R.D.; Popa, D.; Turi, V.; Bordianu, A.; Tasdemir, R.; Craciun, L.M.; et al. The Impact of Medical Physical Training and a Structured Personalized Exercise Training Program on Hemodynamic Parameters and Arterial Stiffness in Pregnant Women. *Biomedicines* **2024**, *12*, 986. https://doi.org/10.3390/biomedicines12050986.
18. Popescu, A.I.; Rata, A.L.; Barac, S.; Popescu, R.; Onofrei, R.R.; Vlad, C.; Vlad, D. Narrative Review of Biological Markers in Chronic Limb-Threatening Ischemia. *Biomedicines* **2024**, *12*, 798. https://doi.org/10.3390/biomedicines12040798.

biomedicines

Review

mTOR Dysregulation, Insulin Resistance, and Hypertension

Silviu Marcel Stanciu [1,†], Mariana Jinga [1], Daniela Miricescu [2,*], Constantin Stefani [3,†], Remus Iulian Nica [4,5], Iulia-Ioana Stanescu-Spinu [6,*], Ileana Adela Vacaroiu [7], Maria Greabu [2] and Silvia Nica [8,9]

1 Department of Internal Medicine and Gastroenterology, Carol Davila University of Medicine and Pharmacy, Central Military Emergency University Hospital, "Dr. Carol Davila", 010825 Bucharest, Romania; silviu.stanciu@umfcd.ro (S.M.S.); mariana.jinga@umfcd.ro (M.J.)
2 Discipline of Biochemistry, Faculty of Dentistry, Carol Davila University of Medicine and Pharmacy, 8 Eroii Sanitari Blvd, 050474 Bucharest, Romania; maria.greabu@umfcd.ro
3 Department of Family Medicine and Clinical Base, Central Military Emergency University Hospital, "Dr. Carol Davila", 010825 Bucharest, Romania; constantin.stefani@umfcd.ro
4 Surgery Department, Central Military Emergency University Hospital, "Dr. Carol Davila", 010825 Bucharest, Romania; remus.nica@umfcd.ro
5 Discipline of General Surgery, Carol Davila University of Medicine and Pharmacy, 8 Eroii Sanotari Blvd, 054474 Bucharest, Romania
6 Discipline of Physiology, Faculty of Dentistry, Carol Davila University of Medicine and Pharmacy, 8 Eroii Sanitari Blvd, 050474 Bucharest, Romania
7 Department of Nephrology, Faculty of Medicine, Carol Davila University of Medicine and Pharmacy, 020021 Bucharest, Romania; ileana.vacaroiu@umfcd.ro
8 Emergency Discipline, University Hospital of Bucharest, 050098 Bucharest, Romania; silvia.nica@umfcd.ro
9 Department of Emergency and First Aid, Carol Davila University of Medicine and Pharmacy, 8 Eroii Sanitari Blvd, 050474 Bucharest, Romania
* Correspondence: daniela.miricescu@umfcd.ro (D.M.); iulia.stanescu@umfcd.ro (I.-I.S.-S.)
† These authors contributed equally to this work.

Abstract: Worldwide, diabetes mellitus (DM) and cardiovascular diseases (CVDs) represent serious health problems associated with unhealthy diet and sedentarism. Metabolic syndrome (MetS) is characterized by obesity, dyslipidemia, hyperglycemia, insulin resistance (IR) and hypertension. The mammalian target of rapamycin (mTOR) is a serine/threonine kinase with key roles in glucose and lipid metabolism, cell growth, survival and proliferation. mTOR hyperactivation disturbs glucose metabolism, leading to hyperglycemia and further to IR, with a higher incidence in the Western population. Metformin is one of the most used hypoglycemic drugs, with anti-inflammatory, antioxidant and antitumoral properties, having also the capacity to inhibit mTOR. mTOR inhibitors such as rapamycin and its analogs everolimus and temsirolimus block mTOR activity, decrease the levels of glucose and triglycerides, and reduce body weight. The link between mTOR dysregulation, IR, hypertension and mTOR inhibitors has not been fully described. Therefore, the main aim of this narrative review is to present the mechanism by which nutrients, proinflammatory cytokines, increased salt intake and renin–angiotensin–aldosterone system (RAAS) dysregulation induce mTOR overactivation, associated further with IR and hypertension development, and also mTOR inhibitors with higher potential to block the activity of this protein kinase.

Keywords: sedentarism; obesity; insulin resistance; protein kinases; mTOR dysregulation; metformin; inhibitors

1. Introduction

Sedentarism, obesity, smoking, older age and male sex are risk factors for diabetes mellitus (DM) and cancer [1]. Diets rich in refined carbohydrates, sugar and processed foods are correlated with an increased risk to develop metabolic syndrome (MetS), DM and cardiovascular diseases (CVDs) [2]. Globally, more than 425 million people have type 2 DM (T2D) [3], representing an alarming public health problem worldwide [4,5]. Globally, one of three deaths is attributed to CVD [6], and it is estimated that 1.56 billion people will develop hypertension by 2025 [7]. MetS also represents a serious health problem worldwide, being characterized by obesity, dyslipidemia, insulin resistance (IR), hyperglycemia and hypertension [8]. The prevalence of MetS in the adult population is between 15 and 25%, with an increasing number every year [9]. Moreover, visceral obesity together with a sedentary life and high-fat intake are important key factors for IR development [10]. Obesity and IR increase every year worldwide [11]. Obesity, especially visceral obesity, represents one of the major risk factors for human primary hypertension, accounting for 65% to 75% [12]. In addition, DM-obese patients with hypertension have a higher rate of developing chronic kidney disease (CKD) [13].

The mammalian target of rapamycin (mTOR) plays an essential role in regulating cell growth, proliferation, survival [14], protein synthesis [15], glucose and lipid metabolism [16]. Moreover, mTOR can regulate blood sugar levels [17]. mTOR dysregulation is correlated with various systemic pathologies including cancer, arthritis, osteoporosis and IR [18]. The main aim of this narrative review is to present the mechanism by which mTOR can induce the development of IR and, further, of hypertension.

2. mTOR Pathway Overview

mTOR is a serine/threonine protein kinase that belongs to the phosphoinositide 3-kinases (PI3K)-related protein kinase families, and is formed by two complexes known as mTOR complex 1 (mTORC1) and mTOR complex 2 (mTORC2) in mammalians [19]. Regarding the structure, both mTOR complexes have some similarities concerning the catalytic subunit, DEP domain-containing mTOR-interacting protein (DEPTOR), and the Tti1/Tti2. mTORC1 has six protein complexes, while mTORC2 has seven [20]. mTORC1 has three core components including mTOR, a regulatory protein associated with mTOR (Raptor), and mammalian lethal with Sec13protein 8, also known as GβL (mLST8) [21]. Moreover, mTORC2 core components include rapamycin-insensitive companion of mTOR (Rictor), stress-activated protein kinase-interacting protein 1 (MSIN1) and protein observed with Rictor 1 and 2 (PROTOR $\frac{1}{2}$) [22]. mTORC1 core proteins include Raptor, mLST8, proline-rich protein kinase B (AKT) substrate (PRAS40) and DEPTOR [23]. Two small G proteins, Ras homolog enriched in the brain (Rheb) and Ras-related GTPases (Rags), are required for activation and localization of mTORC1. Moreover, Rags form two types of heterodimers, Rag-A or Rag-B with Rag-C and Rag-D [24].

Raptor and Rictor act as scaffolds for assembling the two mTOR complexes and as regulators for the binding of substrates [25]. mTORC1 activation occurs via nutrients and AKT, which phosphorylate the tuberous sclerosis complex 2 (TSC2) and inhibit it [26]. TSC refers to the altered gene of tuberous sclerosis complex, an autosomal dominant disease. TSC1 is an important component of the PI3K/AKT/mTOR pathway involved in cell growth, survival, proliferation and autophagy [27].

TSC1/2 regulate mTOR activity [28], and, therefore, their deletion reduces AKT activity [29], being negative regulators of the PI3K/AKT/mTOR signaling pathway together with phosphate and tensin homolog (PTEN) [30]. PTEN, TSC1 and TSC2 inhibit mTOR activity via PI3K/AKT inhibition [31]. Moreover, TSC mutations may affect glucose metabolism and insulin signaling, which can cause mTORC1 activation [32].

Growth factors, insulin, hypoxia, low ATP ratio, tumor necrosis factor alfa (TNF-α), Wnt, leucine, glutamate and arginine induce mTOR activation via different pathways [33], considered the central integrator of several signals [34] in both normal and pathological conditions [35].

Nutrients, energy, oxygen levels, stress and growth factors activate mTORC1 after their binding to tyrosine kinase receptors (RTKs) and further activation of PI3K and AKT, and inhibition of TSC1 and TSC2 [36]. Once activated by phosphorylation, AKT will exert a wide range of functions, such as cell growth, survival and metabolism [37]. AKT stimulates protein synthesis via mTOR activation, phosphorylates and inactivates AKT substrate 160 (AS160) and glycogen synthase kinase 3 (GSK3). Therefore, the inaction of AS160 and GSK3 will induce GLUT4 translocation into the plasma membrane, and glucose will enter the cells [38]. GSK3 is another important member of the PI3K/AKT/mTOR family involved in metabolism, proliferation, insulin signaling and apoptosis [39] (Figure 1).

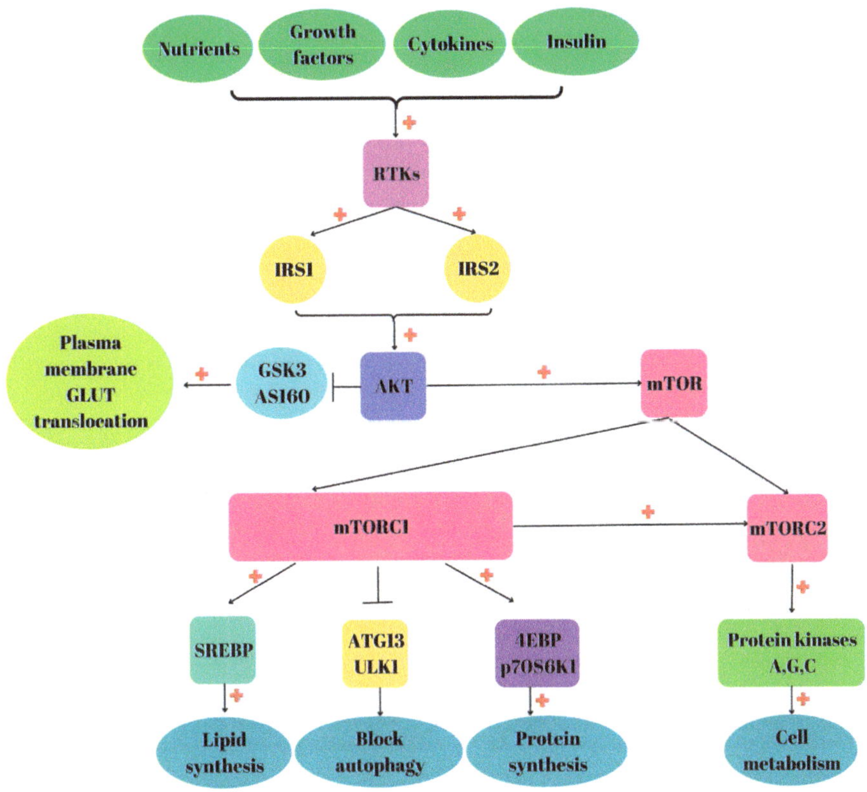

Figure 1. Phosphatidylinositol 3-kinase (PI3K) protein kinases B (AKT)/mammalian target of rapamycin (mTOR) pathway in healthy conditions: Nutrients, growth factors, cytokines and insulin bind to tyrosine kinases receptors (RTKs), leading to insulin receptors substrate 1 or 2 (IRS1/IRS2) activation and further AKT activation by phosphorylation. Once activated, AKT will phosphorylate other protein kinases such as mTOR, composed of the two complexes mTOR complex 1 (mTORC1) and mTOR complex 2 (mTORC2). mTORC1 activates sterol response element binding protein (SREBP) and eukaryotic translation initiator factor 4E binding protein (4EBP) and 70Ka ribosomal protein S56 kinase 1 (p70S6K1), leading to lipid and protein synthesis, respectively. mTORC1 inhibits the activity of unc-51-like kinase 1 (ULK1) and autophagy-related gene 13 (ATG13) blocking autophagy. Inactivation of AKT substrate 160 (AS160) and glycogen synthase 3 (GSK3) induces plasma membrane GLUT translocation. mTORC2 activates other protein kinases such as A, G and C, which positively regulate cellular metabolism. Activation of PI3K/AKT/mTOR will be correlated with cell growth, survival and proliferation. "+" activation.

Protein intake induces mTORC1 activation because amino acids stimulate the Rag GTPases to facilitate the binding to Raptor [40]. Insulin activates both mTORC1 and mTORC2 via PI3K [41]. Furthermore, mTORC1 activation can be performed by resistance exercises, leading to increased synthesis of muscle proteins [42]. Insulin-like growth factor (IGF-1R) and epidermal growth factor receptor (EGFR) regulate mTORC2 [43]. The presence of cytokines, nutrients, energy and hormones, in the cellular environment, induces the recruitment of mTORC1 from the cytoplasm to the lysosome via GTP-bound Rag-A or Rag-B and GTP-bound Rag-C or Rag-D [24].

mTORC1 directly phosphorylates 70 kDa ribosomal protein S6 kinase 1 (p70S6K1) and eukaryotic translation initiation factor 4E binding protein (4EBP) and induces protein synthesis. Moreover, mTORC1 stimulates lipid synthesis through the sterol response element binding protein (SREBP) transcription factor, which satisfies membrane formation during cell growth [44]. In addition, mTORC1 is located at the lysosomal surface, which controls protein synthesis and cellular growth. mTORC2 controls cell metabolism, survival and proliferation via phosphorylation of the protein kinases A, G, C and actin cellular cytoskeleton [45].

mTOR complex plays a key role in liver and adipose tissue lipogenesis via SREBP, considered the master transcriptional regulator of lipogenesis [46]. mTORC1 can phosphorylate various downstream effectors such as p70S6K and regulate mRNA translation [47] and cellular metabolic homeostasis [48]. mTORC1 inhibits autophagy by the phosphorylation of two kinases, unc-51-like kinase 1 (ULK1) and autophagy-related gene 13 (ATG13) [49].

The prolonged mTORC1 activation in the presence of a high-energy diet inhibits IRS via p70S6K blocking GLUTs inside the cells, increasing the blood glucose level, leading to T2D development [50]. In the case of DM patients, a significant downregulation of phosphorylated mTOR and p70S6K had been reported using peripheral blood mononuclear cells (PBMCs) [51].

3. Insulin Resistance Overview

In normal situations, after a meal, the increased plasmatic levels of glucose stimulate the secretion of insulin by pancreatic β cells, promoting carbohydrate uptake by adipose tissue, liver and skeletal muscles [52]. Therefore, in heathy conditions, insulin maintains the normal levels of blood glucose into the body organs by various mechanisms [53]. In the liver and skeletal muscle, insulin stimulates glycogen [54] and triglycerides synthesis [53]. Regarding the lipid metabolism in the adipose tissue, insulin stimulates fatty acids and triglycerides' synthesis and inhibits lipolysis. In the liver and muscles, insulin decreases fatty acid beta-oxidation. The action of insulin in protein metabolism involves stimulation of protein synthesis in the adipose tissue, liver and muscle, by increasing the entry rate of amino acids into the tissue. In muscles, it reduces the degradation rate of proteins [55]. In the diabetic skeletal muscles, genes that encode carbohydrate, energy and amino acids pathways are decreased, including *IRS2*, *mTOR*, *SLC2A4* and *PPARA* [56].

In 1936, Himmsworth introduced the notion of IR, which divided diabetic patients into two categories: insulin sensitive and insulin-insensitive [57]. The incidence of IR in the Western population is around 25–35%, usually associated with obesity and obesity-related complications, being a risk factor for CVD, T2D, infertility, nonalcoholic fatty liver (NAFLD), certain types of cancer [58,59] and kidney dysfunction [60]. IR represents a metabolic disorder characterized by sensitivity to exogenous or endogenous insulin, leading to the body's inability to capture glucose inside the cells [59]. Clinically, IR is also called IR syndrome or syndrome X [61], closely related to MetS [62], and is the first stage of T2D [63].

A very important aspect is that IR can be detected 10–20 years before the hyperglycemia's clinical onset [64]. Moreover, IR can be predicted by several tests including blood glucose detection, serum insulin measurement, the glucose tolerance test and HOMA-R [65]. IR and hyperinsulinemia are characterized by higher levels of serum triglycerides and LDL, and decreased HDL [66]. Another important aspect is that elevated HbA1C between 7 and 10% is positively correlated with macro- and microvascular-T2D diseases [67]. IR is positively associated with visceral obesity, dyslipidemia, microalbuminemia and proinflammatory events [68]. In obese individuals, secretion of IL-1, TNF-α, leptin, adipsin, adiponectin and visfatin contribute to chronic inflammation development [69]. IR is also induced by the release of proinflammatory cytokines, such as TNF-α, with increased concentrations in chronic inflammation [70].

Systemic IR is characterized by ATP overproduction by several mechanisms including mitochondrial dysfunction, AMP-activated protein kinase (AMPK) inhibition, mTOR activation, hyperinsulinemia and hyperglucagonemia [71,72].

The liver, muscles and adipose tissue are affected by IR. Therefore, being insulin-dependent organs, glucose uptake is impaired. In addition, in the liver, insulin loses its capacity to inhibit glycogenolysis and gluconeogenesis [73]. IR is defined by the lack of receptors and GLUTs [74], and represents one of the main markers of T2D associated with lipid metabolism dysregulation. Because the skeletal muscle utilizes around 75–80% of systemic glucose, it presents a crucial role in IR [75]. Studies performed in humans and rodents reported that in skeletal muscles, IR decreases glucose uptake, inhibits glycogen synthesis, and induces hyperglycemia [76]. Additionally, IR and metabolic syndrome lead to muscle mass loss [77]. Thus, skeletal muscle-insulin resistance represents a major pathogenic factor for T2D or type 1 diabetes mellitus (T1D) [78].

In adipocytes, IR is characterized by decreased expression of GLUT4 and also dysregulation regarding secretion of leptin, TNF-α and adiponectin [79]. Adipose tissue-IR directly contributes to liver and muscle IR because higher levels of free fatty acids (FFAs) released would be delivered to these organs [80].

IR and IR syndrome may have several mechanisms as follows: a. genetic abnormalities regarding one or more proteins from the insulin cascade; b. fetal malnutrition; and c. visceral obesity [81]. Regarding T2D, several mechanisms have been postulated, including a lack of GLUTs, IRSs or glucose metabolism enzymes that did not interact with insulin receptors, leading to the inhibition of insulin transport and function [82].

T2D or IR lead to several complications, such as hypertension, atherosclerosis, liver disorders and various types of cancer [83].

4. mTOR Dysregulation and Insulin Resistance

Through its signaling cascade, insulin controls normal growth, metabolism and survival via the activation of PI3K, AKT, mTOR and Mitogen-Activated Protein Kinases (MAPKs). PI3K activation involves the activation of insulin receptor substrate 1 (IRS1), IRS2 and FoxO1 by phosphorylation, playing a key role in nutrient homeostasis and organ survival. IRS1 and IRS2 suppression by AKT inactivation leads to hyperinsulinemia and metabolic inflammation [84]. IRS1 is involved in glucose regulation, including GLUT4 translocation, while IR2 is implicated in adipocyte-fatty acid metabolism [85]. The insulin receptor is a tetramer protein that contains extracellular α subunits and transmembrane β subunits. Insulin or insulin-like growth factors (IGF-1s) bind to insulin receptor α subunits, leading to conformational changes of insulin receptors and dimerization of β subunits [86]. Therefore, IRS dysregulation is involved in metabolic disease initiation and progression [87].

Newgard and his research team reported that rats fed with a high-fat diet and a fat diet supplemented with branched-chain amino acids (BCAAs) develop IR. IR is correlated with chronic phosphorylation of mTOR, c-Jun N-terminal kinase (JNK) and IRS1 [88]. Additionally, BCAA overload leads to IR by mTOR activation [89].

Using primary cultures of rat cortical neurons, Pomytkin and his research team reported that elevated intracellular Ca^{2+} concentrations induced by glutamate and mitochondrial depolarization promote cytotoxicity on IRS, blocking them and further PI3K/AKT/mTOR, stimulating IR development [90].

mTORC1 hyperactivation induces energy metabolism and translation dysregulation, leading to MetS [91]. Excessive consumption of glucose or BCAA chronically activates mTORC1, which further phosphorylates IRS1 at Ser 307 and activates S6K1. This aberrant activation decreases the activity and responsiveness of mTORC1 to insulin, leading to cell IR [92]. Dysregulation of the substrates for insulin receptors plays a key role in IR development, being controlled by more than 50 serine/threonine kinases, with positive or negative impact on insulin sensitivity [93]. In addition, overnutrition mediates obesity and triggers mTOR chronic hyperactivation in various tissues [94], promoting IR, hyperlipidemia, inflammation, stress and vasoconstriction [95]. Elevated FFAs contribute to

IR by activation of IRS1 and further-downstream kinases such as mTOR, p70S6K1 and GSK3 [96]. Excessive alcohol consumption affects mTOR activity via dysregulation of protein synthesis and decreased activity of metabolic enzymes [97]. Long-term treatment with rapamycin disassembles mTORC2, leading to IR [98]. However, den Hartigh and his research team reported in a study conducted on obese male mice that a moderately low dose of rapamycin decreased weight gain and adiposity and improved the metabolic profile regarding triglycerides obesity [99]. Adipose tissue contributes to IR development, being an important source of proinflammatory molecule release such as TNF-α, leptin, IL-6, and anti-inflammatory compounds like adiponectin [100] (Figure 2).

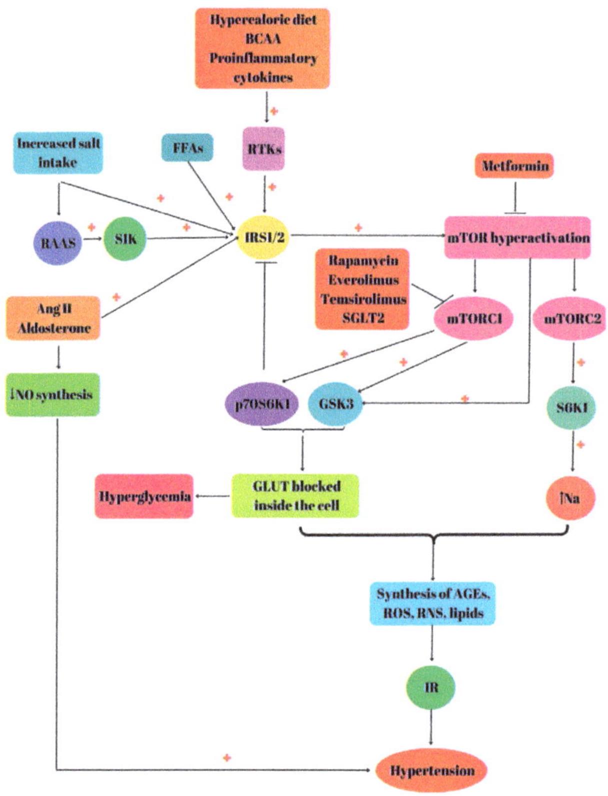

Figure 2. Phosphatidylinositol 3-kinase (PI3K) protein kinase B (AKT)/mammalian target of rapamycin (mTOR) pathway, insulin resistance and hypertension. Hypercaloric diet, branched-chain amino acids (BCAAs), proinflammatory cytokines, free fatty acids (FFAs), increased salt intake, the renin–angiotensin–aldosterone system (RAAS) and salt-inducible kinase (SIK) induce mTOR hyperactivation via RTKs or insulin receptor substrates (IRS1/2). IRS phosphorylation produced by angiotensin II (Ang II) and aldosterone decreases nitric oxide (NO) synthesis. Activation of 70Ka ribosomal protein S6 kinase 1 (p70S6K1) and glycogen synthase 3 (GSK3) inhibits IRS conducing to an increased blood glucose level because GLUT will be blocked inside the cell. mTOR complex 2 (mTORC2) activates serum/glucocorticoid-regulated kinase 1 (SGK1) stimulating Na transport. mTOR over-activation is associated with synthesis of advanced end products (AGEs), reactive oxygen species (ROS), reactive nitrogen species (RNS) and lipids. Metformin has the capacity to inhibit mTOR, while rapamycin, everolimus, temsirolimus and sodium-glucose transporter protein 2 (SGLT2) block mTORC1. All these events will lead to insulin resistance (IR) and further to hypertension. "+" activation; "↓" decrease; "↑" increase.

5. Hyperglycemia, mTOR Dysregulation and Stress

At the beginning of the 20th century, the French chemist Louis Camille Maillard discovered the nonenzymatic and nonoxidative covalent attachment of glucose to proteins, lipids and nucleic acids. Glycoxidation refers to the radical reaction of free and protein-bound sugars. The Amadori rearrangement of the glycated proteins leads to AGEs generation [101]. AGEs can be found in T2D in elevated plasma levels and tend to accumulate in the tissue [89]. Hyperglycemia induces the activation of the polyol pathway, where the first and rate-limiting enzyme aldolase reductase (AR) reduces glucose to sorbitol, with NADPH as a donor of reduction equivalents. Sorbitol dehydrogenase oxidates sorbitol to fructose and NADH [102]. Further, fructose will be metabolized into ketone bodies, triose phosphate or will be transformed under the reaction catalyzed by fructose-3-phosphokinase in carbonyl compounds such as glyoxal, methylglyoxal and 3-deoxyglucose, with the formation of irreversible AGEs [103]. Methylglyoxal is one of the most potent glycating agents and leads to AGEs formation by endogenous, nonenzymatic glycoxidation of proteins, nucleic acids and lipids. Furthermore, methylglyoxal binds to arginine and lysine residues from proteins and also deoxyguanosine from DNA, resulting in the formation of AGEs and DNA adducts [104]. In vivo and in vitro studies revealed that methylglyoxal induces an inflammatory response, cytotoxicity and apoptosis [105]. In addition, the polyol pathway decreases the level of reduced glutathione (GSH) and other intracellular antioxidants because it uses NADPH and deprived glutathione reductase from it [106]. In chronic hyperglycemia, AGEs induce the development of macro- and microvascular complications in both T1D and T2D and enhance the expression of their cognate receptor, RAGE [107,108].

The hexosamine biosynthesis pathway (HBP) represents the link between glucose metabolism and lipid, nucleotide and amino acid metabolisms. Around 2–5% of glucose is converted via HBP to uridine diphosphate N-acetyl glucosamine (UDP-GlcNAc), used for glycolipids, glycoproteins and glycosaminoglycan synthesis, with the implication of fructose-6-phosphate aminotransferase as a rate-limiting enzyme [109]. Hyperglycemia activates the HBP pathway, which acts as an offshoot for glycolysis, leading to vascular damage. Moreover, in hyperglycemic conditions, the glycolysis intermediate fructose-6-phosphate is used to obtain UDP-GlcNAc, utilized as a substrate for acetylation of proteins at serine and threonine residues as O-linked N-acetylglucoseamines. This process of protein acylation is a reversible posttranslational modification that can alter the activity, interaction and function of targeted proteins [110]. Moreover, UDP-GlcNAc induces protein misfolding by interfering with N-linked glycosylation at the level of the endoplasmic reticulum (ER) membrane, leading to ER stress [111] and tumor progression [112].

Inflammation and oxidative stress (OS) are involved in diabetes pathogenesis, both in T1D and T2D, because free radicals damage pancreatic β cells. Sustained hyperglycemia leads to the formation of reactive oxygen species (ROS) and reactive nitrogen species (RNS) [113]. The mitochondrial electron transport chain, xanthine oxidase (XO), nicotinamide dinucleotide phosphate (NADPH) oxidase and uncoupled endothelial nitric oxide synthesis (eNOS) are the main ROS sources in diabetic blood vessels [114]. For example, the reaction of ROS with NO generates peroxynitrite ($ONOO^-$), a powerful oxidant for DNA, lipids and cellular proteins. In this way, NO bioavailability is diminished, which causes endothelial dysfunction. In addition, in diabetes, activation of protein kinase C (PKC) via diacylglycerol (DAG), elevated flux of the HBP, the polyol pathway and increased levels of AGEs contribute to ROS production [115]. Higher levels of DAG activate the PKC pathway, inducing the formation of AGEs [116]. PKC activation is correlated with elevated endothelial inflammation, decreased levels of NO generation and increased expression of vascular endothelial growth factor (VEGF). Once activated, PKC activates MAPK and further PI3K/AKT/mTOR [117]. Taking into consideration all these molecular events, PI3K/AKT/mTOR dysregulation leads to IR, correlated with the synthesis of AGEs, ROS and RNS [88]. Moreover, AGEs, ROS and RNS formation induce stress, protein accumulation, Met S dysfunction and inflammation [90], inducing cell damage of proteins, lipids, sugars and nucleic acids [88] (Figure 3).

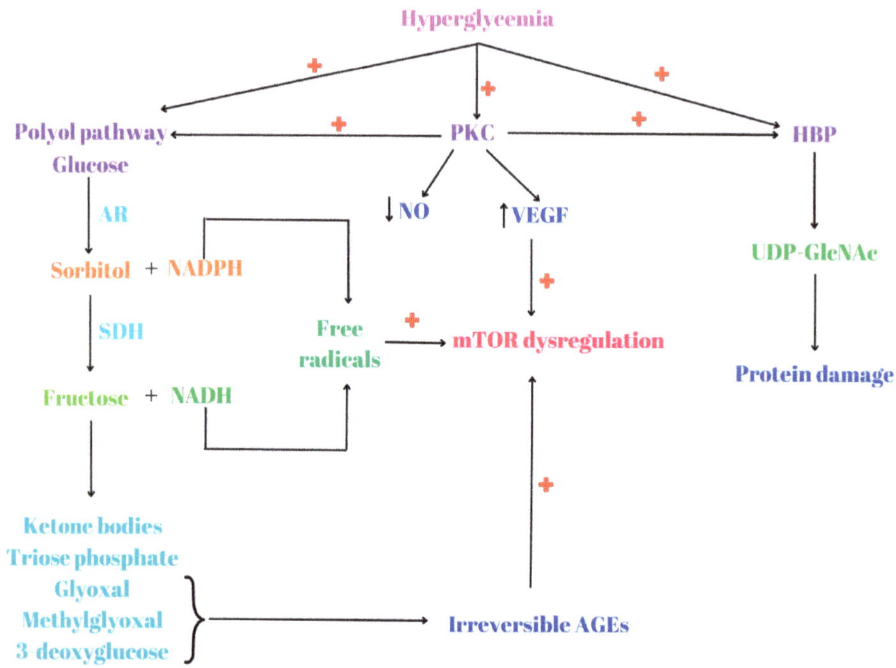

Figure 3. Hyperglycemia is correlated with the activation of the polyol pathway, where glucose is reduced to sorbitol by aldolase reductase (AR) and NADPH. Further, sorbitol will be oxidized to fructose by the enzyme sorbitol dehydrogenase (SDH), and NADH is generated. Fructose will be metabolized into ketone bodies, triose phosphate or carbonylic compounds such as glyoxal, methylglyoxal and 3-deoxyglucose. The last three compounds will contribute to irreversible advanced glycation end product (AGE) formation. NADPH and NADH represent sources for reactive species generation. In hyperglycemic conditions, the hexosamine biosynthesis pathway (HBP) is also activated, leading to the formation of uridine diphosphate N-acetylglucosamine (UDP-GlcNAc), which can induce protein damage. Protein kinase C (PKC) is activated by hyperglycemia, which has the capacity to activate polyol and HBP pathways. PKC activation is associated with decreased levels of nitric oxide (NO) biosynthesis and elevated levels of vascular endothelial growth factor (VEGF). All these molecular events will induce, in the end, mTOR dysregulation. "+" activation; "↑" increase; "↓" decrease.

6. mTOR Dysregulation, Insulin Resistance and Hypertension

Normally, blood pressure represents the product of cardiac output and peripheral vascular resistance. When the systemic blood pressure decreases, kidney-juxtaglomerular cells produce renin, which activates liver angiotensin and produces angiotensin I (Ang I). Furthermore, Ang I will be converted into angiotensin II (Ang II) by angiotensin-converting enzyme (ACE) located in the lungs [118]. In addition, ACE can also be located in endothelial cells [119]. In insulin-target organs, it promotes nitric oxide (NO) and endothelin release, which produce vasodilation and vasoconstriction, respectively, improving glucose distribution [54]. In circulation, Ang II diffuses to the tissues and binds to its main receptors [119], stimulates blood vessel constriction and induces the release of aldosterone from the adrenal glands, leading to sodium reabsorption [118]. In aldosterone-sensitive distal nephrons, together with vasopressin, aldosterone will have synergic effects on the epithelial Na^+ channels (ENaCs) to increase Na reabsorption [120].

Hypertension is often met in patients with hyperglycemia, IR and abdominal obesity. Therefore, diabetic patients will have a 2 to 4 times higher risk of developing CVD [121].

The renin–angiotensin–aldosterone system (RAAS) activation is the primary etiologic event in the development of hypertension in subjects with DM [122]. In humans, higher amounts of salt intake induce alteration of the RAAS system and further IR (Figure 2). Moreover, the release of Ang II from the salt-loading adipose tissue stimulates the synthesis of proinflammatory cytokines, lipogenesis and cardiac hypertrophy and reduces the synthesis of insulin. Studies performed on animals reported that a higher intake of salt leads to diabetes via RAAS activation and salt-inducible kinase (SIK). SIK is a serine/threonine protein kinase that may phosphorylate IRS1, leading to PI3K/AKT/mTOR activation [123].

RAAS leads to hypertension development because Ang II and aldosterone increase IRS phosphorylation at serine residue increasing the PI3K/AKT activity. This molecular event will be correlated with decreased activation of endothelial nitric oxide synthase, leading to reduced NO synthesis [124]. It is well known that insulin stimulates the production of NO from the vascular endothelium. IR induces a decreased production of NO, a key element for CVD development [125]. Endothelial tissue mediates vascular tone, cell growth and the interactions among thrombocytes, leukocytes and the vessel wall. Moreover, the endothelial tissue may synthesize growth factors and thrombo-regulatory molecules [126].

In the cardiovascular system and kidneys, a hypercaloric diet, together with aldosterone, and Ang II promote IR via mTOR-S6K1 activation [127]. IR increases the blood pressure by enhancing tissue Ang II and aldosterone activity and stimulates sympathetic nervous system activity and oxidative stress [126].

Aging is associated with structural and functional modifications of organs, which may lead to senescent endothelial cells, a risk factor for CVD, including hypertension and diabetes [128]. ENaCs play a crucial role in Na^+ homeostasis; therefore, dysregulation leads to many forms of hypertension [129]. mTORC2 regulates serum/glucocorticoid-regulated kinase 1 (SGK1) activity, a key enzyme that stimulates Na^+ transport via insulin and IGF-1 [130]. More than that, mTORC2 is implicated in the regulation of renal tubular Na^+ and K^+ transport [131]. When patients are subjected to pressure overload, the ventricular myocardium switches from fatty acid metabolism to glucose to provide energy. Moreover, subjects with contractile dysfunction of the heart are characterized by myocardial glucose metabolism perturbation leading to glucose-6-phosphate (G6P) accumulation. Further, G6P accumulation activates mTOR [132].

7. Metformin and mTOR Inhibitors

Antidiabetic medications have the property to reduce the oxidative stress induced by hyperglycemia [133]. Metformin is often used for the hypoglycemic effects in T2D. Besides its hypoglycemic property, metformin exerts anti-inflammatory, antioxidant, antitumoral [134–138], antiaging, hepatoprotective, cardioprotective and tissue regenerative effects [139]. Metformin is widely used in pre- and diabetic patients, and also as a PI3K inhibitor, because it has low toxicity [140].

Moreover, metformin inhibits hepatic gluconeogenesis and enhances the peripheral utilization of glucose. More than that, it is considered the first line of treatment against PI3K/AKT/mTOR inhibitors that induce hyperglycemia [141]. Metformin can inhibit respiratory mitochondrial complex I, called NADH: ubiquinone oxidoreductase. At the level of complex I, NADH is oxidized, after being formed in glycolysis, fatty acid β-oxidation and the Krebs cycle. In this way, metformin increases the accumulation of NADH leading to ROS formation, and decreases the synthesis of ATP [142].

Metformin also has the potential to inhibit the mTOR pathway by activating the AMPK, leading to tumor inhibition [143,144]. Moreover, in hepatocytes isolated from rats, at concentrations of 10 to 20 μM, metformin activates AMPK and decreases glycemia via inhibition of hepatic gluconeogenesis [139,145]. It was observed that the administration of metformin for a long term, such as 12 months, decreases the level of C-reactive protein (CRP) in both women and men with impaired glucose tolerance [146]. Furthermore, it increases the survival rate of diabetic patients with advanced pancreatic neuroendocrine tumors [147] and lymphoma [148].

Frequently, mTOR dysregulation is associated with the development of various types of cancer. Therefore, mTOR inhibitors have been tested in this aspect, representing powerful therapeutic agents [149]. In animal studies, Lamming et al. reported that rapamycin inhibits mTORC2, necessary for insulin to suppress hepatic gluconeogenesis [150,151]. Rapamycin analogs such as everolimus and temsirolimus can inhibit only mTORC1 [152]. It is well known that overactivation of mTOR is associated with IR, and caloric restriction and short-term treatment with rapamycin increase glucose uptake and insulin sensitivity [153].

Wang et al. investigated in vivo the effects of evodiamine on IR in obese animals. The study concluded that evodiamine could inhibit the phosphorylation of IRS1, leading to mTOR inhibition and improving glucose tolerance [154]. The results are contradictory because Pereira and his research team illustrated that the treatment of human adipocytes with rapamycin decreases glucose uptake, contributing to IR development [155].

Inhibition of p70S6K1 will improve the life of T2D patients, as it is a downstream effector of mTOR, which mediates glucose homeostasis, protein synthesis, RNA processing, cell growth and apoptosis [156]. Studies performed on knock-out model mice without S6K1 revealed that mTOR inhibition by rapamycin causes hypoinsulinemia and hypersensitivity to insulin [157].

Das and co-workers present new hopes regarding the effects of rapamycin in animal studies. The scientific group observed that treatment with an mTOR inhibitor decreases the level of glucose and triglycerides and reduces body weight. Moreover, the levels of lipid peroxidation were significantly reduced. Rapamycin can inhibit the phosphorylation of mTOR and S6K1 but not of AKT. Administration of rapamycin improves cardiac dysfunction in type 2 diabetic mice [158].

Another glucose-lowering agent, glucagon-like peptide-1 (GLP-1), exerts cardioprotective effects [159,160]. It has been observed that, in the proximal tubular kidney area, sodium-glucose transport protein 2 (SGLT2) inhibitors suppress the gene transcription for glycolysis, gluconeogenesis and the Krebs cycle, blocking the mTORC1 pathway [161].

It is already well known that rapamycin and everolimus inhibit mTORC1. Moreover, studies performed on animals revealed that rapamycin improves health. On the other hand, everolimus enhances immunity in elderly humans without causing side effects [162]. The study conducted on diabetic rats by Zhou et al. reported that rapamycin and metformin significantly ameliorated IR, decreased inflammation, blocked mTOR and induced autophagy [163]. Similar results were obtained by Reifsnyder et al. on type 2 diabetic mice regarding metformin and rapamycin [164], and also only with rapamycin [165].

Rapamycin reduces hyperglycemia, lipid peroxidation, endoplasmic reticulum (ER) stress and dyslipidemia and increases the antioxidant capacity in type 2 diabetic animal studies [166].

The treatment of patients with T2D with acute stroke with metformin also demonstrates its positive effects regarding the neurological function and oxidative stress-related markers [167].

The study performed by Temiz-Resitoglu using hypertensive male rats treated with rapamycin revealed that this mTOR inhibitor normalized the systolic blood pressure. In addition, the activity of ribosomal protein S6 was attenuated in the heart, aorta and kidney [168]. Wang and colleagues reported similar results regarding the effects of rapamycin on early cirrhotic portal hypertension rats [169]. Kumar et al. tested the inhibitory capacity of rapamycin on salt-induced hypertension and kidney injury using Dahl salt-sensitive rats and found that it improved the renal function but did not have good effects on blood pressure [170]. Besides animal studies, promising results come from in vitro studies, where extracts from some vegetables possess anti-obesity and anti-inflammatory properties, and also may block the activity of mTOR [171].

8. Conclusions

Today, diets rich in refined carbohydrates associated with sedentarism lead to obesity, dyslipidemia, IR and also hypertension. The PI3K/AKTmTOR signaling pathway exerts key roles in cell metabolism, controlling growth, proliferation and survival. Normally, mTOR activation can be performed by growth factors, insulin and cytokines that bind to RTKs, leading to AKT and mTOR activation. mTOR hyperactivation is induced by a hypercaloric diet, proinflammatory cytokines, BCAA and dysregulation associated with various systemic pathologies, including IR, cancer and CVD. mTORC1 activates p70S6K1, which will block the IRS conducting to hyperglycemia because GLUT will remain inside the cell. Increased salt intake activates the RAAS system and further PI3K/AKT/mTOR, leading to NO decreased production and hypertension development. In T2D patients, mTOR dysregulation will promote hyperlipidemia, inflammation and vasoconstriction. Metformin is an excellent drug with hypoglycemic, anti-inflammatory and antitumoral properties, also inhibiting mTOR. Studies performed on animals reported that metformin and rapamycin reduced inflammation, hyperlipidemia and hyperglycemia, and induced autophagy by blocking mTOR. Also, everolimus, temsirolimus and SGLT2 block mTORC1, with positive results regarding glucose sensitivity being reported in animal studies.

Taking into consideration all these aspects, mTOR overactivation plays a pivotal role in IR and hypertension pathology. Therefore, detection of mTOR together with other compounds from the PI3K/AKT signaling pathway is important for T2D and T1D patients. Administration of mTOR inhibitors to diabetic patients may decrease the complications of this pathology.

Author Contributions: Conceptualization, D.M., S.M.S., C.S., S.N.; methodology, D.M., S.N., I.-I.S.-S., I.A.V.; software, D.M., R.I.N.; validation, M.J., M.G., S.M.S.; formal analysis, I.A.V.; investigation, D.M., S.N.; resources, C.S., S.M.S., I.-I.S.-S., R.I.N.; data curation, M.J., M.G.; writing—original draft preparation, D.M., S.M.S., I.-I.S.-S.; writing—review and editing, I.-I.S.-S., R.I.N.; visualization, M.J., C.S., I.A.V., S.N., R.I.N.; supervision, M.J., M.G., C.S., S.N., I.-I.S.-S.; project administration, D.M., S.M.S., C.S., S.N.; funding acquisition, S.M.S., I.-I.S.-S. All authors have read and agreed to the published version of the manuscript.

Funding: The publication of this paper was supported by the University of Medicine and Pharmacy Carol Davila, through the institutional program Publish not Perish.

Institutional Review Board Statement: Not applicable.

Informed Consent Statement: Not applicable.

Conflicts of Interest: The authors declare no conflicts of interest.

References

1. Hwangbo, Y.; Lee, E.K. Acute hyperglycemia associated with anti-cancer medication. *Endocrinol. Metab.* **2017**, *32*, 23–29. [CrossRef]
2. Pulakat, L.; Aroor, A.R.; Gul, R.; Sowers, J.R. Cardiac insulin resistance and microRNA modulators. *J. Diabetes Res.* **2012**, *2012*, 654904. [CrossRef] [PubMed]
3. da Silva Rosa, S.C.; Nayak, N.; Caymo, A.M.; Gordon, J.W. Mechanisms of muscle insulin resistance and the cross-talk with liver and adipose tissue. *Physiol. Rep.* **2020**, *8*, e14607. [CrossRef] [PubMed]
4. Narasimhan, A.; Flores, R.R.; Robbins, P.D.; Niedernhofer, L.J. Role of cellular senescence in type II diabetes. *Endocrinology* **2021**, *162*, bqab136. [CrossRef]
5. Akhaphong, B.; Baumann, D.C.; Beetch, M.; Lockridge, A.D.; Jo, S.; Wong, A.; Zemanovic, T.; Mohan, R.; Fondevilla, D.L.; Sia, M. Placental mTOR complex 1 regulates fetal programming of obesity and insulin resistance in mice. *JCI Insight* **2021**, *6*, e149271. [CrossRef]
6. Thomas, M.S.; Calle, M.; Fernandez, M.L. Healthy plant-based diets improve dyslipidemias, insulin resistance, and inflammation in metabolic syndrome. A narrative review. *Adv. Nutr.* **2023**, *14*, 44–54. [CrossRef] [PubMed]
7. Wang, F.; Han, L.; Hu, D. Fasting insulin, insulin resistance and risk of hypertension in the general population: A meta-analysis. *Clin. Chim. Acta* **2017**, *464*, 57–63. [CrossRef]
8. Zheng, Z.-G.; Zhou, Y.-P.; Zhang, X.; Thu, P.M.; Xie, Z.-S.; Lu, C.; Pang, T.; Xue, B.; Xu, D.-Q.; Chen, Y. Anhydroicaritin improves diet-induced obesity and hyperlipidemia and alleviates insulin resistance by suppressing SREBPs activation. *Biochem. Pharmacol.* **2016**, *122*, 42–61. [CrossRef] [PubMed]

9. Natali, A.; Ferrannini, E. Hypertension, insulin resistance, and the metabolic syndrome. *Endocrinol. Metab. Clin.* **2004**, *33*, 417–429. [CrossRef]
10. Roberts, C.K.; Hevener, A.L.; Barnard, R.J. Metabolic syndrome and insulin resistance: Underlying causes and modification by exercise training. *Compr. Physiol.* **2013**, *3*, 1.
11. Lai, Y.; Zhao, A.; Tan, M.; Yang, M.; Lin, Y.; Li, S.; Song, J.; Zheng, H.; Zhu, Z.; Liu, D. DOCK5 regulates energy balance and hepatic insulin sensitivity by targeting mTORC1 signaling. *EMBO Rep.* **2020**, *21*, e49473. [CrossRef]
12. Hall, J.E.; do Carmo, J.M.; da Silva, A.A.; Wang, Z.; Hall, M.E. Obesity-induced hypertension: Interaction of neurohumoral and renal mechanisms. *Circ. Res.* **2015**, *116*, 991–1006. [CrossRef] [PubMed]
13. Arabi, T.; Shafqat, A.; Sabbah, B.N.; Fawzy, N.A.; Shah, H.; Abdulkader, H.; Razak, A.; Sabbah, A.N.; Arabi, Z. Obesity-related kidney disease: Beyond hypertension and insulin-resistance. *Front. Endocrinol.* **2023**, *13*, 1095211. [CrossRef] [PubMed]
14. Sivasubrmanian, S. Fathoming the role of mTOR in diabetes mellitus and its complications. *Curr. Mol. Pharmacol.* **2023**, *16*, 520–529.
15. Ganesan, H.; Balasubramanian, V.; Iyer, M.; Venugopal, A.; Subramaniam, M.D.; Cho, S.-G.; Vellingiri, B. mTOR signalling pathway-A root cause for idiopathic autism? *BMB Rep.* **2019**, *52*, 424. [CrossRef] [PubMed]
16. Vergès, B. mTOR and cardiovascular diseases: Diabetes mellitus. *Transplantation* **2018**, *102*, S47–S49. [CrossRef] [PubMed]
17. Noori, T.; Sureda, A.; Shirooie, S. Role of natural mTOR inhibitors in treatment of diabetes mellitus. *Fundam. Clin. Pharmacol.* **2023**, *37*, 461–479. [CrossRef] [PubMed]
18. Zou, Z.; Tao, T.; Li, H.; Zhu, X. mTOR signaling pathway and mTOR inhibitors in cancer: Progress and challenges. *Cell Biosci.* **2020**, *10*, 31. [CrossRef] [PubMed]
19. Liu, G.Y.; Sabatini, D.M. mTOR at the nexus of nutrition, growth, ageing and disease. *Nat. Rev. Mol. Cell Biol.* **2020**, *21*, 183–203. [CrossRef]
20. Laplante, M.; Sabatini, D.M. mTOR signaling in growth control and disease. *Cell* **2012**, *149*, 274–293. [CrossRef]
21. Saxton, R.A.; Sabatini, D.M. mTOR signaling in growth, metabolism, and disease. *Cell* **2017**, *168*, 960–976. [CrossRef]
22. Burillo, J.; Marqués, P.; Jiménez, B.; González-Blanco, C.; Benito, M.; Guillén, C. Insulin resistance and diabetes mellitus in Alzheimer's disease. *Cells* **2021**, *10*, 1236. [CrossRef] [PubMed]
23. Luo, Q.; Du, R.; Liu, W.; Huang, G.; Dong, Z.; Li, X. PI3K/Akt/mTOR signaling pathway: Role in esophageal squamous cell carcinoma, regulatory mechanisms and opportunities for targeted therapy. *Front. Oncol.* **2022**, *12*, 852383.
24. Gao, Y.; Tian, T. mTOR signaling pathway and gut microbiota in various disorders: Mechanisms and potential drugs in pharmacotherapy. *Int. J. Mol. Sci.* **2023**, *24*, 11811. [CrossRef]
25. Zoncu, R.; Efeyan, A.; Sabatini, D.M. mTOR: From growth signal integration to cancer, diabetes and ageing. *Nat. Rev. Mol. Cell Biol.* **2011**, *12*, 21–35. [CrossRef]
26. Glaviano, A.; Foo, A.S.; Lam, H.Y.; Yap, K.C.; Jacot, W.; Jones, R.H.; Eng, H.; Nair, M.G.; Makvandi, P.; Geoerger, B. PI3K/AKT/mTOR signaling transduction pathway and targeted therapies in cancer. *Mol. Cancer* **2023**, *22*, 138. [CrossRef]
27. Mallela, K.; Kumar, A. Role of TSC1 in physiology and diseases. *Mol. Cell. Biochem.* **2021**, *476*, 2269–2282. [CrossRef] [PubMed]
28. Larsen, L.J.; Møller, L.B. Crosstalk of hedgehog and mTORC1 pathways. *Cells* **2020**, *9*, 2316. [CrossRef] [PubMed]
29. Zhang, H.; Bajraszewski, N.; Wu, E.; Wang, H.; Moseman, A.P.; Dabora, S.L.; Griffin, J.D.; Kwiatkowski, D.J. PDGFRs are critical for PI3K/Akt activation and negatively regulated by mTOR. *J. Clin. Investig.* **2007**, *117*, 730–738. [CrossRef]
30. Ching, C.B.; Hansel, D.E. Expanding therapeutic targets in bladder cancer: The PI3K/Akt/mTOR pathway. *Lab. Investig.* **2010**, *90*, 1406–1414. [CrossRef]
31. Porta, C.; Paglino, C.; Mosca, A. Targeting PI3K/Akt/mTOR signaling in cancer. *Front. Oncol.* **2014**, *4*, 64. [CrossRef] [PubMed]
32. Jurca, C.M.; Kozma, K.; Petchesi, C.D.; Zaha, D.C.; Magyar, I.; Munteanu, M.; Faur, L.; Jurca, A.; Bembea, D.; Severin, E. Tuberous sclerosis, type II diabetes mellitus and the PI3K/AKT/mTOR signaling pathways—Case report and literature review. *Genes* **2023**, *14*, 433. [CrossRef] [PubMed]
33. Lotfimehr, H.; Mardi, N.; Narimani, S.; Nasrabadi, H.T.; Karimipour, M.; Sokullu, E.; Rahbarghazi, R. mTOR signalling pathway in stem cell bioactivities and angiogenesis potential. *Cell Prolif.* **2023**, *56*, e13499. [CrossRef] [PubMed]
34. Deng, C.-Y.; Lv, M.; Luo, B.-H.; Zhao, S.-Z.; Mo, Z.-C.; Xie, Y.-J. The role of the PI3K/AKT/mTOR signalling pathway in male reproduction. *Curr. Mol. Med.* **2021**, *21*, 539–548. [PubMed]
35. Tewari, D.; Patni, P.; Bishayee, A.; Sah, A.N.; Bishayee, A. Natural products targeting the PI3K-Akt-mTOR signaling pathway in cancer: A novel therapeutic strategy. *Semin. Cancer Biol.* **2022**, *80*, 1–17. [CrossRef]
36. Abdo Qaid, E.Y.; Zulkipli, N.N.; Zakaria, R.; Ahmad, A.H.; Othman, Z.; Muthuraju, S.; Sasongko, T.H. The role of mTOR signalling pathway in hypoxia-induced cognitive impairment. *Int. J. Neurosci.* **2021**, *131*, 482–488. [CrossRef] [PubMed]
37. Chen, M.; Chao, B.; Xu, J.; Liu, Z.; Tao, Y.; He, J.; Wang, J.; Yang, H.; Luo, X.; Qi, H. CPT1A modulates PI3K/Akt/mTOR pathway to promote preeclampsia. *Placenta* **2023**, *133*, 23–31. [CrossRef] [PubMed]
38. Sanvee, G.M.; Panajatovic, M.V.; Bouitbir, J.; Krähenbühl, S. Mechanisms of insulin resistance by simvastatin in C2C12 myotubes and in mouse skeletal muscle. *Biochem. Pharmacol.* **2019**, *164*, 23–33. [CrossRef]
39. Nagini, S.; Sophia, J.; Mishra, R. Glycogen synthase kinases: Moonlighting proteins with theranostic potential in cancer. *Semin. Cancer Biol.* **2019**, *56*, 25–36. [CrossRef]
40. Dai, D.-F.; Kang, P.; Bai, H. The mTOR signaling pathway in cardiac aging. *J. Cardiovasc. Aging* **2023**, *3*, 24. [CrossRef]

41. Bodur, C.; Kazyken, D.; Huang, K.; Tooley, A.S.; Cho, K.W.; Barnes, T.M.; Lumeng, C.N.; Myers, M.G., Jr.; Fingar, D.C. TBK1-mTOR signaling attenuates obesity-linked hyperglycemia and insulin resistance. *Diabetes* **2022**, *71*, 2297–2312. [CrossRef] [PubMed]
42. Kido, K.; Sase, K.; Yokokawa, T.; Fujita, S. Enhanced skeletal muscle insulin sensitivity after acute resistance-type exercise is upregulated by rapamycin-sensitive mTOR complex 1 inhibition. *Sci. Rep.* **2020**, *10*, 8509. [CrossRef] [PubMed]
43. Mir, S.A.; Dar, A.; Alshehri, S.A.; Wahab, S.; Hamid, L.; Almoyad, M.A.A.; Ali, T.; Bader, G.N. Exploring the mTOR signalling pathway and its inhibitory scope in cancer. *Pharmaceuticals* **2023**, *16*, 1004. [CrossRef] [PubMed]
44. Wang, H.; Liu, Y.; Wang, D.; Xu, Y.; Dong, R.; Yang, Y.; Lv, Q.; Chen, X.; Zhang, Z. The upstream pathway of mTOR-mediated autophagy in liver diseases. *Cells* **2019**, *8*, 1597. [CrossRef] [PubMed]
45. Melanis, K.; Stefanou, M.-I.; Themistoklis, K.M.; Papasilekas, T. mTOR pathway–a potential therapeutic target in stroke. *Ther. Adv. Neurol. Disord.* **2023**, *16*, 17562864231187770. [CrossRef] [PubMed]
46. Chakrabarti, P.; Kandror, K.V. The role of mTOR in lipid homeostasis and diabetes progression. *Curr. Opin. Endocrinol. Diabetes Obes.* **2015**, *22*, 340–346. [CrossRef] [PubMed]
47. Ding, Y.; Chen, Q. mTOR pathway: A potential therapeutic target for spinal cord injury. *Biomed. Pharmacother.* **2022**, *145*, 112430. [CrossRef] [PubMed]
48. Yang, L.; Zhang, Z.; Wang, D.; Jiang, Y.; Liu, Y. Targeting mTOR signaling in type 2 diabetes mellitus and diabetes complications. *Curr. Drug Targets* **2022**, *23*, 692–710. [CrossRef] [PubMed]
49. Fattahi, S.; Khalifehzadeh-Esfahani, Z.; Mohammad-Rezaei, M.; Mafi, S.; Jafarinia, M. PI3K/Akt/mTOR pathway: A potential target for anti-SARS-CoV-2 therapy. *Immunol. Res.* **2022**, *70*, 269–275. [CrossRef]
50. Ali, M.; Bukhari, S.A.; Lee, H.-W. Upstream signalling of mTORC1 and its hyperactivation in type 2 diabetes (T2D). *BMB Rep.* **2017**, *50*, 601. [CrossRef]
51. Rubie, C.; Zimmer, J.; Lammert, F.; Gross, J.C.; Weber, S.N.; Kruse, B.; Halajda, B.; Wagner, M.; Wagenpfeil, S.; Glanemann, M. MicroRNA-496 and mechanistic target of rapamycin expression are associated with type 2 diabetes mellitus and obesity in elderly people. *Ann. Nutr. Metab.* **2019**, *74*, 279–286. [CrossRef]
52. Lee, S.-H.; Park, S.-Y.; Choi, C.S. Insulin resistance: From mechanisms to therapeutic strategies. *Diabetes Metab. J.* **2022**, *46*, 15–37. [CrossRef] [PubMed]
53. Tsatsoulis, A.; Mantzaris, M.D.; Bellou, S.; Andrikoula, M. Insulin resistance: An adaptive mechanism becomes maladaptive in the current environment—An evolutionary perspective. *Metabolism* **2013**, *62*, 622–633. [CrossRef]
54. Onyango, A.N. Cellular stresses and stress responses in the pathogenesis of insulin resistance. *Oxidative Med. Cell. Longev.* **2018**, *2018*, 4321714. [CrossRef]
55. Dimitriadis, G.; Mitrou, P.; Lambadiari, V.; Maratou, E.; Raptis, S.A. Insulin effects in muscle and adipose tissue. *Diabetes Res. Clin. Pract.* **2011**, *93*, S52–S59. [CrossRef] [PubMed]
56. Wu, C.; Xu, G.; Tsai, S.-Y.A.; Freed, W.J.; Lee, C.-T. Transcriptional profiles of type 2 diabetes in human skeletal muscle reveal insulin resistance, metabolic defects, apoptosis, and molecular signatures of immune activation in response to infections. *Biochem. Biophys. Res. Commun.* **2017**, *482*, 282–288. [CrossRef]
57. Myers, J.; Kokkinos, P.; Nyelin, E. Physical activity, cardiorespiratory fitness, and the metabolic syndrome. *Nutrients* **2019**, *11*, 1652. [CrossRef] [PubMed]
58. Mirabelli, M.; Chiefari, E.; Arcidiacono, B.; Corigliano, D.M.; Brunetti, F.S.; Maggisano, V.; Russo, D.; Foti, D.P.; Brunetti, A. Mediterranean diet nutrients to turn the tide against insulin resistance and related diseases. *Nutrients* **2020**, *12*, 1066. [CrossRef]
59. Tong, C.; Wu, Y.; Zhang, L.; Yu, Y. Insulin resistance, autophagy and apoptosis in patients with polycystic ovary syndrome: Association with PI3K signaling pathway. *Front. Endocrinol.* **2022**, *13*, 1091147. [CrossRef] [PubMed]
60. De Cosmo, S.; Menzaghi, C.; Prudente, S.; Trischitta, V. Role of insulin resistance in kidney dysfunction: Insights into the mechanism and epidemiological evidence. *Nephrol. Dial. Transplant.* **2013**, *28*, 29–36. [CrossRef]
61. Tahapary, D.L.; Pratisthita, L.B.; Fitri, N.A.; Marcella, C.; Wafa, S.; Kurniawan, F.; Rizka, A.; Tarigan, T.J.E.; Harbuwono, D.S.; Purnamasari, D. Challenges in the diagnosis of insulin resistance: Focusing on the role of HOMA-IR and Tryglyceride/glucose index. *Diabetes Metab. Syndr. Clin. Res. Rev.* **2022**, *16*, 102581. [CrossRef] [PubMed]
62. Kosmas, C.E.; Bousvarou, M.D.; Kostara, C.E.; Papakonstantinou, E.J.; Salamou, E.; Guzman, E. Insulin resistance and cardiovascular disease. *J. Int. Med. Res.* **2023**, *51*, 03000605231164548. [CrossRef] [PubMed]
63. Dayi, T.; Ozgoren, M. Effects of the Mediterranean diet on the components of metabolic syndrome. *J. Prev. Med. Hyg.* **2022**, *63*, E56. [PubMed]
64. Perseghin, G.; Petersen, K.; Shulman, G. Cellular mechanism of insulin resistance: Potential links with inflammation. *Int. J. Obes.* **2003**, *27*, S6–S11. [CrossRef] [PubMed]
65. Manaserh, I.H.; Bledzka, K.M.; Junker, A.; Grondolsky, J.; Schumacher, S.M. A cardiac amino-terminal GRK2 peptide inhibits maladaptive adipocyte hypertrophy and insulin resistance during diet-induced obesity. *Basic Transl. Sci.* **2022**, *7*, 563–579. [CrossRef] [PubMed]
66. da Silva, A.A.; do Carmo, J.M.; Li, X.; Wang, Z.; Mouton, A.J.; Hall, J.E. Role of hyperinsulinemia and insulin resistance in hypertension: Metabolic syndrome revisited. *Can. J. Cardiol.* **2020**, *36*, 671–682. [CrossRef] [PubMed]
67. Bar-Tana, J. Type 2 diabetes–unmet need, unresolved pathogenesis, mTORC1-centric paradigm. *Rev. Endocr. Metab. Disord.* **2020**, *21*, 613–629. [CrossRef] [PubMed]

68. Lamounier-Zepter, V.; Ehrhart-Bornstein, M.; Bornstein, S.R. Insulin resistance in hypertension and cardiovascular disease. *Best Pract. Res. Clin. Endocrinol. Metab.* **2006**, *20*, 355–367. [CrossRef]
69. Perrotta, F.; Nigro, E.; Mollica, M.; Costigliola, A.; D'Agnano, V.; Daniele, A.; Bianco, A.; Guerra, G. Pulmonary hypertension and obesity: Focus on adiponectin. *Int. J. Mol. Sci.* **2019**, *20*, 912. [CrossRef]
70. Lee, D.-F.; Kuo, H.-P.; Chen, C.-T.; Wei, Y.; Chou, C.-K.; Hung, J.-Y.; Yen, C.-J.; Hung, M.-C. IKKβ suppression of TSC1 function links the mTOR pathway with insulin resistance. *Int. J. Mol. Med.* **2008**, *22*, 633–638.
71. Ye, J. Mechanism of insulin resistance in obesity: A role of ATP. *Front. Med.* **2021**, *15*, 372–382. [CrossRef] [PubMed]
72. van Niekerk, G.; Christowitz, C.; Engelbrecht, A.-M. Insulin-mediated immune dysfunction in the development of preeclampsia. *J. Mol. Med.* **2021**, *99*, 889–897. [CrossRef] [PubMed]
73. Czech, M.P. Mechanisms of insulin resistance related to white, beige, and brown adipocytes. *Mol. Metab.* **2020**, *34*, 27–42. [CrossRef] [PubMed]
74. Zhang, J.; Feng, Q. Pharmacological effects and molecular protective mechanisms of Astragalus polysaccharides on nonalcoholic fatty liver disease. *Front. Pharmacol.* **2022**, *13*, 854674. [CrossRef] [PubMed]
75. Pan, X.; Liu, C.; Wang, X.; Zhao, M.; Zhang, Z.; Zhang, X.; Wang, C.; Song, G. Resveratrol improves palmitic acid-induced insulin resistance via the DDIT4/mTOR pathway in C2C12 cells. *Mol. Med. Rep.* **2023**, *28*, 181. [CrossRef] [PubMed]
76. Han, X.; Yang, Y.; Liu, S.; Niu, Y.; Shao, H.; Fu, L. Aerobic exercise ameliorates insulin resistance in C57BL/6 J mice via activating Sestrin3. *Biochim. Et Biophys. Acta (BBA)-Mol. Basis Dis.* **2023**, *1869*, 166568. [CrossRef] [PubMed]
77. Nishikawa, H.; Asai, A.; Fukunishi, S.; Nishiguchi, S.; Higuchi, K. Metabolic Syndrome and Sarcopenia. *Nutrients* **2021**, *13*, 3519. [CrossRef] [PubMed]
78. Choi, K.; Kim, Y.-B. Molecular mechanism of insulin resistance in obesity and type 2 diabetes. *Korean J. Intern. Med.* **2010**, *25*, 119. [CrossRef]
79. Szymczak-Pajor, I.; Drzewoski, J.; Śliwińska, A. The molecular mechanisms by which vitamin D prevents insulin resistance and associated disorders. *Int. J. Mol. Sci.* **2020**, *21*, 6644. [CrossRef]
80. Søndergaard, E.; Jensen, M.D. Quantification of adipose tissue insulin sensitivity. *J. Investig. Med.* **2016**, *64*, 989–991. [CrossRef]
81. Lebovitz, H. Insulin resistance: Definition and consequences. *Exp. Clin. Endocrinol. Diabetes* **2001**, *109*, S135–S148. [CrossRef] [PubMed]
82. Meng, X.-H.; Chen, B.; Zhang, J.-P. Intracellular insulin and impaired autophagy in a zebrafish model and a cell model of type 2 diabetes. *Int. J. Biol. Sci.* **2017**, *13*, 985. [CrossRef] [PubMed]
83. Lee, A.Y.; Christensen, S.M.; Duong, N.; Tran, Q.-A.; Xiong, H.M.; Huang, J.; James, S.; Vallabh, D.; Talbott, G.; Rose, M. Sirt3 pharmacologically promotes insulin sensitivity through PI3/AKT/mTOR and their downstream pathway in adipocytes. *Int. J. Mol. Sci.* **2022**, *23*, 3740. [CrossRef] [PubMed]
84. Guo, S. Insulin signaling, resistance, and the metabolic syndrome: Insights from mouse models to disease mechanisms. *J. Endocrinol.* **2014**, *220*, T1. [CrossRef] [PubMed]
85. O'Reilly, C.L.; Uranga, S.; Fluckey, J.D. Culprits or consequences: Understanding the metabolic dysregulation of muscle in diabetes. *World J. Biol. Chem.* **2021**, *12*, 70. [CrossRef] [PubMed]
86. Zheng, M.; Wang, P. Role of insulin receptor substance-1 modulating PI3K/Akt insulin signaling pathway in Alzheimer's disease. *3 Biotech* **2021**, *11*, 179. [CrossRef] [PubMed]
87. Copps, K.; White, M. Regulation of insulin sensitivity by serine/threonine phosphorylation of insulin receptor substrate proteins IRS1 and IRS2. *Diabetologia* **2012**, *55*, 2565–2582. [CrossRef] [PubMed]
88. Newgard, C.B.; An, J.; Bain, J.R.; Muehlbauer, M.J.; Stevens, R.D.; Lien, L.F.; Haqq, A.M.; Shah, S.H.; Arlotto, M.; Slentz, C.A. A branched-chain amino acid-related metabolic signature that differentiates obese and lean humans and contributes to insulin resistance. *Cell Metab.* **2009**, *9*, 311–326. [CrossRef]
89. Bloomgarden, Z. Diabetes and branched-chain amino acids: What is the link? *J. Diabetes* **2018**, *10*, 350–352. [CrossRef]
90. Pomytkin, I.; Krasil'nikova, I.; Bakaeva, Z.; Surin, A.; Pinelis, V. Excitotoxic glutamate causes neuronal insulin resistance by inhibiting insulin receptor/Akt/mTOR pathway. *Mol. Brain* **2019**, *12*, 112. [CrossRef]
91. Morita, M.; Gravel, S.-P.; Chenard, V.; Sikström, K.; Zheng, L.; Alain, T.; Gandin, V.; Avizonis, D.; Arguello, M.; Zakaria, C. mTORC1 controls mitochondrial activity and biogenesis through 4E-BP-dependent translational regulation. *Cell Metab.* **2013**, *18*, 698–711. [CrossRef]
92. Ong, P.S.; Wang, L.Z.; Dai, X.; Tseng, S.H.; Loo, S.J.; Sethi, G. Judicious toggling of mTOR activity to combat insulin resistance and cancer: Current evidence and perspectives. *Front. Pharmacol.* **2016**, *7*, 395. [CrossRef] [PubMed]
93. Aziz, A.U.R.; Farid, S.; Qin, K.; Wang, H.; Liu, B. Regulation of insulin resistance and glucose metabolism by interaction of PIM kinases and insulin receptor substrates. *Arch. Physiol. Biochem.* **2020**, *126*, 129–138. [CrossRef] [PubMed]
94. Granata, S.; Mercuri, S.; Troise, D.; Gesualdo, L.; Stallone, G.; Zaza, G. mTOR-inhibitors and post-transplant diabetes mellitus: A link still debated in kidney transplantation. *Front. Med.* **2023**, *10*, 1168967. [CrossRef] [PubMed]
95. Saha, S.; Fang, X.; Green, C.D.; Das, A. mTORC1 and SGLT2 Inhibitors—A Therapeutic Perspective for Diabetic Cardiomyopathy. *Int. J. Mol. Sci.* **2023**, *24*, 15078. [CrossRef] [PubMed]
96. Den Hartogh, D.J.; Vlavcheski, F.; Giacca, A.; Tsiani, E. Attenuation of free fatty acid (FFA)-induced skeletal muscle cell insulin resistance by resveratrol is linked to activation of AMPK and inhibition of mTOR and p70 S6K. *Int. J. Mol. Sci.* **2020**, *21*, 4900. [CrossRef] [PubMed]

97. Koh, J.-H.; Kim, K.-H.; Park, S.-Y.; Kim, Y.-W.; Kim, J.-Y. PPARδ attenuates alcohol-mediated insulin resistance by enhancing fatty acid-induced mitochondrial uncoupling and antioxidant defense in skeletal muscle. *Front. Physiol.* **2020**, *11*, 749. [CrossRef]
98. Lee, H.-K.; Kwon, B.; Lemere, C.A.; De La Monte, S.; Itamura, K.; Ha, A.Y.; Querfurth, H.W. mTORC2 (Rictor) in Alzheimer's disease and reversal of amyloid-β expression-induced insulin resistance and toxicity in rat primary cortical neurons. *J. Alzheimer's Dis.* **2017**, *56*, 1015–1036. [CrossRef] [PubMed]
99. den Hartigh, L.J.; Goodspeed, L.; Wang, S.A.; Kenerson, H.L.; Omer, M.; O'Brien, K.D.; Ladiges, W.; Yeung, R.; Subramanian, S. Chronic oral rapamycin decreases adiposity, hepatic triglycerides and insulin resistance in male mice fed a diet high in sucrose and saturated fat. *Exp. Physiol.* **2018**, *103*, 1469–1480. [CrossRef]
100. Sharma, A.; Chetty, V. Obesity, hypertension and insulin resistance. *Acta Diabetol.* **2005**, *42*, s3–s8. [CrossRef]
101. Boyer, F.; Vidot, J.B.; Dubourg, A.G.; Rondeau, P.; Essop, M.F.; Bourdon, E. Oxidative stress and adipocyte biology: Focus on the role of AGEs. *Oxidative Med. Cell. Longev.* **2015**, *2015*, 534873. [CrossRef] [PubMed]
102. Kang, Q.; Yang, C. Oxidative stress and diabetic retinopathy: Molecular mechanisms, pathogenetic role and therapeutic implications. *Redox Biol.* **2020**, *37*, 101799. [CrossRef] [PubMed]
103. Ott, C.; Jacobs, K.; Haucke, E.; Santos, A.N.; Grune, T.; Simm, A. Role of advanced glycation end products in cellular signaling. *Redox Biol.* **2014**, *2*, 411–429. [CrossRef] [PubMed]
104. Baver, S.B.; Hope, K.; Guyot, S.; Bjørbaek, C.; Kaczorowski, C.; O'Connell, K.M. Leptin modulates the intrinsic excitability of AgRP/NPY neurons in the arcuate nucleus of the hypothalamus. *J. Neurosci.* **2014**, *34*, 5486–5496. [CrossRef] [PubMed]
105. Chang, W.-C.; Wu, S.-C.; Xu, K.-D.; Liao, B.-C.; Wu, J.-F.; Cheng, A.-S. Scopoletin protects against methylglyoxal-induced hyperglycemia and insulin resistance mediated by suppression of advanced glycation endproducts (AGEs) generation and anti-glycation. *Molecules* **2015**, *20*, 2786–2801. [CrossRef] [PubMed]
106. González, P.; Lozano, P.; Ros, G.; Solano, F. Hyperglycemia and oxidative stress: An integral, updated and critical overview of their metabolic interconnections. *Int. J. Mol. Sci.* **2023**, *24*, 9352. [CrossRef] [PubMed]
107. Stefano, G.B.; Challenger, S.; Kream, R.M. Hyperglycemia-associated alterations in cellular signaling and dysregulated mitochondrial bioenergetics in human metabolic disorders. *Eur. J. Nutr.* **2016**, *55*, 2339–2345. [CrossRef] [PubMed]
108. Pal, R.; Bhadada, S.K. AGEs accumulation with vascular complications, glycemic control and metabolic syndrome: A narrative review. *Bone* **2023**, *176*, 116884. [CrossRef] [PubMed]
109. Wang, Y.; Eshwaran, R.; Beck, S.C.; Hammes, H.-P.; Wieland, T.; Feng, Y. Contribution of the hexosamine biosynthetic pathway in the hyperglycemia-dependent and-independent breakdown of the retinal neurovascular unit. *Mol. Metab.* **2023**, *73*, 101736. [CrossRef]
110. Chatterjee, A.; Eshwaran, R.; Poschet, G.; Lomada, S.; Halawa, M.; Wilhelm, K.; Schmidt, M.; Hammes, H.-P.; Wieland, T.; Feng, Y. Involvement of NDPK-B in glucose metabolism-mediated endothelial damage via activation of the hexosamine biosynthesis pathway and suppression of O-GlcNAcase activity. *Cells* **2020**, *9*, 2324. [CrossRef]
111. Sage, A.T.; Walter, L.A.; Shi, Y.; Khan, M.I.; Kaneto, H.; Capretta, A.; Werstuck, G.H. Hexosamine biosynthesis pathway flux promotes endoplasmic reticulum stress, lipid accumulation, and inflammatory gene expression in hepatic cells. *Am. J. Physiol.-Endocrinol. Metab.* **2010**, *298*, E499–E511. [CrossRef]
112. Vasconcelos-dos-Santos, A.; de Queiroz, R.M.; da Costa Rodrigues, B.; Todeschini, A.R.; Dias, W.B. Hyperglycemia and aberrant O-GlcNAc ylation: Contributions to tumor progression. *J. Bioenerg. Biomembr.* **2018**, *50*, 175–187. [CrossRef] [PubMed]
113. Wronka, M.; Krzemińska, J.; Młynarska, E.; Rysz, J.; Franczyk, B. The influence of lifestyle and treatment on oxidative stress and inflammation in diabetes. *Int. J. Mol. Sci.* **2022**, *23*, 15743. [CrossRef] [PubMed]
114. An, Y.; Xu, B.-T.; Wan, S.-R.; Ma, X.-M.; Long, Y.; Xu, Y.; Jiang, Z.-Z. The role of oxidative stress in diabetes mellitus-induced vascular endothelial dysfunction. *Cardiovasc. Diabetol.* **2023**, *22*, 237. [CrossRef] [PubMed]
115. Luc, K.; Schramm-Luc, A.; Guzik, T.; Mikolajczyk, T. Oxidative stress and inflammatory markers in prediabetes and diabetes. *J. Physiol. Pharmacol.* **2019**, *70*, 809–824.
116. Lima, J.E.; Moreira, N.C.; Sakamoto-Hojo, E.T. Mechanisms underlying the pathophysiology of type 2 diabetes: From risk factors to oxidative stress, metabolic dysfunction, and hyperglycemia. *Mutat. Res./Genet. Toxicol. Environ. Mutagen.* **2022**, *874*, 503437. [CrossRef]
117. Jubaidi, F.F.; Zainalabidin, S.; Taib, I.S.; Abdul Hamid, Z.; Mohamad Anuar, N.N.; Jalil, J.; Mohd Nor, N.A.; Budin, S.B. The role of PKC-MAPK signalling pathways in the development of hyperglycemia-induced cardiovascular complications. *Int. J. Mol. Sci.* **2022**, *23*, 8582. [CrossRef] [PubMed]
118. Adua, E. Decoding the mechanism of hypertension through multiomics profiling. *J. Hum. Hypertens.* **2023**, *37*, 253–264. [CrossRef]
119. Te Riet, L.; van Esch, J.H.; Roks, A.J.; van den Meiracker, A.H.; Danser, A.J. Hypertension: Renin–angiotensin–aldosterone system alterations. *Circ. Res.* **2015**, *116*, 960–975. [CrossRef]
120. Rossier, B.C.; Bochud, M.; Devuyst, O. The hypertension pandemic: An evolutionary perspective. *Physiology* **2017**, *32*, 112–125. [CrossRef]
121. Deedwania, P. Hypertension, dyslipidemia, and insulin resistance in patients with diabetes mellitus or the cardiometabolic syndrome: Benefits of vasodilating β-blockers. *J. Clin. Hypertens.* **2011**, *13*, 52–59. [CrossRef] [PubMed]
122. Hsueh, W.A.; Wyne, K. Renin-angiotensin-aldosterone system in diabetes and hypertension. *J. Clin. Hypertens.* **2011**, *13*, 224–237. [CrossRef] [PubMed]

123. Lee, M.; Sorn, S.R.; Lee, Y.; Kang, I. Salt induces adipogenesis/lipogenesis and inflammatory adipocytokines secretion in adipocytes. *Int. J. Mol. Sci.* **2019**, *20*, 160. [CrossRef] [PubMed]
124. Jia, G.; Sowers, J.R. Hypertension in diabetes: An update of basic mechanisms and clinical disease. *Hypertension* **2021**, *78*, 1197–1205. [CrossRef] [PubMed]
125. Hill, M.A.; Yang, Y.; Zhang, L.; Sun, Z.; Jia, G.; Parrish, A.R.; Sowers, J.R. Insulin resistance, cardiovascular stiffening and cardiovascular disease. *Metabolism* **2021**, *119*, 154766. [CrossRef] [PubMed]
126. Tagi, V.M.; Mainieri, F.; Chiarelli, F. Hypertension in patients with insulin resistance: Etiopathogenesis and management in children. *Int. J. Mol. Sci.* **2022**, *23*, 5814. [CrossRef] [PubMed]
127. Pulakat, L.; DeMarco, V.G.; Whaley-Connell, A.; Sowers, J.R. The impact of overnutrition on insulin metabolic signaling in the heart and the kidney. *Cardiorenal Med.* **2011**, *1*, 102–112. [CrossRef]
128. Hwang, H.J.; Kim, N.; Herman, A.B.; Gorospe, M.; Lee, J.-S. Factors and pathways modulating endothelial cell senescence in vascular aging. *Int. J. Mol. Sci.* **2022**, *23*, 10135. [CrossRef]
129. Gleason, C.E.; Frindt, G.; Cheng, C.-J.; Ng, M.; Kidwai, A.; Rashmi, P.; Lang, F.; Baum, M.; Palmer, L.G.; Pearce, D. mTORC2 regulates renal tubule sodium uptake by promoting ENaC activity. *J. Clin. Investig.* **2015**, *125*, 117–128. [CrossRef]
130. Mansley, M.K.; Wilson, S.M. Dysregulation of epithelial Na+ absorption induced by inhibition of the kinases TORC1 and TORC2. *Br. J. Pharmacol.* **2010**, *161*, 1778–1792. [CrossRef]
131. Kumar, V.; Evans, L.C.; Kurth, T.; Yang, C.; Wollner, C.; Nasci, V.; Zheleznova, N.N.; Bukowy, J.; Dayton, A.; Cowley, A.W., Jr. Therapeutic suppression of mTOR (mammalian target of rapamycin) signaling prevents and reverses salt-induced hypertension and kidney injury in Dahl salt-sensitive rats. *Hypertension* **2019**, *73*, 630–639. [CrossRef] [PubMed]
132. Kundu, B.K.; Zhong, M.; Sen, S.; Davogustto, G.; Keller, S.R.; Taegtmeyer, H. Remodeling of glucose metabolism precedes pressure overload-induced left ventricular hypertrophy: Review of a hypothesis. *Cardiology* **2015**, *130*, 211–220. [CrossRef] [PubMed]
133. Birajdar, S.V.; Mazahir, F.; Alam, M.I.; Kumar, A.; Yadav, A.K. Repurposing and clinical attributes of antidiabetic drugs for the treatment of neurodegenerative disorders. *Eur. J. Pharmacol.* **2023**, *961*, 176117. [CrossRef] [PubMed]
134. Chen, Q.; Zhang, H.; Yang, Y.; Zhang, S.; Wang, J.; Zhang, D.; Yu, H. Metformin attenuates UVA-induced skin photoaging by suppressing mitophagy and the PI3K/AKT/mTOR pathway. *Int. J. Mol. Sci.* **2022**, *23*, 6960. [CrossRef] [PubMed]
135. Ampuero, J.; Romero-Gomez, M. Prevention of hepatocellular carcinoma by correction of metabolic abnormalities: Role of statins and metformin. *World J. Hepatol.* **2015**, *7*, 1105. [CrossRef] [PubMed]
136. Citi, V.; Barresi, E.; Piragine, E.; Spezzini, J.; Testai, L.; Da Settimo, F.; Martelli, A.; Taliani, S.; Calderone, V. Anti-Proliferative Properties of the Novel Hybrid Drug Met-ITC, Composed of the Native Drug Metformin with the Addition of an Isothiocyanate H2S Donor Moiety, in Different Cancer Cell Lines. *Int. J. Mol. Sci.* **2023**, *24*, 16131. [CrossRef] [PubMed]
137. He, X.; Esteva, F.; Ensor, J.; Hortobagyi, G.; Lee, M.-H.; Yeung, S.-C. Metformin and thiazolidinediones are associated with improved breast cancer-specific survival of diabetic women with HER2+ breast cancer. *Ann. Oncol.* **2012**, *23*, 1771–1780. [CrossRef] [PubMed]
138. Pusceddu, S.; Buzzoni, R.; Vernieri, C.; Concas, L.; Marceglia, S.; Giacomelli, L.; Milione, M.; Leuzzi, L.; Femia, D.; Formisano, B. Metformin with everolimus and octreotide in pancreatic neuroendocrine tumor patients with diabetes. *Future Oncol.* **2016**, *12*, 1251–1260. [CrossRef]
139. Shen, Z.; Xue, D.; Wang, K.; Zhang, F.; Shi, J.; Jia, B.; Yang, D.; Zhang, Q.; Zhang, S.; Jiang, H. Metformin exerts an antitumor effect by inhibiting bladder cancer cell migration and growth, and promoting apoptosis through the PI3K/AKT/mTOR pathway. *BMC Urol.* **2022**, *22*, 79. [CrossRef]
140. Hopkins, B.D.; Pauli, C.; Du, X.; Wang, D.G.; Li, X.; Wu, D.; Amadiume, S.C.; Goncalves, M.D.; Hodakoski, C.; Lundquist, M.R. Suppression of insulin feedback enhances the efficacy of PI3K inhibitors. *Nature* **2018**, *560*, 499–503. [CrossRef]
141. Cheung, Y.-M.M.; McDonnell, M.; Hamnvik, O.-P.R. A targeted approach to phosphoinositide-3-kinase/Akt/mammalian target of rapamycin-induced hyperglycemia. *Curr. Probl. Cancer* **2022**, *46*, 100776. [CrossRef] [PubMed]
142. Owen, M.D.; Baker, B.C.; Scott, E.M.; Forbes, K. Interaction between metformin, folate and vitamin B12 and the potential impact on fetal growth and long-term metabolic health in diabetic pregnancies. *Int. J. Mol. Sci.* **2021**, *22*, 5759. [CrossRef] [PubMed]
143. Shen, M.; Yu, H.; Jin, Y.; Mo, J.; Sui, J.; Qian, X.; Chen, T. Metformin facilitates osteoblastic differentiation and M2 macrophage polarization by PI3K/AKT/mTOR pathway in human umbilical cord mesenchymal stem cells. *Stem Cells Int.* **2022**, *2022*, 9498876. [CrossRef]
144. Singh, S.K.; Apata, T.; Singh, S.; McFadden, M.; Singh, R. Clinical implication of metformin in relation to diabetes mellitus and ovarian cancer. *Biomedicines* **2021**, *9*, 1020. [CrossRef] [PubMed]
145. Triggle, C.R.; Mohammed, I.; Bshesh, K.; Marei, I.; Ye, K.; Ding, H.; MacDonald, R.; Hollenberg, M.D.; Hill, M.A. Metformin: Is it a drug for all reasons and diseases? *Metabolism* **2022**, *133*, 155223. [CrossRef] [PubMed]
146. Ala, M.; Ala, M. Metformin for cardiovascular protection, inflammatory bowel disease, osteoporosis, periodontitis, polycystic ovarian syndrome, neurodegeneration, cancer, inflammation and senescence: What is next? *ACS Pharmacol. Transl. Sci.* **2021**, *4*, 1747–1770. [CrossRef] [PubMed]
147. Pusceddu, S.; Vernieri, C.; Di Maio, M.; Marconcini, R.; Spada, F.; Massironi, S.; Ibrahim, T.; Brizzi, M.P.; Campana, D.; Faggiano, A. Metformin use is associated with longer progression-free survival of patients with diabetes and pancreatic neuroendocrine tumors receiving everolimus and/or somatostatin analogues. *Gastroenterology* **2018**, *155*, 479–489.e7. [CrossRef] [PubMed]

148. Wynn, A.; Vacheron, A.; Zuber, J.; Solomon, S.S. Metformin associated with increased survival in type 2 diabetes patients with pancreatic cancer and lymphoma. *Am. J. Med. Sci.* **2019**, *358*, 200–203. [CrossRef] [PubMed]
149. Deblon, N.; Bourgoin, L.; Veyrat-Durebex, C.; Peyrou, M.; Vinciguerra, M.; Caillon, A.; Maeder, C.; Fournier, M.; Montet, X.; Rohner-Jeanrenaud, F. Chronic mTOR inhibition by rapamycin induces muscle insulin resistance despite weight loss in rats. *Br. J. Pharmacol.* **2012**, *165*, 2325–2340. [CrossRef]
150. Lamming, D.W.; Ye, L.; Katajisto, P.; Goncalves, M.D.; Saitoh, M.; Stevens, D.M.; Davis, J.G.; Salmon, A.B.; Richardson, A.; Ahima, R.S. Rapamycin-induced insulin resistance is mediated by mTORC2 loss and uncoupled from longevity. *Science* **2012**, *335*, 1638–1643. [CrossRef]
151. D'Elia, J.A.; Weinrauch, L.A. Hyperglycemia and hyperlipidemia with kidney or liver transplantation: A review. *Biology* **2023**, *12*, 1185. [CrossRef] [PubMed]
152. Blagosklonny, M.V. Once again on rapamycin-induced insulin resistance and longevity: Despite of or owing to. *Aging* **2012**, *4*, 350. [CrossRef]
153. Kezic, A.; Popovic, L.; Lalic, K. mTOR inhibitor therapy and metabolic consequences: Where do we stand? *Oxidative Med. Cell. Longev.* **2018**, *2018*, 2640342. [CrossRef]
154. Wang, T.; Kusudo, T.; Takeuchi, T.; Yamashita, Y.; Kontani, Y.; Okamatsu, Y.; Saito, M.; Mori, N.; Yamashita, H. Evodiamine inhibits insulin-stimulated mTOR-S6K activation and IRS1 serine phosphorylation in adipocytes and improves glucose tolerance in obese/diabetic mice. *PLoS ONE* **2013**, *8*, e83264. [CrossRef] [PubMed]
155. Pereira, M.J.; Palming, J.; Rizell, M.; Aureliano, M.; Carvalho, E.; Svensson, M.K.; Eriksson, J.W. mTOR inhibition with rapamycin causes impaired insulin signalling and glucose uptake in human subcutaneous and omental adipocytes. *Mol. Cell. Endocrinol.* **2012**, *355*, 96–105. [CrossRef]
156. Zhang, N.; Ma, S. Research progress of 70 kDa ribosomal protein S6 kinase (P70S6K) inhibitors as effective therapeutic tools for obesity, type II diabetes and cancer. *Curr. Med. Chem.* **2020**, *27*, 4699–4719. [CrossRef] [PubMed]
157. Tarantino, G.; Capone, D. Inhibition of the mTOR pathway: A possible protective role in coronary artery disease. *Ann. Med.* **2013**, *45*, 348–356. [CrossRef]
158. Das, A.; Durrant, D.; Koka, S.; Salloum, F.N.; Xi, L.; Kukreja, R.C. Mammalian target of rapamycin (mTOR) inhibition with rapamycin improves cardiac function in type 2 diabetic mice: Potential role of attenuated oxidative stress and altered contractile protein expression. *J. Biol. Chem.* **2014**, *289*, 4145–4160. [CrossRef]
159. Wang, J.; Fan, S.; Xiong, Q.; Niu, Y.; Zhang, X.; Qin, J.; Shi, Y.; Zhang, L. Glucagon-like peptide-1 attenuates cardiac hypertrophy via the AngII/AT1R/ACE2 and AMPK/mTOR/p70S6K pathways. *Acta Biochim. Et Biophys. Sin.* **2021**, *53*, 1189–1197. [CrossRef]
160. Patel, S.M.; Kang, Y.M.; Im, K.; Neuen, B.L.; Anker, S.D.; Bhatt, D.L.; Butler, J.; Cherney, D.Z.; Claggett, B.L.; Fletcher, R.A. Sodium-Glucose Cotransporter-2 Inhibitors and Major Adverse Cardiovascular Outcomes: A SMART-C Collaborative Meta-Analysis. *Circulation* **2024**, *149*, 1789–1801. [CrossRef]
161. Schaub, J.A.; AlAkwaa, F.M.; McCown, P.J.; Naik, A.S.; Nair, V.; Eddy, S.; Menon, R.; Otto, E.A.; Demeke, D.; Hartman, J. SGLT2 inhibitors mitigate kidney tubular metabolic and mTORC1 perturbations in youth-onset type 2 diabetes. *J. Clin. Investig.* **2023**, *133*, e164486. [CrossRef]
162. Blagosklonny, M.V. Fasting and rapamycin: Diabetes versus benevolent glucose intolerance. *Cell Death Dis.* **2019**, *10*, 607. [CrossRef] [PubMed]
163. Zhou, W.; Ye, S. Rapamycin improves insulin resistance and hepatic steatosis in type 2 diabetes rats through activation of autophagy. *Cell Biol. Int.* **2018**, *42*, 1282–1291. [CrossRef] [PubMed]
164. Reifsnyder, P.C.; Flurkey, K.; Doty, R.; Calcutt, N.A.; Koza, R.A.; Harrison, D.E. Rapamycin/metformin co-treatment normalizes insulin sensitivity and reduces complications of metabolic syndrome in type 2 diabetic mice. *Aging Cell* **2022**, *21*, e13666. [CrossRef] [PubMed]
165. Reifsnyder, P.C.; Flurkey, K.; Te, A.; Harrison, D.E. Rapamycin treatment benefits glucose metabolism in mouse models of type 2 diabetes. *Aging* **2016**, *8*, 3120. [CrossRef] [PubMed]
166. Gadallah, S.H.; Ghanem, H.M.; Abdel-Ghaffar, A.; Metwaly, F.G.; Hanafy, L.K.; Ahmed, E.K. 4-Phenylbutyric acid and rapamycin improved diabetic status in high fat diet/streptozotocin-induced type 2 diabetes through activation of autophagy. *Arch. Physiol. Biochem.* **2021**, *127*, 235–244. [CrossRef]
167. Zhao, M.; Li, X.W.; Chen, D.Z.; Hao, F.; Tao, S.X.; Yu, H.Y.; Cheng, R.; Liu, H. Neuro-protective role of metformin in patients with acute stroke and type 2 diabetes mellitus via AMPK/mammalian target of rapamycin (mTOR) signaling pathway and oxidative stress. *Med. Sci. Monit. Int. Med. J. Exp. Clin. Res.* **2019**, *25*, 2186. [CrossRef] [PubMed]
168. Temiz-Resitoglu, M.; Guden, D.S.; Senol, S.P.; Vezir, O.; Sucu, N.; Kibar, D.; Yılmaz, S.N.; Tunctan, B.; Malik, K.U.; Sahan-Firat, S. Pharmacological inhibition of mammalian target of rapamycin attenuates deoxycorticosterone acetate salt–induced hypertension and related pathophysiology: Regulation of oxidative stress, inflammation, and cardiovascular hypertrophy in male rats. *J. Cardiovasc. Pharmacol.* **2022**, *79*, 355–367. [CrossRef] [PubMed]
169. Wang, W.; Yan, J.; Wang, H.; Shi, M.; Zhang, M.; Yang, W.; Peng, C.; Li, H. Rapamycin ameliorates inflammation and fibrosis in the early phase of cirrhotic portal hypertension in rats through inhibition of mTORC1 but not mTORC2. *PLoS ONE* **2014**, *9*, e83908. [CrossRef]

170. Kumar, V.; Wollner, C.; Kurth, T.; Bukowy, J.D.; Cowley, A.W., Jr. Inhibition of mammalian target of rapamycin complex 1 attenuates salt-induced hypertension and kidney injury in Dahl salt-sensitive rats. *Hypertension* **2017**, *70*, 813–821. [CrossRef]
171. Kurniawan, R.; Nurkolis, F.; Taslim, N.A.; Subali, D.; Surya, R.; Gunawan, W.B.; Alisaputra, D.; Mayulu, N.; Salindeho, N.; Kim, B. Carotenoids composition of green algae *Caulerpa racemosa* and their antidiabetic, anti-obesity, antioxidant, and anti-inflammatory properties. *Molecules* **2023**, *28*, 3267. [CrossRef]

biomedicines

MDPI

Review

Retinal Imaging-Based Oculomics: Artificial Intelligence as a Tool in the Diagnosis of Cardiovascular and Metabolic Diseases

Laura Andreea Ghenciu [1,2], Mirabela Dima [3,*], Emil Robert Stoicescu [4,5,6], Roxana Iacob [4,7,8], Casiana Boru [9] and Ovidiu Alin Hațegan [9]

1 Department of Functional Sciences, 'Victor Babes' University of Medicine and Pharmacy Timisoara, Eftimie Murgu Square No. 2, 300041 Timisoara, Romania; bolintineanu.laura@umft.ro
2 Center for Translational Research and Systems Medicine, 'Victor Babes' University of Medicine and Pharmacy Timisoara, Eftimie Murgu Square No. 2, 300041 Timisoara, Romania
3 Department of Neonatology, 'Victor Babes' University of Medicine and Pharmacy Timisoara, Eftimie Murgu Square No. 2, 300041 Timisoara, Romania
4 Field of Applied Engineering Sciences, Specialization Statistical Methods and Techniques in Health and Clinical Research, Faculty of Mechanics, 'Politehnica' University Timisoara, Mihai Viteazul Boulevard No. 1, 300222 Timisoara, Romania; stoicescu.emil@umft.ro (E.R.S.); roxana.iacob@umft.ro (R.I.)
5 Department of Radiology and Medical Imaging, 'Victor Babes' University of Medicine and Pharmacy Timisoara, Eftimie Murgu Square No. 2, 300041 Timisoara, Romania
6 Research Center for Pharmaco-Toxicological Evaluations, 'Victor Babes' University of Medicine and Pharmacy Timisoara, Eftimie Murgu Square No. 2, 300041 Timisoara, Romania
7 Doctoral School, "Victor Babes" University of Medicine and Pharmacy Timisoara, Eftimie Murgu Square 2, 300041 Timisoara, Romania
8 Department of Anatomy and Embriology, 'Victor Babes' University of Medicine and Pharmacy Timisoara, 300041 Timisoara, Romania
9 Discipline of Anatomy and Embriology, Medicine Faculty, "Vasile Goldis" Western University of Arad, Revolution Boulevard 94, 310025 Arad, Romania; boru.casiana@uvvg.ro (C.B.); hategan.ovidiu@uvvg.ro (O.A.H.)
* Correspondence: mirabela.dima@umft.ro

Abstract: Cardiovascular diseases (CVDs) are a major cause of mortality globally, emphasizing the need for early detection and effective risk assessment to improve patient outcomes. Advances in oculomics, which utilize the relationship between retinal microvascular changes and systemic vascular health, offer a promising non-invasive approach to assessing CVD risk. Retinal fundus imaging and optical coherence tomography/angiography (OCT/OCTA) provides critical information for early diagnosis, with retinal vascular parameters such as vessel caliber, tortuosity, and branching patterns identified as key biomarkers. Given the large volume of data generated during routine eye exams, there is a growing need for automated tools to aid in diagnosis and risk prediction. The study demonstrates that AI-driven analysis of retinal images can accurately predict cardiovascular risk factors, cardiovascular events, and metabolic diseases, surpassing traditional diagnostic methods in some cases. These models achieved area under the curve (AUC) values ranging from 0.71 to 0.87, sensitivity between 71% and 89%, and specificity between 40% and 70%, surpassing traditional diagnostic methods in some cases. This approach highlights the potential of retinal imaging as a key component in personalized medicine, enabling more precise risk assessment and earlier intervention. It not only aids in detecting vascular abnormalities that may precede cardiovascular events but also offers a scalable, non-invasive, and cost-effective solution for widespread screening. However, the article also emphasizes the need for further research to standardize imaging protocols and validate the clinical utility of these biomarkers across different populations. By integrating oculomics into routine clinical practice, healthcare providers could significantly enhance early detection and management of systemic diseases, ultimately improving patient outcomes. Fundus image analysis thus represents a valuable tool in the future of precision medicine and cardiovascular health management.

Keywords: oculomics; retinal microcirculation; cardiovascular disease; diabetes mellitus; deep learning; artificial intelligence; OCT; OCTA; fundus imaging

1. Introduction

Artificial intelligence (AI) is revolutionizing medicine and diagnostics by enabling more accurate, efficient, and personalized healthcare. AI algorithms, particularly machine learning (ML) and deep learning (DL), can analyze vast amounts of data to identify patterns and make predictions that might be missed by human clinicians [1]. In conjunction with retinal imaging, AI can enhance diagnostic accuracy for various ocular and systemic conditions [2]. Advanced imaging techniques, such as Optical Coherence Tomography (OCT), provide detailed images of the retina, which AI algorithms can analyze to detect early signs of diseases like cardiovascular disease, diabetes mellitus complicated with retinopathy, neurodegenerative diseases, age-related macular degeneration, and glaucoma. AI-driven analysis of retinal images can help in early diagnosis and monitoring of these conditions, facilitating intervention and improved patient outcomes [2,3]. Studies have shown that AI systems can achieve diagnostic performance comparable to that of expert ophthalmologists, thus supporting clinical decision-making and reducing the burden on healthcare systems [1].

Oculomics leverages advanced imaging technologies, genetic information, and data analytics to understand systemic diseases and conditions through ocular biomarkers. The term "oculomics" originates from the combination of "oculo-", referring to the eye, and "-omics", which denotes a comprehensive study of a set of biological molecules. This term was first used in a scientific context in a paper published in 2020 [4]. By analyzing the retina, researchers can detect signs of systemic diseases such as diabetes, cardiovascular diseases, chronic inflammatory diseases and neurodegenerative conditions. The rich vascular structure and neural connections within the eye make it an excellent proxy for detecting early signs of these conditions [2,4].

Cardiovascular diseases (CVDs) are a leading cause of mortality globally, responsible for approximately 17.9 million deaths each year, which accounts for about 32% of all global deaths. The burden of CVD is particularly high in low- and middle-income countries, where over three-quarters of CVD deaths occur. Early detection and management of CVDs are crucial for reducing the associated morbidity and mortality [5]. The retina's microvascular changes can reflect systemic vascular health, allowing for the detection of cardiovascular risk factors like hypertension and diabetes through non-invasive retinal scans [4]. Globally, the prevalence of diabetes has been rising rapidly. As of 2021, approximately 537 million adults aged 20–79 years are living with diabetes, and this number is projected to increase to 783 million by 2045. Early screening for diabetes is crucial for preventing the severe complications associated with the disease. Diabetes is a major cause of blindness, kidney failure, heart attack, stroke, and lower limb amputation. Early screening and detection are essential for managing the disease effectively and reducing its impact on individuals and healthcare systems [6].

Lastly, not only is it relatively straightforward to collect retinal images of a significant number of people, but it is also possible that this new field of study will make use of existing databases like MESA (Multi-ethnic Study of Atherosclerosis) [7], ACCORD (Action to Control Cardiovascular Risk in Diabetes) [8], and ARIC (Atherosclerosis Risk in Communities Study) [9]. Advances in the use of AI and ML approaches to retinal image processing can significantly enhance clinical practice in assessing, predicting, and managing hypertension, CVD, and peripheral arterial disease (PAD).

The aim of this review is to comprehensively examine the emerging field of oculomics, focusing on its potential to revolutionize the diagnosis and management of systemic diseases through the analysis of ocular biomarkers. By integrating advanced imaging technologies, genetic data, and artificial intelligence, oculomics aims to provide a non-invasive, cost-effective, and efficient method for early disease detection and monitoring.

2. Materials and Methods

2.1. Study Design

This review was conducted to evaluate the role of AI in retinal imaging for the diagnosis of cardiovascular and metabolic diseases. The methodology was guided by the Preferred Reporting Items for Systematic Reviews and Meta-Analyses (PRISMA) guidelines, which ensured a structured and transparent approach to the review process [10].

2.2. Indentification and Selection of Studies

A comprehensive search of the peer-reviewed literature was conducted across multiple databases, including PubMed, Scopus, and Google Scholar, to identify studies published in the last 5 years, between January 2019 and May 2024, using both manual and automated searches with MeSH terms. The search strategy was formulated using the Population, Intervention, Comparator, and Outcomes (PICO) framework (Table 1).

Table 1. PICO framework.

PICO	Criteria
Population	Patients at risk of cardiovascular or metabolic diseases (e.g., coronary artery disease, myocardial infarction, hypertension, diabetes)
Intervention	Retinal imaging techniques (fundus photography, OCT, OCTA) analyzed by AI and deep learning models
Comparison	Traditional diagnostic methods such as calcium score, angiography, stress test, clinical biomarkers, and ecocardiography
Outcome	High diagnostic accuracy, sensitivity, and specificity in predicting cardiovascular and metabolic diseases

Initially, research studies were hand-searched in the aforementioned databases using the following keywords: "retinal imaging", "OCT", "OCTA", "fundus photography", "cardiovascular disease", "hypertension", "coronary artery disease", "metabolic disease", and "diabetes mellitus". The same MeSH terms were utilized, alongside their appropriate synonyms and keywords, in combination with Boolean operators (AND, OR); queries were conducted on the title, abstract, keywords, and author keyword fields, utilizing the specified keywords. The search was restricted to journal articles written in English. A methodical and systematic search strategy was employed to identify pertinent scientific papers that investigate the utilization and efficacy of retinal imaging in the diagnosis of cardiovascular and metabolic diseases, according to the PRISMA statement and checklist. The pre-established set of inclusion and exclusion criteria is given in Table 2.

Table 2. Inclusion and exclusion criteria used for this review.

Inclusion Criteria	Exclusion Criteria
Written in English	Articles in other languages
Papers utilizing retinal imaging techniques such as optical coherence tomography (OCT), optical coherence tomography angiography (OCTA), or fundus imaging	Papers with insufficient data for analysis/outcome
Papers focused on the application of AI in retinal imaging for diagnosing cardiovascular and/or metabolic diseases	Review/letters/commentaries/abstracts
Papers published after January 2018	Published before 2018
	Not relevant to the topic

2.3. Data Extraction Process

The lead investigator (L.A.G.) screened the most pertinent publications based on their title, abstract, and a quick glance at the full research manuscript. Abstract screening and the literature database review were then conducted independently by two scientists. All selected articles were added to a Microsoft Excel table with columns for improved subsequent management and organization of the review: title, authors, year and journal of publication, and the specific type of publication. Articles were then structured into cardiovascular or metabolic disease identification and prognosis.

2.4. Overview of Studies Included in the Review

Finally, after the application of the inclusion and exclusion criteria, 37 articles (CVD: 29 articles; Metabolic Diseases: 8 articles) were chosen for the literature review, as they fulfilled all the stated requirements. The process followed for selecting the articles is summarized in the PRISMA diagram (Figure 1).

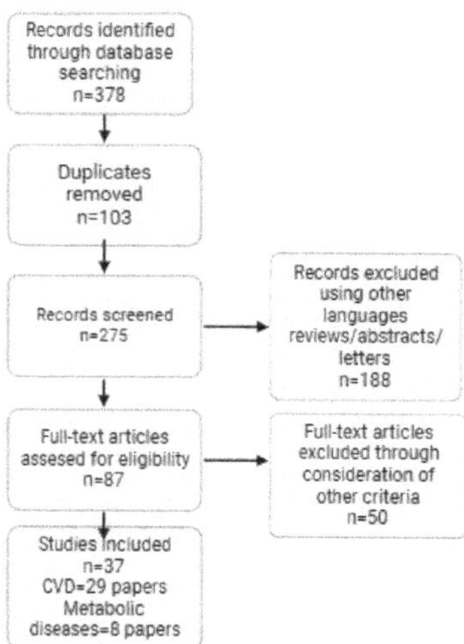

Figure 1. PRISMA flowchart. Created with BioRender.com.

3. Technological Advances in Oculomics

Ideal biomarkers are simple to determine and inexpensive, and ocular imaging has served as the foundation for an AI breakthrough due to its widespread availability and massive worldwide datasets. Color fundus and OCT imaging in ophthalmology provide a wealth of data for neural network training, and developments in multimodal imaging methods and AI have contributed to these developments. Over recent years, there has been an increasing body of data suggesting routine retinal imaging can detect early indicators of several systemic diseases (Figure 2). Thus, retinal vascular variations can aid in predicting cardiac disease and potential risk factors.

Retinal evaluation has been widely used to diagnose hypertension and diabetes mellitus, employing a semiquantitative system of evaluation. Nevertheless, over the last few decades, more accurate, non-invasive tools for assessing microcirculation have emerged.

Retinal biomarkers, for instance ocular imaging techniques, could provide new paths for diagnosis, assessing prognosis, and managing arterial hypertension, heart failure, peripheral arterial disease, and metabolic diseases. When weighed against cardiovascular examination, retinal imaging is more straightforward, more affordable, non-invasive, and can yield high-resolution images of retinal vascularization. Furthermore, retinal vascular alterations can be an indicator of cardiotoxicity caused by medications or environmental exposure, which is a critical feature [1,2,11].

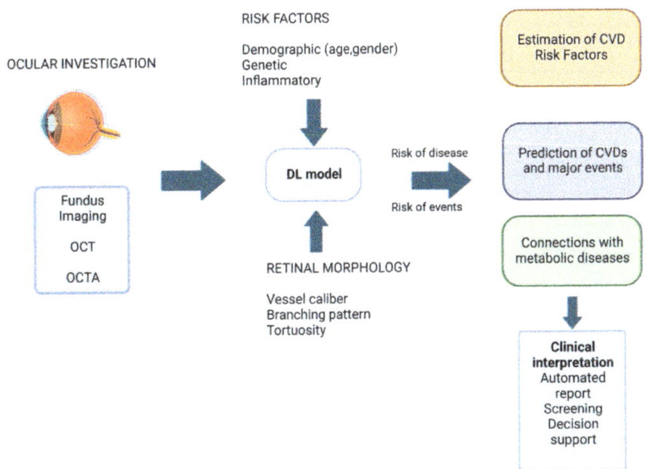

Figure 2. Example of methodology used in medical image analysis. Created with Biorender.

Although invasive, techniques such as fluorescence angiography facilitated the examination of retinal microvessels, while modern approaches, for example, the non-mydriatic video camera and software, permitted extensive analytical investigation of microcirculation [10]. This method and others show promise in prognostic research for cardiovascular illnesses. Further developments include the Retinal Vessel Analyzer (RVA), which investigates dynamic shifts in retinal vessel diameter [12], and scanning laser Doppler flowmetry (SLDF), which evaluates structural and functional capillary characteristics [13]. Adaptive optics retinal imaging devices, initially created for astronomy, have lately been converted for clinical application, resulting in high-resolution images of retinal microcirculation. This method can assess both retinal microvascular variations and endothelial function, but more research is needed to prove its clinical value [14].

OCT and OCTA development and improvement have been the main forces behind oculomics. The advancement of OCT technology from time domain to spectral domain and finally to swept-source has improved resolution, speed, and image quality [15]. OCTA, a readily accessible technology that was developed as an extension of OCT, which uses motion contrast to detect the flow of blood, enables the observation of depth-resolved retinal microvasculature in vivo. Volumetric data segmentation improves viewing of the deep capillary plexus and choroid and makes it easier to identify distinct retinal capillary plexuses at high quality [16]. Numerous retinal biomarkers have been established with the assistance of specific data about the anatomy and circulation of the retina produced by OCT and OCTA, as well as their link with systemic disorders [17]. Multiple imaging techniques are currently being utilized to investigate retinal blood flow patterns and microvascular network properties [18]. These methods depend on current significant advances in computer-based quantitative image analysis technologies. These advanced software programs enable extensive examinations of the morphology of the retinal vessel architecture, including microvascular width, length, quantity, and variations [18]. OCTA is particularly interesting because it provides a three-dimensional picture of retinal blood flow dynamics [19]. Recently published investigations have employed OCTA to connect modifications of retinal capillary networks to characteristics associated with cardiac remodeling [20].

New imaging techniques offer higher resolution, signal-to-noise ratio, and depth than traditional OCT, OCTA, and retinal photography methods. These methods may yield data regarding water content, proteins and lipids, cellular and redox activity, oxygen metabolism, and circulation. Underutilized imaging methods related to oculomics include AO, AO two-photon microscopy, scanning laser ophthalmoscopy, visible-light OCT, localization optoacoustic tomography, and retinal hyperspectral photography [21–24].

Semi-automated identification of retinal arterioles, venules, and the optic nerve head determines retinal microvascular characteristics. Several quantifiable retinal vascular variables can be objectively assessed: retinal caliber, arteriole-to-venule diameter ratio, tortuosity, branching angle, and fractal dimension. The software programs were shown to be extremely reliable and predictable [25].

Prior investigation in animal models of arterial hypertension has demonstrated the significance of alterations in microvascular network architecture in the onset and perpetuation of this disease [26]. The latest research findings on the frequent development of hypertension along with other cardiovascular diseases in individuals with cancer treated with anti-angiogenic medications, which influence microvascular growth and network characteristics, provide additional evidence for the critical role of retinal microcirculation in CVDs.

4. Ocular Biomarkers in Cardiovascular Diseases

4.1. Retinal Morphology Variation in Cardiovascular Disease

Since CVD accounts for about 30% of fatalities globally, it has become more important to create efficient algorithms to identify individuals who are most at risk [4]. Previous research on retinal imaging as an instrument to anticipate CVD risk has mostly focused on conventional risk variables such as age, high blood pressure, and dyslipidemia. Furthermore, researchers have looked into the use of retinal imaging to predict the risk of certain CVD subtypes, such as coronary heart disease and peripheral artery disease. This research has shown that retinal imaging can provide useful insights into CVD risk, expanding the area of risk categorization past traditional markers [7,11].

Research studies have linked retinal features, including arteriolar narrowing and venular widening, to overall mortality and CVD [27]. This suggests that changes in retinal vessels may mirror modifications in peripheral and cerebrovascular flow, shedding light on the role of small vessels in CVD onset and advancement. Tabatabaee et al. discovered that retinal arterial atherosclerosis was closely linked with the degree and extent of coronary artery disease (CAD) utilizing fundus photography [28]. Wong TY et al. discovered an association between retinal arteriolar constriction and the occurrence/development of coronary heart disease (CHD) by analyzing the diameters of each arteriole and venule on retinal images [29]. The predictive relevance of retinal arteriolar narrowing for the onset of hypertension is now thoroughly documented in multiple cohort studies conducted in different areas of the globe and among diverse races [19,30]. A meta-analysis of the majority of these investigations revealed that each decrease in retinal arteriolar diameter by 3 μm correlates with a 10 mmHg increase in blood pressure [31].

Prior research has linked vascular morphology (artery/vein diameter, branching angle, tortuosity, fractal dimension), network variations, and the presence of disease-related retinal characteristics (cotton wool sports, arteriovenous nicking, hemorrhages, microaneurysms) to CVD risk. However, focusing primarily on individual metrics may result in missing vital information and maybe underestimating the retina's total potential to depict cardiovascular health. A broader strategy, such as artificial intelligence, could make better use of the retina's ability as a cardiovascular risk marker.

4.2. Automated Idenfication and Prediction of Cardiovascular Diseases

AI can train on large datasets of retinal images to develop systems that detect and predict CVD risk factors by analyzing retinal features that correlate with cardiovascular health (Table 3). These datasets include labeled images that capture various retinal characteristics like vessel caliber, tortuosity, and the presence of microaneurysms. AI models, particularly deep learning algorithms, learn to recognize patterns and abnormalities associated with CVD. Over time, these systems can accurately predict risks by correlating retinal changes with known cardiovascular conditions, offering a non-invasive tool for early diagnosis and prevention [32].

Retinal aging was recently utilized as a substitute for CVD risk. Nusinovici et al. analyzed the retinal biological age (RetiAGE) using a DL method. They found that RetiAGE, regardless of phenotypic indicators such as impaired levels of creatinine, glucose, C-reactive protein, or chronological age, predicted the occurrence of CVDs [33]. Furthermore, another investigation studied retinal age prediction using retinal photography and discovered that the retinal age gap was strongly linked with arterial stiffness index [34] and stroke [35]. Non-invasive approaches were employed to investigate the relationship between retinal microcirculation, metabolic variables, and CVD prognosis. Previous population-based investigations discovered that narrowing of the retinal arterioles and a widening of the venules were associated with coronary artery disease, heart failure, and stroke, though the results differed by age and gender [29]. Retinal microcirculation studies at a younger age have better predictive potential, especially in females, where microvascular impairment plays a larger role in CVD [30]. The Atherosclerosis Risk in Communities Study is among the most enduring cardiovascular research efforts and has gathered 20 years of data; it concluded that retinal vascular diameter monitoring is an easy, non-invasive method that may anticipate heart failure and undesirable cardiac alterations up to almost two decades in advance, offering important information about long-term cardiovascular health [9]. Comparable outcomes across people with diabetes in the Wisconsin Epidemiologic Study of Diabetic Retinopathy supported this [36]. Nevertheless, a meta-analysis that included six studies assessing retinal vascular caliber and incident stroke for five to twelve years came to the conclusion that larger retinal venular caliber, rather than retinal arteriolar caliber, anticipated stroke [4].

Retinal fundus imaging is being investigated for stroke risk evaluation due to the similarities between retinal and cerebral microcirculations. A binary DL model with VGG19 architecture achieved great accuracy (AUC $\geq$ 0.966). This model received two distinct pre-processed photographs: the first one with contrast normalization and median filtering, and another from U-Net delineation for vascular imaging, with heat maps emphasizing predictive regions [37]. A separate investigation employed Inception-Resnet-v2 to estimate 10-year ischemic CVD risk, with AUCs of 0.976 and 0.876, respectively [38]. A DL system for CVD prediction was created, which includes a hybrid approach that calculates cardiac parameters such as left ventricular mass and left ventricular end-diastolic volume while also predicting myocardial infarction risk [39]. This method employs a multichannel variational autoencoder (mcVAE) and ResNet architecture, which are trained on fundus photographs and cardiac magnetic resonance datasets. The application of statistical analysis on this data yielded an AUC of 0.80, with 0.74 sensitivity and 0.71 specificity to anticipate CAD events.

In another study, researchers created a DL model known as the Deep Learning-Funduscopic Atherosclerosis Score (DL-FAS), which analyzes retinal fundus pictures to anticipate atherosclerosis. Their results demonstrated that retinal pictures could not only identify atherosclerosis but also improve traditional risk stratification values like the Framingham Risk Score when forecasting cardiovascular death. The investigation used a large-sized cohort to investigate the additional benefit of DL-FAS. Importantly, the system had a substantial link with cardiovascular mortality, even in individuals classed as intermediate risk using standard techniques [40]. This is a critical field of research, because standard risk assessments frequently underestimate the danger for individuals with asymptomatic mild atherosclerosis.

Oculomics and genomes may be used in disease diagnosis, including multimodal imaging, non-invasive biomarkers, and other examination results [41,42]. Huang et al. discovered a substantial correlation between particular retinal vascular changes and the chance of developing aneurysms, as well as the outstanding potential of retinal vascular features to predict potential aneurysm risk using a predictive, preventive, and personalized medicine method [42]. According to studies, AI can assess and detect a variety of non-ophthalmologic diseases, including chronic kidney disease, carotid artery atherosclerosis, and several CVD risk factors including blood pressure, body mass index, and hemoglobin A1c. Integrating retinal characteristics into a CVD risk algorithm increased its predicted accuracy more than integrating standard chemical indicators like high-sensitivity C-reactive protein [12].

Table 3. Summary of studies using retinal fundus imaging, optical coherence tomography (OCT), and optical coherence tomography angiography (OCTA) in subjects to identify/predict several types of cardiovascular disease. "Related" indicates that the authors did not publish an AUC value, but their results demonstrated significant connections between retinal changes and outcomes. ** The model achieved these percentages in effectively removing photos not suitable for analysis, ensuring that only high-quality images were considered for accurate evaluation. AO: adaptive optics; AUC: area under the curve; CAD: coronary artery disease; CHF: congestive heart failure; HTN: hypertension; IS: ischemic stroke; MI: myocardial infarction.

Study	Disease	Method	Dataset	Recruitment	Task	Outcome	Results	Sensitivity/Specificity
Aschauer et al., 2021 [43]	CAD	Fundus imaging, OCTA, AO	45 patients	Prospective	Identification	Clinical diagnosis	Related	-
Chang et al., 2020 [40]	CAD	Fundus imaging	15,408 images	Retrospective	Prediction	Atherosclerosis Score	AUC = 0.713	89.1%/40.4%
Cheung et al., 2021 [44]	CAD	Fundus imaging	5309 images	Retrospective	Prediction	Retinal-vessel morphological parameters	Related	-
Huang et al., 2022 [45]	CAD	Fundus imaging	145 patients	Prospective	Prediction	Vascular biomarkers and CAD-RADS	AUC = 0.739	71.1%/69.7%
Lee et al., 2023 [46]	CAD	Fundus imaging	2954 images	Retrospective	Prediction	Clinical diagnosis	AUC = 0.872	87.1%/50.8%
Matuleviciute et al., 2022 [47]	CAD	OCT/ OCTA	184 patients	Retrospective	Prediction	Retinal and choroidal thickness, retinal vascular parameters	Related	-
Nusinovici et al., 2022 [33]	CAD	Fundus imaging	129,236 images	Retrospective	Prediction	Biological age	Related	76%/55%
Ren et al., 2023 [48]	CAD	OCTA	185 patients	Retrospective	Prediction	Clinical diagnosis	AUC = 0.840/0.830	-
Son et al., 2020 [49]	CAD	Fundus imaging	44,184 images	Retrospective	Prediction	Coronary artery calcium score	AUC = 0.832	-
Wang et al., 2019 [50]	CAD	OCTA	316 patients	Prospective	Identification	Clinical diagnosis	Related	-
Cao et al., 2021 [51]	IS	OCTA	86 patients	Retrospective	Identification	Retinal-vessel morphological parameters	Related	-
Duan et al., 2022 [52]	IS	OCTA	60 patients	Retrospective	Identification	Retinal-vessel morphological parameters	Related	-
Liang et al., 2022 [53]	IS	OCTA	268 patients	Retrospective	Identification	Retinal-vessel morphological parameters	Related	-
Molero-Senosiain et al., 2022 [54]	IS	OCT/ OCTA	65 patients	Retrospective	Identification	Retinal-vessel morphological parameters	Related	-
Zhang et al., 2020 [55]	IS	OCTA	150 patients	Retrospective	Prediction	Retinal-vessel morphological parameters	Related	-
Ye et al., 2022 [56]	IS	OCT/ OCTA	66 patients	Retrospective	Identification	Retinal-vessel morphological parameters	Related	-

Table 3. *Cont.*

Study	Disease	Method	Dataset	Recruitment	Task	Outcome	Results	Sensitivity/Specificity
Arnould et al., 2020 [57]	MI	OCTA	30 patients	Prospective	Prediction	Retinal-vessel morphological parameters	Not related	89%
Diaz-Pinto et al., 2022 [39]	MI	Fundus imaging	87,476 participants	Retrospective	Prediction	Cardiac indices	AUC = 0.80	74%/71%
Sideri et al., 2023 [58]	MI	OCTA	165 patients	Prospective	Prediction	Cardiac indices	Related	-
Zhong et al., 2021 [59]	MI	OCTA	218 patients	Prospective	Prediction	Retinal-vessel morphological parameters	AUC = 0.812	65.9%/89%
Rakusiewicz et al., 2021[60]	CHF	OCTA	60 patients	Retrospective	Prediction	Clinical diagnosis	Related	-
Topaloglu et al., 2023 [61]	CHF	OCTA	50 patients	Retrospective	Prediction	Clinical diagnosis	Related	-
Zekavat et al., 2022 [62]	CHF	Fundus imaging	97,895 images	Retrospective	Prediction	Retinal-vessel morphological parameters	Related	97.4%/100% **
Chua et al., 2019 [20]	HTN	Fundus imaging/OCTA	77 patients	Prospective	Prediction	Clinical diagnosis	Related	-
Hua et al., 2019 [63]	HTN	OCTA	97 patients	Prospective	Prediction	Clinical diagnosis	Related	-
Pascual-Prieto et al., 2020 [64]	HTN	OCTA	73 patients	Prospective	Identification	Retinal-vessel morphological parameters	Related	78.3%/66.7% and 56.5%/79.2%
Peng et al., 2020 [65]	HTN	Fundus imaging /OCTA	169 patients	Prospective	Prediction	Retinal-vessel morphological parameters	Related	-
Sargues et al., 2023 [66]	HTN	OCTA	89 patients	Retrospective	Prediction	Retinal-vessel morphological parameters	Related	-
Zeng et al., 2022 [67]	HTN	OCTA	32 patients	Prospective	Identification	Retinal-vessel morphological parameters	Related	-

4.3. Automated Idenfication and Prediction of Cardiovascular Risk Factors

Certain metabolic diseases serve as key indicators of cardiovascular risk, playing a crucial role in assessing and preventing heart disease. Metabolic factors such as hypertension, dyslipidemia, and diabetes are well-established contributors to cardiovascular risk. Meanwhile, individual factors like age, gender, and lifestyle choices, including smoking, diet, and physical activity, also significantly influence cardiovascular outcomes. The importance of these indicators lies in their ability to identify at-risk populations early, enabling targeted interventions that can reduce the incidence and severity of cardiovascular events. When it comes to identifying cardiovascular disease, these biomarkers are vital signs [5–7].

Poplin et al. discovered that deep neural networks may identify various risk variables based on retinal photographs, including age, gender, smoking status, and blood pressure [66]. In Zhu et al.'s study, their model predicted age with a mean absolute error of 3.55 years, which was slightly higher than the error reported by Poplin et al. [68]. Despite this, the model showed an impressive correlation between estimated retinal age and actual chronological age, demonstrating its accuracy in age prediction [35]. In a subsequent study, Vaghefi et al. developed a convolutional neural network for predicting smoking status using just retinal pictures [69]. The studies of Betzler et al. [70] and Korot et al. [71] obtained AUC values of 0.94 and 0.93 for gender as a risk factor. Rim et al. [72] developed a DL-based biomarker predictor model that predicted 10 of the 47 systemic biomarkers tested, with particularly good results for age and sex. These findings indicate that DL can quickly extract further details from fundus images that can help in CVD risk assessment. The paper of Gerrits et al. demonstrates that DL applied to fundus photography effectively predicts important cardiovascular risk factors like age and sex, with moderate success for other cardiometabolic factors (cholesterol, LDL and HDL cholesterol, triglycerides), and, for the first time, attempts to predict glycemic markers (glucose and insulin), though performance was poor [73].

The existence and extent of diabetic retinopathy (DR) are two of the most reliable indicators of CVDs. Studies have shown substantial variation in DR ($p < 0.00001$), age ($p < 0.002$), and gender ($p < 0.039$) among individuals with high coronary artery calcium (CAC) values ($\geq$400), which is considered to be a trustworthy prognostic tool [74]. DR detection was one of the initial proxies used to evaluate CVD using DL. It represents a risk factor and frequently manifests as complications from type 1 and type 2 DM brought on by retinal microcirculation degeneration [20]

4.4. Other Biomarkers in Cardiovascular Assesement

In a previous study, scientists created a RetiCAC system that used CAC as the basis for assessing CVD risk. Despite its usefulness, this research did not compare it to the commonly used QRISK3 score, which limits its relevance in healthcare decisions in the UK [75]. Following this, later research optimized RetiCAC for the UK population, culminating in the development of Reti-CVD. This technique divided participants into three risk groups and revealed substantial patterns in hazard ratios. Reti-CVD revealed a high-risk group of people who had a 10-year CVD risk of more than 10%. Furthermore, when paired with QRISK3, Reti-CVD showed greater prognostic value, especially among individuals in the borderline-QRISK3 group [76].

A significant concern is whether DL algorithms using retinal pictures can replace established cardiovascular indicators such as carotid intima-media thickness. This parameter is a proven indicator of significant cardiac events and is used to detect early atherosclerosis, particularly in intermediate-risk patients [77]. Nevertheless, its assessment is difficult, necessitating specific tools and qualified sonographers. DL systems evaluating fundus images, on the other hand, could provide a simpler approach to predicting cardiovascular risk, perhaps replacing more time-consuming techniques such as carotid intima-media thickness. A DL model was developed by Chang et al. [40] to predict atherosclerotic plaques from retinal imaging, resulting in the Deep Learning Fundus Atherosclerosis Score. This model was found to be an independent predictor of CVD deaths, even when adjusted for the Framingham Risk Score. Their investigation used the Xception framework to create a DL model that predicted atherosclerosis using retinal imaging. Originally developed on retinal imaging and carotid artery sonography data, the model had an AUC of 0.713. Importantly, the system provided additional predictive value beyond what the risk score alone could offer. Another investigation used retinal vascular biomarkers to forecast CAD, and they achieved AUCs greater than 0.692 by collecting characteristics during preliminary processing rather than straight from the retinal images [45]. This suggests that retinal imaging, combined with DL, could enhance CVD risk prediction and potentially improve early intervention strategies by integrating non-invasive retinal assessments with traditional cardiovascular risk models.

5. Linking Automated Prediction and Identification of Metabolic and Cardiovascular Diseases Using AI Models

Cardiovascular disease and diabetic retinopathy are closely linked, as both conditions share common risk factors, making retinal screening a valuable tool for identifying early signs of cardiovascular complications in diabetic patients. Considering the worrying growth in the prevalence of persons with diabetes mellitus and the shortage of qualified retinal specialists, an automated technique utilizing a computer-based examination of the fundus image might lessen the load on health systems in screenings for diabetic retinopathy. As a result, there is a growing interest in the development of automated analysis software that uses AI/DL to analyze fundus photography in individuals with diabetes [78] (Table 4). The IDx-DR system for automatically analyzing and proposing referral or extending screening for DR was cleared by the US FDA in 2018 as the initial AI-enabled diagnostic tool competent for independent assessment [79]. Using a DL model built on the InceptionV3 architecture, analysts were able to identify diabetic macular edema and DR, with an AUC of 0.990 on the MESSIDOR-2 dataset and 0.991 on the EyePACS dataset [32,80]. A further investigation yielded AUCs of 0.94 and 0.95 on MESSIDOR-2 and E-Ophtha datasets, respectively, for DR prognosis by combining a decision tree model with a customized convolutional neural network (CNN) for feature extraction [81]. Employing retinal imaging, a customized CNN obtained a precision of 89% in binary DR classification. Heat maps were used to emphasize significant image areas [82]. Additionally, the findings of Lee et al. [46] demonstrated that fundus images may currently be a cardiovascular risk factor in the diagnosis of CVD and that a multimodal model might perform noticeably better than a single modality model. Their multimodal networks were developed with the help of fundus images and clinical risk factors and showed improvement in the reclassification of both cases and controls [44]. Based on their findings, this strategy might be useful in predicting and preventing chronic disorders like CVDs.

Multiple large-scale studies in diabetic patients have found a correlation between alterations to the retinal microvascular morphology and the extent of both type 1 and type 2 diabetes, though the precise retinal vessel phenotype connected to diabetes is unknown. Meta-analyses have additionally discovered that retinal arteriolar diameters are independently related to body mass index (BMI), metabolic syndrome, and changes in total cholesterol, HDL and LDL cholesterol, and triglycerides [30].

A review of the Maastricht Study discovered a link between the presence of diabetes and wider retinal arteries. The lack of myogenic constriction of retinal arterioles caused by hyperglycemia is hypothesized to lead to arteriolar widening. Chronic hyperglycemia, on the other hand, might cause structural remodeling and arteriolar constriction, particularly when diabetes is paired with CVD [83]. There has been conflicting evidence in recent research on the connection between ocular variables and HbA1c levels. While AI algorithms in retinal imaging are capable of estimating HbA1c, their external reliability is limited [84]. According to OCT investigations, there is a negative association with choroidal thickness [85] and a positive correlation with macular thickness [86]. Significant correlations between HbA1c and foveal avascular zone circularity (FAZc) were discovered in OCTA investigation in diabetic individuals without retinopathy, emphasizing the early stages of microvascular damage [87]. Nonetheless, there is still no solid evidence linking OCTA parameters to long-term HbA1c management.

A recent pilot study addressed cardiovascular risk assessment in a type 2 diabetes mellitus group using DL models using fundus photography. In contrast to prior studies that employed more diverse cohorts, this one used a homogeneous database of diabetic individuals, which enabled more exact model training and a considerable increase in prediction accuracy. The scientists used a conservative prediction technique that combines retinal imaging with additional diagnostic techniques to reduce false negative ratios. This approach ensures that high-risk patients are correctly recognized, eliminating the possibility of missing those who might otherwise be misdiagnosed as low risk [30]. In the investigation of Zhang et al. [88], they developed a fundus image dataset and indicated that DL algorithms may anticipate arterial hypertension, hyperglycemia, and dyslipidemia. Additionally, their findings indicate that using DL for fundus imaging can predict blood erythrocyte characteristics such as hematocrit and mean corpuscular hemoglobin concentration. Earlier research has demonstrated that red blood cell (RBC) characteristics are connected with CVDs such as metabolic syndrome [89] and that impaired RBC characteristics can have negative impacts on retinal artery calibers [90].

In the study of Gulshan regarding retinal fundus pictures from diabetic individuals, a DL algorithm demonstrated great sensitivity and specificity in diagnosing diabetes-related retinopathy. In the first data set, the algorithm achieved 90.3% sensitivity and 98.1% specificity, while in the second data set, it reached 87.0% sensitivity and 98.5% specificity [80]. Several other DL systems have recently demonstrated great sensitivity and specificity (>90%) in diagnosing DR from retinal fundus photography, especially by utilizing high-quality images from freely accessible databases of homogeneous white populations [84,91]. Another study reported that DL models using fundus camera data could predict diabetic retinopathy, with an AUC of 0.75–0.79. For predicting poor blood glucose control, the model achieved an AUC of 0.67–0.73. These results suggest that the model is effective in identifying key cardiovascular and metabolic risk factors in diabetic patients, demonstrating its potential for early, non-invasive risk assessment [92].

Table 4. Summary of studies using retinal fundus imaging, optical coherence tomography (OCT), and optical coherence tomography angiography (OCTA) in subjects to identify/predict several types of cardiovascular disease. "Related" indicates that the authors did not publish an AUC value, but their results demonstrated significant connections between retinal changes and outcomes. AUC: area under the curve; DM: diabetes mellitus; HTN: hypertension.

Study	Disease	Method	Dataset	Recruitment	Task	Outcome	Results	Sensitivity/Specificity
Ale-Chilet et al., 2022 [93]	type I DM	OCTA	425 patients	Prospective	Identification	Clinical diagnosis	AUC = 0.58	-
Barriada et al., 2022 [32]	DM	Fundus Imaging	76 patients	Retrospective	Prediction	Coronary Artery Calcium Score	Related	91% (sensitivity)
Bernal-Morales et al., 2021 [87]	type I DM	OCT/OCTA	593 patients	Prospective	Prediction	Clinical diagnosis	Related	-
Cui et al., 2020 [94]	type II DM	Fluoroscein Angiography/OCTA/Fundus imaging	101 patients	Prospective	Identification	Clinical diagnosis	Related	96.5%/94.7%
DuPont et al., 2024 [95]	type II DM	Fluoroscein Angiography/OCTA	15 patients	Prospective	Prediction	Clinical diagnosis	Related	-
Li et al., 2020 [83]	type II DM/ prediabetes	Fundus imaging	2876 patients	Prospective	Prediction	Clinical diagnosis/risk variables	Related	-
Torabi et al., 2019 [85]	type II DM	OCT	115 patients	Prospective	Prediction	Choroidal thickness	Related	-
Zhang et al., 2020 [88]	HTN Hyperglycemia, dyslipidemia	Fundus imaging	625 patients	Prospective	Prediction	Clinical diagnosis/risk variables	AUC = 0.766; AUC = 0.880; AUC = 0.703	-

6. Artificial Intelligence-Driven Development of Automated Retinal Vessel Measurement Models

The development of AI-based software for retinal vessel measurement represents a breakthrough in the precise and efficient analysis of retinal vasculature. These tools utilize advanced machine learning algorithms to automatically measure retinal vessel calibers, including parameters like arteriolar and venular diameters, branching patterns, and tortuosity. Certain changes and variations in retinal vessels may be closely connected to the development of cardiovascular diseases and major cardiovascular events [96] (Table 5). By automating these processes, AI reduces the variability and potential errors associated with manual measurements, enhancing the accuracy of diagnosis and longitudinal studies. This technology also allows for large-scale screening programs, where retinal images can be quickly analyzed to identify early signs of systemic diseases like hypertension, diabetes, and atherosclerosis. Furthermore, integrating AI into retinal vessel analysis provides the potential to uncover new biomarkers [97]. This automated approach not only speeds up the analysis but also enables more consistent and reproducible results across diverse populations and clinical settings, making it a valuable tool in preventive healthcare and personalized medicine.

Table 5. Connections between retinal characteristics and systemic diseases.

Retinal Parameter	Variation	Associated Outcome
Retinal Arteriolar Tortuosity	Increased	Linked with current blood pressure and early kidney disease
	Decreased	Associated with current blood pressure and ischemic heart disease
Retinal Venular Tortuosity	Increased	Connected to current blood pressure
Retinal Vascular Fractal Dimension	Increased	Related to acute lacunar stroke
	Decreased	Correlates with current blood pressure, lacunar and incident stroke
	Suboptimal	Associated with chronic kidney disease and coronary heart disease
Retinal Arteriolar Branching Angle	Increased	Associated with current blood pressure
Retinal Arteriolar Branching Asymmetry Ratio	Decreased	Linked to current blood pressure
Retinal Arteriolar Length-to-Diameter Ratio	Decreased	Connected to current blood pressure, hypertension, and stroke
Retinal Arteriolar Branching Coefficient	Decreased	Associated with ischemic heart disease
Retinal Arteriolar Optimal Parameter	Increased	Linked to peripheral vascular disease

Tapp et al. were the first to investigate retinal microcirculation by applying fully automated software in a large sample size. They discovered that narrower retinal arteriolar diameters were substantially related to increased systolic and diastolic blood pressure. Wider venular diameters were associated with higher arterial stiffness, as evaluated by pulse wave velocity. The connections remained after accounting for additional risk variables for CVD. Retinal arteriolar tortuosity was likewise strongly associated with higher blood pressure, but venular tortuosity had a lesser relationship [98]. This shows that the structural integrity of the retinal microcirculation may indicate underlying cardiovascular stress.

The Singapore I Vessel Assessment – Deep Learning System (SIVA-DLS) is a completely automated DL model that Cheung et al. created. It achieves coefficients of correlation ranging from 0.82 to 0.95 when juxtaposed with traditional measurements, and it accurately predicts central retinal artery and vein equivalents. SIVA-DLS measures of retinal vessel diameters have been demonstrated to exceed manual measurements in their high correlation with CVD events and various risk variables [44].

7. Traditional Diagnostic Methods for Cardiovascular Diseases Versus AI Retinal-Based Approaches

CVDs have long been diagnosed using well-established methods such as electrocardiograms (ECGs), echocardiography, coronary angiography, and stress tests [99]. These tools have proven highly effective in identifying heart conditions, but they have limitations when compared to emerging AI-driven retinal imaging techniques. ECG and stress testing are cornerstones for diagnosing ischemic heart disease. According to a meta-analysis of over 20,000 patients from 147 studies, ECG stress testing has a 68% sensitivity and a 77% specificity in identifying CAD [100]. However, these tests are generally more effective when patients are symptomatic, which may lead to missed opportunities for early detection in asymptomatic individuals. Stress tests also come with the risk of false positives, which can result in unnecessary procedures [101,102]. In contrast, AI-based retinal imaging offers a non-invasive, more accessible approach to detecting early vascular changes linked to cardiovascular risk, even in asymptomatic individuals. AI can analyze subtle patterns in retinal vessels, potentially identifying risks earlier than other traditional diagnostic methods. Echocardiography provides detailed structural information and is crucial for diagnosing heart failure and valvular disease. The analysis of eighteen papers revealed that echocardiography had a high specificity (96%) and sensitivity (92%) for diagnosing acute heart failure [103]. A study conducted a meta-analysis of 20 studies to assess the diagnostic accuracy of brain natriuretic peptide (BNP) for heart failure, comparing it to atrial natriuretic peptide (ANP) and using echocardiographic or clinical criteria as reference standards. BNP is a highly accurate diagnostic marker for heart failure, showing greater sensitivity and specificity compared to ANP, with a pooled diagnostic odds ratio of 30.9 against clinical criteria [104]. Non-invasive coronary CT angiography [105] and calcium scoring [106] are valuable for assessing coronary artery disease and atherosclerosis with high sensitivity and specificity (80%/67% and 90%/40%) but are costly and involve radiation exposure. Despite significant advancements in AI and even with comparable specificity and sensitivity, traditional diagnostic methods continue to be the gold standard for diagnosing cardiovascular disease (Table 6).

Table 6. Comparison of retinal investigation methods with state-of-the-art diagnostic tools for cardiovascular and metabolic diseases.

Disease	Retinal Investigation	Comparison
CAD	Fundus Imaging, OCTA	Comparable AUC and sensitivity to current deep learning-based predictive models for CAD, such as coronary angiography and calcium scoring models with AUC > 0.8 [40,43–50,105,106].
IS	Fundus Imaging, OCTA	Moderate accuracy for ischemic stroke risk prediction compared to established methods like carotid intima-media thickness measurement and brain MRI, which have higher specificity and sensitivity. Retinal imaging offers additional predictive value but often has lower AUC [51–56,107,108].
MI	Fundus Imaging, OCTA	Some retinal imaging models show high accuracy in predicting myocardial infarction risk, comparable to traditional methods like ECG and cardiac MRI, with AUC values competitive with advanced predictive models [39,57,100,109].
CHF	Automated Retinal Vessel Measurement, OCTA	High correlation with cardiovascular events and risk factors. Shows promise as a non-invasive tool for early detection, with comparable performance to echocardiography and brain natriuretic peptide testing [60–62,103,104].
HTN	Fundus Imaging, OCTA	Slightly lower AUC compared to ambulatory blood pressure monitoring. However, retinal vessel analysis correlates well with cardiovascular risk factors, suggesting potential in improving predictive accuracy [20,63–67,110].
DM	Fundus Imaging, OCTA, Fluorescein Angiography	High sensitivity and specificity in detecting retinal complications of DM, comparable to clinical grading by ophthalmologists [32,88,93,94,111].
Hyperlipidemia	Fundus Imaging	Moderate predictive accuracy for dyslipidemia when using retinal imaging. Studies show that retinal imaging can predict lipid abnormalities but with slightly lower specificity compared to blood lipid panel tests [88,112].

8. Challenges and Future Perspectives

Oculomics is not solely limited to imaging techniques; there are various additional non-invasive biomarkers, and many others are still to be found. Tears include a few hundred different proteins and inflammatory mediators, and an analysis may be performed using minimally invasive procedures. Researchers are currently in the clinical evaluation phase and must guarantee that implementing oculomics in screening does not jeopardize safety, prejudice, or public trust. The goal is to improve outcomes, reduce medical expenses, and give patients a better quality of life. To establish confidence among patients, we must encourage standardization, investigate generalizability and algorithmic bias, and push international collaboration toward harmonized techniques. Oculomics research faces significant challenges, particularly regarding standardization and clinical utility. The lack of standardized imaging equipment and algorithms complicates data comparison, as different machines produce varying results. Moreover, translating research findings into clinical practice remains uncertain, with questions about how these findings will benefit patients and who will bear the costs [113]. This uncertainty is often referred to as the "translational valley of death", where promising discoveries struggle to find practical application [4,30,68].

Another major concern is data sharing and privacy. Retinal images, now classified as protected health information, are difficult to share across institutions due to strict privacy regulations. This has stalled the initial excitement around using big data in oculomics. Researchers are exploring solutions, such as generative adversarial networks (GANs), which modify retinal images to protect patient identity while still allowing AI to learn from the data. Despite advancements in AI, clinicians remain crucial in designing relevant studies and interpreting results, ensuring that new technologies are effectively integrated into patient care [30,66,68].

9. Novel Contributions

This study shows the potential of AI-driven retinal imaging to improve the prediction and diagnosis of cardiovascular and metabolic diseases. A key contribution is the demonstration of how retinal imaging, traditionally used for ophthalmological assessments, can serve as a comprehensive and non-invasive diagnostic tool for systemic diseases. Unlike conventional methods, which often rely on invasive procedures or broad clinical metrics, AI-based retinal analysis can detect subtle microvascular changes linked to conditions like CAD, myocardial infarction, and DM. This innovative use of retinal biomarkers offers a new dimension in risk assessment, enabling earlier and more precise detection. The AI models in this study achieve high AUC values, sensitivity, and specificity, outperforming conventional risk assessment tools in certain cases.

One of the most significant innovations of this study is the potential for large-scale application in clinical settings. Retinal imaging, using techniques such as fundus photography and OCT, is already widely available and routinely used in ophthalmic exams. By integrating AI-based analysis into these imaging tools, healthcare providers can leverage existing infrastructure to screen for cardiovascular and metabolic diseases on a large scale. This approach offers a non-invasive and accessible solution, making it possible to implement widespread screening programs in primary care settings without the need for specialized equipment or invasive procedures.

The innovation of AI-driven retinal imaging lies in its ability to analyze vast amounts of data quickly and efficiently, making it suitable for large population-based screenings. With further research and standardization, the integration of retinal oculomics into routine clinical practice has the potential to revolutionize the early detection and management of systemic diseases. By addressing these gaps in current healthcare approaches, the study lays the groundwork for a transformative shift in how cardiovascular and metabolic diseases are diagnosed, making this a promising contribution to both research and clinical practice.

10. Conclusions

This article highlights the transformative potential of oculomics in diagnosing and managing systemic diseases through retinal biomarkers. By leveraging advanced imaging techniques like OCT and OCTA, combined with AI-driven analysis, oculomics can provide early, non-invasive detection of cardiovascular and metabolic diseases. Recent studies have demonstrated that AI models analyzing retinal images can accurately predict CAD, ischemic stroke, and myocardial infarction, with high AUC values ranging from 0.71 to 0.97 and sensitivities between 71% and 89%. Retinal imaging has also shown its capability in detecting diabetic retinopathy and predicting DM-associated complications. Advanced DL algorithms applied to fundus photography have demonstrated high sensitivity and specificity, comparable to clinical grading by ophthalmologists. The findings suggest that retinal imaging can reveal subtle changes in microvascular structure associated with conditions such as DM and CVD, offering a powerful tool for risk assessment. Moreover, AI models demonstrated high accuracy in predicting cardiovascular risk factors from retinal images. The integration of oculomics into clinical practice could revolutionize personalized medicine, allowing for earlier intervention and improved patient outcomes. However, further research is needed to standardize imaging protocols and ensure the clinical utility of these biomarkers across diverse populations.

Author Contributions: Conceptualization, L.A.G.; methodology, E.R.S.; software, E.R.S.; formal analysis, R.I.; investigation, R.I.; writing—original draft preparation, O.A.H. and C.B.; writing—review and editing, M.D.; visualization, O.A.H. and M.D.; supervision, L.A.G. All authors have read and agreed to the published version of the manuscript.

Funding: We would like to acknowledge VICTOR BABES UNIVERSITY OF MEDICINE AND PHARMACY TIMISOARA for their support in covering the costs of publication for this research paper.

Institutional Review Board Statement: Not applicable.

Informed Consent Statement: Not applicable.

Data Availability Statement: No new data were created.

Conflicts of Interest: The authors declare no conflicts of interest.

References

1. Basu, K.; Sinha, R.; Ong, A.; Basu, T. Artificial Intelligence: How Is It Changing Medical Sciences and Its Future? *Indian J. Dermatol.* **2020**, *65*, 365. [CrossRef] [PubMed]
2. Li, H.; Cao, J.; Grzybowski, A.; Jin, K.; Lou, L.; Ye, J. Diagnosing Systemic Disorders with AI Algorithms Based on Ocular Images. *Healthcare* **2023**, *11*, 1739. [CrossRef] [PubMed]
3. Zhu, Y.; Salowe, R.; Chow, C.; Li, S.; Bastani, O.; O'Brien, J.M. Advancing Glaucoma Care: Integrating Artificial Intelligence in Diagnosis, Management, and Progression Detection. *Bioengineering* **2024**, *11*, 122. [CrossRef] [PubMed]
4. Wagner, S.K.; Fu, D.J.; Faes, L.; Liu, X.; Huemer, J.; Khalid, H.; Ferraz, D.; Korot, E.; Kelly, C.; Balaskas, K.; et al. Insights into Systemic Disease through Retinal Imaging-Based Oculomics. *Transl. Vis. Sci. Technol.* **2020**, *9*, 6. [CrossRef]
5. Muharram, F.R.; Multazam, C.E.C.Z.; Mustofa, A.; Socha, W.; Andrianto; Martini, S.; Aminde, L.; Yi-Li, C. The 30 Years of Shifting in The Indonesian Cardiovascular Burden—Analysis of The Global Burden of Disease Study. *J. Epidemiol. Glob. Health* **2024**, *14*, 193–212. [CrossRef]
6. Magliano, D.; Boyko, E.J. *IDF Diabetes Atlas*, 10th ed.; International Diabetes Federation: Brussels, Belgium, 2021; ISBN 978-2-930229-98-0.
7. Blaha, M.J.; DeFilippis, A.P. Multi-Ethnic Study of Atherosclerosis (MESA): JACC Focus Seminar 5/8. *J. Am. Coll. Cardiol.* **2021**, *77*, 3195–3216. [CrossRef]
8. ACCORD Study Group; Buse, J.B.; Bigger, J.T.; Byington, R.P.; Cooper, L.S.; Cushman, W.C.; Friedewald, W.T.; Genuth, S.; Gerstein, H.C.; Ginsberg, H.N.; et al. Action to Control Cardiovascular Risk in Diabetes (ACCORD) Trial: Design and Methods. *Am. J. Cardiol.* **2007**, *99*, 21i–33i. [CrossRef]
9. Chandra, A.; Seidelmann, S.B.; Claggett, B.L.; Klein, B.E.; Klein, R.; Shah, A.M.; Solomon, S.D. The Association of Retinal Vessel Calibres with Heart Failure and Long-term Alterations in Cardiac Structure and Function: The Atherosclerosis Risk in Communities (ARIC) Study. *Eur. J. Heart Fail.* **2019**, *21*, 1207–1215. [CrossRef]

10. Page, M.J.; McKenzie, J.E.; Bossuyt, P.M.; Boutron, I.; Hoffmann, T.C.; Mulrow, C.D.; Shamseer, L.; Tetzlaff, J.M.; Akl, E.A.; Brennan, S.E.; et al. The PRISMA 2020 Statement: An Updated Guideline for Reporting Systematic Reviews. *BMJ* **2021**, *372*, n71. [CrossRef]
11. Wong, T.Y.; Klein, R.; Couper, D.J.; Cooper, L.S.; Shahar, E.; Hubbard, L.D.; Wofford, M.R.; Sharrett, A.R. Retinal Microvascular Abnormalities and Incident Stroke: The Atherosclerosis Risk in Communities Study. *The Lancet* **2001**, *358*, 1134–1140. [CrossRef]
12. Seifert, B.-U.; Vilser, W. Retinal Vessel Analyzer (Rva)—Design and Function. *Biomed. Tech. Eng.* **2002**, *47*, 678–681. [CrossRef] [PubMed]
13. Harazny, J.M.; Ritt, M.; Baleanu, D.; Ott, C.; Heckmann, J.; Schlaich, M.P.; Michelson, G.; Schmieder, R.E. Increased Wall:Lumen Ratio of Retinal Arterioles in Male Patients with a History of a Cerebrovascular Event. *Hypertension* **2007**, *50*, 623–629. [CrossRef] [PubMed]
14. Rizzoni, D.; Mengozzi, A.; Masi, S.; Agabiti Rosei, C.; De Ciuceis, C.; Virdis, A. New Noninvasive Methods to Evaluate Microvascular Structure and Function. *Hypertension* **2022**, *79*, 874–886. [CrossRef] [PubMed]
15. Ghenciu, L.A.; Șișu, A.M.; Stoicescu, E.R.; Dănilă, A.-I.; Iacob, R.; Săndesc, M.-A.; Hațegan, O.A. Thyroid Eye Disease and Glaucoma: A Cross-Sectional Study Comparing Clinical Characteristics and Disease Severity. *Medicina* **2024**, *60*, 1430. [CrossRef]
16. Spaide, R.F.; Fujimoto, J.G.; Waheed, N.K.; Sadda, S.R.; Staurenghi, G. Optical Coherence Tomography Angiography. *Prog. Retin. Eye Res.* **2018**, *64*, 1–55. [CrossRef]
17. Mukherjee, C.; Al-Fahad, Q.; Elsherbiny, S. The Role of Optical Coherence Tomography in Therapeutics and Conditions, Which Primarily Have Systemic Manifestations: A Narrative Review. *Ther. Adv. Ophthalmol.* **2019**, *11*, 251584141983115. [CrossRef]
18. DeBuc, D.C.; Rege, A.; Smiddy, W.E. Use of XyCAM RI for Noninvasive Visualization and Analysis of Retinal Blood Flow Dynamics During Clinical Investigations. *Expert Rev. Med. Devices* **2021**, *18*, 225–237. [CrossRef]
19. Bakker, E.; Dikland, F.A.; Van Bakel, R.; Andrade De Jesus, D.; Sánchez Brea, L.; Klein, S.; Van Walsum, T.; Rossant, F.; Farías, D.C.; Grieve, K.; et al. Adaptive Optics Ophthalmoscopy: A Systematic Review of Vascular Biomarkers. *Surv. Ophthalmol.* **2022**, *67*, 369–387. [CrossRef]
20. Chua, J.; Le, T.; Sim, Y.C.; Chye, H.Y.; Tan, B.; Yao, X.; Wong, D.; Ang, B.W.Y.; Toh, D.; Lim, H.; et al. Relationship of Quantitative Retinal Capillary Network and Myocardial Remodeling in Systemic Hypertension. *J. Am. Heart Assoc.* **2022**, *11*, e024226. [CrossRef]
21. Zhang, P.; Wahl, D.J.; Mocci, J.; Miller, E.B.; Bonora, S.; Sarunic, M.V.; Zawadzki, R.J. Adaptive Optics Scanning Laser Ophthalmoscopy and Optical Coherence Tomography (AO-SLO-OCT) System for In Vivo Mouse Retina Imaging. *Biomed. Opt. Express* **2023**, *14*, 299. [CrossRef]
22. Mujat, M.; Ferguson, R.D.; Hammer, D.X.; Patel, A.H.; Iftimia, N. High-Resolution Retinal Imaging: Technology Overview and Applications. *Photonics* **2024**, *11*, 522. [CrossRef]
23. Luís Dean-Ben, X.; Razansky, D. Localization Optoacoustic Tomography. *Light Sci. Appl.* **2018**, *7*, 18004. [CrossRef] [PubMed]
24. Saeed, A.; Hadoux, X.; Van Wijngaarden, P. Hyperspectral Retinal Imaging Biomarkers of Ocular and Systemic Diseases. *Eye* **2024**, *6*, 2. [CrossRef]
25. Arnould, L.; Meriaudeau, F.; Guenancia, C.; Germanese, C.; Delcourt, C.; Kawasaki, R.; Cheung, C.Y.; Creuzot-Garcher, C.; Grzybowski, A. Using Artificial Intelligence to Analyse the Retinal Vascular Network: The Future of Cardiovascular Risk Assessment Based on Oculomics? A Narrative Review. *Ophthalmol. Ther.* **2023**, *12*, 657–674. [CrossRef] [PubMed]
26. Levy, B.I.; Schiffrin, E.L.; Mourad, J.-J.; Agostini, D.; Vicaut, E.; Safar, M.E.; Struijker-Boudier, H.A.J. Impaired Tissue Perfusion: A Pathology Common to Hypertension, Obesity, and Diabetes Mellitus. *Circulation* **2008**, *118*, 968–976. [CrossRef] [PubMed]
27. Wong, T.Y. Quantitative Retinal Venular Caliber and Risk of Cardiovascular Disease in Older Persons: The Cardiovascular Health Study. *Arch. Intern. Med.* **2006**, *166*, 2388. [CrossRef]
28. Tabatabaee, A.; Asharin, M.; Dehghan, M.; Pourbehi, M.; Nasiri-Ahmadabadi, M.; Assadi, M. Retinal Vessel Abnormalities Predict Coronary Artery Diseases. *Perfusion* **2013**, *28*, 232–237. [CrossRef]
29. Wong, T.Y.; Klein, R.; Sharrett, A.R.; Duncan, B.B.; Couper, D.J.; Tielsch, J.M.; Klein, B.E.K.; Hubbard, L.D. Retinal Arteriolar Narrowing and Risk of Coronary Heart Disease in Men and Women: The Atherosclerosis Risk in Communities Study. *JAMA* **2002**, *287*, 1153–1159. [CrossRef]
30. Hanssen, H.; Streese, L.; Vilser, W. Retinal Vessel Diameters and Function in Cardiovascular Risk and Disease. *Prog. Retin. Eye Res.* **2022**, *91*, 101095. [CrossRef]
31. Chew, S.K.H.; Xie, J.; Wang, J.J. Retinal Arteriolar Diameter and the Prevalence and Incidence of Hypertension: A Systematic Review and Meta-Analysis of Their Association. *Curr. Hypertens. Rep.* **2012**, *14*, 144–151. [CrossRef]
32. Barriada, R.G.; Simó-Servat, O.; Planas, A.; Hernández, C.; Simó, R.; Masip, D. Deep Learning of Retinal Imaging: A Useful Tool for Coronary Artery Calcium Score Prediction in Diabetic Patients. *Appl. Sci.* **2022**, *12*, 1401. [CrossRef]
33. Nusinovici, S.; Rim, T.H.; Yu, M.; Lee, G.; Tham, Y.-C.; Cheung, N.; Chong, C.C.Y.; Da Soh, Z.; Thakur, S.; Lee, C.J.; et al. Retinal Photograph-Based Deep Learning Predicts Biological Age, and Stratifies Morbidity and Mortality Risk. *Age Ageing* **2022**, *51*, afac065. [CrossRef]
34. Zhu, Z.; Chen, Y.; Wang, W.; Wang, Y.; Hu, W.; Shang, X.; Liao, H.; Shi, D.; Huang, Y.; Ha, J.; et al. Association of Retinal Age Gap with Arterial Stiffness and Incident Cardiovascular Disease. *Stroke* **2022**, *53*, 3320–3328. [CrossRef] [PubMed]
35. Zhu, Z.; Hu, W.; Chen, R.; Xiong, R.; Wang, W.; Shang, X.; Chen, Y.; Kiburg, K.; Shi, D.; He, S.; et al. Retinal Age Gap as a Predictive Biomarker of Stroke Risk. *BMC Med.* **2022**, *20*, 466. [CrossRef] [PubMed]

36. Klein, R.; Klein, B.E.K.; Moss, S.E.; Wong, T.Y.; Sharrett, A.R. Retinal Vascular Caliber in Persons with Type 2 Diabetes: The Wisconsin Epidemiological Study of Diabetic Retinopathy: XX. *Ophthalmology* **2006**, *113*, 1488–1498. [CrossRef] [PubMed]
37. Lim, G.; Lim, Z.W.; Xu, D.; Ting, D.S.W.; Wong, T.Y.; Lee, M.L.; Hsu, W. Feature Isolation for Hypothesis Testing in Retinal Imaging: An Ischemic Stroke Prediction Case Study. *Proc. AAAI Conf. Artif. Intell.* **2019**, *33*, 9510–9515. [CrossRef]
38. Szegedy, C.; Ioffe, S.; Vanhoucke, V.; Alemi, A. Inception-v4, Inception-ResNet and the Impact of Residual Connections on Learning. *Proc. AAAI Conf. Artif. Intell.* **2017**, *31*, 1. [CrossRef]
39. Diaz-Pinto, A.; Ravikumar, N.; Attar, R.; Suinesiaputra, A.; Zhao, Y.; Levelt, E.; Dall'Armellina, E.; Lorenzi, M.; Chen, Q.; Keenan, T.D.L.; et al. Predicting Myocardial Infarction through Retinal Scans and Minimal Personal Information. *Nat. Mach. Intell.* **2022**, *4*, 55–61. [CrossRef]
40. Chang, J.; Ko, A.; Park, S.M.; Choi, S.; Kim, K.; Kim, S.M.; Yun, J.M.; Kang, U.; Shin, I.H.; Shin, J.Y.; et al. Association of Cardiovascular Mortality and Deep Learning-Funduscopic Atherosclerosis Score Derived from Retinal Fundus Images. *Am. J. Ophthalmol.* **2020**, *217*, 121–130. [CrossRef]
41. Chaitanuwong, P.; Singhanetr, P.; Chainakul, M.; Arjkongharn, N.; Ruamviboonsuk, P.; Grzybowski, A. Potential Ocular Biomarkers for Early Detection of Alzheimer's Disease and Their Roles in Artificial Intelligence Studies. *Neurol. Ther.* **2023**, *12*, 1517–1532. [CrossRef]
42. Huang, Y.; Li, C.; Shi, D.; Wang, H.; Shang, X.; Wang, W.; Zhang, X.; Zhang, X.; Hu, Y.; Tang, S.; et al. Integrating Oculomics with Genomics Reveals Imaging Biomarkers for Preventive and Personalized Prediction of Arterial Aneurysms. *EPMA J.* **2023**, *14*, 73–86. [CrossRef] [PubMed]
43. Aschauer, J.; Aschauer, S.; Pollreisz, A.; Datlinger, F.; Gatterer, C.; Mylonas, G.; Egner, B.; Hofer, D.; Steiner, I.; Hengstenberg, C.; et al. Identification of Subclinical Microvascular Biomarkers in Coronary Heart Disease in Retinal Imaging. *Transl. Vis. Sci. Technol.* **2021**, *10*, 24. [CrossRef] [PubMed]
44. Cheung, C.Y.; Xu, D.; Cheng, C.-Y.; Sabanayagam, C.; Tham, Y.-C.; Yu, M.; Rim, T.H.; Chai, C.Y.; Gopinath, B.; Mitchell, P.; et al. A Deep-Learning System for the Assessment of Cardiovascular Disease Risk via the Measurement of Retinal-Vessel Calibre. *Nat. Biomed. Eng.* **2020**, *5*, 498–508. [CrossRef] [PubMed]
45. Huang, F.; Lian, J.; Ng, K.-S.; Shih, K.; Vardhanabhuti, V. Predicting CT-Based Coronary Artery Disease Using Vascular Biomarkers Derived from Fundus Photographs with a Graph Convolutional Neural Network. *Diagnostics* **2022**, *12*, 1390. [CrossRef] [PubMed]
46. Lee, Y.C.; Cha, J.; Shim, I.; Park, W.-Y.; Kang, S.W.; Lim, D.H.; Won, H.-H. Multimodal Deep Learning of Fundus Abnormalities and Traditional Risk Factors for Cardiovascular Risk Prediction. *Npj Digit. Med.* **2023**, *6*, 14. [CrossRef]
47. Matulevičiūtė, I.; Sidaraitė, A.; Tatarūnas, V.; Veikutienė, A.; Dobilienė, O.; Žaliūnienė, D. Retinal and Choroidal Thinning—A Predictor of Coronary Artery Occlusion? *Diagnostics* **2022**, *12*, 2016. [CrossRef]
48. Ren, Y.; Hu, Y.; Li, C.; Zhong, P.; Liu, H.; Wang, H.; Kuang, Y.; Fu, B.; Wang, Y.; Zhao, H.; et al. Impaired Retinal Microcirculation in Patients with Non-Obstructive Coronary Artery Disease. *Microvasc. Res.* **2023**, *148*, 104533. [CrossRef]
49. Son, J.; Shin, J.Y.; Chun, E.J.; Jung, K.-H.; Park, K.H.; Park, S.J. Predicting High Coronary Artery Calcium Score from Retinal Fundus Images with Deep Learning Algorithms. *Transl. Vis. Sci. Technol.* **2020**, *9*, 28. [CrossRef]
50. Wang, J.; Jiang, J.; Zhang, Y.; Qian, Y.W.; Zhang, J.F.; Wang, Z.L. Retinal and Choroidal Vascular Changes in Coronary Heart Disease: An Optical Coherence Tomography Angiography Study. *Biomed. Opt. Express* **2019**, *10*, 1532. [CrossRef]
51. Cao, Y.; Yan, J.; Zhan, Z.; Liang, Y.; Han, Z. Macula Structure and Microvascular Changes in Recent Small Subcortical Infarct Patients. *Front. Neurol.* **2021**, *11*, 615252. [CrossRef]
52. Duan, H.; Xie, J.; Zhou, Y.; Zhang, H.; Liu, Y.; Tang, C.; Zhao, Y.; Qi, H. Characterization of the Retinal Microvasculature and FAZ Changes in Ischemic Stroke and Its Different Types. *Transl. Vis. Sci. Technol.* **2022**, *11*, 21. [CrossRef] [PubMed]
53. Liang, Y.; Liu, B.; Xiao, Y.; Zeng, X.; Wu, G.; Du, Z.; Fang, Y.; Hu, Y.; Yang, X.; Yu, H. Retinal Neurovascular Changes in Patients with Ischemic Stroke Investigated by Optical Coherence Tomography Angiography. *Front. Aging Neurosci.* **2022**, *14*, 834560. [CrossRef] [PubMed]
54. Molero-Senosiain, M.; Vidal-Villegas, B.; Pascual-Prieto, J.; Valor-Suarez, C.; Saenz-Frances, F.; Santos-Bueso, E. Correlation Between Retrograde Trans-Synaptic Degeneration of Ganglion Cells and Optical Coherence Tomography Angiography Following Ischemic Stroke. *Cureus* **2021**, *13*, e19788. [CrossRef] [PubMed]
55. Zhang, Y.; Shi, C.; Chen, Y.; Wang, W.; Huang, S.; Han, Z.; Lin, X.; Lu, F.; Shen, M. Retinal Structural and Microvascular Alterations in Different Acute Ischemic Stroke Subtypes. *J. Ophthalmol.* **2020**, *2020*, 1–10. [CrossRef]
56. Ye, C.; Kwapong, W.R.; Tao, W.; Lu, K.; Pan, R.; Wang, A.; Liu, J.; Liu, M.; Wu, B. Characterization of Macular Structural and Microvascular Changes in Thalamic Infarction Patients: A Swept-Source Optical Coherence Tomography–Angiography Study. *Brain Sci.* **2022**, *12*, 518. [CrossRef]
57. Arnould, L.; Guenancia, C.; Azemar, A.; Alan, G.; Pitois, S.; Bichat, F.; Zeller, M.; Gabrielle, P.-H.; Bron, A.M.; Creuzot-Garcher, C.; et al. The EYE-MI Pilot Study: A Prospective Acute Coronary Syndrome Cohort Evaluated with Retinal Optical Coherence Tomography Angiography. *Investig. Opthalmology Vis. Sci.* **2018**, *59*, 4299. [CrossRef]
58. Sideri, A.-M.; Kanakis, M.; Katsimpris, A.; Karamaounas, A.; Brouzas, D.; Petrou, P.; Papakonstaninou, E.; Droutsas, K.; Kandarakis, S.; Giannopoulos, G.; et al. Correlation Between Coronary and Retinal Microangiopathy in Patients with STEMI. *Transl. Vis. Sci. Technol.* **2023**, *12*, 8. [CrossRef]
59. Zhong, P.; Hu, Y.; Jiang, L.; Peng, Q.; Huang, M.; Li, C.; Kuang, Y.; Tan, N.; Yu, H.; Yang, X. Retinal Microvasculature Changes in Patients with Coronary Total Occlusion on Optical Coherence Tomography Angiography. *Front. Med.* **2021**, *8*, 708491. [CrossRef]

60. Rakusiewicz, K.; Kanigowska, K.; Hautz, W.; Ziółkowska, L. The Impact of Chronic Heart Failure on Retinal Vessel Density Assessed by Optical Coherence Tomography Angiography in Children with Dilated Cardiomyopathy. *J. Clin. Med.* **2021**, *10*, 2659. [CrossRef]
61. Topaloglu, C.; Bekmez, S. Retinal Vascular Density Change in Patients with Heart Failure. *Photodiagnosis Photodyn. Ther.* **2023**, *42*, 103621. [CrossRef]
62. Zekavat, S.M.; Raghu, V.K.; Trinder, M.; Ye, Y.; Koyama, S.; Honigberg, M.C.; Yu, Z.; Pampana, A.; Urbut, S.; Haidermota, S.; et al. Deep Learning of the Retina Enables Phenome- and Genome-Wide Analyses of the Microvasculature. *Circulation* **2022**, *145*, 134–150. [CrossRef] [PubMed]
63. Hua, D.; Xu, Y.; Zeng, X.; Yang, N.; Jiang, M.; Zhang, X.; Yang, J.; He, T.; Xing, Y. Use of Optical Coherence Tomography Angiography for Assessment of Microvascular Changes in the Macula and Optic Nerve Head in Hypertensive Patients without Hypertensive Retinopathy. *Microvasc. Res.* **2020**, *129*, 103969. [CrossRef] [PubMed]
64. Pascual-Prieto, J.; Burgos-Blasco, B.; Ávila Sánchez-Torija, M.; Fernández-Vigo, J.I.; Arriola-Villalobos, P.; Barbero Pedraz, M.A.; García-Feijoo, J.; Martínez-de-la-Casa, J.M. Utility of Optical Coherence Tomography Angiography in Detecting Vascular Retinal Damage Caused by Arterial Hypertension. *Eur. J. Ophthalmol.* **2020**, *30*, 579–585. [CrossRef] [PubMed]
65. Peng, Q.; Hu, Y.; Huang, M.; Wu, Y.; Zhong, P.; Dong, X.; Wu, Q.; Liu, B.; Li, C.; Xie, J.; et al. Retinal Neurovascular Impairment in Patients with Essential Hypertension: An Optical Coherence Tomography Angiography Study. *Investig. Opthalmology Vis. Sci.* **2020**, *61*, 42. [CrossRef]
66. Remolí Sargues, L.; Monferrer Adsuara, C.; Castro Navarro, V.; Navarro Palop, C.; Montero Hernández, J.; Cervera Taulet, E. Swept-Source Optical Coherence Tomography Angiography Automatic Analysis of Microvascular Changes Secondary to Systemic Hypertension. *Eur. J. Ophthalmol.* **2023**, *33*, 1452–1458. [CrossRef]
67. Zeng, R.; Garg, I.; Bannai, D.; Kasetty, M.; Katz, R.; Park, J.Y.; Lizano, P.; Miller, J.B. Retinal Microvasculature and Vasoreactivity Changes in Hypertension Using Optical Coherence Tomography-Angiography. *Graefes Arch. Clin. Exp. Ophthalmol.* **2022**, *260*, 3505–3515. [CrossRef]
68. Poplin, R.; Varadarajan, A.V.; Blumer, K.; Liu, Y.; McConnell, M.V.; Corrado, G.S.; Peng, L.; Webster, D.R. Prediction of Cardiovascular Risk Factors from Retinal Fundus Photographs via Deep Learning. *Nat. Biomed. Eng.* **2018**, *2*, 158–164. [CrossRef]
69. Vaghefi, E.; Yang, S.; Hill, S.; Humphrey, G.; Walker, N.; Squirrell, D. Detection of Smoking Status from Retinal Images; a Convolutional Neural Network Study. *Sci. Rep.* **2019**, *9*, 7180. [CrossRef]
70. Betzler, B.K.; Yang, H.H.S.; Thakur, S.; Yu, M.; Quek, T.C.; Soh, Z.D.; Lee, G.; Tham, Y.-C.; Wong, T.Y.; Rim, T.H.; et al. Gender Prediction for a Multiethnic Population via Deep Learning Across Different Retinal Fundus Photograph Fields: Retrospective Cross-Sectional Study. *JMIR Med. Inform.* **2021**, *9*, e25165. [CrossRef]
71. Korot, E.; Pontikos, N.; Liu, X.; Wagner, S.K.; Faes, L.; Huemer, J.; Balaskas, K.; Denniston, A.K.; Khawaja, A.; Keane, P.A. Predicting Sex from Retinal Fundus Photographs Using Automated Deep Learning. *Sci. Rep.* **2021**, *11*, 10286. [CrossRef]
72. Rim, T.H.; Lee, G.; Kim, Y.; Tham, Y.-C.; Lee, C.J.; Baik, S.J.; Kim, Y.A.; Yu, M.; Deshmukh, M.; Lee, B.K.; et al. Prediction of Systemic Biomarkers from Retinal Photographs: Development and Validation of Deep-Learning Algorithms. *Lancet Digit. Health* **2020**, *2*, e526–e536. [CrossRef] [PubMed]
73. Gerrits, N.; Elen, B.; Craenendonck, T.V.; Triantafyllidou, D.; Petropoulos, I.N.; Malik, R.A.; De Boever, P. Age and Sex Affect Deep Learning Prediction of Cardiometabolic Risk Factors from Retinal Images. *Sci. Rep.* **2020**, *10*, 9432. [CrossRef] [PubMed]
74. Budoff, M.J.; Raggi, P.; Beller, G.A.; Berman, D.S.; Druz, R.S.; Malik, S.; Rigolin, V.H.; Weigold, W.G.; Soman, P. Noninvasive Cardiovascular Risk Assessment of the Asymptomatic Diabetic Patient. *JACC Cardiovasc. Imaging* **2016**, *9*, 176–192. [CrossRef] [PubMed]
75. Tseng, R.M.W.W.; Rim, T.H.; Cheung, C.Y.; Wong, T.Y. Artificial Intelligence Using the Eye as a Biomarker of Systemic Risk. In *Artificial Intelligence in Ophthalmology*; Grzybowski, A., Ed.; Springer International Publishing: Cham, Switzerland, 2021; pp. 243–255, ISBN 978-3-030-78600-7.
76. Tseng, R.M.W.W.; Rim, T.H.; Shantsila, E.; Yi, J.K.; Park, S.; Kim, S.S.; Lee, C.J.; Thakur, S.; Nusinovici, S.; Peng, Q.; et al. Validation of a Deep-Learning-Based Retinal Biomarker (Reti-CVD) in the Prediction of Cardiovascular Disease: Data from UK Biobank. *BMC Med.* **2023**, *21*, 28. [CrossRef]
77. Touboul, P.-J. Intima-Media Thickness of Carotid Arteries. In *Frontiers of Neurology and Neuroscience*; Alonso, A., Hennerici, M.G., Meairs, S., Eds.; S. Karger AG: Basel, Switzerland, 2015; Volume 36, pp. 31–39, ISBN 978-3-318-02790-7.
78. Simó, R.; Bañeras, J.; Hernández, C.; Rodríguez-Palomares, J.; Valente, F.; Gutierrez, L.; González-Alujas, T.; Ferreira, I.; Aguadé-Bruix, S.; Montaner, J.; et al. Diabetic Retinopathy as an Independent Predictor of Subclinical Cardiovascular Disease: Baseline Results of the PRECISED Study. *BMJ Open Diabetes Res. Care* **2019**, *7*, e000845. [CrossRef]
79. Grzybowski, A.; Rao, D.P.; Brona, P.; Negiloni, K.; Krzywicki, T.; Savoy, F.M. Diagnostic Accuracy of Automated Diabetic Retinopathy Image Assessment Softwares: IDx-DR and Medios Artificial Intelligence. *Ophthalmic Res.* **2023**, *66*, 1286–1292. [CrossRef]
80. Gulshan, V.; Peng, L.; Coram, M.; Stumpe, M.C.; Wu, D.; Narayanaswamy, A.; Venugopalan, S.; Widner, K.; Madams, T.; Cuadros, J.; et al. Development and Validation of a Deep Learning Algorithm for Detection of Diabetic Retinopathy in Retinal Fundus Photographs. *JAMA* **2016**, *316*, 2402. [CrossRef]
81. Breiman, L.; Friedman, J.H.; Olshen, R.A.; Stone, C.J. *Classification And Regression Trees*, 1st ed.; Routledge: London, UK, 2017; ISBN 978-1-315-13947-0.

82. Shetkar, A.; Mai, C.K.; Yamini, C. Diabetic Symptoms Prediction Through Retinopathy. In *Machine Learning Technologies and Applications*; Mai, C.K., Reddy, A.B., Raju, K.S., Eds.; Algorithms for Intelligent Systems; Springer: Singapore, 2021; pp. 13–20, ISBN 978-981-334-045-9.
83. Li, W.; Schram, M.T.; Berendschot, T.T.J.M.; Webers, C.A.B.; Kroon, A.A.; Van Der Kallen, C.J.H.; Henry, R.M.A.; Schaper, N.C.; Huang, F.; Dashtbozorg, B.; et al. Type 2 Diabetes and HbA1c Are Independently Associated with Wider Retinal Arterioles: The Maastricht Study. *Diabetologia* **2020**, *63*, 1408–1417. [CrossRef]
84. Ting, D.S.W.; Cheung, C.Y.-L.; Lim, G.; Tan, G.S.W.; Quang, N.D.; Gan, A.; Hamzah, H.; Garcia-Franco, R.; San Yeo, I.Y.; Lee, S.Y.; et al. Development and Validation of a Deep Learning System for Diabetic Retinopathy and Related Eye Diseases Using Retinal Images from Multiethnic Populations with Diabetes. *JAMA* **2017**, *318*, 2211. [CrossRef]
85. Torabi, H.; Saberi Isfeedvajani, M.; Ramezani, M.; Daryabari, S.-H. Choroidal Thickness and Hemoglobin A1c Levels in Patients with Type 2 Diabetes Mellitus. *J. Ophthalmic Vis. Res.* **2019**, *14*, 285–290. [CrossRef]
86. Subrayan, V.; Menon, S.; Peyman, M.; Loo Voon Pei, A. Correlation between Optical Coherence Tomography-Derived Macular Measurements and Glycosylated Haemoglobin, Age, Visual Acuity and Diabetes Duration in Patients with Type 2 Diabetes Mellitus. *Int. J. Diabetes Dev. Ctries.* **2015**, *35*, 385–388. [CrossRef]
87. Bernal-Morales, C.; Alé-Chilet, A.; Martín-Pinardel, R.; Barraso, M.; Hernández, T.; Oliva, C.; Vinagre, I.; Ortega, E.; Figueras-Roca, M.; Sala-Puigdollers, A.; et al. Optical Coherence Tomography Angiography in Type 1 Diabetes Mellitus. Report 4: Glycated Haemoglobin. *Diagnostics* **2021**, *11*, 1537. [CrossRef] [PubMed]
88. Zhang, L.; Yuan, M.; An, Z.; Zhao, X.; Wu, H.; Li, H.; Wang, Y.; Sun, B.; Li, H.; Ding, S.; et al. Prediction of Hypertension, Hyperglycemia and Dyslipidemia from Retinal Fundus Photographs via Deep Learning: A Cross-Sectional Study of Chronic Diseases in Central China. *PLoS ONE* **2020**, *15*, e0233166. [CrossRef] [PubMed]
89. Wu, S.; Lin, H.; Zhang, C.; Zhang, Q.; Zhang, D.; Zhang, Y.; Meng, W.; Zhu, Z.; Tang, F.; Xue, F.; et al. Association between Erythrocyte Parameters and Metabolic Syndrome in Urban Han Chinese: A Longitudinal Cohort Study. *BMC Public Health* **2013**, *13*, 989. [CrossRef]
90. Liew, G.; Wang, J.J.; Rochtchina, E.; Wong, T.Y.; Mitchell, P. Complete Blood Count and Retinal Vessel Calibers. *PLoS ONE* **2014**, *9*, e102230. [CrossRef]
91. Gargeya, R.; Leng, T. Automated Identification of Diabetic Retinopathy Using Deep Learning. *Ophthalmology* **2017**, *124*, 962–969. [CrossRef]
92. Babenko, B.; Mitani, A.; Traynis, I.; Kitade, N.; Singh, P.; Maa, A.Y.; Cuadros, J.; Corrado, G.S.; Peng, L.; Webster, D.R.; et al. Detection of Signs of Disease in External Photographs of the Eyes via Deep Learning. *Nat. Biomed. Eng.* **2022**, *6*, 1370–1383. [CrossRef]
93. Alé-Chilet, A.; Bernal-Morales, C.; Barraso, M.; Hernández, T.; Oliva, C.; Vinagre, I.; Ortega, E.; Figueras-Roca, M.; Sala-Puigdollers, A.; Esquinas, C.; et al. Optical Coherence Tomography Angiography in Type 1 Diabetes Mellitus—Report 2: Diabetic Kidney Disease. *J. Clin. Med.* **2021**, *11*, 197. [CrossRef]
94. Cui, Y.; Zhu, Y.; Wang, J.C.; Lu, Y.; Zeng, R.; Katz, R.; Vingopoulos, F.; Le, R.; Laíns, I.; Wu, D.M.; et al. Comparison of Widefield Swept-Source Optical Coherence Tomography Angiography with Ultra-Widefield Colour Fundus Photography and Fluorescein Angiography for Detection of Lesions in Diabetic Retinopathy. *Br. J. Ophthalmol.* **2021**, *105*, 577–581. [CrossRef]
95. DuPont, M.; Arthur, E.; Shihab, Y.; Kenny, M.; Ravichandran, S.; Parsons-Wingerter, P.; Vyas, R.; Murray, M.C.; Predovic, M.; Lim, S.; et al. Use of VESsel GENeration with Optical Coherence Tomography Angiography and Fluorescein Angiography for Detection and Quantification of Vascular Changes in Mild and Moderate Diabetic Retinopathy. *Life* **2024**, *14*, 893. [CrossRef]
96. Cheung, C.Y.; Ikram, M.K.; Sabanayagam, C.; Wong, T.Y. Retinal Microvasculature as a Model to Study the Manifestations of Hypertension. *Hypertension* **2012**, *60*, 1094–1103. [CrossRef] [PubMed]
97. Wong, T. Computer-Assisted Measurement of Retinal Vessel Diameters in the Beaver Dam Eye Study*1methodology, Correlation between Eyes, and Effect of Refractive Errors. *Ophthalmology* **2004**, *111*, 1183–1190. [CrossRef] [PubMed]
98. Tapp, R.J.; Owen, C.G.; Barman, S.A.; Welikala, R.A.; Foster, P.J.; Whincup, P.H.; Strachan, D.P.; Rudnicka, A.R. For the UK Biobank Eye and Vision Consortium Associations of Retinal Microvascular Diameters and Tortuosity with Blood Pressure and Arterial Stiffness: United Kingdom Biobank. *Hypertension* **2019**, *74*, 1383–1390. [CrossRef] [PubMed]
99. Rubiś, P.P. Cardiac Disease: Diagnosis, Treatment, and Outcomes. *J. Pers. Med.* **2022**, *12*, 1212. [CrossRef]
100. Detrano, R.; Gianrossi, R.; Froelicher, V. The Diagnostic Accuracy of the Exercise Electrocardiogram: A Meta-Analysis of 22 Years of Research. *Prog. Cardiovasc. Dis.* **1989**, *32*, 173–206. [CrossRef]
101. Hendel, R.C.; Jabbar, A.Y.; Mahata, I. Initial Diagnostic Evaluation of Stable Coronary Artery Disease: The Need for a Patient-Centered Strategy. *J. Am. Heart Assoc.* **2017**, *6*, e006863. [CrossRef]
102. Krittayaphong, R.; Muenkaew, M.; Chiewvit, P.; Ratanasit, N.; Kaolawanich, Y.; Phrommintikul, A.; CORE Investigators. Electrocardiographic Predictors of Cardiovascular Events in Patients at High Cardiovascular Risk: A Multicenter Study. *J. Geriatr. Cardiol.* **2019**, *16*, 630–638. [CrossRef]
103. Lv, Q.; Tang, G.; Zhang, N.; Yu, D.; Sun, H. The Specificity and Accuracy of Echocardiography in Diagnosing Acute Heart Failure: A Systematic Review and Meta-Analysis. *Altern. Ther. Health Med.* 2024; *Epub ahead of print.*
104. Doust, J.A.; Glasziou, P.P.; Pietrzak, E.; Dobson, A.J. A Systematic Review of the Diagnostic Accuracy of Natriuretic Peptides for Heart Failure. *Arch. Intern. Med.* **2004**, *164*, 1978–1984. [CrossRef]

105. Gorenoi, V.; Schönermark, M.P.; Hagen, A. CT Coronary Angiography vs. Invasive Coronary Angiography in CHD. *GMS Health Technol. Assess.* **2012**, *8*, Doc02. [CrossRef]
106. Neves, P.O.; Andrade, J.; Monção, H. Coronary Artery Calcium Score: Current Status. *Radiol. Bras.* **2017**, *50*, 182–189. [CrossRef]
107. Sahoo, R.; Krishna, M.V.; Subrahmaniyan, D.K.S.; Dutta, T.K.; Elangovan, S. Common carotid intima-media thickness in acute ischemic stroke: A case-control study. *Neurol. India* **2009**, *57*, 627–630. [CrossRef] [PubMed]
108. Tedyanto, E.H.; Tini, K.; Pramana, N.A.K. Magnetic Resonance Imaging in Acute Ischemic Stroke. *Cureus* **2022**, *14*, e27224. [CrossRef] [PubMed]
109. Feng, L.; Yang, Z.; Chen, S.; Wan, J. Diagnostic value of myocardial stress detection based on feature tracking MRI in patients with acute myocardial infarction. *J. Thorac. Dis.* **2022**, *14*, 3454–3461. [CrossRef] [PubMed]
110. Lee, E.M. When and how to use ambulatory blood pressure monitoring and home blood pressure monitoring for managing hypertension. *Clin. Hypertens* **2024**, *30*, 10. [CrossRef]
111. Teoh, C.S.; Wong, K.H.; Xiao, D.; Wong, H.C.; Zhao, P.; Chan, H.W.; Yuen, Y.S.; Naing, T.; Yogesan, K.; Koh, V.T.C. Variability in Grading Diabetic Retinopathy Using Retinal Photography and Its Comparison with an Automated Deep Learning Diabetic Retinopathy Screening Software. *Healthcare* **2023**, *11*, 1697. [CrossRef]
112. Shin, J.H.; Cheong, J.I.; Cheuh, H.W.; Yoo, J.H. Limitations of Current Screening Methods for Lipid Disorders in Korean Adolescents and a Proposal for an Effective Detection Method: A Nationwide, Cross-Sectional Study. *Ann. Pediatr. Endocrinol. Metab.* **2020**, *25*, 265–271. [CrossRef]
113. Ghenciu, L.A.; Hațegan, O.A.; Stoicescu, E.R.; Iacob, R.; Șișu, A.M. Emerging Therapeutic Approaches and Genetic Insights in Stargardt Disease: A Comprehensive Review. *Int. J. Mol. Sci.* **2024**, *25*, 8859. [CrossRef]

biomedicines

MDPI

Systematic Review

The Triglyceride/HDL Ratio as a Surrogate Biomarker for Insulin Resistance

Petru Baneu [1,2,3], Cristina Văcărescu [2,3,4,*], Simona-Ruxanda Drăgan [2,3,4], Liviu Cirin [1], Alexandra-Iulia Lazăr-Höcher [1,3], Andreea Cozgarea [1,5], Adelina-Andreea Faur-Grigori [3], Simina Crișan [2,3,4], Dan Gaiță [2,3,4], Constantin-Tudor Luca [2,3,4] and Dragoș Cozma [2,3,4]

1 Doctoral School, "Victor Babes" University of Medicine and Pharmacy, 300041 Timisoara, Romania; petru.baneu@umft.ro (P.B.); liviu.cirin@umft.ro (L.C.); alexandra.hocher@umft.ro (A.-I.L.-H.); andreea.cozgarea@umft.ro (A.C.)

2 Department of Cardiology, "Victor Babes" University of Medicine and Pharmacy, 2 Eftimie Murgu Square, 300041 Timisoara, Romania; simona.dragan@umft.ro (S.-R.D.); simina.crisan@umft.ro (S.C.); dan.gaita@umft.ro (D.G.); constantin.luca@umft.ro (C.-T.L.); dragos.cozma@umft.ro (D.C.)

3 Institute of Cardiovascular Diseases Timisoara, 13A Gheorghe Adam Street, 300310 Timisoara, Romania; andreeaadelinafaur@yahoo.com

4 Research Center of the Institute of Cardiovascular Diseases Timisoara, 13A Gheorghe Adam Street, 300310 Timisoara, Romania

5 County Clinical Emergency Hospital of Sibiu, 550245 Sibiu, Romania

* Correspondence: cristina.vacarescu@umft.ro

Abstract: Given the widespread occurrence of insulin resistance, a key factor in metabolic syndrome and a distinct condition altogether, there is a clear need for effective, surrogate markers. The triglyceride-to-high-density lipoprotein (TG/HDL) ratio stands out as a viable option, indicative of changes in lipid metabolism associated with insulin resistance, offering a cost-effective and straightforward alternative to traditional, more complex biomarkers. This review, in line with PRISMA guidelines, assesses the TG/HDL ratio's potential as an indirect indicator of insulin resistance. Analysing 32 studies over 20 years, involving 49,782 participants of diverse ethnic backgrounds, including adults and children, this review primarily uses a cross-sectional analysis with the Homeostatic Model Assessment for Insulin Resistance (HOMA-IR) to gauge insulin resistance. It reveals the TG/HDL ratio's varied predictive power across ethnicities and sexes, with specific thresholds providing greater accuracy for Caucasians, Asians, and Hispanics over African Americans and for men over women. Valid across different weights and ages, for adults and children, it suggests average cutoffs of 2.53 for women and 2.8 for men. The analysis supports the TG/HDL ratio as a simple, accessible marker for insulin resistance, though it advises further research on tailored cutoffs reflecting ethnic and gender differences.

Keywords: TG/HDL ratio; insulin resistance; surrogate biomarker; metabolic syndrome

1. Introduction

Insulin resistance (IR) is a widespread health concern worldwide, with precise global prevalence figures being challenging to pinpoint due to variations in diagnostic criteria and population studies. It is most associated with obesity and is a core component of metabolic syndrome (MS) [1,2]. Even though this association is completely justified, IR is starting to take shape as a separate entity. Recently, the TOFI (thin-outside-fat-inside) phenotype has been used to describe lean individuals with a disproportionate amount of visceral fat, who are insulin-resistant [1]. On the other hand, the MHO phenotype (metabolically healthy obese) represents a unique subset of euglycemic individuals who bear significant amounts of subcutaneous adipose tissue but display favorable lipid profiles, an absence of systemic inflammation, and normal liver function [2]. Therefore, IR, MS, and obesity are evidently intertwined and interdependent but not superposable. Thus, search on the dedicated biomarkers of IR is more prevalent than ever.

Despite this obvious and urgent necessity, quantifying IR has proven to be a significant challenge in clinical and research settings due to the complexity of its underlying mechanisms and the lack of a universally accepted measurement standard [1–3]. Traditional direct methods, such as the hyperinsulinemic–euglycemic clamp technique, are often deemed impractical for routine clinical use, owing to their invasiveness, technical complexity, and resource-intensive nature. Consequently, the medical community has sought alternative, indirect biomarkers that could serve as surrogates for assessing insulin sensitivity.

HOMA-IR (Homeostatic Model Assessment for Insulin Resistance) and FPI (Fasting Plasma Insulin) are both commonly used as surrogate markers for assessing IR with a strong predictive power, high specificity, and sensitivity. Nonetheless, even though they are more feasible than the hyperinsulinemic–euglycemic clamp technique, they are still cumbersome in daily practice [2–5]. Therefore, the search for simpler biomarkers to be integrated into a standard examination continues unabated.

The triglyceride-to-high-density lipoprotein (TG/HDL) ratio has been proposed as an indirect marker of IR. This is because the metabolic processes that result in IR also lead to changes in lipid metabolism, which are reflected in the levels of serum triglycerides and HDL cholesterol [2]. A brief dive into the pathophysiology of IR reveals that one of the physiological functions of insulin is to inhibit the release of free fatty acids from adipose tissue and promote the storage of triglycerides in adipocytes [4]. However, in IR, this regulatory mechanism is impaired. Firstly, an increased rate of unchecked lipolysis leads to an accelerated release of free fatty acids (FFAs) into the bloodstream [4]. Consequently, the liver, inundated with excess FFAs, increases triglyceride production, packaging them into very low-density lipoprotein (VLDL) particles, resulting in hypertriglyceridemia. On the other hand, IR also augments the catabolism of HDL particles, partly due to the heightened activity of hepatic lipase, an enzyme that hydrolyzes HDL triglycerides and phospholipids, leading to smaller and less stable HDL particles that are more rapidly cleared from circulation [4,6]. Additionally, IR impairs the synthesis of apolipoprotein A-I (ApoA-I), a primary structural protein of HDL. Finally, IR alters the structural characteristics of HDL, making it more prone to oxidative stress, negatively affecting its protective properties [3,4,6]. The resulting lipid profile, characterized by elevated triglycerides and reduced HDL cholesterol, can be succinctly represented by the TG/HDL ratio.

The unequivocal simplicity and accessibility of these two biomarkers have encouraged the pursuit of defining the exact predictive capability, limitations, and peculiarities of this ratio over the last two decades.

This systematic review has as the main objective of assessing the feasibility of utilizing the TG/HDL ratio as a surrogate marker for IR.

2. Materials and Methods

The methodology for selecting studies in this review adhered to the PRISMA (Preferred Reporting Items for Systematic Reviews and Meta-Analyses) guidelines, being registered on the PROSEPRO platform, with the following code: CRD42024545597. The process entailed an extensive bibliographic examination using databases such as the PubMed database and Google Scholar, using "TG/HDL ratio" and "insulin resistance" as keywords.

2.1. Eligibility Criteria

The inclusion criteria were represented by prospective or retrospective observational studies that included nondiabetic adults or children and that were aimed at quantifying the predictive value the TG/HDL ratio as a surrogate marker of IR. The IR was measured utilizing the gold standard test—the hyperinsulinemic–euglycemic clamp technique or other consecrated surrogate markers for IR.

2.2. Electronic Search and Study Selection

The determination of the most relevant articles was based on a thorough evaluation of their titles, the content of their abstracts, and a preliminary review of the complete manuscripts. Articles that were not in English, publications that were only available as abstracts, and redundant entries were systematically excluded from this review.

A total of 32 scientific papers were selected and included in this review. The studies are listed in Tables 1 and 2, along with the test of IR utilized, the TG/HDL ratio for women and men, respectively, the BMI (Body Mass Index) of the participants, and the number of participants. Tabel 1 comprises the studies that enlisted less than 1000 participants, whereas Tabel 2 displays those with studies with more than 1000 participants.

Table 1. The 22 studies with less than 1000 participants included in this review.

Study	Test for IR	Cutoff TG/HDL Women	Cutoff TG/HDL Men	Number of Participants	BMI of Participants
McLaughlin et al., 2003 [7]	Steady-state plasma glucose concentration during the insulin suppression test	3	3	258	Overweight
McLaughlin et al., 2005 [8]	Steady-state plasma glucose concentration during the insulin suppression test	3.5	3.5	449	Normal
Summer et al., 2005 [9]	Steady-state plasma glucose concentration during the insulin suppression test	3	3	125	Overweight
Bovet et al., 2006 [10]	HOMA-IR	3.5	3.5	630	Overweight
Karelis et al., 2007 [11]	Hyperinsulinemic–euglycemic clamp and HOMA-IR	-	-	131	Overweight or obese
Quijada et al., 2008 [12]	HOMA-IR and QUICKI (Quantitative insulin sensitivity check index)	3.5	3.5	67	Variable
Kim-Dorner et al., 2009 [13]	HOMA-IR	-	-	149	Variable
Chiang et al., 2011 [14]	HOMA-IR	-	-	812	Overweight or obese
Gonzalez-Chavez et al., 2011 [15]	HOMA-IR	3	3	177	Variable
Gasevic et al., 2012 [16]	HOMA-IR	-	-	784	Variable
He et al., 2014 [17]	HOMA-IR	-	-	533	Normal
Hirschler et al., 2014 [18]	HOMA-IR	-	-	501	Variable
Maturu et al., 2015 [19]	Frequently sampled IV glucose tolerance test (FSIVGTT)	-	-	41	Overweight or obese
Zhou et al., 2016 [20]	HOMA-IR	-	-	379	Variable
Iwani et al., 2016 [21]	HOMA-IR	2.48	2.48	271	Overweight or obese
Borrayo et al., 2018 [22]	HOMA-IR	3	-	253	Variable

Table 1. *Cont.*

Study	Test for IR	Cutoff TG/HDL Women	Cutoff TG/HDL Men	Number of Participants	BMI of Participants
Pantoja-Torres et al., 2019 [23]	HOMA-IR	-	-	118	Normal
Behiry et al., 2019 [24]	HOMA-IR	1.36	1.36	90	Overweight or obese
Garcia et al., 2019 [25]	HOMA-IR	2.22	2.22	201	Overweight or obese
Yeh et al., 2019 [26]	HOMA-IR	2.197	2.2	398	Variable
Demiral et al., 2021 [27]	HOMA-IR	-	-	159	Overweight or obese
Sowndarya et al., 2021 [28]	HOMA-IR	-	-	71	Normal

Table 2. The 11 studies with more than 1000 participants included in this review.

Study	Test for IR	Cutoff TG/HDL Women	Cutoff TG/HDL Men	Number of Participants	BMI of Participants
Li et al., 2008 [29]	Fasting serum insulin (FSI)	3.2	3.2	2652	Variable
Glueck et al., 2009 [30]	HOMA-IR	-	-	1724	Variable
Summer et al., 2010 [31]	HOMA-IR	-	2.5	1903	Variable
Giannini et al., 2011 [32]	HOMA-IR	2.27	2.27	1452	Overweight or obese
Kim et al., 2012 [33]	HOMA-IR	-	-	7623	Variable
Kang et al., 2012 [34]	HOMA-IR	-	-	8411	Variable
Salazar et al., 2012 [35]	HOMA-IR and fasting serum insulin (FSI)	2.5	3.5	1566	Variable
Murguia-Romero et al., 2013 [36]	HOMA-IR and QUICKI	2.5	3.5	2244	Variable
Von Bibra et al., 2017 [37]	HOMA-IR and QUICKI	1.9	2.8	1932	Variable
Gong et al., 2021 [38]	HOMA-IR	-	-	10,132	Variable

The PRISMA diagram below illustrates the search strategy employed, along with the filters that were applied (Figure 1).

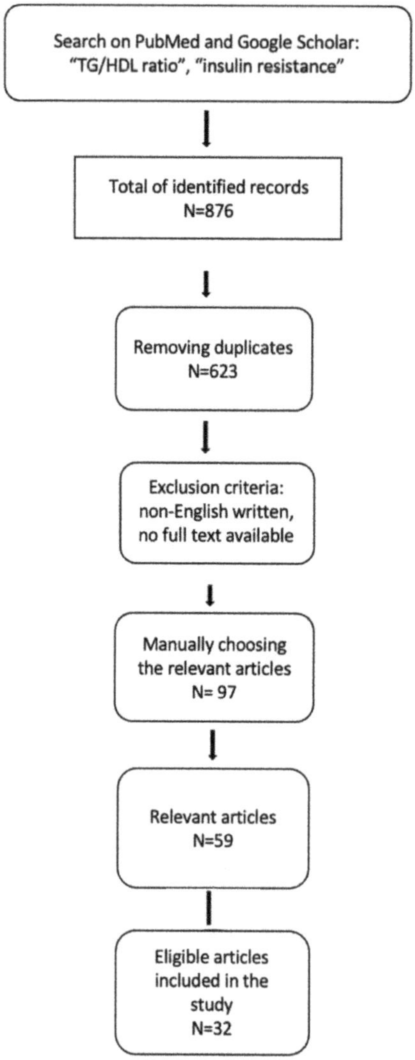

Figure 1. Search strategy employed in this review.

3. Results

3.1. Overview

3.1.1. Participant Numbers and Demographics

Over the course of two decades, spanning from 2003 to 2023, our review encompassed 32 studies involving a cumulative total of 49,782 participants. The scope of these studies varied considerably, ranging from a minimal cohort of 61 children to a substantial assembly of 10,132 adults. Within this spectrum, 7 studies specifically investigated pediatric subpopulations, whereas 25 studies primarily focused on adult demographics. Distinct studies targeted gender-specific populations, with three dedicated to female participants, one to male participants, and the remainder incorporating a gender-inclusive approach.

3.1.2. Ethnic and Racial Diversity

The studies examined a wide array of subpopulations including, but not limited to, Caucasians, African Americans, Asians, and Hispanics.

3.1.3. Classification of Study Types

Predominantly, the research methodologies employed were of a cross-sectional nature, with 24 such studies conducted. Additional methodological approaches included clinical transversal observational studies and retrospective cohorts.

3.1.4. Statistical Methods

The analytical techniques employed across the studies were diverse. Notably, the Receiver Operating Characteristic (ROC) curve analysis was utilized in 17 studies with an Area Under Curve (AUC) exceeding 0.7, which signified a reasonable predictive capacity. The odds ratio (OR) analysis was another prevalent method, which was applied in 12 studies.

The Homeostatic Model Assessment for Insulin Resistance (HOMA-IR) emerged as the predominant metric for assessing IR in 28 studies. It assesses IR and quantifies the beta-cell function by integrating fasting blood glucose and fasting insulin levels [39]. Its simplicity and non-invasiveness are the reasons for its widespread acceptance and use in most scientific scenarios [39]. Fasting serum insulin (FSI) is another marker that measures the concentration of insulin in the blood after an overnight fast. Despite being straightforward, it does not provide a complete picture of insulin sensitivity, which generally restricts its applicability [40,41]. The third test found was the quantitative insulin sensitivity check index (QUICKI), which is derived from fasting blood glucose and fasting insulin levels and is considered both reliable and simple [42]. The steady-state plasma glucose concentration during an insulin suppression test is a more direct and invasive method, providing an accurate assessment of IR, but it is less commonly used due to its complexity, even in studies [43,44]. The frequently sampled intravenous glucose tolerance test (FSIVGTT) involves administering a glucose injection, followed by frequent blood sampling, to measure glucose and insulin levels over time, with the data then analyzed using the minimal model analysis to estimate insulin sensitivity. This is probably the most time-consuming and labor-intensive method [45,46]. Lastly, the hyperinsulinemic–euglycemic clamp technique represents the gold standard for measuring insulin sensitivity and assessing insulin resistance. By inserting concomitant intravenous lines, insulin and glucose are infused, with the measurement of the glucose infusion rate (GIR), which reflects the amount of glucose necessary to maintain euglycemia under hyperinsulinemic conditions. This rate is directly proportional to insulin sensitivity. This method is also labor-intensive, costly, and requires significant expertise [47,48].

3.1.5. Body Mass Index (BMI) of Participants

The studies exhibited a wide range of participant BMIs, from those classified as overweight or obese (13) to individuals of normal weight (4). Most of the studies did not have the BMI as an exclusion criterion, but with no exception, this parameter was noted.

3.2. Comorbidities and Chronic Treatment

In the total of 32 studies included in our review, no patient was on medications that could interfere with the lipid parameters. Moreover, the participants were free of known major diseases, such as heart disease, peripheral vascular disease, liver disease, thyroid and other endocrine diseases, or neoplasms. In only one of the studies, 20% of the subjects were reported to have hypertension [9].

3.3. Ethnicity and Gender

In 2003, McLaughlin et al. were the first to mention a correlation between the TG/HDL ratio and IR in overweight nondiabetic patients. They utilized a cutoff of 3.0 for the

TG/HDL ratio, finding a AUC-ROC of 0.781 (CI 95%). Despite this encouraging percentage, this study had several limitations that have been briefly noted in the literature: the patient cohort consisted mostly of Caucasians, with only 1% African Americans, and did not differentiate based on gender, neglecting normal-weight subjects, who can also be affected by IR [7]. Two years later, in 2005, the same team further explored this issue by conducting another study involving twice as many healthy, nondiabetic individuals [8]. Gender, BMI, and age were reported to bear no statistical significance, and the cutoff utilized this time was 3.5, which has been described as indicative of IR. During the same year, Summer et al. published an article focusing on the utility of the TG/HDL ratio in predicting IR in a population of African Americans. The number of patients was relatively small—125—but the results were unequivocal: the AUC-ROC for a TG/HDL of >3 was just 0.56 ± 0.05 (CI 95%) [9].

The Asian subpopulations were examined in the years that followed, with 7 studies focusing on South Korean, Japanese, Chinese, Malaysian, and Taiwanese populations, totaling 18,158 adults and 271 children [14,17,20,21,26,33,34,49]. The TG/HDL ratio was generally portraited as a capable surrogate marker of IR, with several observations that deserve to be noted: Chiang et al. in 2011 found that additional clinical factors such as gender, waist circumferences, and ALT levels can augment the diagnostic accuracy, while Kang et al. and Kim et al., one year later, noted that the TG/HDL ratio is linearly associated with IR independently of waist circumference in both genders [14,26,33,34]. Zhou et al. and Iwani et al. also advocated for the predictive value of the TG/HDL ratio for IR, without insisting on differences based on gender or anthropometric elements [20,21]. In contrast, He et al., in 2014, published an article with Chinese adult participants and found that the TG/HDL ratio was adequate for discriminating IR mainly in non-obese women [17].

The Hispanic population received separate attention in research studies. Either with varied ethnic subgroups or by solely enlisting Hispanic participants, several papers have conveyed that the TG/HDL ratio is a useful tool for predicting IR [15,22,23,29,35,36]. In 2008, Li et al. addressed the question of ethnicity, finding no relevant difference in the OR of the three separate subpopulations of their study, non-Hispanic whites, non-Hispanic blacks, and Mexican Americans, respectively, with the TG/HDL ratio of >3.5 showing a considerable predictive value for IR. After adjustments for potential confounding effects, the prevalence ratio of hyperinsulinemia was 2.16 (95% confidence interval [CI], 1.74 to 2.08) when using a single cutoff point of 3.5 and 2.23 (95% CI, 1.83 to 2.72) when using race/ethnicity-specific cutoff points of 3.0 for non-Hispanic whites and Mexican Americans and 2.0 for non-Hispanic blacks for the TG/HDL-C ratio. The AUC-ROC of the TG/HDL-C ratio for predicting hyperinsulinemia was 0.77 (95% CI, 0.74 to 0.79); 0.75 (95% CI, 0.69 to 0.77); and 0.74 (95% CI, 0.69 to 0.76) for non-Hispanic whites, non-Hispanic blacks, and Mexican Americans, respectively [29]. Gonzalez et al., Salazar et al., and Murguia-Romero et al. conducted studies focusing only on the Hispanic subpopulation, demonstrating the predictive power of the TG/HDL ratio and proposing various cutoff values, either as one common number regardless of gender or with variations based on it [15,35,36]. In 2018, Borrayo et al. focused on a subpopulation of Hispanic women, reporting strong predictive values for a TG/HDL ratio of >3 both in non-obese and obese subjects with an OR of 3.27 (95% CI) and 4.7 (95% CI), respectively [22]. In 2019, Pantoja-Torres et al. highlighted that the TG/HDL ratio could be used for assessing IR in euthyroid normal-weight adults [23].

3.4. Gender Particularities

Gender-specific differences have also emerged as a significant factor to be taken into consideration. In 2007, Karelis et al. analyzed 131 overweight or obese nondiabetic women, concluding that the TG/HDL ratio alone could serve as a reliable tool in identifying women with IR, mainly in the obese, post-menopausal subpopulations [11]. Eight years later, Maturu et al. stated that the TG/HDL-C ratio is a poor predictor of IR in African American women [19]. In contrast, in 2018, Borrayo et al. focused on a subpopulation of Hispanic women, reporting strong predictive values for a TG/HDL ratio of >3 both in non-obese and obese subjects, with odds ratios of 3.27 (95% CI) and 4.7 (95% CI), respectively [22]. He et al. evaluated a subpopulation of Chinese subjects segregated by gender and BMI, reporting a predictive TG/HDL ratio only for the group of non-obese women with an AUC-ROC of 0.718 (95% CI) [17].

3.5. Children Particularities

The pediatric population has been examined separately. The 7 studies that were included in our review spanned over a period of 13 years and included children between 5 and 18 years of age, with various ethnic backgrounds (Caucasian, Asian, Hispanic, African American, and Egyptian) [12,18,21,24,25,27,32]. Atotal of 6 of these studies concluded that the TG/HDL ratio has a significative predictive value for IR in pediatric populations, regardless of gender, age, or ethnicity, with a reported OR of 2.58 by Hirschler et al. and 2.47 by Iwani et al. [18,21]. The AUC-ROC found by Giannini et al. was 0.706 [32]. Behiry et al. stated that a TG/HDL ratio of $\geq$1.36 had 85.7% sensitivity and 66.7% specificity, while Garcia et al. found an AUC-ROC of 0.729 for a TG/HDL ratio above 2.22 [24,25]. Quijada et al.'s work (2008) was the only study that depicted a lack of correlation of the TG/GHDL ratio with insulin sensitivity indexes like HOMA or QUICKI but demonstrated that a significant proportion of obese children, those with hypertension and those with MS, exhibited a TG/HDL-C ratio of 3.5 or higher [12].

3.6. TG/HDL Ratio Cutoff Values

One important aspect in clinical practice is represented by TG/HDL ratio cutoff values. In 50% of the studies, specific cutoff values were proposed by the authors, with the rest having used the TG/HDL ratio as a continuous variable. In the case where exact numbers were attributed to the ratio, it was either a general one for the entire subpopulation, or several cutoffs were recommended in functions of race or gender. The lowest ratio was 1.36 for both genders in children, as proposed by Behiry et al. in 2019 [24]. The highest one was 3,5 for both genders, as was postulated in 3 separate studies between 2005 and 2008 [8,10,12]. The median cutoff value for women was 2.53, whereas the median one for men was 2.8. In 2008, Li et al. addressed the question of ethnicity, finding no relevant difference in the OR of the 3 separate subpopulations of their study, non-Hispanic whites, non-Hispanic blacks, and Mexican Americans, respectively, with the TG/HDL ratio, when using ethnicity-specific cutoff points, of 3.0 for Caucasians and Mexican Americans and 2.0 for African Americans [29].

3.7. The Triad TG/HDL, IR, and BMI

In most of the studies, when a statistical analysis was used to filter the altering effects of the BMI as a confounding factor for the predictability of the TG/HDL ratio for IR, an independent correlation was indeed reported. On the other hand, Gong et al., in 2021, described an inverse correlation between the TG/HDL ratio and the BMI, the strongest association being in subjects with a BMI of 18.5–24 [38]. Pantoja-Torres et al. concentrated only on normal weight healthy adults in demonstrating the predictive value of the TG/HDL ratio [23]. Yeh et al., in 2019, reported the opposite: the TG/HDL ratio was higher as the BMI value increased [26]. Borrayo et al., in 2018, described the TG/HDL ratio as a capable predictive biomarker for IR in both overweight/obese and normal weight women [22]. He at al., in 2014, concluded that the discriminatory power of the TG/HDL ratio for IR differs by the gender and obesity index in the normo-glycemic Chinese population, and the TG/HDL ratio could discriminate IR in non-obese and normoglycemic women [17].

4. Discussion

4.1. TG/HDL Ratio and Ethnicity

It is a known fact that differences between the lipid profiles in African American populations in contrast with the Caucasian population exist. Genetic, dietary, lifestyle, socioeconomic, and environmental factors are implied [50]. Moreover, research indicates that the activity of lipoprotein lipase (LPL) tends to be stronger in African Americans compared to Caucasians [51]. LPL is a critical enzyme in lipid metabolism, playing a significant role in the hydrolysis of triglycerides in lipoproteins into free fatty acids and glycerol, thereby facilitating the clearance of triglycerides from the bloodstream. In addition, African Americans often have higher average HDL cholesterol levels compared to Caucasians [50]. This difference is observed across various age groups and genders. Several studies within African American populations by Summer et al. and Kim-Dormer et al. have confirmed the disparities in the ratio's effectiveness, indicating a weaker association in contrast to Caucasian cohorts [13,31]. This disparity was further explored by Bovet et al. and others, who expanded the ethnic spectrum, incorporating Africans, mixed ethnic groups, and non-Africans, thereby reinforcing the concept that metabolic markers cannot be universally applied without considering ethnic-specific thresholds [10,31]. Even so, not all the studies including African Americans point towards the idea that the TG/HDL ratio is an inappropriate surrogate marker for IR in this subpopulation. Large studies, such as the one published by Li et al. comprising 2652 adults, reported a favorable predictive value across all evaluated ethnic groups (Caucasians, Hispanics, and African Americans) [29]. Moreover, the largest one, enlisting more than 10,000 subjects of various ethnic origins, including more than 20% African Americans, concluded that the TG/HDL ratio is positively associated with IR in a nonlinear interaction pattern. In regards to the discrepancies noted among the African American populations in comparison to Caucasians, Asians, or Hispanics, lower cutoffs of 2.5 or even 2.0 appear to be more appropriate [38].

4.2. TG/HDL Ratio and Gender

Another possible altering factor is gender. Women, particularly in the premenopausal age, are known to have more favorable lipid profiles, which can evidently decrease the sensitivity and specificity of the TG/HDL ratio. If the women are of African American ethnicity, the effect may become cumulative, necessitating adjusted cutoffs between 1.5 and 2.0. Several means exist to augment the predictive value of the ratio in certain subpopulations. One approach is the addition of anthropometric data or other biomarkers, as demonstrated by Chiang et al., who managed to increase the AUC-ROC from 0.66 to 0.77 by including gender, ALT levels, and waist circumference [13]. Another possibility is to use other indirect biomarkers for IR, such as the triglyceride–glucose index, which also shows promising predictive capabilities [25,52,53].

4.3. Overall Predictive Value of TG/HDL Ratio

In half of the articles reviewed, the TG/HDL ratio was reported to present an AUC-ROC above 0.7 (threshold marked by the red line in Figure 2) in cases of mixed subpopulations or Caucasians. Similar conclusions can be drawn regarding the subpopulations of Hispanics and Asians. However, in African Americans, the results were less reassuring. Considering that a value between 0.5–0.7 is labelled as fair discrimination, with good discrimination being seen only in the interval of 0.8–0.9, by analyzing Figure 2, the fact that only 2 of the 17 studies having used this statistical method have ratios equal to or above 0.8 indicates that additional parameters could be useful in order the enhance the predictive value of the TG/HDL ratio.

4.4. TG/HDL Ratio Cutoff Values

Probably the most difficult task lies in establishing the proper TG/HDL cutoff, as in half the reviewed studies, no value was even proposed. Considering the mean values obtained from the 17 studies that did discuss this issue, TG/HDL ratios above 2.5 for women and above 2.8 for men seem appropriate for all populations other than African Americans. In the case of the latter, ratios above 1.5 for women and 2 for men, respectively, can be proposed, with further research being needed for a better calibration of the biomarker.

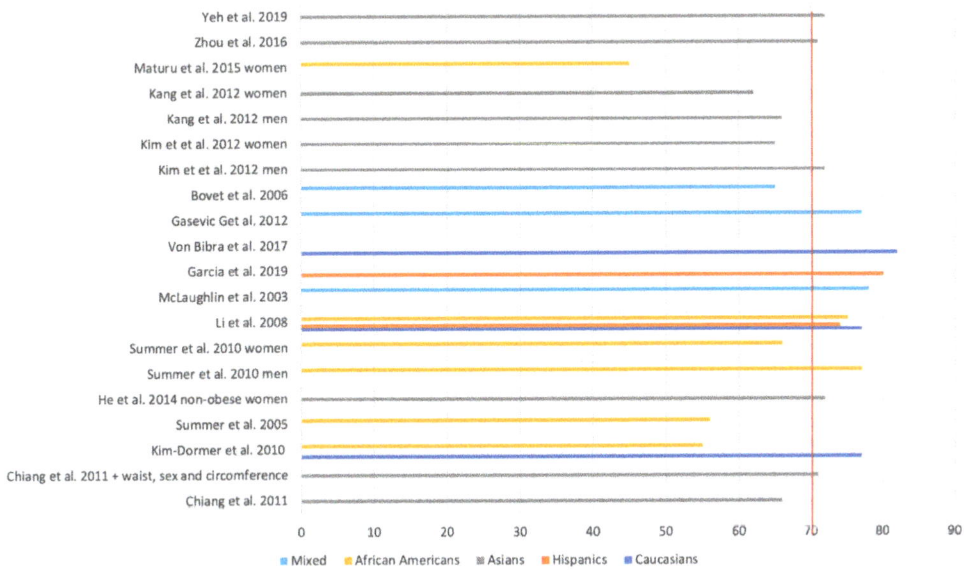

Figure 2. AUC-ROC for the predictive value of the TG/HDL ratio [7,9,10,13,14,16,17,19,20,25,29,31,33,34,37,38].

4.5. TG/HDL Ratio and Children

Regarding the applicability to children, the studies evaluated in this review strongly conclude towards a valuable predictive power of the TG/HDL ratio as a surrogate biomarker for IR in overweight or obese patients, regardless of age, sex, or ethnicity. A deeper assessment of the capability of this ratio in normal weight children would be appropriate to be able to extend its use.

4.6. TG/HDL Ratio and Obesity

As previously mentioned, IR has taken shape as a separate entity, being also able to promote obesity in normal weight subjects and not only act as a repercussion of it. Studies, like the one published by Gong et al. in 2021, validated the predictive value of the TG/HDL ratio for IR in normal weight patients [38,54–65].

4.7. TG/HDL Ratio and Lipoprotein(a)

Lipoprotein(a) (Lp(a)) is a solid risk factor for cardiovascular diseases, with values that seem to be constant throughout one's lifetime, which are largely unaffected by lifestyle changes [66–72]. Despite consistent efforts invested in pharmacological means of lowering it, there is currently no clinically applicable solution. Lately, a peculiar inverse relationship has been observed in a few studies between Lp(a) levels and IR [72]. To the best of our knowledge, the reasons for this are unknown. Several hypotheses have been proposed to explain this. Some suggest that Lp(a) might exert anti-inflammatory or antioxidative effects in certain contexts, potentially mitigating some of the pathways that lead to IR. Others base this situation on genetic factors [73]. As the levels of Lp(a) are primarily genetically determined, this might explain why its relationship with IR can vary across different studies and populations, in either direction. It is worth mentioning that this inverse association is not widely accepted as a general fact, being contradicted by other studies. Moreover, one study by Tian et al. from 2023, which compared two groups of patients with carotid plaque separated into stable and unstable, found that subjects from the latter group displayed significantly higher levels of both Lp(a) and the TG/HDL ratio than those from the former [74]. Therefore, more research is warranted for a better understanding of the pathophysiological role of Lp(a) in the context of IR. Additionally, considering the importance of Lp(a) in the sphere of cardiovascular disease and the strong correlation between IR and cardiovascular risk, further research is needed to assess the role of Lp(a) and the TG/HDL ratio as combined risk predictors in specific situations, as seen in the above-mentioned article.

4.8. TG/HDL Ratio and Apolipoprotein B

Apolipoprotein B (ApoB) is a crucial protein component of various lipoproteins, including very low-density lipoproteins (VLDLs), intermediate-density lipoproteins (IDLs), and low-density lipoproteins (LDLs). It plays an essential role in the assembly and secretion of these lipoproteins from the liver into the bloodstream [6]. Elevated ApoB levels, indicative of a high concentration of atherogenic lipoprotein particles, are strongly associated with an increased risk in cardiovascular diseases [74]. In individuals with insulin resistance (IR), the presence of high ApoB levels, combined with other dyslipidemic components such as elevated triglycerides (TGs) and reduced high-density lipoprotein cholesterol (HDL-C), significantly elevates the risk of atherosclerosis and related cardiovascular events [74]. Additionally, incorporating apolipoprotein A-I (ApoA-I), a key component of HDL-C, into the calculation provides the ApoB/ApoA-I ratio, offering insights into the balance between atherogenic and protective HDL particles [6,74]. When considered alongside the TG/HDL-C ratio, which reflects the balance between triglycerides and HDL cholesterol, these two ratios together provide a comprehensive view of lipid abnormalities and cardiovascular risk in subjects with IR.

4.9. General Considerations

We would like to emphasize the utmost importance of using standardized pre-test protocols. Patients should undergo a fasting period of 8–12 h before blood sample collection, avoid alcohol and high-fat meals for at least 24 h prior, and discontinue medications that might interfere with lipid levels, as advised by a healthcare provider in accordance with the specific context [75].

Finally, we strongly believe that, apart from the automated determination of lipid levels, the cold flotation test should not be routinely performed in order to prevent procedural variability and provide consistent and reproducible results, using an easily available, simple, and cost-effective method [76].

5. Conclusions

Our article represents the first paper to offer an overview of the feasibility of using the TG/HDL ratio as a surrogate biomarker for IR, highlighting both its strengths and limits, in various subpopulations, since its first mentioning in the literature to the present day. As in recent years, IR has been associated with a varied spectrum of pathologies from Alzheimer's disease and depression to oncologic conditions and a whole plethora of cardiovascular diseases The utility of determining IR becomes of utmost importance and easily expands beyond the domain of metabolic disorders [66–71].

The TG/HDL ratio demonstrates significant predictive values for IR, including for non-obese individuals, thereby challenging the conventional association of IR solely with obesity. Moreover, the TG/HDL ratio demonstrates potential as a valuable predictive tool in pediatric populations, indicating its broader applicability beyond adult cohorts.

The mean cutoffs found in the studies were 2.53 for women and 2.8 for men, and this is what we recommend as the limit for raising awareness and conducting further investigations.

Nevertheless, its effectiveness varies across ethnic groups, also presenting gender-specific differences, with specific cutoff values enhancing its precision in certain populations. It demonstrates greater accuracy for Caucasians, Asians, and Hispanics over African Americans and for men over women. Despite its strengths, the AUC-ROC never virtually surpassing the 0.8 upper limit conveys that the predictive capabilities of the TG/HDL ratio leave room for improvement and seems to be more effective when considered alongside other markers and patient-specific factors.

Further research to integrate, in daily practice, cheap and readily available surrogate biomarkers as the TG/HDL ratio is needed to better calibrate their predictive power.

Author Contributions: Conceptualization, P.B., C.V., S.-R.D. and D.C.; methodology, P.B., C.V., S.-R.D. and D.C.; software, P.B., L.C., A.C. and C.V.; validation, S.-R.D. and D.C.; formal analysis, P.B., A.C., A.-I.L.-H., C.V., S.-R.D. and D.C.; investigation, P.B., C.V., S.-R.D. and D.C.; resources, P.B., A.-I.L.-H. and C.V.; data curation, S.-R.D., L.C. and D.C.; writing—original draft preparation, P.B., C.V., S.C. and D.C.; writing—review and editing P.B., C.V. and A.-A.F.-G.; visualization, P.B., C.V., A.-A.F.-G. and D.C.; supervision, S.C., C.V., D.G. and C.-T.L.; project administration, P.B., C.V., S.-R.D. and D.C.; funding acquisition, S.-R.D., D.G. and D.C. All authors have read and agreed to the published version of the manuscript.

Funding: This research received no external funding. For internal funding, we would like to acknowledge the Victor Babes University of Medicine and Pharmacy Timisoara for their support in covering the costs of publication for this research paper.

Institutional Review Board Statement: Not applicable.

Informed Consent Statement: Not applicable.

Data Availability Statement: Data sharing is not applicable.

Conflicts of Interest: The authors declare no conflicts of interest.

References

1. Salmón-Gómez, L.; Catalán, V.; Frühbeck, G.; Gómez-Ambrosi, J. Relevance of body composition in phenotyping the obesities. *Rev. Endocr. Metab. Disord.* **2023**, *24*, 809–823. [CrossRef]
2. Caleyachetty, R.; Thomas, G.N.; Toulis, K.A.; Mohammed, N.; Gokhale, K.M.; Balachandran, K.; Nirantharakumar, K. Metabolically Healthy Obese and Incident Cardiovascular Disease Events among 3.5 Million Men and Women. *J. Am. Coll. Cardiol.* **2017**, *70*, 1429–1437. [CrossRef] [PubMed]
3. Huang, P.L. A comprehensive definition for metabolic syndrome. *Dis. Model. Mech.* **2009**, *2*, 231–237. [CrossRef] [PubMed] [PubMed Central]
4. Colantoni, A.; Bucci, T.; Cocomello, N.; Angelico, F.; Ettorre, E.; Pastori, D.; Lip, G.Y.; Del Ben, M.; Baratta, F. Lipid-based insulin-resistance markers predict cardiovascular events in metabolic dysfunction associated steatotic liver disease. *Cardiovasc. Diabetol.* **2024**, *23*, 175. [CrossRef]
5. Alberti, K.G.; Eckel, R.H.; Grundy, S.M.; Zimmet, P.Z.; Cleeman, J.I.; Donato, K.A.; Fruchart, J.C.; James, W.P.; Loria, C.M.; Smith, S.C., Jr.; et al. Harmonizing the metabolic syndrome: A joint interim statement of the International Diabetes Federation Task Force on Epidemiology and Prevention; National Heart, Lung, and Blood Institute; American Heart Association; World Heart Federation; International Atherosclerosis Society; and International Association for the Study of Obesity. *Circulation* **2009**, *120*, 1640–1645. [CrossRef] [PubMed]
6. Cui, D.-Y.; Zhang, C.; Chen, Y.; Qian, G.-Z.; Zheng, W.-X.; Zhang, Z.-H.; Zhang, Y.; Zhu, P. Associations between non-insulin-based insulin resistance indices and heart failure prevalence in overweight/obesity adults without diabetes mellitus: Evidence from the NHANES 2001–2018. *Lipids Health Dis.* **2024**, *23*, 123. [CrossRef]
7. McLaughlin, T.; Abbasi, F.; Cheal, K.; Chu, J.; Lamendola, C.; Reaven, G. Use of metabolic markers to identify overweight individuals who are insulin resistant. *Ann. Intern. Med.* **2003**, *139*, 802–809. [CrossRef] [PubMed]
8. McLaughlin, T.; Reaven, G.; Abbasi, F.; Lamendola, C.; Saad, M.; Waters, D.; Simon, J.; Krauss, R.M. Is there a simple way to identify insulin-resistant individuals at increased risk of cardiovascular disease? *Am. J. Cardiol.* **2005**, *96*, 399–404. [CrossRef] [PubMed]
9. Sumner, A.E.; Finley, K.B.; Genovese, D.J.; Criqui, M.H.; Boston, R.C. Fasting triglyceride and the triglyceride-HDL cholesterol ratio are not markers of insulin resistance in African Americans. *Arch. Intern. Med.* **2005**, *165*, 1395–1400. [CrossRef] [PubMed]
10. Bovet, P.; Faeh, D.; Gabriel, A.; Tappy, L. The prediction of insulin resistance with serum triglyceride and high-density lipoprotein cholesterol levels in an East African population. *Arch. Intern. Med.* **2006**, *166*, 1236–1237. [CrossRef] [PubMed]
11. Karelis, A.D.; Pasternyk, S.M.; Messier, L.; St-Pierre, D.H.; Lavoie, J.M.; Garrel, D.; Rabasa-Lhoret, R. Relationship between insulin sensitivity and the triglyceride-HDL-C ratio in overweight and obese postmenopausal women: A MONET study. *Appl. Physiol. Nutr. Metab.* **2007**, *32*, 1089–1096. [CrossRef] [PubMed]
12. Quijada, Z.; Paoli, M.; Zerpa, Y.; Camacho, N.; Cichetti, R.; Villarroel, V.; Arata-Bellabarba, G.; Lanes, R. The triglyceride/HDL-cholesterol ratio as a marker of cardiovascular risk in obese children; association with traditional and emergent risk factors. *Pediatr. Diabetes* **2008**, *9*, 464–471. [CrossRef] [PubMed]

13. Kim-Dorner, S.J.; Deuster, P.A.; Zeno, S.A.; Remaley, A.T.; Poth, M. Should triglycerides and the triglycerides to high-density lipoprotein cholesterol ratio be used as surrogates for insulin resistance? *Metabolism* **2010**, *59*, 299–304. [CrossRef] [PubMed]
14. Chiang, J.-K.; Lai, N.-S.; Chang, J.-K.; Koo, M. Predicting insulin resistance using the triglyceride-to-high-density lipoprotein cholesterol ratio in Taiwanese adults. *Cardiovasc. Diabetol.* **2011**, *10*, 93. [CrossRef]
15. González-Chávez, A.; Simental-Mendía, L.E.; Elizondo-Argueta, S. Elevated triglycerides/HDL-cholesterol ratio associated with insulin resistance. *Cir. Cir.* **2011**, *79*, 126–131. [PubMed]
16. Gasevic, D.; Frohlich, J.; Mancini, G.B.; Lear, S.A. The association between triglyceride to high-density-lipoprotein cholesterol ratio and insulin resistance in a multiethnic primary prevention cohort. *Metabolism* **2012**, *61*, 583–589. [CrossRef] [PubMed]
17. He, J.; He, S.; Liu, K.; Wang, Y.; Shi, D.; Chen, X. The TG/HDL-C Ratio Might Be a Surrogate for Insulin Resistance in Chinese Nonobese Women. *Int. J. Endocrinol.* **2014**, *2014*, 105168. [CrossRef] [PubMed] [PubMed Central]
18. Hirschler, V.; Maccallini, G.; Sanchez, M.; Gonzalez, C.; Molinari, C. Association between triglyceride to HDL-C ratio and insulin resistance in indigenous Argentinean children. *Pediatr. Diabetes* **2014**, *16*, 606–612. [CrossRef] [PubMed]
19. Maturu, A.; DeWitt, P.; Kern, P.A.; Rasouli, N. The triglyceride to high-density lipoprotein cholesterol (TG/HDL-C) ratio as a predictor of β-cell function in African American women. *Metabolism* **2015**, *64*, 561–565. [CrossRef] [PubMed]
20. Zhou, M.; Zhu, L.; Cui, X.; Feng, L.; Zhao, X.; He, S.; Ping, F.; Li, W.; Li, Y. The triglyceride to high-density lipoprotein cholesterol (TG/HDL-C) ratio as a predictor of insulin resistance but not of β cell function in a Chinese population with different glucose tolerance status. *Lipids Health Dis.* **2016**, *15*, 104. [CrossRef]
21. Iwani, N.A.; Jalaludin, M.Y.; Zin, R.M.; Fuziah, M.Z.; Hong, J.Y.; Abqariyah, Y.; Mokhtar, A.H.; Wan Nazaimoon, W.M. Triglyceride to HDL-C Ratio is Associated with Insulin Resistance in Overweight and Obese Children. *Sci. Rep.* **2017**, *7*, 40055. [CrossRef] [PubMed] [PubMed Central]
22. Borrayo, G.; Basurto, L.; González-Escudero, E.; Diaz, A.; Vázquez, A.; Sánchez, L.; Hernández-González, G.O.; Barrera, S.; Degollado, J.A.; Córdova, N.; et al. Tg/Hdl-C Ratio as Cardio-Metabolic Biomarker even in Normal Weight Women. *Acta Endocrinol.* **2018**, *14*, 261–267. [CrossRef] [PubMed] [PubMed Central]
23. Pantoja-Torres, B.; Toro-Huamanchumo, C.J.; Urrunaga-Pastor, D.; Guarnizo-Poma, M.; Lazaro-Alcantara, H.; Paico-Palacios, S.; Del Carmen Ranilla-Seguin, V.; Benites-Zapata, V.A.; Insulin Resistance and Metabolic Syndrome Research Group. High triglycerides to HDL-cholesterol ratio is associated with insulin resistance in normal-weight healthy adults. *Diabetes Metab. Syndr.* **2018**, *13*, 382–388. [CrossRef] [PubMed]
24. Behiry, E.G.; El Nady, N.M.; AbdEl Haie, O.M.; Mattar, M.K.; Magdy, A. Evaluation of TG-HDL Ratio Instead of HOMA Ratio as Insulin Resistance Marker in Overweight and Children with Obesity. *Endocr. Metab. Immune Disord. Drug Targets* **2019**, *19*, 676–682. [CrossRef] [PubMed]
25. García, A.G.; Urbina Treviño, M.V.; Villalpando Sánchez, D.C.; Aguilar, C.A. Diagnostic accuracy of triglyceride/glucose and triglyceride/HDL index as predictors for insulin resistance in children with and without obesity. *Diabetes Metab. Syndr.* **2019**, *13*, 2329–2334. [CrossRef] [PubMed]
26. Yeh, W.-C.; Tsao, Y.-C.; Li, W.-C.; Tzeng, I.-S.; Chen, L.-S.; Chen, J.-Y. Elevated triglyceride-to-HDL cholesterol ratio is an indicator for insulin resistance in middle-aged and elderly Taiwanese population: A cross-sectional study. *Lipids Health Dis.* **2019**, *18*, 176. [CrossRef]
27. Demiral, M. A novel diagnostic tool in determining insulin resistance in obese children: Triglyceride/HDL ratio. *J. Surg. Med.* **2021**, *5*, 1144–1147. [CrossRef]
28. Sowndarya, K.; Joseph, J.A.; Shenoy, A. Evaluation of triglyceride/high-density lipoprotein ratio as a surrogate marker for insulin resistance in healthy young males. *J. Nat. Sci. Biol. Med.* **2021**, *12*, 213–217. [CrossRef]
29. Li, C.; Ford, E.S.; Meng, Y.X.; Mokdad, A.H.; Reaven, G.M. Does the association of the triglyceride to high-density lipoprotein cholesterol ratio with fasting serum insulin differ by race/ethnicity? *Cardiovasc. Diabetol.* **2008**, *7*, 4. [CrossRef] [PubMed] [PubMed Central]
30. Glueck, C.J.; Khan, N.A.; Umar, M.; Uppal, M.S.; Ahmed, W.; Morrison, J.A.; Goldenberg, N.; Wang, P. Insulin Resistance and Triglycerides. *J. Investig. Med.* **2009**, *57*, 874–881. [CrossRef] [PubMed]
31. Sumner, A.E.; Harman, J.L.; Buxbaum, S.G.; Miller, B.V., 3rd; Tambay, A.V.; Wyatt, S.B.; Taylor, H.A.; Rotimi, C.N.; Sarpong, D.F. The triglyceride/high-density lipoprotein cholesterol ratio fails to predict insulin resistance in African-American women: An analysis of Jackson Heart Study. *Metab. Syndr. Relat. Disord.* **2010**, *8*, 511–514. [CrossRef] [PubMed] [PubMed Central]
32. Giannini, C.; Santoro, N.; Caprio, S.; Kim, G.; Lartaud, D.; Shaw, M.; Pierpont, B.; Weiss, R. The triglyceride-to-HDL cholesterol ratio: Association with insulin resistance in obese youths of different ethnic backgrounds. *Diabetes Care* **2011**, *34*, 1869–1874. [CrossRef] [PubMed] [PubMed Central]
33. Kim, J.S.; Kang, H.T.; Shim, J.Y.; Lee, H.R. The association between the triglyceride to high-density lipoprotein cholesterol ratio with insulin resistance (HOMA-IR) in the general Korean population: Based on the National Health and Nutrition Examination Survey in 2007–2009. *Diabetes Res. Clin. Pract.* **2012**, *97*, 132–138. [CrossRef] [PubMed]
34. Kang, H.T.; Yoon, J.H.; Kim, J.Y.; Ahn, S.K.; Linton, J.A.; Koh, S.B.; Kim, J.K. The association between the ratio of triglyceride to HDL-C and insulin resistance according to waist circumference in a rural Korean population. *Nutr. Metab. Cardiovasc. Dis.* **2012**, *22*, 1054–1060. [CrossRef] [PubMed]

35. Salazar, M.R.; Carbajal, H.A.; Espeche, W.G.; Leiva Sisnieguez, C.E.; Balbín, E.; Dulbecco, C.A.; Aizpurúa, M.; Marillet, A.G.; Reaven, G.M. Relation among the plasma triglyceride/high-density lipoprotein cholesterol concentration ratio, insulin resistance, and associated cardio-metabolic risk factors in men and women. *Am. J. Cardiol.* **2012**, *109*, 1749–1753. [CrossRef] [PubMed]
36. Murguía-Romero, M.; Jiménez-Flores, J.R.; Sigrist-Flores, S.C.; Espinoza-Camacho, M.A.; Jiménez-Morales, M.; Piña, E.; Méndez-Cruz, A.R.; Villalobos-Molina, R.; Reaven, G.M. Plasma triglyceride/HDL-cholesterol ratio, insulin resistance, and cardiometabolic risk in young adults. *J. Lipid Res.* **2013**, *54*, 2795–2799. [CrossRef] [PubMed] [PubMed Central]
37. von Bibra, H.; Saha, S.; Hapfelmeier, A.; Müller, G.; Schwarz, P.E.H. Impact of the Triglyceride/High-Density Lipoprotein Cholesterol Ratio and the Hypertriglyceremic-Waist Phenotype to Predict the Metabolic Syndrome and Insulin Resistance. *Horm. Metab. Res.* **2017**, *49*, 542–549. [CrossRef] [PubMed]
38. Gong, R.; Luo, G.; Wang, M.; Ma, L.; Sun, S.; Wei, X. Associations between TG/HDL ratio and insulin resistance in the US population: A cross-sectional study. *Endocr. Connect.* **2021**, *10*, 1502–1512. [CrossRef] [PubMed] [PubMed Central]
39. Matthews, D.R.; Hosker, J.P.; Rudenski, A.S.; Naylor, B.A.; Treacher, D.F.; Turner, R.C. Homeostasis model assessment: Insulin resistance and beta-cell function from fasting plasma glucose and insulin concentrations in man. *Diabetologia* **1985**, *28*, 412–419. [CrossRef]
40. Calle, E.E.; Thun, M.J.; Petrelli, J.M.; Rodriguez, C.; Heath, C.W., Jr. Body-mass index and mortality in a prospective cohort of, U.S. adults. *N. Engl. J. Med.* **1999**, *341*, 1097–1105. [CrossRef]
41. Ferrannini, E.; Natali, A.; Bell, P.; Cavallo-Perin, P.; Lalic, N.; Mingrone, G. Insulin resistance and hypersecretion in obesity. *J. Clin. Investig.* **1997**, *100*, 1166–1173. [CrossRef]
42. Katz, A.; Nambi, S.S.; Mather, K.; Baron, A.D.; Follmann, D.A.; Sullivan, G.; Quon, M.J. Quantitative insulin sensitivity check index: A simple, accurate method for assessing insulin sensitivity in humans. *J. Clin. Endocrinol. Metab.* **2000**, *85*, 2402–2410. [CrossRef]
43. Shen, S.W.; Reaven, G.M.; Farquhar, J.W. Comparison of impedance to insulin-mediated glucose uptake in normal subjects and in subjects with latent diabetes. *J. Clin. Investig.* **1970**, *49*, 2151–2160. [CrossRef]
44. Harano, Y.; Kosugi, K.; Hyosu, T.; Suzuki, M.; Hidaka, H.; Uno, S.; Ishitani, F.; Shibahara, S.; Shibata, S.; Shichiri, M. Measurement of the insulin sensitivity index by the glucose clamp procedure in nonobese and moderately obese Japanese subjects. *Diabetologia* **1981**, *20*, 159–167. [CrossRef]
45. Bergman, R.N.; Ider, Y.Z.; Bowden, C.R.; Cobelli, C. Quantitative estimation of insulin sensitivity. *Am. J. Physiol.* **1979**, *236*, E667–E677. [CrossRef]
46. Pacini, G.; Bergman, R.N. MINMOD: A computer program to calculate insulin sensitivity and pancreatic responsivity from the frequently sampled intravenous glucose tolerance test. *Comput. Methods Programs Biomed.* **1986**, *23*, 113–122. [CrossRef]
47. DeFronzo, R.A.; Tobin, J.D.; Andres, R. Glucose clamp technique: A method for quantifying insulin secretion and resistance. *Am. J. Physiol. Endocrinol. Metab.* **1979**, *237*, E214–E223. [CrossRef]
48. Ferrannini, E.; Mari, A. How to measure insulin sensitivity. *J. Hypertens.* **1998**, *16*, 895–906. [CrossRef]
49. Squillace, N.; Lorenzini, P.; Lapadula, G.; Bandera, A.; Cozzi-Lepri, A.; Rusconi, S.; Puoti, M.; Castagna, A.; Antinori, A.; Gori, A.; et al. Triglyceride/HDL ratio and its impact on the risk of diabetes mellitus development during ART. *J. Antimicrob. Chemother.* **2016**, *71*, 2663–2669. [CrossRef] [PubMed]
50. Bentley, A.R.; Rotimi, C.N. Interethnic Differences in Serum Lipids and Implications for Cardiometabolic Disease Risk in African Ancestry Populations. *Glob. Heart* **2017**, *12*, 141–150. [CrossRef] [PubMed] [PubMed Central]
51. Sumner, A.E.; Vega, G.L.; Genovese, D.J.; Finley, K.B.; Bergman, R.N.; Boston, R.C. Normal triglyceride levels despite insulin resistance in African Americans: Role of lipoprotein lipase. *Metabolism* **2005**, *54*, 902–909. [CrossRef] [PubMed]
52. Holven, K.B.; Roeters van Lennep, J. Sex differences in lipids: A life course approach. *Atherosclerosis* **2023**, *384*, 117270. [CrossRef] [PubMed]
53. Bertoluci, M.C.; Quadros, A.S.; Sarmento-Leite, R.; Schaan, B.D. Insulin resistance and triglyceride/HDLc index are associated with coronary artery disease. *Diabetol. Metab. Syndr.* **2010**, *2*, 11. [CrossRef] [PubMed]
54. Cordero, A.; Laclaustra, M.; León, M.; Casasnovas, J.A.; Grima, A.; Luengo, E.; Ordoñez, B.; Bergua, C.; Bes, M.; Pascual, I.; et al. Comparison of serum lipid values in subjects with and without the metabolic syndrome. *Am. J. Cardiol.* **2008**, *102*, 424–428. [CrossRef] [PubMed]
55. Moriyama, K. Associations Between the Triglyceride to High-Density Lipoprotein Cholesterol Ratio and Metabolic Syndrome, Insulin Resistance, and Lifestyle Habits in Healthy Japanese. *Metab. Syndr. Relat. Disord.* **2020**, *18*, 260–266. [CrossRef] [PubMed]
56. Paulmichl, K.; Hatunic, M.; Højlund, K.; Jotic, A.; Krebs, M.; Mitrakou, A.; Porcellati, F.; Tura, A.; Bergsten, P.; Forslund, A.; et al. Modification and Validation of the Triglyceride-to-HDL Cholesterol Ratio as a Surrogate of Insulin Sensitivity in White Juveniles and Adults without Diabetes Mellitus: The Single Point Insulin Sensitivity Estimator (SPISE). *Clin. Chem.* **2016**, *62*, 1211–1219. [CrossRef] [PubMed]
57. Young, K.A.; Maturu, A.; Lorenzo, C.; Langefeld, C.D.; Wagenknecht, L.E.; Chen, Y.I.; Taylor, K.D.; Rotter, J.I.; Norris, J.M.; Rasouli, N. The triglyceride to high-density lipoprotein cholesterol (TG/HDL-C) ratio as a predictor of insulin resistance, β-cell function, and diabetes in Hispanics and African Americans. *J. Diabetes Complicat.* **2018**, *33*, 118–122. [CrossRef] [PubMed] [PubMed Central]
58. Salazar, M.R.; A Carbajal, H.; Espeche, W.G.; A Dulbecco, C.; Aizpurúa, M.; Marillet, A.G.; Echeverría, R.F.; Reaven, G.M. Relationships among insulin resistance, obesity, diagnosis of the metabolic syndrome and cardio-metabolic risk. *Diab. Vasc. Dis. Res.* **2011**, *8*, 109–116. [CrossRef] [PubMed]

59. Ren, X.; Chen, Z.A.; Zheng, S.; Han, T.; Li, Y.; Liu, W.; Hu, Y. Association between Triglyceride to HDL-C Ratio (TG/HDL-C) and Insulin Resistance in Chinese Patients with Newly Diagnosed Type 2 Diabetes Mellitus. *PLoS ONE* **2016**, *11*, e0154345. [CrossRef] [PubMed] [PubMed Central]
60. Flores-Guerrero, J.L.; Been, R.A.; Shalaurova, I.; Connelly, M.A.; van Dijk, P.R.; Dullaart, R.P.F. Triglyceride/HDL cholesterol ratio and lipoprotein insulin resistance Score: Associations with subclinical atherosclerosis and incident cardiovascular disease. *Clin. Chim. Acta* **2024**, *553*, 117737. [CrossRef] [PubMed]
61. Girona, J.; Amigó, N.; Ibarretxe, D.; Plana, N.; Rodríguez-Borjabad, C.; Heras, M.; Ferré, R.; Gil, M.; Correig, X.; Masana, L. HDL Triglycerides: A New Marker of Metabolic and Cardiovascular Risk. *Int. J. Mol. Sci.* **2019**, *20*, 3151. [CrossRef] [PubMed] [PubMed Central]
62. Babic, N.; Valjevac, A.; Zaciragic, A.; Avdagic, N.; Zukic, S.; Hasic, S. The Triglyceride/HDL Ratio and Triglyceride Glucose Index as Predictors of Glycemic Control in Patients with Diabetes Mellitus Type 2. *Med. Arch.* **2019**, *73*, 163–168. [CrossRef] [PubMed] [PubMed Central]
63. Pacifico, L.; Bonci, E.; Andreoli, G.; Romaggioli, S.; Di Miscio, R.; Lombardo, C.V.; Chiesa, C. Association of serum triglyceride-to-HDL cholesterol ratio with carotid artery intima-media thickness, insulin resistance and nonalcoholic fatty liver disease in children and adolescents. *Nutr. Metab. Cardiovasc. Dis.* **2014**, *24*, 737–743. [CrossRef] [PubMed]
64. Hadaegh, F.; Khalili, D.; Ghasemi, A.; Tohidi, M.; Sheikholeslami, F.; Azizi, F. Triglyceride/HDL-cholesterol ratio is an independent predictor for coronary heart disease in a population of Iranian men. *Nutr. Metab. Cardiovasc. Dis.* **2008**, *19*, 401–408. [CrossRef] [PubMed]
65. Kannel, W.B.; Vasan, R.S.; Keyes, M.J.; Sullivan, L.M.; Robins, S.J. Usefulness of the triglyceride-high-density lipoprotein versus the cholesterol-high-density lipoprotein ratio for predicting insulin resistance and cardiometabolic risk (from the Framingham Offspring Cohort). *Am. J. Cardiol.* **2008**, *101*, 497–501. [CrossRef] [PubMed] [PubMed Central]
66. Shishehbor, M.H.; Hoogwerf, B.J.; Lauer, M.S. Association of Triglyceride–to–HDL Cholesterol Ratio with Heart Rate Recovery. *Diabetes Care* **2004**, *27*, 936–941. [CrossRef] [PubMed]
67. Salazar, M.R.; Carbajal, H.A.; Espeche, W.G.; Aizpurúa, M.; Maciel, P.M.; Reaven, G.M. Identification of cardiometabolic risk: Visceral adiposity index versus triglyceride/HDL cholesterol ratio. *Am. J. Med.* **2014**, *127*, 152–157. [CrossRef] [PubMed]
68. Abbasi, F.; Reaven, G.M. Comparison of two methods using plasma triglyceride concentration as a surrogate estimate of insulin action in nondiabetic subjects: Triglycerides × glucose versus triglyceride/high-density lipoprotein cholesterol. *Metabolism* **2011**, *60*, 1673–1676. [CrossRef] [PubMed]
69. Suleiman, R.R.; Salih, S.F.; Abdullah, B.I.; Ibrahim, I.H.; Saeed, Z.A. Triglyceride Glucose Index, its Modified Indices, and Triglyceride HDL-C Ratio as Predictor Markers of Insulin Resistance in Prediabetic Individuals. *Med. J. Babylon* **2023**, *20*, 268–273. [CrossRef]
70. Reaven, G.; McLaughlin, T. Why the plasma TG/HDL-C concentration ratio does not predict insulin resistance in African Americans. *Arch. Intern. Med.* **2006**, *166*, 249. [CrossRef] [PubMed]
71. Abbasi, F.; Shiffman, D.; Tong, C.H.; Devlin, J.J.; McPhaul, M.J. Insulin Resistance Probability Scores for Apparently Healthy Individuals. *J. Endocr. Soc.* **2018**, *2*, 1050–1057. [CrossRef] [PubMed] [PubMed Central]
72. Wang, H.; Fan, J.L. Association between lipoprotein(a) and insulin resistance in Chinese adults: Results from the China health and nutrition survey. *Front. Endocrinol.* **2023**, *14*, 1234140. [CrossRef] [PubMed] [PubMed Central]
73. Huhtala, M.; Rönnemaa, T.; Tertti, K. Insulin Resistance Is Associated with an Unfavorable Serum Lipoprotein Lipid Profile in Women with Newly Diagnosed Gestational Diabetes. *Biomolecules* **2023**, *13*, 470. [CrossRef] [PubMed]
74. Tian, Y.; Lu, L.; Zhang, Y.; Wei, J. The value of Lp(a) and TG/HDLC in peripheral blood to assess the stability of carotid plaque in patients with ischemic stroke. *Brain Behav.* **2024**, *14*, e3355. [CrossRef] [PubMed] [PubMed Central]
75. Zhang, Y.; Wang, R.; Fu, X.; Song, H. Non-insulin-based insulin resistance indexes in predicting severity for coronary artery disease. *Diabetol. Metab. Syndr.* **2022**, *14*, 191. [CrossRef] [PubMed]
76. McNamara, J.R.; Schaefer, E.J. Automated enzymatic standardized lipid analyses for plasma and lipoprotein fractions. *Clin. Chim. Acta* **1987**, *166*, 1845–1850. [CrossRef]

biomedicines

MDPI

Article

Urinary and Serum Amino Acids May Be Associated with Podocyte, Proximal Tubule, and Renal Endothelial Injury in Early Diabetic Kidney Disease in Type 2 Diabetes Mellitus Patients

Maria Mogos [1,2,3], Oana Milas [1,2,3,*], Carmen Socaciu [3,4], Andreea Iulia Socaciu [5], Adrian Vlad [2,3,6], Florica Gadalean [1,2,3], Flaviu Bob [1,2,3], Octavian Marius Cretu [7,8], Anca Suteanu-Simulescu [1,2,3], Mihaela Glavan [1,2,3], Lavinia Balint [1,2,3], Silvia Ienciu [1,2,3], Iuliana-Lavinia Iancu [1,2,3], Dragos Catalin Jianu [2,3,9,10], Sorin Ursoniu [3,11,12] and Ligia Petrica [1,2,3,10,11]

1 Department of Internal Medicine II—Division of Nephrology, "Victor Babes" University of Medicine and Pharmacy, Eftimie Murgu Sq. No. 2, 300041 Timisoara, Romania; maria.mogos@umft.ro (M.M.); gadalean.florica@umft.ro (F.G.); bob.flaviu@umft.ro (F.B.); anca.simulescu@umft.ro (A.S.-S.); patruica.mihaela@umft.ro (M.G.); lavinia.balint@umft.ro (L.B.); ioana.ienciu@umft.ro (S.I.); iuliana.alioani@umft.ro (I. L.I.); petrica.ligia@umft.ro (L.P.)

2 County Emergency Hospital Timisoara, 300723 Timisoara, Romania; vlad.adrian@umft.ro (A.V.); jianu.dragos@umft.ro (D.C.J.)

3 Centre for Molecular Research in Nephrology and Vascular Disease, Faculty of Medicine, "Victor Babes" University of Medicine and Pharmacy, Eftimie Murgu Sq. No. 2, 300041 Timisoara, Romania; carmen.socaciu@usamvcluj.ro (C.S.); sursoniu@umft.ro (S.U.)

4 Research Center for Applied Biotechnology and Molecular Therapy BIODIATECH, SC Proplanta, Str. Trifoiului 12G, 400478 Cluj-Napoca, Romania

5 Department of Occupational Health, University of Medicine and Pharmacy "Iuliu Haţieganu", Str. Victor Babes 8, 400347 Cluj-Napoca, Romania; andreea.socaciu@umfcluj.ro

6 Department of Internal Medicine II—Division of Diabetes and Metabolic Diseases, "Victor Babes" University of Medicine and Pharmacy, Eftimie Murgu Sq. No. 2, 300041 Timisoara, Romania

7 Department of Surgery I–Division of Surgical Semiology I, "Victor Babes" University of Medicine and Pharmacy, Eftimie Murgu Sq. No. 2, 300041 Timisoara, Romania; octavian.cretu@umft.ro

8 Emergency Clinical Municipal Hospital Timisoara, 300079 Timisoara, Romania

9 Department of Neurosciences—Division of Neurology, "Victor Babes" University of Medicine and Pharmacy, Eftimie Murgu Sq. No. 2, 300041 Timisoara, Romania

10 Centre for Cognitive Research in Neuropsychiatric Pathology (Neuropsy-Cog), Faculty of Medicine, "Victor Babes" University of Medicine and Pharmacy, Eftimie Murgu Sq. No. 2, 300041 Timisoara, Romania

11 Center for Translational Research and Systems Medicine, Faculty of Medicine, "Victor Babes" University of Medicine and Pharmacy, Eftimie Murgu Sq. No. 2, 300041 Timisoara, Romania

12 Department of Functional Sciences III, Division of Public Health and History of Medicine, "Victor Babes" University of Medicine and Pharmacy, Eftimie Murgu Sq. No. 2, 300041 Timisoara, Romania

* Correspondence: milas.oana@umft.ro

Abstract: Background/Objectives: The pathogenesis of diabetic kidney disease (DKD) is complex and multifactorial. Because of its complications and reduced number of diagnostic biomarkers, it is important to explore new biomarkers with possible roles in the early diagnosis of DKD. Our study aims to investigate the pattern of previously identified metabolites and their association with biomarkers of endothelial dysfunction, proximal tubule (PT) dysfunction, and podocyte injury. **Methods**: A total of 110 participants, comprising 20 healthy individuals and 90 patients divided in three groups were enrolled in the study: normoalbuminuria, microalbuminuria, and macroalbuminuria. Untargeted and targeted metabolomic methods were employed to assess urinary and serum biomarkers, as well as indicators of endothelial dysfunction, podocyte damage, and PT dysfunction through ELISA techniques. **Results**: Our research uncovered specific metabolites that exhibit varying levels across different sub-groups. Notably, glycine serves as a distinguishing factor between group C and the normoalbuminuric group. Furthermore, glycine is correlated with endothelial

 https://doi.org/10.3390/biomedicines13030675

markers, especially VCAM. We observed a gradual decrease in kynurenic acid levels from group C to group P3; this biomarker also demonstrates an inverse relationship with both p-selectin and VCAM. Additionally, tryptophan levels decline progressively from group C to group P3, accompanied by a negative correlation with p-selectin and VCAM. Urinary tiglylglycine also differentiates among the patient groups, with concentrations decreasing as the condition worsens. It shows a strong positive correlation with nephrin, podocalyxin, KIM1, and NAG. **Conclusions**: In conclusion, glycine, tiglylglycine, kynurenic acid and tryptophan may be considered putative biomarkers for early diagnosis of DKD and T2DM progression.

Keywords: diabetic kidney disease; biomarkers; metabolites; endothelial dysfunction; proximal tubule damage; podocyte injury

1. Introduction

Diabetic kidney disease (DKD) is characterized by increased levels of albumin in the urine, decreased glomerular filtration rate (GFR), or a combination of both. It is a complication arising from type 2 diabetes mellitus (T2DM) and represents the leading cause of chronic kidney disease, potentially progressing to end-stage renal disease [1]. As a result of the rising population of individuals diagnosed with DM, there has been a significant increase in both the incidence and prevalence of DKD. The International Diabetes Federation estimates that this figure will grow from 10.5% in 2021 to 12.2% by the year 2045 [2,3]. As highlighted in numerous earlier research efforts, DKD is a multifaceted condition characterized by diverse pathogenic mechanisms [1,4,5]. Chronic hyperglycaemia is marked by persistent high blood sugar levels, which can cause harm to the glomerular filtration barrier. This damage extends to endothelial cells, the glomerular basement membrane, and podocytes. The filtration barrier is essential for filtering out substances such as water and solutes while retaining albumin. Deterioration of podocytes, alterations in the glomerular basement membrane, and mesangial expansion lead to the development of nodular sclerosis. This condition may also be linked with arterial hyalinosis and tubulointerstitial fibrosis in more advanced stages. Consequently, these changes result into the onset of microalbuminuria, which can eventually progress to macroalbuminuria [5].

As previously noted, the rise in DKD patients can be attributed to the absence of early indicators for the condition. In recent years, a developing collection of studies has emerged and emphasize serum and urine metabolites, along with initial biomarkers associated with podocytes, endothelium, and proximal tubules.

Our ongoing research is centred on the role of specific metabolites: tryptophan (TRP), kynurenic acid (KA), L-acetylcarnitine (LAC), glycine (Gly), tiglylglycine (Tyg), and taurine (Tau) at the levels of podocytes, tubules, and endothelial cells.

The aim of this study is to illustrate the potential connections between amino acids, identified through both untargeted ultra-high-performance liquid chromatography coupled with electrospray-ionization quadrupole time-of-flight mass spectrometry (UHPLC-QTOF-ESI+-MS) and targeted methods utilizing pure standards, and biomarkers indicative of podocyte injury, renal proximal tubule dysfunction, and endothelial dysfunction.

2. Materials and Methods

2.1. Patients and Compliance with Ethical Standards

This study was designed as a pilot and cross-sectional study, and it was conducted in the Nephrology Department and in the Diabetes and Metabolic Diseases Department,

County Emergency Hospital, Timisoara, Romania from July 2021 to April 2022. After approval of the Ethics Committee for Scientific Research of "Victor Babes" University of Medicine and Pharmacy Timisoara (no. 28/02.09.2020) and the Ethics Committee for Scientific Research of "Pius Brinzeu" County Emergency Hospital Timisoara (no. 296/06.04.2022), 110 participants were included in this study, from which 20 were healthy control subjects and 90 were patients with long-standing T2DM. Based on UACR, we stratified the 90 patients with T2DM in three equal subgroups of 30 patients each: subgroup P1 (UACR < 30 mg/g), P2 (UACR: 30–300 mg/g), and P3 (UACR > 300 mg/g). As an inclusion criterion, we selected patients with T2DM, with a duration of minimum five years. In addition, hospitalized patients enrolled in the study were non-critically ill, and the samples were collected after initial biological investigations. Patients with T2DM with poor control of diabetes (HbA1c > 10%), active infections, neoplasia, glomerular disease, end-stage renal disease, and T1DM were excluded from the study. At the time of screening, all patients had received treatment with angiotensin-converting enzyme inhibitors (e.g., Perindopril) or angiotensin receptor blockers (e.g., Candesartan, Irbesarta) for at least 10 years, as well as oral antidiabetic agents, insulin, and/or statins. Written informed consent was obtained from all participants, and to maintain the confidentiality, we used numerical codes for each sample.

2.2. *The Preparation of Samples*

The blood samples were collected via venipuncture and transferred into sterile vacutainers that did not contain anticoagulants, while urine samples were placed in sterile vials. These specimens were preserved at −80 °C until analysis. For the preparation, 0.8 mL of a mixture consisting of pure HPLC-grade methanol and acetonitrile was added to each 0.2 mL of serum and urine separately. The mixtures were vortexed to precipitate proteins, subjected to ultrasonication, and then stored at −20 °C for 24 h to enhance protein precipitation. Following centrifugation, the supernatant was collected and filtered through nylon filters. It was then transferred into glass microvials before being loaded into the autosampler of the UHPLC system for injection. Furthermore, the supernatant was moved into an autosampler vial for HPLC-MS analysis. Quality control (QC) samples were also obtained and utilized as representative generic samples; these QC samples were injected at both the beginning and end of the experiment, as well as after every tenth injection during the analysis of study samples [6,7].

2.3. *Analytical Methods*

2.3.1. UHPLC-QTOF-ESI+-MS Analysis

The metabolomic analysis was conducted utilizing ultra-high-performance liquid chromatography in combination with electrospray ionization–quadrupole-time of flight–mass spectrometry (UHPLC-QTOF-ESI+-MS). This was achieved using a ThermoFisher Scientific UHPLC Ultimate 3000 system, which featured a quaternary pump, a Dionex delivery system, and mass spectrometry detection equipment from MaXis Impact (Bruker Daltonics). Metabolites were separated on an Acclaim C18 column (5 μm, 2.1 × 100 mm, with a pore size of 30 nm from Thermo Scientific, Waltham, MA, USA) maintained at 28 °C. The mobile phase comprised 0.1% formic acid in water (component A) and 0.1% formic acid in acetonitrile (component B). The total elution time was established at 20 min, with flow rates set at 0.3 mL/min for serum samples and 0.8 mL/min for urine samples.

For serum samples, the gradient was as follows: from 90% to 85% A over the first three minutes, then from 85% to 50% A between three to six minutes, followed by a decrease from 50% to 30% A during the next two minutes (six to eight minutes), transitioning from 30% to 5% A from eight to twelve minutes, and finally ramping back up to 90% A by the end of twenty minutes. In contrast, the gradient for urine samples started similarly with a shift from 90% to 85% A over three minutes, then reduced from 85% to 30% A during the next three minutes, followed by a decline from 30% to10% A over two minutes. This was held isocratic until twelve minutes before increasing back up to 90% by twenty minutes.

An injection volume of five millilitres was utilized while maintaining a column temperature of 25 °C. Several quality control (QC) samples obtained from each group were analysed simultaneously for calibration purposes. An internal standard solution of Doxorubicin hydrochloride (m/z = 581.3209) at a concentration of 0.5 mg/mL was added alongside the QC samples.

The mass spectrometry parameters included a positive ionization mode (ESI+), calibration with sodium formate, a capillary voltage set at 3500 V, a nebulizing gas pressure maintained at 2.8 bar, a drying gas flow rate of 12 L/min, and a drying temperature regulated at 300 °C. The mass-to-charge ratio values targeted for separation ranged between 60 and 600 Daltons. Instrument control and data processing were managed via specialized software: TofControl version 3.2, HyStar version 3.2, Data Analysis version 4.2 (Bruker Daltonics, Billerica, MA, USA), alongside Chromeleon™ 6.8 Chromatography Data System (CDS) Software.

2.3.2. ELISA Technique

The ELISA technique was utilized in order to assess the urinary biomarkers of endothelial dysfunction, such as V-CAM1 (Catalogue Nr. E-EL-H5587 Elabscience, sensitivity—0.94 ng/mL; detection range—1.56–100 ng/mL; coefficient of variance (CV) < 10%); and p-selectin (Catalogue Nr. E-EL-H6180 Elabscience, sensitivity—18.75 pg/mL; detection range—31.25–2000 pg/mL; coefficient of variance (CV) < 10%); biomarkers of podocyte injury, such as nephrine and podocalyxin (Catalogue Nr. E-EL-H2360 Elabscience, sensitivity—0.1 ng/mL; detection range—0.16–10 ng/mL; coefficient of variance (CV) < 10%); and of proximal tubule dysfunction, such as KIM-1 (Catalogue Nr. E-EL-H6029 Elabscience; sensitivity—4.69 pg/mL; detection range—7.81–500 pg/mL; CV < 10%) and NAG (Catalogue Nr. E-EL-H0898 Elabscience; sensitivity—0.94 ng/mL; detection range—1.56–100 ng/mL; CV < 10%).

2.4. The Integration of the Results and Statistical Analysis

The present study builds upon earlier research by focusing on the identification and correlation of specific metabolites with markers of dysfunction in endothelial cells, proximal tubules, and podocytes. To achieve these findings, our initial review [6] involved collecting samples from patients diagnosed with diabetic kidney disease (DKD) and conducting statistical analyses utilizing both untargeted multivariate and univariate metabolomic methods. This analysis included a multivariate comparison between controls (group C) and all patients (the overall group P) based on the final data matrices. The differentiation between these two groups was illustrated through Fold Change, Volcano test results, Partial Least Squares Discriminant Analysis (PLSDA), and Variable Importance in Projection (VIP) values, which incorporated cross-validation parameters. Subsequently, we employed a Random Forest-based prediction test to compute p-values. Receiver Operating Characteristic (ROC) curves along with area under the curve values were derived from biomarker analysis. In the second phase, univariate analysis facilitated comparisons among subgroups P1–P3 against group C using one-way ANOVA, PLSDA, Random Forest techniques, and Heatmaps. Consequently, several potential biomarkers indicative of differentiation were identified.

In our follow-up investigation [7], we focused on 5 to 10 distinct molecules found in serum or urine and utilized the intensity of mass spectrometry peaks to compare various patient groups, such as between groups C and P, or among subgroups P1 to P3. For quantitative assessment, we identified particular biomarkers and constructed calibration curves using pure standards.

All the information outlined previously enabled us to identify metabolites that may be valuable for the early detection of DKD, including glycine, its derivative tiglylglycine, kynurenic acid, and tryptophan. Furthermore, we examined their relationships with proximal tubular, podocyte, and endothelial markers.

3. Results

3.1. Clinical Features and Biological Results

Table 1 presents the data resulting from history and the clinical examination, the common biological parameters, and those resulting from the ELISA assay and UHPLC-QTOF-ESI+-MS techniques. The data are presented as means ± standard deviations (SDs). The comparison between group C and patients was realized using the one-way ANOVA with Bonferroni correction, a chi-squared test, and a Kruskal–Wallis test, whereas the comparison between subgroups, namely C vs. P1, P1 vs. P2 and P2 vs. P3, was carried out by applying Student's *t*-test, the chi-squared test, and a Mann–Whitney test.

Table 1. Demographic data, clinical parameters, and biological results of healthy controls and of patients with type 2 DM divided into three stages: normoalbuminuria (P1), microalbuminuria (P2), and macroalbuminuria (P3).

	Healthy Subjects (C = 20)	Normoalbuminuria (P1 = 30)	Microalbuminuria (P2 = 30)	Macroalbuminuria (P3 = 30)
		clinical parameters		
Age (years)	68.0 ± 3.9	68.5 ± 4.9	69.6 ± 5.0	69.4 ± 3.9
Sex (%)				
M	14 (70.0%)	16 (53.3%)	17 (56.7%)	21 (70.0%)
F	6 (30.0%)	14 (46.7%)	13 (43.3%)	9 (30.0%)
Duration of DM (years)	0 (0–0) # ▲	12 (10–17)	16 (14–22) ‡	22 (18–26)
BMI (kg/m^2)	24.8 ± 4.4 # ▲	30.0 ± 4.5	31.5 ± 4.0	31.0 ± 5.3
Retinopathy (%)	0 (0.0%) ◊ ▲	5 (16.7%)	10 (33.3%) ¶	24 (80.0%)
Neuropathy (%)	0 (0.0%) # ▲	13 (43.3%)	15 (50.0%)	16 (53.3%)
		biological parameters		
Cholesterol (mg/dL)	132.5 ± 24.6 ▲	164.1 ± 53.5	166.8 ± 57.7 ‡	199.5 ± 48.1
HDLc (mg/dL)	45 (35–48)	46 (41–52)	44 (34–52)	45 (36–52)
LDLc (mg/dL)	68 (65–88) Δ	87 (65–114)	95 (62–120)	97 (70–137)
Triglycerides	98 (92–101) ◊ ▲	142 (105–172)	146 (112–203) ‡	188 (160–281)
HbA1c (%)	5.0 ± 0.2 # ▲	7.2 ± 0.9 *	8.2 ± 1.4	8.4 ± 1.1
eGFR (mL/min/1.73 m^2)	84 (81–88) # ▲	78 (73–83) □	67 (64–73) ¶	48 (42–56)
UA	11 (9–14) ◊ ▲	15 (11–22) □	69 (51–167) ¶	483 (263–1572)
UCr	93 (77–131)	89 (53–116)	100 (66–115)	70 (52–90)
uACR (mg/g)	11 (10–14) # ▲	20 (13–26) □	98 (61–155) ¶	925 (416–1391)
		markers of proximal tubular dysfunction		
KIM-1 (pg/g)	43 (26–46) # ▲	80 (67–94) □	140 (125–152) ¶	408 (321–458)
NAG (ng/g)	3 (2–3) ◊ ▲	3 (2-5) □	11 (11–18) ‡	17 (17–18)
		markers of endothelial damage		
U P-selectin	0 (0–0) # ▲	1 (1–1) □	3 (3–4) ¶	7 (5–7)
S P-selectin	1 (0–1) # ▲	1 (1–1) □	4 (4–5) ¶	8 (7–9)
U VCAM1 (pg/g)	2 (2–3) # ▲	5 (4–9) □	11 (9–12) ¶	16 (13–18)
S VCAM1 (pg/g)	10 (9–11) ◊ ▲	11 (11–12) □	15 (14–16) ¶	21 (19–24)

Table 1. *Cont.*

	Healthy Subjects (C = 20)	Normoalbuminuria (P1 = 30)	Microalbuminuria (P2 = 30)	Macroalbuminuria (P3 = 30)
		markers of podocyte damage		
Podocalixin (mg/g)	0 (0–0) # ▲	1 (1–1) □	4 (3–4) ¶	8 (7–9)
Nephrin (ng/g)	0 (0–0) ▲	0 (0–0) □	0 (0–0) ¶	0 (0–0)
		METABOLITES		
s Glycine	217 (200–229) ▲	199 (169–204)	185 (169–199)	184 (170–187)
s Taurine	87 (83–93)	85 (82–90)	87 (76–91)	83 (78–87)
s KA	6 (4–6) ◊ ▲	4 (3–6)	4 (3–5)	4 (3–5)
s AC	5 (4–7)	6 (4–7)	5 (4–6)	5 (4–6)
s TRP	57 (48–67) ◊	51 (41–59)	52 (33–62)	48 (37–62)
u Glycine	12 (9–14) Δ	10 (7–14)	8 (6–12)	7 (5–13)
u Tiglylglycine	5 (4–6) ▲	4 (3–6)	4 (3–5) ¶	2 (1–3)
u Taurine	8 (6–10)	9 (7–10)	8 (6–11)	9 (8–14)
u KA	0 (0–0) Δ	0 (0–1)	0 (0–0)	0 (0–1)
u AC	0 (0–0)	0 (0–0)	0 (0–0)	0 (0–1)
u TRP	7 (4–10) ◊ ▲	4 (3–6) □	12 (6–16)	16 (10–21)

Continuous data presented as means ± SD or as median (interquartile range) as appropriate. p-value based on one-way ANOVA with Bonferroni correction, chi-squared test, Kruskal–Wallis test; significance of C vs. P1: # $p < 0.001$; ◊ $p > 0.001$ and $p < 0.05$; significance of P1 vs. P2: □ $p < 0.001$; * $p > 0.001$ and $p < 0.05$; significance of P2 vs. P3: ¶ $p < 0.001$; ‡ $p > 0.001$ and $p < 0.05$; significance of C vs. P1 vs. P2 vs. P3: ▲ $p < 0.001$; Δ $p > 0.001$ and $p < 0.05$; BMI: body mass index; DM: diabetes mellitus; HbA1C: glycated hemoglobin; eGFR: estimated glomerular filtration rate; UA: urinary albumin; UCr: urinary creatinine; uACR: urinary albumin/creatinine ratio; KIM-1: kidney injury molecule-1; NAG: N-acetyl-β-(D)-glucosaminidase; U P-selectin: urinary p-selectin; S P-selectin: serum p-selectin; U VCAM-1: urinary vascular cell adhesion molecule-1; S VCAM-1: serum vascular cell adhesion molecule-1; s Glycine: serum glycine; s Taurine: serum taurine; sKA: serum kinurenic acid, sAC: serum acetylcarnitine; sTRP: serum tryptophan; u glycine: urinary glycine; u tiglyglycine: urinary tiglylglycine; u taurine: urinary taurine; u KA: urinary kinurenic acid; u AC: urinary acetylcarnitine; u TRP: urinary tryptophan.

3.2. *Correlation of Serum Metabolites with Markers of Endothelial Damage*

3.2.1. Univariable Linear Regression Analysis

First, we employed the univariable linear regression analysis to identify metabolites associated with DKD, particularly those that distinguish between subgroups. The results indicated that serum glycine, serum KA, and serum TRP exhibited negative correlations with all markers related to proximal tubules, endothelial cells, and podocytes. Furthermore, we found a negative correlation between urinary glycine and urinary tiglylglycine, while a positive correlation was observed between urinary TRP and the aforementioned markers.

3.2.2. Multivariable Linear Regression Analysis

The subsequent phase in identifying predictive models for metabolites involves multivariable linear regression analysis, which demonstrates a strong correlation between Tiglylglycine and P-selectin, podocalixin, and KIM-1.

3.3. *The Impact of Tubular, Endothelial, and Podocyte Damage Biomarkers in DKD*

3.3.1. Kidney Injury Molecule-1

Kidney injury molecule-1 (KIM-1) is characterized as a type I transmembrane protein that is absent in healthy kidneys but emerges in the renal proximal tubule following injury. Van Timmeren MM et al. outline various mechanisms through which the buildup of proteins results in tubular blockage and mechanical strain, which subsequently activates tubular cells and stimulates the synthesis of KIM-1. Additionally, another mechanism is noted in diabetic patients, where tubular cells are activated by a harmful infiltrate, leading to the production of pro-inflammatory factors and dysfunction in the tubulointerstitial segment [8].

Our findings indicate increased levels of KIM1 among the different patient groups, particularly within the normoalbuminuric cohort, a conclusion that aligns with previous research concerning early DKD [9–11], data that can be found in Table 1.

3.3.2. N-Acetyl-β-D-glucosaminidase

N-acetyl-β-D-glucosaminidase (NAG) is an enzyme found in lysosomes, which is primarily located in the proximal tubules of the kidneys and excreted in minimal amounts through urine [12]. Injury to the epithelial cells within the proximal tubule leads to an excessive buildup of NAG. Furthermore, since NAG plays a role in carbohydrate metabolism, it is suggested that higher concentrations of NAG result from the exposure of proximal tubular cells to increased glucose levels [13].

Our study evaluated and found significantly higher levels of NAG in patients categorized as group P3 when compared to group P1, with notable statistical significance in P1 (see Table 1).

The findings were similarly reported by Quinghua Huang et al., who noted that the urinary NAG-to-creatinine ratio serves as a significant predictor, as well as by Mohammadi Karakani et al., regarding the assessment of urinary enzymes. Additionally, Miyachi E. et al. focused on the activity of urinary angiotensin-converting enzyme in patients with T2DM, while Skrha J et al., conducted a six-year follow-up study examining the correlation between NAG levels and albuminuria [14–17]. Collectively, these studies highlighted that levels of urine NAG rise with the progression of nephropathy, demonstrating a significant distinction between early and advanced DKD, particularly showing elevated NAG levels in patients exhibiting macroalbuminuria.

3.3.3. Nephrin

Nephrin is a protein that spans across membranes and plays a crucial role in the area between the foot processes of podocytes in the kidney. In cases of hyperglycaemia-affecting podocytes, there is an alteration in nephrin regulation, resulting in nephrinuria, particularly observed in patients with normal albumin levels [18].

We observed elevated nephrin levels in patients with diabetes when compared to healthy individuals (data presented in Table 1). This particular biomarker has received limited research attention, but we identified several studies that address its role in diabetic mice versus their healthy counterparts. Of interest, several references include Kandasamy's work on nephrin as an early indicator of glomerular injury, as well as studies by Chang et al., focusing on DKD in FVB/NJ Akita mice. Additionally, Ganesh Veluri et al. and Irena Kostovska et al., highlighted that urinary nephrin serves as a more sensitive and specific marker for diabetic nephropathy than microalbuminuria, finding significant nephrin levels in both groups of individuals with T2DM compared to healthy controls [18–21].

3.3.4. P-Selectin

Patients suffering from type 2 diabetes mellitus experience systemic inflammation that may result in kidney damage. This inflammatory response causes an influx of monocytes and lymphocytes into the renal tissue, which in turn release pro-inflammatory cytokines, chemokines, and adhesion molecules such as VCAM and P-selectin [22].

Our research on p-selectin indicated a gradual rise in urinary levels of this biomarker, progressing from the P1 group to the P3 group. Similar patterns for this marker were observed in studies by Feng Wang et al., which examined the clinical significance of plasma CD146 and p-selectin, as well as by Khalid al Rubeean et al., who investigated IL-18, VCAM, and P-selectin as early biomarkers [22,23].

3.3.5. Podocalixin

The upper surface of glomerular podocytes comprises a transmembrane protein known as podocalixin (PCX). In cases where podocyte function is impaired, this protein can leak into the urine. Consequently, elevated concentrations of PCX have been detected in the urine of individuals with diabetes [24].

Podocalyxin demonstrated statistical significance in our analysis, particularly when comparing the P1 group to the C group and within the subgroups P2-P3, consistent with findings from other studies. Hui Xie et al. noted that PCX is a positive marker, Hara M. et al., identified it as an early indicator, Vestra M. et al., linked it to podocyte injury in diabetic nephropathy, and Weil E. et al., discussed its role in podocyte detachment and reduced glomerular capillary function. These studies indicated a correlation between urinary PCX levels and UACR levels, as well as elevated urinary PCX levels in patients who exhibited normal urinary albumin values [25–28].

3.3.6. VCAM1

VCAM1 is yet another molecule that plays a role in the adhesion of leukocytes to endothelial cells, facilitating the gathering of leukocytes during inflammatory responses. In summary, there is an elevated expression of VCAM in the kidneys of individuals diagnosed with DN [29]. Numerous studies indicate that VCAM is linked to the progression of diabetic kidney disease in individuals with diabetes, aligning with our findings [30,31].

3.4. Interpretation of Data Subsequent to Statistical Evaluation

- Serum Glycine

In Table 1, it is evident that glycine differentiates between group C and the normoalbuminuric group, as well as between the P1 group and the P2-P3 groups, with levels declining as diabetic kidney disease advances. Additionally, it can be noted that glycine shows a correlation with endothelial markers, particularly VCAM, achieving a statistically significant value ($p < 0.001$) as it is shown in Table 2.

Table 2. Univariable linear regression analysis of serum and urine samples.

Dependent Variable	Independent Variable	R^2	Coef β	*p* Value
s Glyc	p-selectin	0.067	−3.14	0.006
	VCAM1	0.069	−2.01	0.005
s Taurine	p-selectin	0.020	−0.80	0.138
	VCAM1	0.010	−0.35	0.296
s KA	p-selectin	0.099	−0.12	0.000
	VCAM1	0.061	−0.06	0.008
s AC	p-selectin	0.000	−0.005	0.928
	VCAM1	0.003	−0.02	0.553
s TRP	p-selectin	0.003	−0.29	0.548
	VCAM1	0.007	−0.27	0.372
u Glyc	Nephrin	0.039	−0.68	0.037
	Podocalixin	0.025	−0.36	0.097
	KIM1	0.054	−0.01	0.014
	NAG	0.027	−0.16	0.081
u Tiglyglycine	Nephrin	0.156	−0.57	0.000
	Podocalixin	0.120	−0.33	0.000
	KIM1	0.178	−0.00	0.000
	NAG	0.051	−0.09	0.017

Table 2. *Cont.*

Dependent Variable	Independent Variable	R^2	Coef β	*p* Value
u Taurine	Nephrin	0.005	0.19	0.428
	Podocalixin	0.031	0.30	0.065
	KIM1	0.040	0.00	0.034
	NAG	0.032	0.13	0.059
u KA	Nephrin	0.001	0.00	0.681
	Podocalixin	0.032	0.01	0.057
	KIM1	0.023	0.00	0.111
	NAG	0.027	0.00	0.084
u AC	Nephrin	0.039	0.03	0.036
	Podocalixin	0.052	0.02	0.015
	KIM1	0.036	0.01	0.045
	NAG	0.098	0.01	0.000
u TRP	Nephrin	0.019	0.72	0.148
	Podocalixin	0.044	0.72	0.027
	KIM1	0.052	0.01	0.015
	NAG	0.035	0.28	0.047

KIM-1: kidney injury molecule-1; NAG: N-acetyl-β-(D)-glucosaminidase; P-selectin: p-selectin; VCAM-1: vascular cell adhesion molecule-1; s Glycine: serum glycine; s Taurine: serum taurine; sKA: serum kinurenic acid, sAC: serum acetylcarnitine; sTRP: serum tryptophan; u glycine: urinary glycine; u tiglyglycine: urinary tiglylglycine; u taurine: urinary taurine; u KA: urinary kinurenic acid; u AC: urinary acetylcarnitine; u TRP: urinary tryptophan.

- Serum TRP and kinurenic acid

Our findings indicated a gradual decline in tryptophan levels from group C to group P3, along with a negative correlation observed with p-selectin and VCAM. Additionally, we noted a clear distinction between healthy individuals and those in the normoalbuminuric group.

Also, in our article, we observed a gradual reduction in S KA from group C to group P3, with a clear distinction noted between group C and normoalbuminuric patients. Additionally, in Table 2 is highlighted that this biomarker exhibits an inverse correlation with p-selectin and VCAM, as evidenced by highly significant *p*-values ($p < 0.001$ for p-selectin and $p < 0.05$ for VCAM).

- Urinary Glycine

In urine, glycine demonstrated significant variations among the subgroups from group C to group P3. It demonstrates strong negative correlation with nephrin, while showing a weaker correlation with podocalyxin and N-acetyl-β-D-glucosaminidase (NAG).

In our examination, we observe noteworthy levels of this metabolite that effectively distinguish between different patient groups, with diminished concentrations noted as the condition progresses. Moreover, this metabolite shows a strong positive correlation with various markers of podocytes and proximal tubules, including nephrin, podocalyxin, KIM1, and NAG.

- Urinary TRP

TRP is a metabolite that has been the subject of extensive research. In urine, TRP effectively distinguishes group C from group P1, as well as group P2 with group P3, due to a notable reduction in concentration levels observed in normoalbuminuric group, achieving statistical significance. It is important to note that group P1 indicates markedly low values, which subsequently increase threefold in groups P2 and P3 in comparison to group P1.

Additionally, we identified a strong and positive relationship involving podocalyxin, KIM1, and NAG.

- Urinary Tiglylglycine

In our examination, we observe noteworthy levels of this metabolite that effectively distinguish between different patient groups, with diminished concentrations noted as the condition progresses. Moreover, this metabolite shows a strong positive correlation with various markers of podocytes and proximal tubules, including nephrin, podocalyxin, KIM1, and NAG, as it can be seen in Table 3.

Table 3. Urinary tiglylglycine; p-selectin, podocalixin, kidney injury molecule-1, significance of urinary tiglylglycine, and correlation with p-selectin, podocalixin, KIM-1 ($p < 0.01$).

	Dependent Variable	R^2	Coef β	*p* Value
U Tiglylglycine	P-selectin	0.2143	−1.49	0.0000
	Podocalixin	0.2143	1.47	0.0000
	KIM1	0.2143	−0.01	0.0000

4. Discussion

In our study the presence of glycine, kynurenic acid, and tryptophan in serum indicates their potential role as biomarkers for renal endothelial dysfunction. Moreover, in urine, all metabolites—including glycine, tiglylglycine, and tryptophan—correlated with indicators of podocyte injury and proximal tubular dysfunction.

4.1. Serum Indicators of Endothelial Injury in Initial Stages of DKD

4.1.1. Serum Glycine May Be a Marker of Endothelial Dysfunction in Early DKD

Glycine, categorized as a "nonessential" amino acid that the body can produce from serine, has been consistently linked to a negative correlation with T2DM. Research indicates that individuals who are nondiabetic but exhibit insulin resistance or impaired glucose tolerance show decreased levels of circulating glycine. This reduction is also observed in nondiabetic children of parents diagnosed with T2DM. A similar pattern of diminished plasma glycine concentrations is present in cases of obesity, where overweight and obese individuals have lower circulating glycine levels compared to their lean counterparts. Moreover, longitudinal studies conducted over periods ranging from 1 to 19 years reveal that lower glycine levels are inversely related to insulin resistance and serve as predictors for the development of T2DM [32].

4.1.2. Serum TRP and Serum KA as Possible Biomarkers Indicating Renal Endothelial Injury in the Initial Stages of DKD

The biological implications of the kynurenine pathway activation in the context of progressive DKD are still not fully understood. Tryptophan undergoes metabolism through the kynurenine pathway, resulting in the formation of oxidized NAD. Since a reduction in NAD levels significantly contributes to the development of renal diseases, it is likely that many metabolites produced in the kynurenine pathway are redirected toward the NAD pathway to restore cellular NAD levels. Interestingly, manipulating indoleamine 2,3-dioxygenase (IDO) activity has led to conflicting results in various animal studies. For instance, the inhibition of IDO using 1-methyltryptophan exacerbated crescentic glomerulonephritis in renal tissues, which implies that the activation of IDO may exert an anti-inflammatory effect. Conversely, both the overexpression of IDO and the administration of IDO agonists appeared to alleviate renal damage in mice with IgA nephropathy. Additionally, a different preclinical investigation indicated that IDO activation could stimulate Wnt/β-catenin signalling, thereby promoting kidney fibrosis. While we cannot fully reconcile these opposing results due to lack of data deriving from human studies, the variability in the animal models utilized in these studies may help explain these inconsistencies [33].

4.2. Biomarkers Indicating Podocyte Injury and Proximal Tubule Dysfunction Evaluated Through Urine Analysis

4.2.1. The Role of Urinary Glycine in Podocyte Injury and Proximal Tubule Dysfunction

Decreased glycine may be a secondary consequence of excessive free fatty acid (FFA) and branched-chain amino acids (BCAAs) metabolism. FFA metabolism can lead to an accumulation of β-oxidation intermediates (such as acyl-CoA esters). These are conjugated with glycine via the activity of acyl-CoA/glycine-*N*-acyltransferase, which is responsible for the transesterification of acyl-CoA esters with glycine to produce acyl-glycines. Acyl-glycine is membrane permeable and is readily excreted in the urine, thus serving as a mechanism for the elimination of excess β-oxidation intermediates. Similarly, BCAA catabolism byproducts also conjugate to glycine in the liver for excretion. Therefore, circulating glycine could be consumed to facilitate excretion of waste products associated with elevated FFAs and BCAAs. Indeed, in a rat model of obesity, a BCAA-restricted diet causes an increase in circulating glycine concentrations, demonstrating an inverse relationship between BCAA availability and circulating glycine levels. The BCAA-restricted diet restores acyl-glycines in the urine and the urinary acyl-glycine levels are linearly related to skeletal muscle glycine concentrations. These pathways have recently been reviewed. Regardless of the mechanism(s), it is important to note that the low circulating glycine levels in prediabetes/T2D are reflected in peripheral tissues and, to a lesser extent, in the brain, where key actions may be exerted on blood glucose control [34].

4.2.2. Urinary Tiglylglycine

Tiglylglycine is a metabolite that appears in urine under certain pathological conditions. Its production is associated with metabolic disorders involving BCAA metabolism, particularly isoleucine catabolism. Isoleucine is a branched-chain amino acid metabolized in the mitochondria through several enzymatic steps. During its breakdown, isoleucine is converted to tiglyl-CoA, a critical intermediate. Normally, tiglyl-CoA is further metabolized by the enzyme enoyl-CoA hydratase in the β-oxidation pathway. If there is a defect in this pathway (e.g., a deficiency in enzymes like methylcrotonyl-CoA carboxylase or propionyl-CoA carboxylase), tiglyl-CoA accumulates. The accumulated tiglyl-CoA is detoxified through conjugation with glycine, forming tiglylglycine, which is then excreted in urine [35].

However, a case report describes an adult with beta-ketothiolase deficiency who developed diabetic ketoacidosis. This case highlights the importance of considering inherited metabolic disorders in the differential diagnosis of diabetic ketoacidosis, although such situations are rare. In conclusion, although tiglylglycine is not commonly associated with diabetes, monitoring its levels may be relevant in identifying rare metabolic disorders that may coexist or influence diabetes management [36].

4.3. A Concise Summary of the Clinical Significance of Metabolites

As it was mentioned by Imenshahidi, M., Gannon MC, and González-Ortiz M., glycine supplementation has been shown to enhance several aspects of metabolic syndrome, such as diabetes, obesity, hyperlipidemia, and hypertension by increasing insulin secretion. Looking ahead, glycine could play a crucial role in the clinical management of individuals suffering from metabolic syndrome [37–39].

A study conducted by Tomoko Inubushi et al. indicated that the administration of L-TRP to diabetic mice reduces the increase in glucose levels in blood and alleviates the strain on insulin secretion from beta cells [40].

To reduce misinterpretation of these substances and evaluate the clinical role, it is essential to conduct prospective randomized controlled trials.

The research presents a number of limitations: first it is a cross-sectional study, which means it cannot determine a causal relationship between our results and the clinical parameters. Second, the variability of the biological parameters (glycemia, lipids), could have introduced a bias in the interpretation of data. Third, the number of patients was limited.

Nevertheless, our study possesses certain strengths. To our knowledge, this is the first study that identifies tiglylglycine as a possible biomarker for DKD. Additionally, through statistical analysis, we demonstrated that this metabolite holds significance in effectively differentiating between various patient subgroups and exhibits robust correlations with markers related to proximal tubules and podocytes.

5. Conclusions

In this study, we utilized LC-UHPLC techniques to analyse the trend in serum and urine metabolites, aiming to identify the distinctions between control groups and various patient subgroups with diabetic kidney disease, with a specific focus on the normoalbuminuric subgroup. Our findings indicated several metabolites that may serve as putative biomarkers for early DKD, including glycine, kynurenic acid, tryptophan, and tiglylglycine.

Author Contributions: Conceptualisation, M.M., F.G. and L.P.; methodology, M.M., F.G., L.P. and A.V.; software, O.M. and A.S.-S.; validation, C.S., A.I.S., M.G., S.I. and L.B.; formal analysis, C.S. and A.I.S.; investigation, M.M., C.S., L.P., F.G., A.V., M.G. and I.-L.I.; resources, C.S. and L.P.; data curation, L.P. and C.S.; writing—original draft preparation, M.M.; writing—review and editing, C.S., L.P., F.G. and C.S.; visualisation, M.M., F.G., L.P., F.B., O.M.C. and D.C.J.; supervision, M.M., F.G. and L.P.; project administration, M.M., C.S., F.G. and L.P.; S.U., statistical analysis. All authors have read and agreed to the published version of the manuscript.

Funding: This research was funded by "Victor Babes" University of Medicine and Pharmacy, Timisoara, Romania, through doctoral grant GD 2020 to M.M.

Institutional Review Board Statement: The protocol of the study has received approval by the Ethics Committee for Scientific Research of "Victor Babes" University of Medicine and Pharmacy Timisoara number 28/02.09.2020 and "Pius Brinzeu" County Emergency Hospital Timisoara number 296/06.04.2022.

Informed Consent Statement: Informed consent was obtained from all subjects involved in this study.

Data Availability Statement: The data that support the findings of this study are available from the corresponding author upon reasonable request.

Acknowledgments: We would like to acknowledge "Victor Babes" University of Medicine and Pharmacy Timisoara for their support in covering the costs of publication for this research paper.

Conflicts of Interest: The authors declare no conflicts of interest.

References

1. Rustiasari, U.J.; Roelofs, J.J. The role of platelets in diabetic kidney disease. *Int. J. Mol. Sci.* **2022**, *23*, 8270. [CrossRef] [PubMed] [PubMed Central]
2. International Diabetes Federation. *IDF Diabetes Atlas: Global, Regional and Country-Level Diabetes Prevalence Estimates for 2021 and Projections for 2045*; Elsevier: Amsterdam, The Netherlands, 2022.
3. Hoogeveen, E. The epidemiology of diabetic kidney disease. *Kidney Dial.* **2022**, *2*, 433–442. [CrossRef]
4. Hirata, K.; Shikata, K.; Matsuda, M.; Akiyama, K.; Sugimoto, H.; Kushiro, M.; Makino, H. Increased expression of selectins in kidneys of patients with diabetic nephropathy. *Diabetologia* **1998**, *41*, 185–192. [CrossRef] [PubMed]

5. Kravets, I.; Mallipattu, S.K. The role of podocytes and podocyte-associated biomarkers in diagnosis and treatment of diabetic kidney disease. *J. Endocr. Soc.* **2020**, *4*, bvaa029. [CrossRef] [PubMed] [PubMed Central]
6. Mogos, M.; Socaciu, C.; Socaciu, A.I.; Vlad, A.; Gadalean, F.; Bob, F.; Milas, O.; Cretu, O.M.; Suteanu-Simulescu, A.; Glavan, M.; et al. Metabolomic Investigation of Blood and Urinary Amino Acids and Derivatives in Patients with Type 2 Diabetes Mellitus and Early Diabetic Kidney Disease. *Biomedicines* **2023**, *11*, 1527. [CrossRef] [PubMed] [PubMed Central]
7. Mogos, M.; Socaciu, C.; Socaciu, A.I.; Vlad, A.; Gadalean, F.; Bob, F.; Milas, O.; Cretu, O.M.; Suteanu-Simulescu, A.; Glavan, M.; et al. Biomarker Profiling with Targeted Metabolomic Analysis of Plasma and Urine Samples in Patients with Type 2 Diabetes Mellitus and Early Diabetic Kidney Disease. *J. Clin. Med.* **2024**, *13*, 4703. [CrossRef] [PubMed] [PubMed Central]
8. van Timmeren, M.M.; van den Heuvel, M.C.; Bailly, V.; Bakker, S.J.; van Goor, H.; Stegeman, C.A. Tubular kidney injury molecule-1 (KIM-1) in human renal disease. *J. Pathol.* **2007**, *212*, 209–217. [CrossRef] [PubMed]
9. Nauta, F.L.; Boertien, W.E.; Bakker, S.J.; van Goor, H.; van Oeveren, W.; de Jong, P.E.; Bilo, H.; Gansevoort, R.T. Glomerular and tubular damage markers are elevated in patients with diabetes. *Diabetes Care* **2011**, *34*, 975–981. [CrossRef] [PubMed] [PubMed Central]
10. Chaudhary, K.; Phadke, G.; Nistala, R.; Weidmeyer, C.E.; McFarlane, S.I.; Whaley-Connell, A. The emerging role of biomarkers in diabetic and hypertensive chronic kidney disease. *Curr. Diab Rep.* **2010**, *10*, 37–42. [CrossRef]
11. Rossing, P. Promotion, prediction and prevention of progression of nephropathy in type 1 diabetes mellitus. *Diabet. Med.* **1998**, *15*, 900–919. [CrossRef] [PubMed]
12. Siddiqui, K.; Al-Malki, B.; George, T.P.; Nawaz, S.S.; Rubeaan, K.A. Urinary N-acetyl-beta-d-glucosaminidase (NAG) with neutrophil gelatinase-associated lipocalin (NGAL) improves the diagnostic value for proximal tubule damage in diabetic kidney disease. *3 Biotech* **2019**, *9*, 66. [CrossRef] [PubMed] [PubMed Central]
13. Novak, R.; Salai, G.; Hrkac, S.; Vojtusek, I.K.; Grgurevic, L. Revisiting the role of NAG across the continuum of kidney disease. *Bioengineering* **2023**, *10*, 444. [CrossRef] [PubMed] [PubMed Central]
14. Huang, Q.; Fei, X.; Zhan, H.; Gong, J.; Zhou, J.; Zhang, Y.; Ye, X.; Song, Y.; Ma, J.; Wu, X. Urinary N-acetyl-β-d-glucosaminidase-creatine ratio is a valuable predictor for advanced diabetic kidney disease. *J. Clin. Lab. Anal.* **2023**, *37*, e24769. [CrossRef] [PubMed] [PubMed Central]
15. Mohammadi-Karakani, A.; Asgharzadeh-Haghighi, S.; Ghazi-Khansari, M.; Hosseini, R. Determination of urinary enzymes as a marker of early renal damage in diabetic patients. *J. Clin. Lab. Anal.* **2007**, *21*, 413–417. [CrossRef] [PubMed] [PubMed Central]
16. Miyauchi, E.; Hosojima, H.; Morimoto, S. Urinary angiotensin-converting enzyme activity in type 2 diabetes mellitus: Its relationship to diabetic nephropathy. *Acta Diabetol.* **1995**, *32*, 193–197. [CrossRef]
17. Skrha, J.; Haas, T.; Sperl, M.; Stibor, V.; Stolba, P. A six-year follow-up of the relationship between N-acetyl-beta-glucosaminidase and albuminuria in relation to retinopathy. *Diabet. Med.* **1991**, *8*, 817–821. [CrossRef] [PubMed]
18. Veluri, G.; Mannangatti, M. Urinary nephrin is a sensitive marker to predict early onset of nephropathy in type 2 diabetes mellitus. *J. Lab. Physicians* **2022**, *14*, 497–504. [CrossRef] [PubMed] [PubMed Central]
19. Kandasamy, Y.; Smith, R.; Lumbers, E.R.; Rudd, D. Nephrin—A biomarker of early glomerular injury. *Biomark. Res.* **2014**, *2*, 21. [CrossRef] [PubMed] [PubMed Central]
20. Chang, J.H.; Paik, S.Y.; Mao, L.; Eisner, W.; Flannery, P.J.; Wang, L.; Tang, Y.; Mattocks, N.; Hadjadj, S.; Goujon, J.-M.; et al. Diabetic kidney disease in FVB/NJ Akita mice: Temporal pattern of kidney injury and urinary nephrin excretion. *PLoS ONE* **2012**, *7*, e33942. [CrossRef] [PubMed] [PubMed Central]
21. Kostovska, I.; Tosheska-Trajkovska, K.; Topuzovska, S.; Cekovska, S.; Spasovski, G.; Kostovski, O.; Labudovic, D. Urinary nephrin is earlier, more sensitive and specific marker of diabetic nephropathy than microalbuminuria. *J. Med. Biochem.* **2020**, *39*, 83–90. [CrossRef] [PubMed] [PubMed Central]
22. Wang, F.; Xing, T.; Wang, N.; Liu, L. Clinical significance of plasma CD146 and P-selectin in patients with type 2 diabetic nephropathy. *Cytokine* **2012**, *57*, 127–129. [CrossRef] [PubMed]
23. Al-Rubeaan, K.; Nawaz, S.S.; Youssef, A.M.; Al Ghonaim, M.; Siddiqui, K. IL-18, VCAM-1 and P-selectin as early biomarkers in normoalbuminuric type 2 diabetes patients. *Biomark. Med.* **2019**, *13*, 467–478. [CrossRef] [PubMed]
24. Xie, Y.; Jin, D.; Qiu, H.; Lin, L.; Sun, S.; Li, D.; Sha, F.; Zhou, W.; Jia, M. Assessment of urinary podocalyxin as an alternative marker for urinary albumin creatinine ratio in early stage of diabetic kidney disease in older patients. *Nefrologia* **2022**, *42*, 664–670. [CrossRef] [PubMed]
25. Ye, H.; Bai, X.; Gao, H.; Li, L.; Wu, C.; Sun, X.; Zhang, C.; Shen, Y.; Zhang, J.; Lu, Z. Urinary podocalyxin positive-element occurs in the early stage of diabetic nephropathy and is correlated with a clinical diagnosis of diabetic nephropathy. *J. Diabetes Complicat.* **2014**, *28*, 96–100. [CrossRef] [PubMed]
26. Hara, M.; Yamagata, K.; Tomino, Y.; Saito, A.; Hirayama, Y.; Ogasawara, S.; Kurosawa, H.; Sekine, S.; Yan, K. Urinary podocalyxin is an early marker for podocyte injury in patients with diabetes: Establishment of a highly sensitive ELISA to detect urinary podocalyxin. *Diabetologia* **2012**, *55*, 2913–2919. [CrossRef] [PubMed] [PubMed Central]

27. Dalla Vestra, M.; Masiero, A.; Roiter, A.M.; Saller, A.; Crepaldi, G.; Fioretto, P. Is podocyte injury relevant in diabetic nephropathy? Studies in patients with type 2 diabetes. *Diabetes* **2003**, *52*, 1031–1035. [CrossRef] [PubMed]
28. Weil, E.J.; Lemley, K.V.; Mason, C.C.; Yee, B.; Jones, L.I.; Blouch, K.; Lovato, T.; Richardson, M.; Myers, B.D.; Nelson, R.G. Podocyte detachment and reduced glomerular capillary endothelial fenestration promote kidney disease in type 2 diabetic nephropathy. *Kidney Int.* **2012**, *82*, 1010–1017. [CrossRef] [PubMed] [PubMed Central]
29. Lim, A.K.H.; Tesch, G.H. Inflammation in diabetic nephropathy. *Diabetes* **2012**, *65*, 2311–2321. [CrossRef]
30. Liu, J.J.; Yeoh, L.Y.; Sum, C.F.; Tavintharan, S.; Ng, X.W.; Liu, S.; Lee, S.B.; Tang, W.E.; Lim, S.C. Vascular cell adhesion molecule-1, but not intercellular adhesion molecule-1, is associated with diabetic kidney disease in Asians with type 2 diabetes. *J. Diabetes Complicat.* **2015**, *29*, 707–712. [CrossRef] [PubMed]
31. Thakur, V.; Nargis, S.; Gonzalez, M.; Pradhan, S.; Terreros, D.; Chattopadhyay, M. Role of glycyrrhizin in the reduction of inflammation in diabetic kidney disease. *Nephron* **2017**, *137*, 137–147. [CrossRef] [PubMed]
32. Yan-Do, R.; Duong, E.; Manning Fox, J.E.; Dai, X.; Suzuki, K.; Khan, S.; Bautista, A.; Ferdaoussi, M.; Lyon, J.; Wu, X.; et al. A glycine-insulin autocrine feedback loop enhances insulin secretion from human β-cells and is impaired in type 2 diabetes. *Diabetes* **2016**, *65*, 2311–2321. [CrossRef] [PubMed]
33. Liu, J.J.; Ching, J.; Wee, H.N.; Liu, S.; Gurung, R.L.; Lee, J.; Zheng, H.; Lee, L.S.; Ang, K.; Shao, Y.M.; et al. Plasma tryptophan-kynurenine pathway metabolites and risk for progression to end-stage kidney disease in patients with type 2 diabetes. *Diabetes Care* **2023**, *46*, 2223–2231. [CrossRef] [PubMed] [PubMed Central]
34. Alves, A.; Bassot, A.; Bulteau, A.-L.; Pirola, L.; Morio, B. Glycine Metabolism and Its Alterations in Obesity and Metabolic Diseases. *Nutrients* **2019**, *11*, 1356. [CrossRef] [PubMed]
35. Bennett, M.J.; Powell, S.; Swartling, D.J.; Gibson, K.M. Tiglylglycine excreted in urine in disorders of isoleucine metabolism and the respiratory chain measured by stable isotope dilution GC-MS. *Clin. Chem.* **1994**, *40*, 1879–1883. [CrossRef] [PubMed]
36. Zhen, X.M.; Twigg, S.M.; Wu, T.; Tabet, E.; McGill, M.J.; Constantino, M.; Mallawaarachchi, A.; Luo, C.; Thillainadesan, S.; Rahman, Y.; et al. Diabetic ketoacidosis in an adult with beta-ketothiolase deficiency (BKD) involving a novel ACAT1 variant: First report of established diabetes in BKD and a review of the literature. *Clin. Diabetes Endocrinol.* **2024**, *10*, 17. [CrossRef] [PubMed] [PubMed Central]
37. Imenshahidi, M.; Hossenzadeh, H. Effects of glycine on metabolic syndrome components: A review. *J. Endocrinol. Investig.* **2022**, *45*, 927–939. [CrossRef]
38. Gannon, M.C.; Nuttall, J.A.; Nuttall, F.Q. The metabolic response to ingested glycine. *Am. J. Clin. Nutr.* **2002**, *76*, 1302–1307. [CrossRef] [PubMed]
39. González-Ortiz, M.; Medina-Santillán, R.; Martínez-Abundis, E.; von Drateln, C.R. Effect of glycine on insulin secretion and action in healthy first-degree relatives of type 2 diabetes mellitus patients. *Horm. Metab. Res.* **2001**, *33*, 358–360. [CrossRef] [PubMed]
40. Inubushi, T.; Kamemura, N.; Oda, M.; Sakurai, J.; Nakaya, Y.; Harada, N.; Suenaga, M.; Matsunaga, Y.; Ishidoh, K.; Katunuma, N. L-tryptophan suppresses rise in blood glucose and preserves insulin secretion in type-2 diabetes mellitus rats. *J. Nutr. Sci. Vitaminol.* **2012**, *58*, 415–422. [CrossRef] [PubMed]

biomedicines

Review

Narrative Review of Biological Markers in Chronic Limb-Threatening Ischemia

Alexandra Ioana Popescu [1], Andreea Luciana Rata [2], Sorin Barac [3,*], Roxana Popescu [4], Roxana Ramona Onofrei [5], Cristian Vlad [6] and Daliborca Vlad [6]

1 Pharmacology Department, Doctoral School, "Victor Babes" University of Medicine and Pharmacy, 300041 Timisoara, Romania; alexandra_popescu2007@yahoo.com
2 Surgical Emergencies Department, "Victor Babes" University of Medicine and Pharmacy, 300041 Timisoara, Romania; rataandreealuciana@gmail.com
3 Vascular Surgery Department, "Victor Babes" University of Medicine and Pharmacy, 300041 Timisoara, Romania
4 Cell and Molecular Biology Department, "Victor Babes" University of Medicine and Pharmacy, 300041 Timisoara, Romania; popescu.roxana@umft.ro
5 Department of Rehabilitation, Physical Medicine and Rheumatology, Research Center for Assessment of Human Motion, Functionality and Disability, "Victor Babes" University of Medicine and Pharmacy, 300041 Timisoara, Romania; onofrei.roxana@umft.ro
6 Pharmacology Department, "Victor Babes" University of Medicine and Pharmacy, 300041 Timisoara, Romania; vlad.cristian@umft.ro (C.V.); vlad.daliborca@umft.ro (D.V.)
* Correspondence: sorinbarac@gmail.com; Tel.: +40-748-331-276

Abstract: Background: Chronic limb-threatening ischemia (CLTI), the advanced stage of peripheral arterial disease, is diagnosed in the presence of ischemic rest pain, non-healing ulcers, or gangrene. Several studies have demonstrated that inflammation and endothelial dysfunction are some of the main substrates of CLTI. Methods: A narrative review was conducted and reported according to PRISMA guidelines. Three databases were searched—Web of Science, Medline, and EMBASE—for the studies assessing CLTI and the biological markers related to it. Results: We included 22 studies, and all the markers identified (C-reactive protein, D-dimers, fibrinogen, cytokines, IL-6, TNF-α, ICAM-1 (Intracellular Adhesion Molecule-1), VCAM-1 (Vascular Cell Adhesion Molecule-1), neutrophile-to-lymphocytes ratio (NLR), IL-8, Pentraxin-3, neutrophil gelatinase-associated lipocalin (NGAL), calprotectin, E-selectin, P-selectin, neopterin, High-Mobility Group Box-1 protein (HGMB-1), Osteoprotegerin (OPG) and Sortilin) were positively associated with advanced CLTI, with major limb or major cardiovascular events in these patients. Conclusions: All the studied markers had increased values in patients with CLTI, especially when associated with diabetes mellitus, proving a very important association between diabetes and major limb or cardiovascular events in these patients. There is a need for more studies to validate these markers in terms of diagnosis or prognosis in CLTI patients and in trying to find new medical strategies that target inflammation or endothelial dysfunction in these patients.

Keywords: chronic limb-threatening ischemia; biological markers; inflammatory markers; endothelial dysfunction

1. Introduction

Peripheral arterial disease (PAD) incidence has increased significantly in the last few years. Most patients are asymptomatic for long periods of time, but at least 10% will progress toward chronic limb-threatening ischemia (CLTI) or will present per primam in this stage of the disease. The modifiable risk factors for PAD and CLTI are smoking, diabetes mellitus, arterial hypertension, chronic kidney disease, sedentary lifestyle, and obesity. Despite the best medical treatment and the progress made in correcting the risk factors, CLTI is still associated with higher morbidity and mortality. Untreated, CLTI leads to an approximately 25% major amputation rate 1 year after the diagnosis [1].

CLTI guidelines published in 2019 [2] proposed that the definition of CLTI should include a broader spectrum and a more heterogenous group of patients, with different ischemia degrees and a higher major amputation risk.

Ischemic rest pain is usually described as affecting the forefoot and is usually aggravated by the decubitus position; for the diagnosis, the pain should be present for more than 2 weeks and associated with one or more abnormal parameters: ankle–brachial index < 0.4, ankle pressure < 50 mmHg in absolute value, hallux pressure under 30 mmHg in absolute value, a transcutaneous oxygen pressure under 30 mmHg, and a flat or weakly pulsating wave curve (equivalent to a third degree of ischemia in the WIfI classification) [3].

The primary process that leads to atherosclerosis is represented by endothelial dysfunction, and the organism is trying to counterbalance it through the activation of progenitor endothelial cells to produce vascular repair.

Inflammation plays a key role in PAD and CLTI, but its mediators are not clearly defined [4,5]. The role of inflammatory biomarkers in the atherosclerotic process has been extensively analyzed, both in experimental and clinical studies. Although inflammatory mediators such as IL-6, TNF-α, and C-reactive protein (CRP) were identified as predictors for major cardiovascular events, randomized studies demonstrated opposite results, which justifies a more thorough analysis of these markers in CLTI.

It is well known that in the early stages of the atherosclerotic process, endothelial dysfunction leads to the production of increased quantities of inflammatory cytokines (IL1β, IL6, CRP, MCP-1—monocyte chemoattractant protein-1), proteases (matrix metalloproteinase—MMP), extracellular vesicles, and adhesion molecules (P-selectin, E-selectin, ICAM—Intracellular Adhesion Molecule, VCAM—Vascular Cell Adhesion Molecule), which contributes to monocyte attraction and is secondary to intima infiltration. However, compared with coronary artery disease, these mechanisms are not widely studied for CLTI [6].

The aim of our review was to summarize the most important markers studied so far in CLTI, keeping in mind that algorithms derived from these markers can lead to prediction models in PAD, CLTI, and major amputations, or can estimate the risk for major cardiovascular events in patients with CLTI.

2. Materials and Methods

We performed an electronic medical database search—of Web of Science, MEDLINE, and Embase—in which we included English-language articles from January 1956 to November 2023. We also analyzed the references in every article. The terms we used were: critical limb ischemia, chronic limb-threatening ischemia, lower-limb ischemia, inflammatory markers, C-reactive protein (CRP), D-dimers, fibrinogen, cytokines, interleukin-6 (IL-6), Tumor Necrosis Factor-α (TNF-α), Intracellular Adhesion Molecule-1 (ICAM-1), Vascular Cell Adhesion Molecule-1 (VCAM-1), neutrophile-to-lymphocytes ratio (NLR), Interleukin 8 (IL-8), Pentraxin-3 (PTX-3), neutrophil gelatinase-associated lipocalin (NGAL), calprotectin, E-selectin, P-selectin, neopterin, High-Mobility Group Box-1 protein (HGMB-1), Osteoprotegerin (OPG) and Sortilin (SORT) (Figure 1).

The search results were imported into EPPI-Reviewer 6 for duplicate removal and study selection. After this step, titles and abstracts were independently reviewed by two investigators (A.I.P and A.L.R.). Full-text articles were then read, and we collected data on the study type, methods, participants, outcomes, and results of every different study. All disagreements were solved by discussion between all the authors.

This review will focus on the association of the above markers with chronic limb-threatening ischemia in terms of prediction, progression, major cardiovascular events in these patients, and major limb events, but it will also emphasize other specific findings when considered useful to clinical

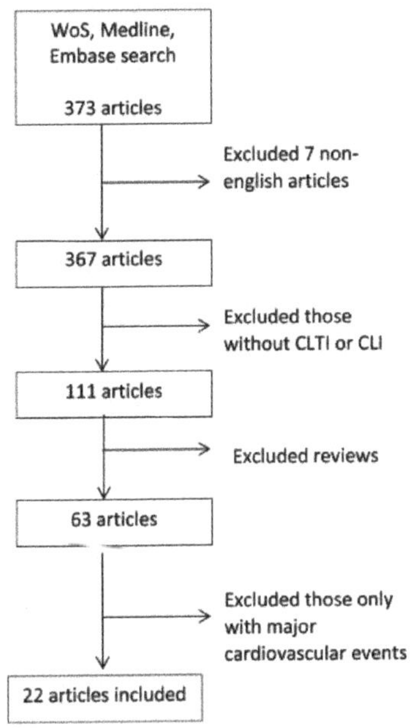

Figure 1. PRISMA flow diagram.

practice.

3. Results

When speaking of chronic threatening limb ischemia, we are speaking of the following marker categories: markers of thrombosis, markers of lipid metabolism, markers of tissue remodeling and angiogenesis, inflammatory markers, markers of endothelial activation and dysfunction, and markers of oxidative stress.

We have attempted to synthesize the most important markers and highlight the most relevant studies related to CLTI.

3.1. C-Reactive Protein (CRP)

C-reactive protein (CRP) was identified in 222 studies for PAD in general and in 8 studies for CLTI. CRP is an acute-phase reactant, and its plasma concentration can increase up to 1000-fold in the acute phase of the pathology [7]. The predictive association between CRP and coronary heart disease has been extensively demonstrated. Different studies have demonstrated that CRP contributes to inflammation at the level of atheroma plaque and is actively involved in early atherogenesis [8]. hs-CRP (high-sensitivity CRP) is known as a predictive factor of myocardial infarction [9,10], stroke, and peripheral arterial disease [11–13].

Patients with peripheral arterial disease have elevated levels of hs-CRP, and it appears to be predictive of disease progression, as measured by the ankle–brachial index, and the severity of functional impairment [14].

Nardella et al. [15] conducted a prospective non-randomized study of 264 patients in which they identified the relationship between baseline CRP levels and the incidence of major cardiovascular events (MACEs) and major lower-limb events (MALEs) in diabetic patients with CLTI. They identified elevated CRP levels with poor post-revascularization outcomes in patients with CLTI and diabetes. Moreover, 15.9% of patients developed MACEs within the first year after revascularization and all had elevated serum CRP values. Likewise, 30.7% of patients developed MACEs 1 year after revascularization and, again, serum CRP levels were significantly elevated. The authors concluded from multivariate logistic regressions that in patients with critical ischemia, elevated CRP values are an independent determinant of MALEs and MACEs after revascularization.

Husakova J. et al. [16] studied risk factors for major amputations in patients with diabetic ulcers and CLTI treated with autologous cell therapy. Their study included 113 patients divided into two groups—those with and those without major amputation. The group with major amputation had significantly increased CRP levels compared to the group without major amputation (22.7 vs. 10.7 mg/L).

Another study led by Fujii M. retrospectively studied 30 patients with CLTI and forefoot osteomyelitis and recommends, as the first therapeutic intention, debridement and infection clearance if a CRP level greater than 40 mg/L is identified [17].

Biscetti et al. [18] studied the association between the levels of the most important inflammatory cytokines and the presence of diabetes mellitus in a group of 299 patients, as well as the results of these markers after endovascular procedures in patients with diabetes mellitus and CLTI. They identified increased levels of CRP values in association with a negative postoperative outcome in patients, with an association between CLTI and diabetes.

In a prospective study of 71 patients with Fontaine stage II-IV PAD, Tschopl et al. [19] studied the role and values of various known hemostatic factors that may be associated with an increased risk of thrombosis and identified that patients with restenosis of atherosclerotic lesions had higher CRP values at 3–6 months after PTA (25.4 +/− 46.7 versus 7.9 +/− 6.9 mg/L, $p < 0.05$).

Also, another observational study of 116 patients, of which 46% had CLTI, showed increased serum values in these patients compared to patients without CLTI (37.53 ± 46.61 mg/L vs. 9.18 ± 26.12 mg/L, $p = 0.000$) [20].

3.2. D-Dimers

D-dimers are a degradation product of cross-linked fibrin and are a marker of coagulation system activation. They are a marker of fibrinolysis and are often associated with thrombosis processes [21,22]. Vidula et al. [23] reported a relation between D-dimer levels and mortality in patients with PAD, as well as higher levels 1–2 years before death. Elevated D-dimer levels have been associated with a risk of subsequent venous or arterial thrombotic events, especially in patients with pre-existing vascular disease [22,24].

Tschopl et al. also studied D-dimer output in Fontaine stage II-IV patients and found significantly increased D-dimer values at 1 h, 24, and 48 h, respectively, after PTA in a group of 71 patients [19].

In a systematic review including 10 studies and 2420 patients, other authors demonstrated that increased D-dimer levels are associated with a two-fold increased risk of developing major cardiovascular events in patients with PAD [24].

3.3. Fibrinogen

Fibrinogen is a glycoprotein with an extremely important role in several physiological and biochemical processes. It is expressed primarily in hepatocytes, and its synthesis is regulated by acute-phase proteins. Thus, fibrinogen is an acute-phase reactant because its synthesis is increased during inflammation, in the acute phase, its plasma concentration can exceed 7 g/L [25]. Fibrinogen synthesis is stimulated by cytokines in activated megakaryocytes and plays a key role as an acute-phase reactant. Thus, fibrinogen is considered a key molecule in the inflammation and coagulation cascade and is involved in the pathogenesis of the atherosclerotic process and the development of atherothrombotic complications [26].

In their study, Tschopl et al. [19] demonstrated significantly increased fibrinogen values 48 h after PTA. Another phenomenon demonstrated by them is that patients who experienced post-revascularization restenosis showed increased values of this marker, both initially and 3–6 months after PTA.

In an observational prospective study on 116 patients, Ferreira et al. [20] demonstrated that patients with CLTI had increased serum fibrinogen levels compared to patients without CLTI (466.18 ± 208.07 mg/dL vs. 317.37 ± 79.42 mg/dL, $p = 0.000$).

In a study of 108 CLTI patients led by Pedrinelli et al. [27], who studied the association between mortality rate and plasma fibrinogen levels in CLTI patients who died during the first 6 months of follow-up, extremely elevated plasma fibrinogen values were identified. Also, in a Cox-multivariate regression analysis, only plasma fibrinogen had an independent predictive value for mortality.

3.4. Interleukin-6 (IL-6)

Interleukin-6 (IL-6) was discovered in 1986 and is a member of the pro-inflammatory cytokine family; it induces the expression of proteins responsible for the acute phase of inflammation and plays an important role in cell differentiation and the proliferation of non-immune cells [28]. IL-6 also plays an important role in the acquired immune response by stimulating antibody production and the development of effector T-cells [28].

An important element to note about IL-6 that is directly related to critical ischemia is that an immediate expression of IL-6 is generated in response to environmental stressors such as infection or tissue injury. Withdrawal of the source of stress on the host will lead to a decrease in the activation of the IL-6-mediated negative regulatory system cascade, with degradation of IL-6 mRNA via regenerase-1 leading to a termination of IL-6 production. A variety of circumstances related to the vascular wall, such as oxidative stress and vascular injury, can lead to increased IL-6 secretion [29]. There is also a strong association between circulating IL-6 levels and the risk of major cardiovascular events [30–32].

Nardella et al. demonstrated in a prospective study of 264 patients that elevated IL-6 levels are associated with poor outcomes in diabetic patients with critical ischemia after revascularization [15].

Gremmels et al. [33] investigated several markers with a role in the occurrence of major cardiovascular events or major amputations. IL-6 was found to be significantly elevated in patients who reached one of the above points, leading to the conclusion that inflammatory markers play a role in predicting the risk of major cardiovascular events in patients with critical ischemia.

3.5. Tumor Necrosis Factor-α (TNF-α)

Tumor Necrosis Factor-α (TNF-α) is a multifunctional cytokine that has been implicated as a mediator of various physiological and pathophysiological events, including cell survival, growth, differentiation, apoptosis, inflammation, and angiogenesis [34].

Two receptors with high affinity for TNF-α are TNF-α-Receptor-1 (TNF-α-R-1, known as p55) and TNF-α-Receptor -2 (TNF-α-R-2, known as p75), with roles in regulating processes in critical ischemia [34].

Caicedo et al. [35] studied TNF-α in 35 patients with CLTI and found increased levels ($\geq$8.1) in 68.6% of patients and concluded that this marker is very important in the progression of ischemia, especially in diabetic patients.

Also, Biscetti et al. [18] showed in 299 patients with BTK disease that TNF-α is associated with worse vascular outcomes in patients with CLTI and diabetes mellitus.

3.6. Intracellular Adhesion Molecule—1 (ICAM-1) and Vascular Cell Adhesion Molecule—1 (VCAM-1)

Soluble Intracellular Adhesion Molecule-1 (ICAM-1), also known as CD54, encodes a cell surface glycoprotein that mediates leukocyte stationary adhesion and transmigration and can be regulated during tissue reperfusion. A study led by Foussard et al. [36] demonstrated that impaired limb reperfusion was associated with increased endothelial activation of ICAM-1 expression and impaired perfusion of capillaries that are smaller in diameter than a leukocyte when it interacts with leukocytes.

VCAM-1 is expressed in endothelial cells in response to cytokines, mediates the adhesion of leukocytes, including lymphocytes and monocytes, and is associated with vascular inflammation. VCAM-1 also plays a key role in leukocyte–endothelial cell signal translation and in the development of atherosclerosis [37]. Regarding the relationship between VCAM-1 and PAD, patients with PAD are more likely to have increased circulating levels of soluble adhesion molecules [38].

When searching the databases, we did not specifically find the association between the two molecules and CLTI specifically. However, we have identified various studies related to PAD in general and the association with the 2 molecules. Lee et al. [39] identified elevated serum levels and tissue expression of VCAM-1 as increased in patients with PAD and advanced chronic kidney disease.

Another study by Edlinger et al. [40] on 126 patients, of whom 51 with PAD manifestations and 75 without a history of PAD, demonstrated increased VCAM-1 values in patients with PAD, 1352 pg/mL vs. 953 pg/mL) and concluded that VCAM-1 is a marker that accurately identifies the severity of the systemic atherosclerotic process.

3.7. Neutrophile-to-Lymphocytes Ratio (NLR)

Over the last 10 years, this ratio seems to have become an extremely important marker. It is calculated as the simple ratio of neutrophils to lymphocytes measured in peripheral blood and is a marker that shows two sides of the immune system: the innate side due to neutrophils and the acquired side given by lymphocytes [41].

Neutrophils are responsible for the first line of immune response by chemotaxis, phagocytosis, and the release of oxidative reactive species, granular proteins, and cytokines [42]. NLR has been associated with high mortality in patients with critical ischemia [42].

We found 26 articles and selected 11 that addressed chronic limb-threatening ischemia.

A retrospective study of 268 patients who were not scheduled to receive either surgical or endovascular treatment but only a conservative treatment showed that patients with a ratio greater than 4.63 did not respond positively to drug treatment of the pathology [43].

Gary T. et al. [44] demonstrated in another retrospective study of 2121 patients with PAD at various stages that the neutrophil/lymphocyte ratio was significantly increased in patients with CLTI (usually around 3.95).

Another retrospective study of 195 patients in which NLR was associated with critical ischemia showed that at 1-year follow-up, patients with NLR over 8 had higher in-hospital mortality. In terms of major amputation events, an NLR ≥ 6 was associated with a higher frequency (adjusted HR: 2.804, 95% CI: 1.292–6.088, $p = 0.009$) [45].

Spark et al. [46], in a prospective study of 149 patients with an average follow-up period of 8.7 months, identified that increased NLR was identified in a group of patients with critical ischemia at risk of developing major amputation-type events.

3.8. Interleukin-8 (IL-8)

IL-8, also known as neutrophil chemotactic factor, was first discovered in 1987; its primary role is to induce chemotaxis in neutrophils to the damaged tissue [47]. The main cellular sources of IL-8 are typically monocytes and macrophages, with IL-8 playing a primary role in the recruitment of monocytes and neutrophils—promoters of the acute inflammatory response. A functional feature of IL-8 is that it remains for a very long time at the site of acute inflammation, sometimes even weeks; this contrasts with other inflammatory cytokines that disappear within hours. IL-8 is very sensitive to anti-oxidants, which greatly reduce IL-8 gene expression, and has an important role in vascular diseases, where ischemia-induced oxidative stress is both a marker of disease and a potential target for therapy [48,49].

In a study comparing critical ischemic patients with PTA vs. diagnostic angiography (25 vs. 20 patients), baseline IL-8 levels pre- and post-procedurally demonstrated that IL-8 values were not significantly different between the two groups, and at 1 year, 45% of the PTAs failed, but there was no significant correlation with the inflammatory markers [50].

Another observational, prospective study of 119 patients, including 45 with CLTI, which analyzed histopathological samples from the sartorius muscle of 26 patients, demonstrated significant associations with increased IL-8 levels in these patients [51].

3.9. Pentraxin-3 (PTX3)

PTX3 is an inflammatory phase glycoprotein from the same family as CRP. It appears to be localized in atheroma plaque [52]. The synthesis of PTX3 is stimulated in endothelial cells, macrophages, myeloid cells, and dendritic cells by cytokines, endotoxins such as bacterial products, IL-1, and TNF. PTX3 is localized in the atheroma plaque and plays an important role in modulating the procoagulant activity of endothelial cells [53].

A literature review demonstrated the association of the presence of elevated PTX-3 values with the severity of peripheral arterial disease but did not specifically discuss critical ischemia [5].

A retrospective study of 12 patients demonstrated the association of PAD severity with PTX-3 values, and the authors extend the idea that this marker could be used in relation to the Rutherford classification to determine PAD severity [54].

3.10. Calprotectin and Neutrophil Gelatinase-Associated Lipocalin (NGAL)

Calprotectin is a complex protein that, in the presence of calcium, is capable of binding transition metals such as iron, zinc, and manganese, thus offering complex antimicrobial activity [55]. An association has been identified between increased circulating levels of calprotectin and the risk of developing cardiovascular events or amputation in patients with symptomatic BAP [5]. Saenz-Pipaon et al. [5] studied 331 Fontaine II-IV patients (serum levels) and 413 Fontaine 0–1 patients (plasma levels). They analyzed human femoral plaque and identified that calprotectin levels were 64% lower in plasma than in serum. In PAD patients, the risk of major limb events and major cardiovascular events was associated with 1.8-fold higher serum values for calprotectin [55].

NGAL is a polypeptide released by damaged nephron tubular cells, which is also expressed in atheromatous plaque and is implicated in the development of cardiovascular disease. Various studies have shown that increased levels of NGAL are correlated with the severity of coronary heart disease [56] and are also seen in obese and diabetic patients and correlate with increased CRP levels [57].

3.11. E-Selectin (CD 62)

The leukocyte–endothelial cell adhesion molecule represents an adhesion molecule expressed only in cytokine-activated endothelial cells. Like other selectins, it plays an important role in inflammation, being vital for the recruitment of progenitor stem cells required for the neovascularization of ischemic tissue. Animal studies have shown that E-selectin is vital for neovascularization and tissue repair [58].

A major focus is now on preclinical studies using mesenchymal stem cells enhanced with soluble E-selectin to enhance ischemic tissue repair and regeneration in animal models. In 2022, Quiroz et al. [59] created a viral vector to overexpress E-selectin on mesenchymal cells in order to increase their therapeutic profile; they concluded that the new "supercharged" cells grow faster and induce functional recovery, angiogenesis, and tissue repair in CLTI murine models.

A study of 157 patients with PAD and 206 in the control group that analyzed genetic polymorphism demonstrated that E-selectin was independently associated with PAD, and synergistic effects were identified, resulting in a genetic profile that significantly influences the increased risk of CLTI [60].

Another prospective study of 175 patients with PAD (one group with intermittent claudication and one group with CLTI) who underwent endovascular intervention procedures demonstrated that patients with E-selectin values above 44.9 mg/dl had a 1.9-fold adjusted risk of restenosis (95% CI 1.09 to 3.30) [61].

3.12. Neopterin

Neopterin is a pyrazino–pyrimidine compound that may play an important role in the pathogenesis and progression of coronary artery disease and peripheral arterial disease by regulating bioavailability and the proliferation and differentiation of hematopoietic stem cells [62].

Some studies have demonstrated the association of neopterin with ABI and increased mortality in patients with vascular calcifications undergoing angiography [63].

Despite all the above markers, neopterin has been studied more extensively in relation to CLTI. Neopterin levels were also found to predict vascular adverse events in patients with CLTI, making this molecule a very useful marker of atherosclerotic disease [64].

Signorelli et al. [65] investigated neopterin levels in three groups of patients (control group, symptomatic PAD, and asymptomatic PAD) and demonstrated that mean plasma levels were higher in symptomatic (9.4 ± 4.6 nmol/L) and asymptomatic (7.4 ± 4.0 nmol/L) patients compared to control patients (5.3 ± 3.2 nmol/L).

Another observational study of 259 patients with critical ischemia studied neopterin levels in diabetic vs. non-diabetic patients and found increased levels in diabetic patients (31 vs. 21 mmol/L, $p < 0.01$) [66].

3.13. High-Mobility Group Box-1 (HMGB-1)

This is a nuclear protein that regulates gene expression and induces an inflammatory response during vascular injury, but it also plays a role in activating the pro-inflammatory response after it is released passively by necrotic cells or actively secreted by mock immune cells such as endothelial cells [67]. Moreover, the hs-CRP-induced release of HMGB-1 induces, amplifies, and extends the inflammatory process surrounding the atherosclerotic injury. Further, HMBG-1 causes the secretion of inflammatory molecules such as IL-6 and TNF-α by neutrophils and macrophages. In diabetic patients, this protein promotes chronic inflammation and neovascularization, is directly correlated with HbA1c levels, and is present in the retina of diabetic retinopathy patients [68].

Nardella et al. [15] studied the relationship between baseline biomarker levels and the incidence of MACEs (major adverse cardiac events) and MALEs (major adverse limb events) in diabetic patients with CLTI and identified that increased levels correlate with poor post-revascularization outcomes.

A prospective observational study of 201 CLTI patients who required revascularization benefited from HGMB-1 determination, and the aim of the study was to assess the association of HGMB-1 with MACEs or MALEs after revascularization. Patients who developed limb-related events or major cardiovascular events after revascularization had higher HGMB-1 serum levels: 7.5 ng/mL vs. 4.9 ng/mL ($p < 0.01$) for cardiovascular events and 7.2 ng/mL vs. 4.8 ng/mL ($p < 0.01$) for limb events [69].

3.14. Osteoprotegerin (OPG)

This is a member of the TNF family of receptors involved in bone turnover, and recent studies have shown that it is an important molecule in the atherosclerotic process and contributes to the calcification of small vessels in diabetic patients. OPG expression is induced by HMBG-1 in osteoblasts and attaches to osteoclasts and osteoblasts during endochondral ossification [70].

Current studies have generated quite controversial results. At this point, its role and relationship with inflammatory markers in diabetic patients with peripheral artery disease is quite unclear, and further investigations are needed [71].

All the studies demonstrated that increased levels of OPG correlate with poor outcomes in diabetic patients with CLTI after revascularization [15,72].

Giovannini et al. [73], in a retrospective observational study that analyzed OPG levels in 1393 diabetic patients with and without PAD, demonstrated that OPG levels were significantly higher in PAD vs. non-PAD patients (6.54 ± 7.76 pmol/L vs. 2.98 ± 2.01 pmol/L) and that OPG levels also correlated positively with the clinical severity of PAD.

3.15. Sortilin

Sortilin is a protein that is mainly expressed in hepatocytes; it takes part in the sorting of intracellular proteins between the Golgi network and endocytosomes. The sortilin membrane acts as a receptor for circulating LDL and promotes its integration into hepatocytes via a receptor-dependent mechanism. Following the discovery of the link with the atherosclerotic process, key roles in cytokine release or expression in platelets have also been discovered. It is also involved in LDL uptake by macrophages and the progression of inflammatory mechanisms during the process of atheroma plaque formation as well as its progression [74,75].

Nardella et al. [15] also demonstrated in 264 patients that increased levels of sortilin correlate with poor outcomes in diabetic patients with CLTI after revascularization.

All our findings are summarized in Table 1.

Table 1. Summary of biological markers found in CLTI.

Study	Author	Marker(s)	Population	Findings
Development of a biomarker panel for assessing cardiovascular risk in diabetic patients with chronic limb-threatening ischemia (CLTI): a prospective study	Nardella et al., 2023 [15]	CRP, IL-6, HMGB-1, OPG, Sortilin	264 CLTI patients	Increased levels correlate with poor outcomes in diabetic patients with CLTI after revascularization
Factors Influencing the Risk of Major Amputation in Patients with Diabetic Foot Ulcers Treated by Autologous Cell Therapy	Husakova et al., 2022 [16]	CRP	113 patients with diabetic foot ulcers	Increased levels of CRP in the group that suffered major amputation than in the group that did not
Inflammatory Cytokines Associated with Failure of Lower-Extremity Endovascular Revascularization (LER): A Prospective Study of a Population With Diabetes. Diabetes Care	Biscetti et al., 2019 [18]	CRP, TNF-α	299 patients	Elevated CRP levels in patients with worse vascular outcomes in patients with diabetes TNF-α is associated with worse vascular outcomes especially in diabetic patients
Role of hemostatic risk factors for restenosis in peripheral arterial occlusive disease after transluminal angioplasty	Tschopl et al., 1997 [19]	CRP, D-dimers, Fibrinogen	71 patients	Restenotic patients had higher CRP levels at 3 and 6 months after PTA Increased levels of D-dimers at 1, 24 and 48 h after PTA Fibrinogen levels higher 48 h after PTA. Restenotic patients had higher plasma fibrinogen levels at follow-up. Patients with III/IV stages had significantly higher fibrinogen values
Inflammation and Loss of Skeletal Muscle Mass in Chronic Limb Threatening Ischemia	Ferreira et al., 2023 [20]	CRP, Fibrinogen	116 patients, 46% with CLTI	Increased CRP serum levels vs. non-CLTI patients CLTI patients had increased fibrinogen levels than non-CLTI patients
Fibrinogen and mortality in chronic critical limb ischemia	Pedrinelli et al., 1999 [27]	Fibrinogen	108 patients, 78 with CLTI	48 deceased patients from CLTI group, with increased fibrinogen values in the first 6 months on follow-up and in a Cox-multivariate analysis only plasma fibrinogen had an independent predictive value
A Pro-Inflammatory Biomarker-Profile Predicts Amputation-Free Survival in Patients with Severe Limb Ischemia	Gremmels et al., 2019 [33]	IL-6	108 patients	Il-6 values were higher in patients that reached a major endpoint (death and/or major amputation)
The Inflammatory Pattern of Chronic Limb-Threatening Ischemia in Muscles: The TNF-α Hypothesis	Caicedo et al., 2022 [35]	TNF-α	35 patients	Increased levels in 68.6% of patients and concluded that the marker is important in the progression of ischemia, especially in diabetic patients
Expression of Vascular Cell Adhesion Molecule-1 in Peripheral Artery Disease is Enriched in Patients with Advanced Kidney Disease	Lee et al., 2021 [39]	VCAM-1	51 patients	Elevated levels
Critical limb ischemia patients clinically improving with medical treatment have lower neutrophil-to-lymphocyte and platelet-to-lymphocyte ratios	Erdoğan et al., 2021 [43]	NLR	268 patients	Patients with NLR higher that 4.64 did not respond to medical treatment
Neutrophil-to-lymphocyte ratio and its association with critical limb ischemia in PAOD patients	Gary et al., 2013 [44]	NLR	2121 patients	Increased values in patients with CLTI
Neutrophil-to-lymphocyte ratio associated with an increased risk of mortality in patients with critical limb ischemia	Su et al., 2021 [47]	NLR	195 patients	Increase levels associated with major cardiovascular or major limb events
An elevated neutrophil-lymphocyte ratio independently predicts mortality in chronic critical limb ischemia	Spark et al., 2010 [46]	NLR	149 patients	Elevated levels in patients with higher risk at developing major adverse limb events
Inflammation Is a Histological Characteristic of Skeletal Muscle in Chronic Limb Threatening Ischemia	Ferreira et al., 2024 [51]	IL-8	119 patients	Higher serum levels

Table 1. *Cont.*

Study	Author	Marker(s)	Population	Findings
Relationship of Inflammatory Biomarkers with Severity of Peripheral Arterial Disease	Igari et al., 2016 [54]	PTX3	89 patients	PTX3 highly correlated with the severity of the disease
Lipocalin-2 and Calprotectin Potential Prognosis Biomarkers in Peripheral Arterial Disease	Saenz-Pipaon et al., 2022 [55]	Calprotectin and lipocalin-2	331 patients	High serum levels associated with major limb and major cardiovascular events in CLTI patients
Pro-inflammatory genetic profiles in subjects with peripheral arterial occlusive disease and critical limb ischemia	Flex A. et al., 2007 [60]	E-selectin	157 patients	E-selectin polymorphism associated with CLTI
E-Selectin and restenosis after femoropopliteal angioplasty: prognostic impact of the Ser128Arg genotype and plasma levels	Mlekusch et al. 2004 [61]	E-selectin	175 patients	High values associated with restenosis risk in CLTI patients
Inflammatory mediators are associated with 1-year mortality in critical limb ischemia	Barani et al., 2005 [76]	Neopterin	256 patients	Associated with 1-year mortality in CLTI patients
Are there differences of inflammatory bio-markers between diabetic and non-diabetic patients with critical limb ischemia?	Bertz et al., 2006 [66]	Neopterin	259 patients	High values in diabetic patients with CLTI
Serum high mobility group box-1 levels associated with cardiovascular events after lower extremity revascularization: a prospective study of a diabetic population	Rando et al., 2022 [69]	HGMB-1	201 patients	High serum levels in CLTI patients that developed limb related events or major cardiovascular events
Osteoprotegerin concentration is associated with the presence and severity of peripheral arterial disease in type 2 diabetes mellitus	Demková K. et al., 2018 [72]	OPG	165 patients	High levels associated with the severity of CLTI

Also, in Table 2, we detail the mechanisms and effects of these markers, as well as the specific method for laboratory determination.

Table 2. Summary of actions and effects of the studied markers.

Biomarker	Marker Type	Action and Effects	Methods for Identification
CRP	Inflammatory	- Inhibits the nitric oxide and Increases endothelin-1 production contributing to endothelial dysfunction (it impairs endothelial-dependent vascular relaxation) - Contributes also to thrombus formation - Induces leukocyte recruitment into atherosclerotic tissue	Immunoturbidimetric determination
D-dimers	Thrombotic	- Increases fibrin turnover	Coagulometry
Fibrinogen	Thrombotic	- Pro-inflammatory	Coagulometry
Interleukin-6	Inflammatory	- Pro-inflammatory cytokine, released by leukocytes and stromal cells	Chemiluminescence
Tumor Necrosis Factor	Inflammatory	- Inflammatory factor probably through upregulating the transcytosis of LDL across endothelial cells and retaining the LDL-particles in vessel walls [77]	ELISA Technique
ICAM-1 and VCAM-1	Inflammatory	- Endothelial adhesion - Inflammatory molecules	Immunoassay determination Flow-cytometric method ELISA Technique
NLR	inflammatory	- Neutrophils may make atherosclerotic plaque more vulnerable and secrete inflammatory mediators	Flow-cytometric method, spectrophotometry
Interleukin-8	Inflammatory	- It is involved by recruiting inflammatory cells into the atherosclerotic plaques	Chemiluminescence ELISA Technique
Pentraxin-3	Inflammatory	- Similar to CRP, being a cognate molecule of CRP - Regulatory role in inflammation and extracellular matrix organization and remodeling [78]	Immunoturbidimetric determination

Table 2. *Cont.*

Biomarker	Marker Type	Action and Effects	Methods for Identification
Calprotectin and NGAL	Inflammatory	- Pro-inflammatory	ELISA Technique
E-selectin	Inflammatory	- Adhesion molecule mediating leukocyte extravasation	Multiplex immunoassay determination Flow-cytometric method ELISA Technique
Neopterin	Inflammatory	- Is a metabolite of guanosine triphosphate with proinflammatory action	Immunoenzymatic assay
HMGB-1	Inflammatory	- Mediates inflammation	ELISA Technique
Osteoprotegerin (OPG)	Inflammatory	- Acts in endothelial dysfunction as a proinflammatory and pro-calcification marker	ELISA Technique
Sortilin	Inflammatory	- Arterial wall inflammation and calcification	Flow-cytometric method

4. Discussions

The atherosclerotic process begins with endothelial dysfunction based on the concurrent action of multiple risk factors (hypertension, diabetes, obesity, high LDL, chronic kidney disease, or other inflammatory diseases) [5]. Following damage to the vascular endothelium, a series of pro-inflammatory cytokines (IL6, CRP), extracellular vesicles, a series of proteases, and adhesion molecules (E-selectin, ICAM, VCAM) are released, which recruit monocytes and infiltrate the vascular lining [18]. Another phenomenon occurring currently is the activation of environmental factors that contribute to atheroma plaque progression through macrophage polarization. An important role is also played by extracellular vesicles of thrombocytic origin, which play an extremely important role in thrombosis phenomena in the atheroma plaque in the context of exposure to procoagulant factors. Thrombotic phenomena in turn lead to increased levels of biomarkers such as CRP, ICAM, VCAM, interleukin family, or vascular smooth muscle cells (VSMCs) [79].

Peripheral arterial disease, and in particular its end stage, CLTI, is associated with significant morbidity, mortality, and a serious impairment of quality of life. CLTI is often accompanied by atherosclerotic processes in all vascular beds, and this association presents a significant risk of ischemic events and death in these patients, much more than the single impairment in other vascular beds [5].

Currently, PAD risk assessment is performed only on clinical classifications and an ABI basis and is not highly specific, especially in patients with concomitant diabetes mellitus (where we know all too well of the presence of false-positive ABI values due to massive calcifications of infragenicular vessels).

In this context, PAD is an often-underestimated pathology, especially in patients with diabetes, thus leading to the need for early diagnostic and prognostic markers.

Not all markers presented have sufficient studies to be considered diagnostic or prognostic markers in CLTI. Of those we present, CRP, fibrinogen, D-dimer, IL-6, IL-8, and NLR have multiple studies that demonstrate their value. We consider that the others need further studies to prove their involvement in the atherosclerosis process and the possibility of their inclusion as diagnostic or prognostic markers for major cardiac events or events related to the performance of revascularization procedures.

Besides the markers studied and presented in this review, it would be more important to pay attention to extracellular vesicles and micro-RNAs that would show an effect in PAD and CLTI.

There is not enough information in the literature related to biomarkers present in CLTI, but the discovery of these links would clearly contribute to the discovery of new diagnostic and therapeutic methods for these patients.

There are several studies focusing on the identification of some types of microRNAs in CLTI, such as miR-1827, miR-323b-5p, miR-4739, and miR-27b, which are significantly elevated in the serum of these patients. It is also worth studying the interaction between other circulating elements and micro-RNAs in different stages of atherosclerosis [80].

Another important phenomenon that needs to be discussed when speaking about atherosclerosis and CLTI relates to the extremely important role that the innate and adaptive immune system appears to play in this process. The attraction of cytokines and the expression of adhesion molecules seem to trigger a cascade response of immune cells, which leads to the nucleation of a lesion in the vascular wall that may subsequently develop into an atherosclerotic plaque. In addition, dendritic cells, macrophages, and T cells (all belonging to the immune system) appear to play a role in the development of the atheroma plaque. Furthermore, along the way, these cells undergo apoptosis and must be eliminated, leading to secondary necrosis and the formation of a necrotic core in the plaque. Programmed cell death at this level can also lead to the progression of atherosclerosis. Plaque development is favored by the tipping of the scales toward autoimmune cell recruitment and continued macrophage proliferation [81].

Atherosclerotic disease is considered to have a multifactorial etiology that includes both genetic determinism and the action of environmental factors [82].

There is current evidence of the importance of genetic factors through various population studies, with an estimated heritability of PAD of approximately 20–58% [83]. There are currently a number of genes that are involved in atherosclerosis: genes that are involved in lipid metabolism (*APOB* on chromosome 2p24.1), genes involved in inflammatory mechanisms in the vascular wall (IL6 gene located on 7p15.3), genes involved in blood pressure regulation (*ACE* genes), genes involved in the function of Vascular Smooth Muscle Cells, genes involved in the maintenance of vascular homeostasis, or genes that contribute to the process of atherothrombosis. The discovery of the genes involved in the pathophysiological mechanisms of BAP is a step toward finding an early diagnosis as well as a complete and effective treatment of this pathology [84].

5. Conclusions

This review gathered data on inflammatory markers with a role in peripheral arterial disease in general and critical ischemia in particular, noting that the search did not identify exact associations between inflammatory markers and what current guidelines define as critical ischemia.

Therefore, we believe that further studies are needed to identify the targeted feasibility of using inflammatory markers in the diagnosis, prognosis, and treatment of critical ischemia in practice.

Thus, we need studies to identify different risk classes according to the value of the markers and to identify the disease prognosis according to the evolution of these markers. Also, we need to identify these markers in the clinical staging of the disease in the post-revascularization phase, both in terms of events related to the revascularized limb and in terms of major cardiac events.

Author Contributions: Conceptualization, A.I.P., A.L.R. and S.B.; methodology, A.I.P., A.L.R.; software, C.V.; validation, D.V., R.P. and A.L.R.; formal analysis, R.R.O. and S.B.; investigation, A.I.P. and A.L.R.; resources, R.R.O., A.I.P. and A.L.R.; data curation, A.I.P., S.B. and A.L.R.; writing—original draft preparation, A.I.P.; writing—review and editing, A.L.R.; visualization, A.I.P., A.L.R., S.B., R.R.O., R.P., C.V. and D.V.; supervision, D.V. and R.P.; project administration, A.I.P. and A.L.R. All authors have read and agreed to the published version of the manuscript.

Funding: We would like to acknowledge "Victor Babes" University of Medicine and Pharmacy Timisoara for their support in covering the costs of publication for this research paper.

Conflicts of Interest: The authors declare no conflicts of interest.

References

1. Abu Dabrh, A.M.; Steffen, M.W.; Undavalli, C.; Asi, N.; Wang, Z.; Elamin, M.B.; Conte, M.S.; Murad, M.H. The Natural History of Untreated Severe or Critical Limb Ischemia. *J. Vasc. Surg.* **2015**, *62*, 1642–1651.e3. [CrossRef] [PubMed]
2. Conte, M.S.; Bradbury, A.W.; Kolh, P.; White, J.V.; Dick, F.; Fitridge, R.; Mills, J.L.; Ricco, J.-B.; Suresh, K.R.; Murad, M.H.; et al. Global Vascular Guidelines on the Management of Chronic Limb-Threatening Ischemia. *Eur. J. Vasc. Endovasc. Surg.* **2019**, *58*, S1–S109.e33. [CrossRef] [PubMed]
3. Mills, J.L.; Conte, M.S.; Armstrong, D.G.; Pomposelli, F.B.; Schanzer, A.; Sidawy, A.N.; Andros, G. The Society for Vascular Surgery Lower Extremity Threatened Limb Classification System: Risk Stratification Based on Wound, Ischemia, and Foot Infection (WIfI). *J. Vasc. Surg.* **2014**, *59*, 220–234.e2. [CrossRef]
4. Brevetti, G.; Giugliano, G.; Brevetti, L.; Hiatt, W.R. Inflammation in Peripheral Artery Disease. *Circulation* **2010**, *122*, 1862–1875. [CrossRef]
5. Saenz-Pipaon, G.; Martinez-Aguilar, E.; Orbe, J.; Gonzalez Miqueo, A.; Fernandez-Alonso, L.; Paramo, J.A.; Roncal, C. The Role of Circulating Biomarkers in Peripheral Arterial Disease. *Int. J. Mol. Sci.* **2021**, *22*, 3601. [CrossRef] [PubMed]
6. Hayek, S.S.; MacNamara, J.; Tahhan, A.S.; Awad, M.; Yadalam, A.; Ko, Y.-A.; Healy, S.; Hesaroieh, I.; Ahmed, H.; Gray, B.; et al. Circulating Progenitor Cells Identify Peripheral Arterial Disease in Patients With Coronary Artery Disease. *Circ. Res.* **2016**, *119*, 564–571. [CrossRef] [PubMed]
7. Gabay, C.; Kushner, I. Acute-Phase Proteins and Other Systemic Responses to Inflammation. *N. Engl. J. Med.* **1999**, *340*, 448–454. [CrossRef] [PubMed]
8. Pepys, M.B.; Rowe, I.F.; Baltz, M.L. C-Reactive Protein: Binding to Lipids and Lipoproteins. *Int. Rev. Exp. Pathol.* **1985**, *27*, 83–111. [PubMed]
9. Ridker, P.M.; Hennekens, C.H.; Buring, J.E.; Rifai, N. C-Reactive Protein and Other Markers of Inflammation in the Prediction of Cardiovascular Disease in Women. *N. Engl. J. Med.* **2000**, *342*, 836–843. [CrossRef]
10. Koenig, W.; Sund, M.; Fröhlich, M.; Fischer, H.-G.; Löwel, H.; Döring, A.; Hutchinson, W.L.; Pepys, M.B. C-Reactive Protein, a Sensitive Marker of Inflammation, Predicts Future Risk of Coronary Heart Disease in Initially Healthy Middle-Aged Men. *Circulation* **1999**, *99*, 237–242. [CrossRef]
11. Ridker, P.M.; Buring, J.E.; Shih, J.; Matias, M.; Hennekens, C.H. Prospective Study of C-Reactive Protein and the Risk of Future Cardiovascular Events Among Apparently Healthy Women. *Circulation* **1998**, *98*, 731–733. [CrossRef] [PubMed]
12. Ridker, P.M.; Cushman, M.; Stampfer, M.J.; Tracy, R.P.; Hennekens, C.H. Plasma Concentration of C-Reactive Protein and Risk of Developing Peripheral Vascular Disease. *Circulation* **1998**, *97*, 425–428. [CrossRef] [PubMed]
13. Ridker, P.M.; Stampfer, M.J.; Rifai, N. Novel Risk Factors for Systemic AtherosclerosisA Comparison of C-Reactive Protein, Fibrinogen, Homocysteine, Lipoprotein(a), and Standard Cholesterol Screening as Predictors of Peripheral Arterial Disease. *JAMA* **2001**, *285*, 2481–2485. [CrossRef] [PubMed]
14. McDermott, M.M.; Greenland, P.; Green, D.; Guralnik, J.M.; Criqui, M.H.; Liu, K.; Chan, C.; Pearce, W.H.; Taylor, L.; Ridker, P.M.; et al. D-Dimer, Inflammatory Markers, and Lower Extremity Functioning in Patients With and Without Peripheral Arterial Disease. *Circulation* **2003**, *107*, 3191–3198. [CrossRef] [PubMed]
15. Nardella, E.; Biscetti, F.; Rando, M.M.; Cecchini, A.L.; Nicolazzi, M.A.; Rossini, E.; Angelini, F.; Iezzi, R.; Eraso, L.H.; Dimuzio, P.J.; et al. Development of a Biomarker Panel for Assessing Cardiovascular Risk in Diabetic Patients with Chronic Limb-Threatening Ischemia (CLTI): A Prospective Study. *Cardiovasc. Diabetol.* **2023**, *22*, 136. [CrossRef]
16. Husakova, J.; Bem, R.; Fejfarova, V.; Jirkovska, A.; Woskova, V.; Jarosikova, R.; Lovasova, V.; Jude, E.B.; Dubsky, M. Factors Influencing the Risk of Major Amputation in Patients with Diabetic Foot Ulcers Treated by Autologous Cell Therapy. *J. Diabetes Res.* **2022**, *2022*, 3954740. [CrossRef]
17. Fujii, M.; Terashi, H.; Yokono, K.; Armstrong, D.G. The Degree of Blood Supply and Infection Control Needed to Treat Diabetic Chronic Limb-Threatening Ischemia with Forefoot Osteomyelitis. *J. Am. Podiatr. Med. Assoc.* **2021**, *111*. [CrossRef]
18. Biscetti, F.; Ferraro, P.M.; Hiatt, W.R.; Angelini, F.; Nardella, E.; Cecchini, A.L.; Santoliquido, A.; Pitocco, D.; Landolfi, R.; Flex, A. Inflammatory Cytokines Associated With Failure of Lower-Extremity Endovascular Revascularization (LER): A Prospective Study of a Population With Diabetes. *Diabetes Care* **2019**, *42*, 1939–1945. [CrossRef]
19. Tschöpl, M.; Tsakiris, D.A.; Marbet, G.A.; Labs, K.-H.; Jäger, K. Role of Hemostatic Risk Factors for Restenosis in Peripheral Arterial Occlusive Disease After Transluminal Angioplasty. *Arterioscler. Thromb. Vasc. Biol.* **1997**, *17*, 3208–3214. [CrossRef]
20. Ferreira, J.; Carneiro, A.; Vila, I.; Silva, C.; Cunha, C.; Longatto-Filho, A.; Mesquita, A.; Cotter, J.; Mansilha, A.; Correia-Neves, M.; et al. Inflammation and Loss of Skeletal Muscle Mass in Chronic Limb Threatening Ischemia. *Ann. Vasc. Surg.* **2023**, *88*, 164–173. [CrossRef]
21. Lee F Gerald, R.; Lowe Gordon, D.O.; Rumley Ann, A.J.F. Fibrin D-Dimer, Haemostatic Factors and Peripheral Arterial Disease. *Thromb. Haemost.* **1995**, *74*, 828–832. [CrossRef]
22. Komarov, A.L.; Panchenko, E.P.; Dobrovolsky, A.B.; Karpov, Y.A.; Deev, A.D.; Titaeva, E.V.; Davletov, K.K.; Eshkeeva, A.R.; Markova, L.A. D-Dimer and Platelet Aggregability Are Related to Thrombotic Events in Patients with Peripheral Arterial Occlusive Disease. *Eur. Heart J.* **2002**, *23*, 1309–1316. [CrossRef] [PubMed]
23. Vidula, H.; Tian, L.; Liu, K.; Criqui, M.H.; Ferrucci, L.; Pearce, W.H.; Greenland, P.; Green, D.; Tan, J.; Garside, D.B.; et al. Biomarkers of Inflammation and Thrombosis as Predictors of Near-Term Mortality in Patients with Peripheral Arterial Disease: A Cohort Study. *Ann. Intern. Med.* **2008**, *148*, 85–93. [CrossRef] [PubMed]

24. Kleinegris, M.C.F.; ten Cate, H.; ten Cate-Hoek, A.J. D-Dimer as a Marker for Cardiovascular and Arterial Thrombotic Events in Patients with Peripheral Arterial Disease. *Thromb. Haemost.* **2013**, *110*, 233–243. [CrossRef] [PubMed]
25. Surma, S.; Banach, M. Fibrinogen and Atherosclerotic Cardiovascular Diseases—Review of the Literature and Clinical Studies. *Int. J. Mol. Sci.* **2021**, *23*, 193. [CrossRef]
26. Ernst, E.; Resch, K.L. Fibrinogen as a Cardiovascular Risk Factor. *Ann. Intern. Med.* **1993**, *118*, 956–963. [CrossRef]
27. Pedrinelli, R.; Dell Omo, G.; Barchielli, A.; Berchiolli, R.; Melillo, E.; Mariani, M.; Balbarini, A.; Ferrari, M. Fibrinogen and Mortality in Chronic Critical Limb Ischaemia. *J. Intern. Med.* **1999**, *245*, 75–81. [CrossRef] [PubMed]
28. Uciechowski, P.; Dempke, W.C.M. Interleukin-6: A Masterplayer in the Cytokine Network. *Oncology* **2020**, *98*, 131–137. [CrossRef]
29. Esmon, C.T. Role of Coagulation Inhibitors in Inflammation. *Thromb. Haemost.* **2001**, *86*, 51–56. [CrossRef]
30. Ridker, P.M.; Rifai, N.; Stampfer, M.J.; Hennekens, C.H. Plasma Concentration of Interleukin-6 and the Risk of Future Myocardial Infarction Among Apparently Healthy Men. *Circulation* **2000**, *101*, 1767–1772. [CrossRef]
31. Danesh, J.; Kaptoge, S.; Mann, A.G.; Sarwar, N.; Wood, A.; Angleman, S.B.; Wensley, F.; Higgins, J.P.T.; Lennon, L.; Eiriksdottir, G.; et al. Long-Term Interleukin-6 Levels and Subsequent Risk of Coronary Heart Disease: Two New Prospective Studies and a Systematic Review. *PLoS Med.* **2008**, *5*, e78. [CrossRef]
32. Sattar, N.; Murray, H.M.; Welsh, P.; Blauw, G.J.; Buckley, B.M.; Cobbe, S.; de Craen, A.J.M.; Lowe, G.D.; Jukema, J.W.; Macfarlane, P.W.; et al. Are Markers of Inflammation More Strongly Associated with Risk for Fatal Than for Nonfatal Vascular Events? *PLoS Med.* **2009**, *6*, e1000099. [CrossRef] [PubMed]
33. Gremmels, H.; Teraa, M.; de Jager, S.C.A.; Pasterkamp, G.; de Borst, G.J.; Verhaar, M.C. A Pro-Inflammatory Biomarker-Profile Predicts Amputation-Free Survival in Patients with Severe Limb Ischemia. *Sci. Rep.* **2019**, *9*, 10740. [CrossRef] [PubMed]
34. Naldini, A.; Carraro, F. Role of Inflammatory Mediators in Angiogenesis. *Curr. Drug Targets-Inflamm. Allergy* **2005**, *4*, 3–8. [CrossRef] [PubMed]
35. Caicedo, D.; Alvarez, C.V.; Perez-Romero, S.; Devesa, J. The Inflammatory Pattern of Chronic Limb-Threatening Ischemia in Muscles: The TNF-α Hypothesis. *Biomedicines* **2022**, *10*, 489. [CrossRef] [PubMed]
36. Foussard, N.; Rouault, P.; Cornuault, L.; Bourguignon, C.; Grouthier, V.; Chapouly, C.; Gadeau, A.-P.; Couffinhal, T.; Renault, M.-A. ICAM1 Expression by the Microvasculature Impairs Capillary Perfusion Which Compromises Hind Limb Ischemia Recovery in Diabetic Mice. *Arch. Cardiovasc. Dis. Suppl.* **2023**, *15*, 184–185. [CrossRef]
37. González-Amaro, R.; Sanchez-Madrid, F. Cell Adhesion Molecules: Selectins and Integrins. *Crit. Rev. Immunol.* **1999**, *19*, 389–429. [PubMed]
38. Tsakiris, D.A.; Tschöpl, M.; Jäger, K.; Haefeli, W.E.; Wolf, F.; Marbet, G.A. Circulating Cell Adhesion Molecules and Endothelial Markers before and after Transluminal Angioplasty in Peripheral Arterial Occlusive Disease. *Atherosclerosis* **1999**, *142*, 193–200. [CrossRef]
39. Lee, P.-T.; Liao, I.-C.; Lee, C.-H.; Hsu, L.-W.; Liu, P.-Y. Expression of Vascular Cell Adhesion Molecule-1 in Peripheral Artery Disease Is Enriched in Patients with Advanced Kidney Disease. *Acta Cardiol. Sin.* **2021**, *37*, 591.
40. Edlinger, C.; Lichtenauer, M.; Wernly, B.; Pistulli, R.; Paar, V.; Prodinger, C.; Krizanic, F.; Thieme, M.; Kammler, J.; Jung, C.; et al. Disease-Specific Characteristics of Vascular Cell Adhesion Molecule-1 Levels in Patients with Peripheral Artery Disease. *Heart Vessel.* **2019**, *34*, 976–983. [CrossRef]
41. Song, M.; Graubard, B.I.; Rabkin, C.S.; Engels, E.A. Neutrophil-to-Lymphocyte Ratio and Mortality in the United States General Population. *Sci. Rep.* **2021**, *11*, 464. [CrossRef] [PubMed]
42. Mortaz, E.; Alipoor, S.D.; Adcock, I.M.; Mumby, S.; Koenderman, L. Update on Neutrophil Function in Severe Inflammation. *Front. Immunol.* **2018**, *9*, 411381. [CrossRef]
43. Erdoğan, S.B.; Selçuk, Ü.N.; Baştopçu, M.; Arslanhan, G.; Çakmak, A.Y.; Kuplay, H.; Mete, E.M.T.; Aka, S.A. Critical Limb Ischemia Patients Clinically Improving with Medical Treatment Have Lower Neutrophil-to-Lymphocyte and Platelet-to-Lymphocyte Ratios. *Vascular* **2021**, *29*, 920–926. [CrossRef]
44. Gary, T.; Pichler, M.; Belaj, K.; Hafner, F.; Gerger, A.; Froehlich, H.; Eller, P.; Pilger, E.; Brodmann, M. Neutrophil-to-Lymphocyte Ratio and Its Association with Critical Limb Ischemia in PAOD Patients. *PLoS ONE* **2013**, *8*, e56745. [CrossRef] [PubMed]
45. Su, M.-I.; Liu, C.-W. Neutrophil-to-Lymphocyte Ratio Associated with an Increased Risk of Mortality in Patients with Critical Limb Ischemia. *PLoS ONE* **2021**, *16*, e0252030. [CrossRef]
46. Spark, J.I.; Sarveswaran, J.; Blest, N.; Charalabidis, P.; Asthana, S. An Elevated Neutrophil-Lymphocyte Ratio Independently Predicts Mortality in Chronic Critical Limb Ischemia. *J. Vasc. Surg.* **2010**, *52*, 632–636. [CrossRef]
47. Hedges, J.C.; Singer, C.A.; Gerthoffer, W.T. Mitogen-Activated Protein Kinases Regulate Cytokine Gene Expression in Human Airway Myocytes. *Am. J. Respir. Cell Mol. Biol.* **2000**, *23*, 86–94. [CrossRef]
48. Murphy, P.M.; Tiffany, H.L. Cloning of Complementary DNA Encoding a Functional Human Interleukin-8 Receptor. *Science* **1991**, *253*, 1280–1283. [CrossRef]
49. DeForge, L.E.; Preston, A.M.; Takeuchi, E.; Kenney, J.; Boxer, L.A.; Remick, D.G. Regulation of Interleukin 8 Gene Expression by Oxidant Stress. *J. Biol. Chem.* **1993**, *268*, 25568–25576. [CrossRef]
50. Parmar, J.H.; Aslam, M.; Standfield, N.J. Percutaneous Transluminal Angioplasty of Lower Limb Arteries Causes a Systemic Inflammatory Response. *Ann. Vasc. Surg.* **2009**, *23*, 569–576. [CrossRef]

51. Ferreira, J.; Afonso, J.; Longatto-Filho, A.; Roque, S.; Carneiro, A.; Vila, I.; Silva, C.; Cunha, C.; Mesquita, A.; Cotter, J.; et al. Inflammation Is a Histological Characteristic of Skeletal Muscle in Chronic Limb Threatening Ischemia. *Ann. Vasc. Surg.* **2024**, *99*, 10–18. [CrossRef] [PubMed]
52. Garlanda, C.; Bottazzi, B.; Bastone, A.; Mantovani, A. Pentraxins at the Crossroads between Innate Immunity, Inflammation, Matrix Deposition, and Female Fertility. *Annu. Rev. Immunol.* **2004**, *23*, 337–366. [CrossRef] [PubMed]
53. Napoleone, E.; Di Santo, A.; Bastone, A.; Peri, G.; Mantovani, A.; de Gaetano, G.; Donati, M.B.; Lorenzet, R. Long Pentraxin PTX3 Upregulates Tissue Factor Expression in Human Endothelial Cells. *Arterioscler. Thromb. Vasc. Biol.* **2002**, *22*, 782–787. [CrossRef] [PubMed]
54. Igari, K.; Kudo, T.; Toyofuku, T.; Inoue, Y. Relationship of Inflammatory Biomarkers with Severity of Peripheral Arterial Disease. *Int. J. Vasc. Med.* **2016**, *2016*, 6015701. [CrossRef] [PubMed]
55. Saenz-Pipaon, G.; Ravassa, S.; Larsen, K.L.; Martinez-Aguilar, E.; Orbe, J.; Rodriguez, J.A.; Fernandez-Alonso, L.; Gonzalez, A.; Martín-Ventura, J.L.; Paramo, J.A.; et al. Lipocalin-2 and Calprotectin Potential Prognosis Biomarkers in Peripheral Arterial Disease. *Eur. J. Vasc. Endovasc. Surg.* **2022**, *63*, 648–656. [CrossRef] [PubMed]
56. Oberoi, R.; Bogalle, E.P.; Matthes, L.A.; Schuett, H.; Koch, A.-K.; Grote, K.; Schieffer, B.; Schuett, J.; Luchtefeld, M. Lipocalin (LCN) 2 Mediates Pro-Atherosclerotic Processes and Is Elevated in Patients with Coronary Artery Disease. *PLoS ONE* **2015**, *10*, e0137924. [CrossRef]
57. Wang, Y.; Lam, K.S.L.; Kraegen, E.W.; Sweeney, G.; Zhang, J.; Tso, A.W.K.; Chow, W.-S.; Wat, N.M.S.; Xu, J.Y.; Hoo, R.L.C.; et al. Lipocalin-2 Is an Inflammatory Marker Closely Associated with Obesity, Insulin Resistance, and Hyperglycemia in Humans. *Clin. Chem.* **2007**, *53*, 34–41. [CrossRef] [PubMed]
58. Mazo, I.B.; Gutierrez-Ramos, J.-C.; Frenette, P.S.; Hynes, R.O.; Wagner, D.D.; von Andrian, U.H. Hematopoietic Progenitor Cell Rolling in Bone Marrow Microvessels: Parallel Contributions by Endothelial Selectins and Vascular Cell Adhesion Molecule 1. *J. Exp. Med.* **1998**, *188*, 465–474. [CrossRef]
59. Quiroz, H.J.; Valencia, S.F.; Shao, H.; Li, Y.; Ortiz, Y.Y.; Parikh, P.P.; Lassance-Soares, R.M.; Vazquez-Padron, R.I.; Liu, Z.-J.; Velazquez, O.C. E-Selectin-Overexpressing Mesenchymal Stem Cell Therapy Confers Improved Reperfusion, Repair, and Regeneration in a Murine Critical Limb Ischemia Model. *Front. Cardiovasc. Med.* **2022**, *8*, 826687. [CrossRef]
60. Flex, A.; Gaetani, E.; Angelini, F.; Sabusco, A.; Chillà, C.; Straface, G.; Biscetti, F.; Pola, P.; Castellot Jr, J.J.; Pola, R. Pro-Inflammatory Genetic Profiles in Subjects with Peripheral Arterial Occlusive Disease and Critical Limb Ischemia. *J. Intern. Med.* **2007**, *262*, 124–130. [CrossRef]
61. Mlekusch, W.; Exner, M.; Schillinger, M.; Sabeti, S.; Mannhalter, C.; Minar, E.; Wagner, O. E-Selectin and Restenosis after Femoropopliteal Angioplasty: Prognostic Impact of the Ser128Arg Genotype and Plasma Levels. *Thromb. Haemost.* **2004**, *91*, 171–179. [CrossRef] [PubMed]
62. Shirai, R.; Sato, K.; Yamashita, T.; Yamaguchi, M.; Okano, T.; Watanabe-Kominato, K.; Watanabe, R.; Matsuyama, T.; Ishibashi-Ueda, H.; Koba, S.; et al. Neopterin Counters Vascular Inflammation and Atherosclerosis. *J. Am. Heart Assoc.* **2024**, *7*, e007359. [CrossRef] [PubMed]
63. Gur, D.O.; Gur, O.; Guzel, S.; Akyuz, A.; Gurkan, S.; Alpsoy, S.; Gulec, N.S.; Koc, F. Inflammatory Mediators across the Spectrum of Ankle-Brachial Index. *J. Atheroscler. Thromb.* **2019**, *26*, 351–361.
64. Pacileo, M.; Cirillo, P.; De Rosa, S.; Chiariello, M. Neopterin Is Not Only a Marker of Inflammation but Might Be an Active Effector in Diabetic Patients with Critical Limb Ischemia. *Int. Angiol.* **2008**, *27*, 269. [PubMed]
65. Signorelli, S.S.; Anzaldi, M.; Fiore, V.; Candido, S.; Di Marco, R.; Mangano, K.; Quattrocchi, C.; Neri, S. Neopterin: A Potential Marker in Chronic Peripheral Arterial Disease. *Mol. Med. Rep.* **2013**, *7*, 1855–1858. [CrossRef] [PubMed]
66. Bertz, L.; Barani, J.; Gottsäter, A.; Nilsson, P.M. Are There Differences of Inflammatory Bio-Markers between Diabetic and Non-Diabetic Patients with Critical Limb Ischemia? *Int. Angiol.* **2006**, *25*, 370. [PubMed]
67. Kawahara, K.; Biswas, K.K.; Unoshima, M.; Ito, T.; Kikuchi, K.; Morimoto, Y.; Iwata, M.; Tancharoen, S.; Oyama, Y.; Takenouchi, K.; et al. C-Reactive Protein Induces High-Mobility Group Box-1 Protein Release through Activation of P38MAPK in Macrophage RAW264.7 Cells. *Cardiovasc. Pathol.* **2008**, *17*, 129–138. [CrossRef] [PubMed]
68. Nogueira-Machado, J.A.; Volpe, C.M.D.O.; Veloso, C.A.; Chaves, M.M. HMGB1, TLR and RAGE: A Functional Tripod That Leads to Diabetic Inflammation. *Expert. Opin. Ther. Targets* **2011**, *15*, 1023–1035. [CrossRef] [PubMed]
69. Rando, M.M.; Biscetti, F.; Cecchini, A.L.; Nardella, E.; Nicolazzi, M.A.; Angelini, F.; Iezzi, R.; Eraso, L.H.; Dimuzio, P.J.; Pitocco, D.; et al. Serum High Mobility Group Box-1 Levels Associated with Cardiovascular Events after Lower Extremity Revascularization: A Prospective Study of a Diabetic Population. *Cardiovasc. Diabetol.* **2022**, *21*, 214. [CrossRef]
70. Harper, E.; Forde, H.; Davenport, C.; Rochfort, K.D.; Smith, D.; Cummins, P.M. Vascular Calcification in Type-2 Diabetes and Cardiovascular Disease: Integrative Roles for OPG, RANKL and TRAIL. *Vascul Pharmacol.* **2016**, *82*, 30–40. [CrossRef]
71. Biscetti, F.; Straface, G.; Pitocco, D.; Angelini, F.; Tinelli, G.; Landolfi, R.; Flex, A. Fibroblast Growth Factor 23 Serum Level in Type 2 Diabetic Italian Subjects with Peripheral Arterial Disease and Critical Limb Ischemia. *Eur. Rev. Med. Pharmacol. Sci.* **2016**, *20*, 4048–4054. [PubMed]
72. Demkova, K.; Kozarova, M.; Malachovska, Z.; Javorský, M.; Tkáč, I. Osteoprotegerin Concentration Is Associated with the Presence and Severity of Peripheral Arterial Disease in Type 2 Diabetes Mellitus. *Vasa* **2018**, *47*, 131–135. [CrossRef] [PubMed]
73. Giovannini, S.; Tinelli, G.; Biscetti, F.; Straface, G.; Angelini, F.; Pitocco, D.; Mucci, L.; Landolfi, R.; Flex, A. Serum High Mobility Group Box-1 and Osteoprotegerin Levels Are Associated with Peripheral Arterial Disease and Critical Limb Ischemia in Type 2 Diabetic Subjects. *Cardiovasc. Diabetol.* **2017**, *16*, 99. [CrossRef] [PubMed]

74. Mortensen, M.B.; Kjolby, M.; Gunnersen, S.; Larsen, J.V.; Palmfeldt, J.; Falk, E.; Nykjaer, A.; Bentzon, J.F. Targeting Sortilin in Immune Cells Reduces Proinflammatory Cytokines and Atherosclerosis. *J. Clin. Investig.* **2014**, *124*, 5317–5322. [CrossRef] [PubMed]
75. Patel, K.M.; Strong, A.; Tohyama, J.; Jin, X.; Morales, C.R.; Billheimer, J.; Millar, J.; Kruth, H.; Rader, D.J. Macrophage Sortilin Promotes LDL Uptake, Foam Cell Formation, and Atherosclerosis. *Circ. Res.* **2015**, *116*, 789–796. [CrossRef] [PubMed]
76. Barani, J.; Nilsson, J.-Å.; Mattiasson, I.; Lindblad, B.; Gottsäter, A. Inflammatory Mediators Are Associated with 1-Year Mortality in Critical Limb Ischemia. *J. Vasc. Surg.* **2005**, *42*, 75–80. [CrossRef] [PubMed]
77. Zhang, Y.; Yang, X.; Bian, F.; Wu, P.; Xing, S.; Xu, G.; Li, W.; Chi, J.; Ouyang, C.; Zheng, T.; et al. TNF-α Promotes Early Atherosclerosis by Increasing Transcytosis of LDL across Endothelial Cells: Crosstalk between NF-KB and PPAR-γ. *J. Mol. Cell Cardiol.* **2014**, *72*, 85–94. [CrossRef] [PubMed]
78. Garlanda, C.; Bottazzi, B.; Magrini, E.; Inforzato, A.; Mantovani, A. PTX3, a Humoral Pattern Recognition Molecule, in Innate Immunity, Tissue Repair, and Cancer. *Physiol. Rev.* **2018**, *98*, 623–639. [CrossRef] [PubMed]
79. Piechocki, M.; Przewłocki, T.; Pieniążek, P.; Trystuła, M.; Podolec, J.; Kabłak-Ziembicka, A. A Non-Coronary, Peripheral Arterial Atherosclerotic Disease (Carotid, Renal, Lower Limb) in Elderly Patients—A Review: Part I—Epidemiology, Risk Factors, and Atherosclerosis-Related Diversities in Elderly Patients. *J. Clin. Med.* **2024**, *13*, 1471. [CrossRef]
80. Ring, A.; Ismaeel, A.; Wechsler, M.; Fletcher, E.; Papoutsi, E.; Miserlis, D.; Koutakis, P. MicroRNAs in Peripheral Artery Disease: Potential Biomarkers and Pathophysiological Mechanisms. *Ther. Adv. Cardiovasc. Dis.* **2022**, *16*, 17539447221096940. [CrossRef]
81. Roy, P.; Orecchioni, M.; Ley, K. How the Immune System Shapes Atherosclerosis: Roles of Innate and Adaptive Immunity. *Nat. Rev. Immunol.* **2022**, *22*, 251–265. [CrossRef] [PubMed]
82. Shemirani, A.-H.; Zsóri, K.S.; Javor, A.; Csiki, Z. Genetics in Peripheral Artery Disease. In *Peripheral Arterial Disease*; Sareen, N., Ojha, A., Eds.; IntechOpen: Rijeka, Croatia, 2018; Chapter 8; ISBN 978-1-78984-218-0.
83. Belkin, N.; Damrauer, S.M. Peripheral Arterial Disease Genetics: Progress to Date and Challenges Ahead. *Curr. Cardiol. Rep.* **2017**, *19*, 131. [CrossRef] [PubMed]
84. Butnariu, L.I.; Gorduza, E.V.; Florea, L.; Țarcă, E.; Moisă, Ș.M.; Tradafir, L.M.; Cojocaru, E.; Luca, A.-C.; Stătescu, L.; Bădescu, M.C. The Genetic Architecture of the Etiology of Lower Extremity Peripheral Artery Disease: Current Knowledge and Future Challenges in the Era of Genomic Medicine. *Int. J. Mol. Sci.* **2022**, *23*, 10481. [CrossRef] [PubMed]

biomedicines

MDPI

Article

Predictors of Diabetic Retinopathy in Type 2 Diabetes: A Cross-Sectional Study

Adriana Ivanescu [1,2], Simona Popescu [1,3,*], Radu Ivanescu [2], Monica Potra [1] and Romulus Timar [1,3]

[1] Second Department of Internal Medicine, "Victor Babes" University of Medicine and Pharmacy, 300041 Timisoara, Romania; adriana.ivanescu@umft.ro (A.I.); monica.rusu@umft.ro (M.P.); timar.romulus@umft.ro (R.T.)

[2] Opticlass Ophtalmology Clinic, 300012 Timisoara, Romania

[3] Department of Diabetes, "Pius Brinzeu" Emergency Hospital, 300723 Timisoara, Romania

* Correspondence: popescu.simona@umft.ro

Abstract: Background: Type 2 diabetes mellitus (T2DM) represents one of the most impacting health issues of the modern era, as it is associated with an extensive range of comorbidities. Diabetic retinopathy (DR) is one the utmost severe diabetes complications as it is one of the major causes of vision loss among these patients. Our present research aims to evaluate the most frequent risk factors related to the occurrence of DR in T2DM patients. Method: This study consisted of a research group of 302 participants, priorly diagnosed with T2DM, that were evaluated for the most important risk factors related to the occurrence of DR. Results: Patients had a median age of 64 years, 48% of them being women, with a 12-year median duration of DM and presenting a deficient glycaemic control echoed by a median HbA1C value of 7.5%. From the total number of participants, the total prevalence of DR in different stages of severity was 34.8% with a 95% CI. Statistically significant values were found regarding DM duration ($p = 0.007$), HbA1c > 7.2% ($p = 0.001$) and patients aged over 67 years ($p = 0.0035$), all these parameters being directly linked to DR. Conclusions: Older patients with T2DM that have a longer disease duration and simultaneous comorbidities present a higher risk of DR development, consequently a stringent management of these pathologies is needed.

Keywords: type 2 diabetes mellitus; diabetic retinopathy; risk factors; quality of life

1. Introduction

Type 2 diabetes mellitus (T2DM) is a chronic and progressive cardio-metabolic disorder, ranking among the primary causes of morbidity, disability, and mortality worldwide. According to the International Diabetes Federation (IDF), the global prevalence of diabetes mellitus (DM) was 463 million in 2019 and is projected to reach 700 million by 2045 [1]. Diabetic retinopathy (DR), a prevalent and severe microvascular complication of DM, is a leading cause of blindness among the adult population. In recent years, we noticed an important increase in both the prevalence of DR and the rates of blindness caused by it, representing a significant threat to the quality of life for diabetic patients. With a growing global population, longer lifespans for those with DM, and lifestyle changes elevating DM risk, the medical and economic burden of DR is expected to continue rising. This situation requires the urgent need for comprehensive eye care and extensive treatment strategies to address this pressing public health challenge [2,3].

Despite the decrease in the proportion of diabetic individuals developing proliferative diabetic retinopathy (PDR) and severe vision loss from 1980 to 2008 in populations with better diabetes control, there has been a significant increase in the prevalence of visual impairment and blindness caused by DR between 1990 and 2015. This trend, highlighted by the Vision Loss Expert Group of the Global Burden of Disease Study, is primarily attributed to the rising prevalence of T2DM [4].

Routine eye exams and timely interventions, coupled with systemic management of blood glucose, hypertension, and dyslipidaemia, are vital for reducing vision loss related to DM. Advances in technology and the rise of biologic treatments offer promising new and effective options to achieve this purpose. Nevertheless, the most crucial strategy for preventing ocular complications in diabetic patients remains maintaining strict glycaemic control [5,6].

Additional risk factors for DR encompass dyslipidaemia, high body mass index (BMI), puberty, pregnancy, and cataract surgery. Yet, clinical investigations in diabetic patients have unveiled substantial diversity in the onset and severity of DR, not fully attributable to all these established risk factors. Clinicians acknowledge that not all individuals with poor glycaemic control or uncontrolled blood pressure develop DR. Conversely, some patients with well-maintained glycaemic levels and no hypertension might still experience its onset. Considering these aspects, genetic factors might be involved in this variability. Still, further research is needed to confirm their impact on this pathology, with a future better understanding of DR [4].

The purpose of this this study was to evaluate the main conventional risk factors associated with the occurrence of DR in patients with T2DM.

2. Materials and Methods

2.1. Study Design and Population

This cross-sectional, non-interventional study was conducted at the Outpatient Diabetes Care Facility Centre of the Pius Brinzeu County Emergency Hospital Timisoara between 21 May 2024 to 24 June 2024. From a total of 573 patients that attended their prescheduled visits at the Diabetes Care Center, we enrolled a final number of 302 participants (145 females, 157 males), while 157 patients declined to participate in this research for personal reasons and 114 of them did not meet the inclusion criteria or were excluded due to the presence of any of the undermentioned general or ocular health status. Exclusion criteria referred to severe cognitive impairment or psychiatric disorders that prevented patients from providing informed consent, other medical pathologies that required hospitalisation on the duration of the study or institutionalised patients. Also, exclusion criteria referred to ophthalmologic diseases that impede proper fundus examination (advanced cataract and significant vitreous haemorrhage) or other retinal diseases that interfere with a proper classification of diabetic retinopathy by altering retinal structure (high myopia, retinal detachment, significant epiretinal membranes). Informed consent was obtained from all participants, none of them being involved in the development of this study. This research process was performed according to the Declaration of Helsinki (2013 version) and was approved by the Ethics Committee of the Emergency County Hospital "Pius Brinzeu" Timișoara (approval no. 467, approved on 20 May 2024)

Selected patients were above 18 years of age and have been priorly diagnosed with T2DM. Study participants had a median age of 64 years [57; 70] and a median T2DM duration of 12 years [6; 17]. Patients underwent the standardised general evaluation that is performed by their physician at each visit and also a comprehensive eye exam performed by an ophthalmologist. Study protocol included the assessment and evaluation of demographic characteristics, anthropometric indexes, diabetes mellitus profile and metabolic control, general comorbidities, ocular diabetes complications and smoker status.

2.2. Data Collection and Medical Assessment

Demographic data regarding all patients were obtained from their medical chart. Biological parameters were assessed by performing a full blood panel for all patients during their scheduled visit in the Diabetes Care Center. Diagnosis of T2DM was priorly made by the presence of a fasting plasma glucose level > 7.0 mmol/L (126 mg/dL), a 2-h post load plasma glucose > 11.1 mmol/L (200 mg/dL) or HbA1c level above 6.5% (48 mmol/mol). Disease duration was defined as the number of years passed from DM diagnosis to the date of inclusion in this study.

Anthropometric data, such as height and weight, were measured for each patient. BMI was calculated using the metric system, by dividing the weight measured in kg by squared height measured in meters. According to World Health Organization (WHO), we considered patients with BMI above 25 kg/m^2 to be overweight, while those with BMI equal or above 30 kg/m^2 were diagnosed with obesity.

Blood pressure was measured for all participants using an aneroid sphygmomanometer. Hypertension was considered at a systolic blood pressure above or equal to 140 mmHg and/or diastolic blood pressure values above or equal to 90 mmHg. Presence of cardiovascular disease (CVD), meaning coronary heart disease, strokes or peripheral arterial disease was noted according to patients' medical history.

Diabetic neuropathy was diagnosed by performing nerve conduction velocity (NCV) and with the usage of the Michigan Neuropathy Screening Instrument (MNSI). A positive diagnosis was considered with a MNSI clinical score above 2.5, a questionnaire score above 7 or overall score above 9.5 and a NCV less than 40 m/s.

Chronic kidney disease (CKD) was diagnosed by analysing the creatinine-based estimate of glomerular filtration rate (eGFR) and albumin/creatinine ratio (ACR).

Presence of dyslipidaemia was noted according to lipid panel values. Smoker status was self-reported.

A comprehensive fundus examination with pupil dilation was performed on all patients by a trained ophthalmologist. Presence of cataract or previous cataract surgery with intraocular lens implantation (IOL) was noted. Examination of the central and peripheral retina included assessing the following findings: microaneurysms or retinal haemorrhage, cotton wool spots, hard exudates and macular oedema. Regarding retinal vasculature, the following aspects were evaluated: venous beading (VB), intraretinal microvascular abnormalities (IRMA) and neovascularisation of the optic disc (NVE) or elsewhere in the retina (NVE). Those findings were the basis for DR and diabetic maculopathy (DME) diagnosis, according to the Early Treatment Diabetic Retinopathy Study Design (ETDRS) guidelines. DR was classified as follows: nonproliferative diabetic retinopathy (NPDR) with mild NPDR (at least one microaneurysm), moderate NPDR (microaneurysms or haemorrhages, exudates, cotton wool spots, VB, IRMA) and severe NPDR (microaneurysms or haemorrhages present in all four retinal quadrants, IRMA in at least one quadrant and VB in two or more quadrants) and proliferative diabetic retinopathy (PDR) which was defined by the presence NVE and preretinal or vitreous haemorrhage. DME was considered when exudates or retinal thickening were found within at least one disc diameter from the fovea. Intraocular pressure (IOP) was measured for all patients after the instillation of an anaesthetic and a drop of fluorescein dye by using Perkins handheld applanation tonometer.

2.3. Statistical Analysis

Statistical data were gathered and analysed by using MedCalc R Statistical Software, the 22.016 version, developed by MedCalc Software Ltd. in Ostend, Belgium. This software may be accessed at https://www.medcalc.org (accessed on 30 May 2024) and was used in May 2024. The analysed cohorts were depicted by using median and interquartile range (continuous variables with non-parametric distribution) and minimum and maximum values. The categorical variables are presented by absolute and relative (percentages) frequencies. In order to evaluate the statistical significance of differences in central tendency indicators between the evaluated groups, we used unpaired Student's *t*-test for comparing the arithmetic means of the parametric variables between two groups, Mann–Whitney-U tests for comparing two medians, ANOVA test to analyse the variation of the mean values between more than two groups, respectively, Kruskal–Wallis test to study the variation of the median values between more than two groups.

Regarding the assessment of statistically significant differences between percentages, we performed chi-square tests (for comparison of two proportions) and chi-square for trend (for comparison between more than two proportions). Spearman's correlation coefficient was used to evaluate the strength and direction of the associations between the numerical variables.

To investigate the adjusted strength, direction and significance of the associations between more than two numerical variables, multivariate logistic regression models were built, while to evaluate the association between numerical (independent) and dichotomous (dependent) variables, multivariate logistic regression models were applied.

"Receiver-Operating Characteristics" (ROC) analyses were conducted in order to appraise the performance of continuous variables as predictive factors for a dichotomous outcome. The prediction threshold was considered the Youden's index (the point which maximizes the sum of sensitivity and specificity of the test), while the evaluated variables were considered as valid predictors if the area under the ROC curve was significantly higher than 0.5.

The sample size was a priori calculated to provide a confidence level (1-a) of 0.95 in parallel with a statistical power (1-b) of 0.80 for the study's primary outcome.

In the present research, we provided a 95% confidence interval and considered the threshold of statistical significance at a *p*-value lower than 0.05.

3. Results

This study included a final number of 302 participants, with a median age of 64 years, 48% being women (145 individuals). Patients had a median duration of DM of 12 years, with an inadequate glycaemic control reflected by the median HbA1C value of 7.5%. Most of the study population presented several comorbidities like diabetic polyneuropathy, hypertension, CVD, CKD and dyslipidaemia. The main characteristics of the whole study group are exhibited in Table 1.

Table 1. Characteristics of the studied group.

Variable	Value
Number of patients	302
Women Nr (%) [a]	145 (48.0%)
Age (years) [b]	64 [57; 70]
DM duration (years) [b]	12 [6; 17]
BMI (Kg/m^2) [b]	27 [25; 30.8]
HbA1c (%)[b]	7.5 [7; 8]
Mean IOP (mmHg) [b]	15 [13; 17]
IOP right eye (mmHg) [b]	14 [12; 16]
IOP left eye (mmHg) [b]	16 [14; 18]
Cataract or IOL implant Nr (%) [a]	61 (20.2%)
DR Nr (%) [a]	105 (34.8%)
Hypertension Nr (%) [a]	212 (69.5%)
CVD Nr (%) [a]	236 (78.2%)
Diabetic polyneuropathy Nr (%) [a]	191 (63.3%)
CKD Nr (%) [a]	84 (27.8%)
Dyslipidaemia Nr (%) [a]	150 (49.7%)
Smoker status Nr (%) [a]	59 (19.5%)

Notes: [a] categorical variables are presented by absolute frequency (percentage) in the sample. [b] continuous variables (with non-Gaussian distribution) are indicated by their median (interquartile range); Abbreviations: DM, diabetes mellitus; BMI, body mass index; HbA1C, haemoglobin A1c; IOP, intraocular pressure; IOL, intraocular lens; DR, diabetic retinopathy; CVD, cardiovascular disease; CKD, chronic kidney disease.

In our study group, DR was found in 105 patients, representing a prevalence of 34.8% [28.4–42.1%], 95% CI (Figure 1). According to the ophthalmologic evaluation, most of these patients presented proliferative diabetic retinopathy (PDR) 32.4%, 27.6% presented severe nonproliferative diabetic retinopathy (NPDR), 21% individuals had moderate NPDR, while only 19% of the study group presented a mild stage of NPDR (Figure 2).

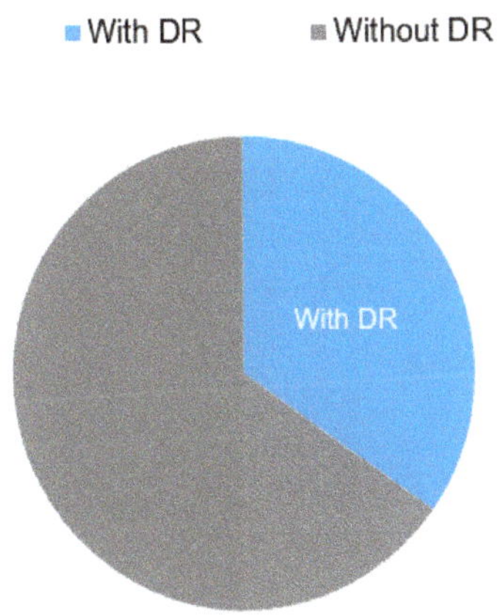

Figure 1. The prevalence of DR.

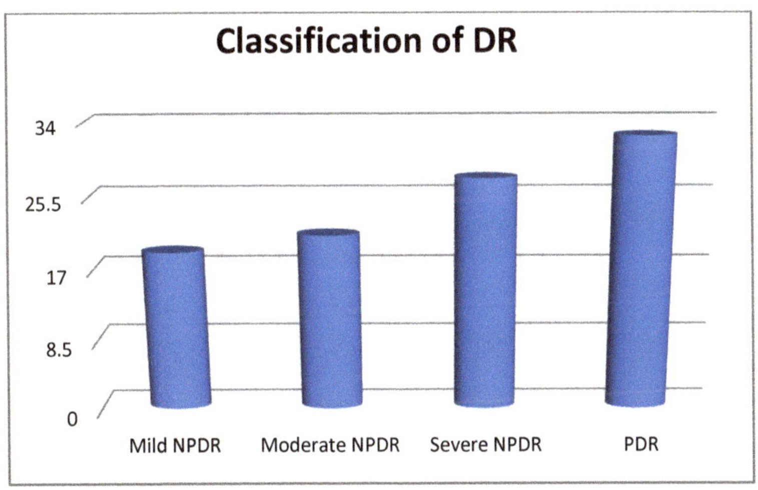

Figure 2. The classification of DR.

In diabetic patients with DR (Table 2) gender distribution was almost equal, with 47.6% women, patients presented a mean age of 66 years old. The mean DM duration was 15 years, while HbA1C median value was 8% [7.5–8.8%]. The majority of these patients were overweight (mean BMI 28.3 Kg/m^2) and presented mostly cardiovascular comorbidities (hypertension 78.1% and CVD 86.7%), but also diabetic polyneuropathy (71.4%) and dyslipidaemia (59%). Presence of DME was found in 18.1% of patients with DR, while intraocular pressure was within normal range in this subgroup (mean IOP 15.5 mmHg). Smoking status was self-reported among 25.7% of patients.

Table 2. Characteristics of patients with DR.

Variable	Value
Number of patients	105
Women Nr (%) [a]	50 (47.6%)
Age (years) [b]	66 [59; 73]
DM duration (years) [b]	15 [7.9; 20]
BMI (Kg/m^2) [b]	28.3 [25.7; 31]
HbA1c (%) [b]	8 [7.5; 8.8]
Mean IOP (mmHg) [b]	15.5 [14; 17.5]
IOP right eye (mmHg) [b]	15 [14; 17]
IOP left eye (mmHg) [b]	16 [14; 18]
Cataract or IOL implant Nr (%) [a]	22 (21%)
DME Nr (%) [a]	19 (18.1%)
Hypertension Nr (%) [a]	82 (78.1%)
CVD Nr (%) [a]	91 (86.7%)
Diabetic polyneuropathy Nr (%) [a]	75 (71.4%)
CKD Nr (%) [a]	41 (39.1%)
Dyslipidaemia [a]	62 (59.0%)
Smoker status Nr (%) [a]	27 (25.7%)
Argon laser photocoagulation Nr (%) [a]	56 (53.3%)

Notes: [a] categorical variables are presented by absolute frequency (percentage) in the sample. [b] continuous variables (with non-Gaussian distribution) are indicated by their median (interquartile range). Abbreviations: DM, diabetes mellitus; BMI, body mass index; HbA1C, haemoglobin A1c; IOP, intraocular pressure; IOL, intraocular lens; DME, diabetic macular oedema; DR, diabetic retinopathy; CVD, cardiovascular disease; CKD, chronic kidney disease.

Regarding the severity of DR, a higher HbA1c value was associated with a more severe DR (from 7.1% in mild NDPR to 8.9% in PDR; $p < 0.0001$). In addition, a longer DM duration was associated with a more severe DR (from 8 years in mild NPDR to 20 years in PDR; $p < 0.0001$). No significant association between patients age and the severity of DR was found. The relationship between the severity of DR and studied parameters is presented in Table 3.

Table 3. Characteristics of people with DR depending on the severity of DR.

Parameter	Mild NPDR	Moderate NPDR	Severe NPDR	PDR	*p* *
HbA1c (%) [b]	7.1 [7; 7.45]	8 [7.5; 8.6]	8 [7.45; 8.2]	8.9 [8; 9.1]	<0.0001
DM duration (years) [b]	8 [5; 10]	5 [3; 11.5]	15.5 [12.5; 20]	20 [15; 23]	<0.0001
Age (years) [b]	68 [60.5; 72]	69 [58.2; 75.7]	64.5 [56; 70.5]	64.5 [60; 73]	0.51

Notes: Numerical variables with non-Gaussian distribution are indicated by their median (interquartile range); Results are presented as median (interquartile range). *p*-value was calculated using Kruskal–Wallis test. Abbreviations: HbA1C, haemoglobin A1c; DM, diabetes mellitus; NPDR, nonproliferative diabetic retinopathy. [b] Continuous variable; * ANOVA: Kruskal-Wallis test.

The presence of DR was associated with a significantly higher diabetes duration (15 vs. 12 years; $p = 0.0076$; Mann–Whitney test), HbA1c (8.0 vs. 7.2 percentage points; $p < 0.0001$; Figure 3), BMI (28.3 vs. 27 kg/m; $p = 0.0064$) and age (66 vs. 63 years; $p = 0.037$; Figure 4). No significant association was found between DR and IOP values, as illustrated in Table 4.

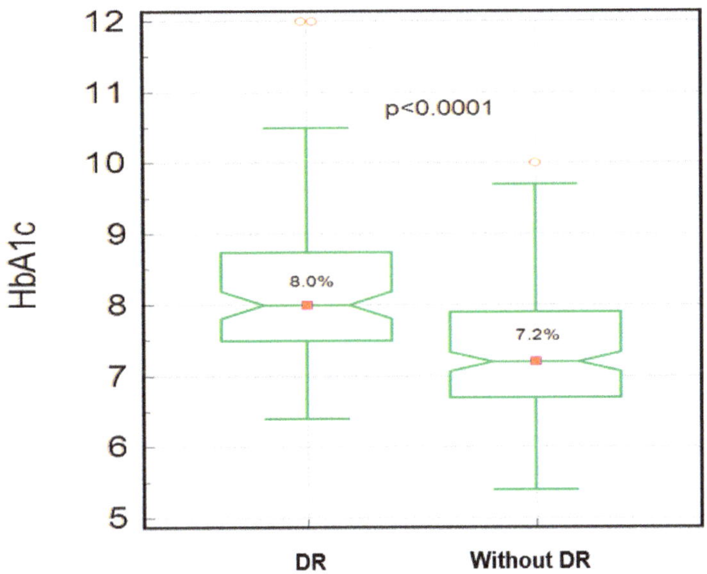

Figure 3. The median value of HbA1c in patients with DR vs. without DR.

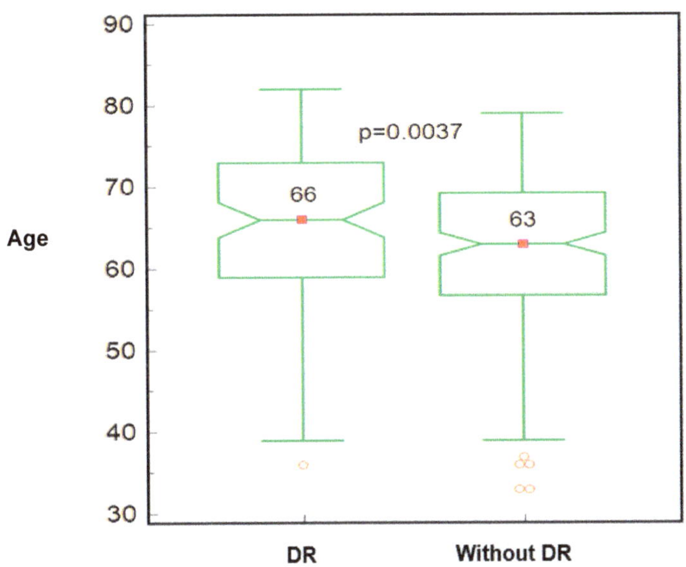

Figure 4. Median age value for patients with DR vs. without DR.

Considering the fact that the majority of the patients included in this study are elderly, we also evaluated the presence of cataract, as it represents the most frequent ocular pathology found among this age group. No significant differences were found between patients with vs. without DR (Table 5).

Table 4. Comparison between patients with and without DR.

Variable	With DR			Without DR			
	n	Median	Average Rank	*n*	Median	Average Rank	*p* [a]
DM duration	105	15.0000	169.8524	197	12.0000	141.7183	0.0076
HbA1c	105	8.0000	199.0190	197	7.2000	126.1726	<0.0001
BMI	105	28.2828	170.2476	197	27.0000		0.0064
IOP OD	105	14.0000	121.7476	197	13.5000	109.2863	0.1530
IOP OS	105	16.0000	156.3095	197	16.0000	148.9365	0.4821
Age	105	66.0000	171.4619	197	63.0000	140.8604	0.0037

Notes: [a] Mann–Whitney test. Abbreviations: DM, diabetes mellitus; IOP, intraocular pressure.

Table 5. Comparison between patients with and without DR regarding associated cataract.

	DR	Without DR	*p* *	Chi-Squared
Cataract Nr (%) [a]	22 (21%)	39 (19.8%)	0.8120	0.0565

Notes: * Chi-squared test. [a] Numerical values with non-Gaussian distribution. Results are presented in percentage from total. Abbreviations: DR, diabetic retinopathy.

To evaluate the adjusted impact of HbA1c, age and DM duration on the development of DR, we built a multivariate logistic regression model. In this model, we identified that increases in HbA1c value and age significantly enhanced the risk of DR occurrence (Table 6). This model explained 25.29% of the factors involved in the development of DR in patients with T2DM.

Table 6. Predictors for DR development in patients with T2DM.

Variable	Odds Ratio	95% CI
HbA1c	2.6624	1.9309 to 3.6710
Age	1.0500	1.0184 to 1.0826
DM duration	1.0182	0.9859 to 1.0515

Nagelkerke $R^2 = 0.2529$. Significance level $p < 0.0001$.

To evaluate the prediction performance of HbA1c in the development of DR, ROC analysis was performed. The results pointed out that HbA1c value is a valid predictor for the development of DR (AUROC = 0.741; $p = 0.001$), having the best prediction threshold, according to the Youden's method at a HbA1c value higher than 7.2%, corresponding to a sensitivity of 83.81% and associated specificity of 56.35% (Figure 5).

Another valid predictor for the development of DR in patients with Type 2 DM was patient's age, with a threshold of > 67 years, corresponding to a sensitivity of 46.47% and specificity of 70.05% (AUROC = 0.601; $p = 0.004$; Figure 6).

Regarding DM duration, as stated by the ROC curve parameters (AUROC = 0.593, $p = 0.007$), DM duration over 13 years was associated with a sensitivity of 56.19% and specificity of 60.91% (Figure 7).

Most T2DM patients, including the population of this study, exhibit a various number of comorbidities that significantly impact their quality of life by also subsequently increasing their potential risk of developing DR. As shown in Table 7, the presence of other diabetes complications or comorbidities (hypertension, CVD, CKD and dyslipidaemia) were associated with a higher risk of DR occurrence (Figure 8), while no significant differences were found regarding polyneuropathy or smoking.

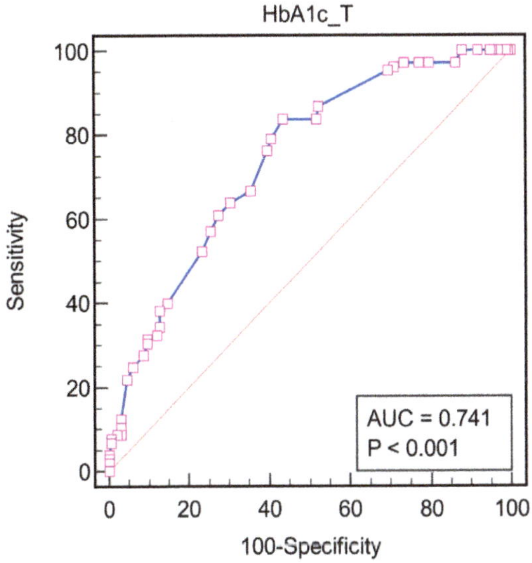

Figure 5. Receiver operating characteristics analysis for HbA1c as a predictor for DR. Associated criterion: HbA1c > 7.2%, AUC = 0.741; Youden index J: 0.4015 95%, CI: 0.688 to 0.790; Sensitivity: 83.81%, z statistic = 8.417; Specificity: 56.36%, $p < 0.0001$. The squares represent individual data points, the blue line represents the ROC curve and the red diagonal line is the reference line that represents a model with no discriminative ability.

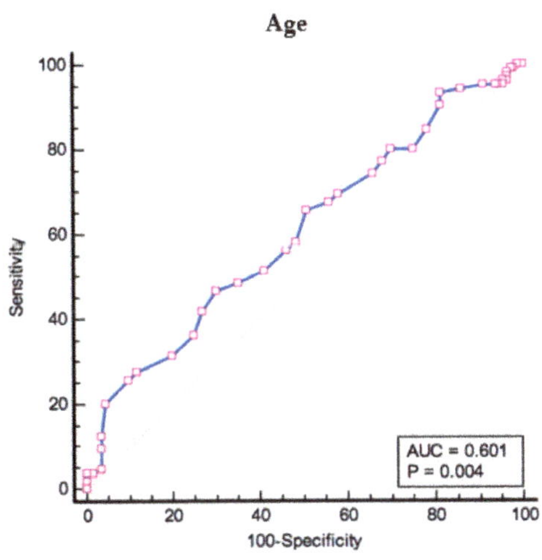

Figure 6. Receiver operating characteristics analysis for patient's age as a predictor for DR. Associated criterion: Age > 67 years, AUC = 0.601; Youden index J: 0.1672 95%, CI: 0.544 to 0.657; Sensitivity: 46.67%, z statistic = 2.916; Specificity: 70.05%, $p = 0.0035$. The squares represent individual data points, the blue line represents the ROC curve and the dotted red diagonal line is the reference line that represents a model with no discriminative ability.

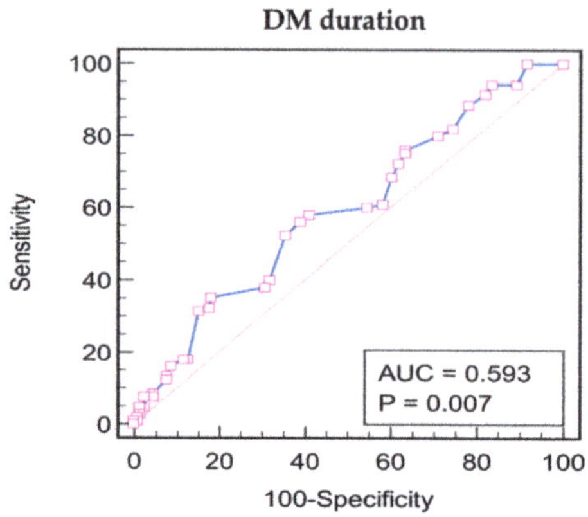

Figure 7. Receiver operating characteristics analysis for patient's DM duration as a predictor for DR. Associated criterion: DM duration > 13years, AUC = 0.593; Youden index J: 0.1710 95%, CI: 0.535 to 0.649; Sensitivity: 56.19%, z statistic = 2.719; Specificity: 60.91%, p = 0.0065. The squares represent individual data points, the blue line represents the ROC curve and the red diagonal line is the reference line that represents a model with no discriminative ability.

Table 7. The probability of DR occurrence depending on the presence of various diseases.

Comorbidity	OR	95% CI	Z Statistic	Significance Level
HTA	1.8375	1.0618 to 3.1797	2.174	p = 0.0297
CVD	2.3310	1.2221 to 4.4462	2.569	p = 0.0102
Polyneuropathy	1.7026	1.0215 to 2.8379	2.042	p = 0.0412
CKD	2.2943	1.3672 to 3.8502	3.144	p = 0.0017
Dyslipidaemia	1.8275	1.1299 to 2.9558	2.458	p = 0.0140
Smoker status	1.7740	0.9945 to 3.1647	1.941	p = 0.0522

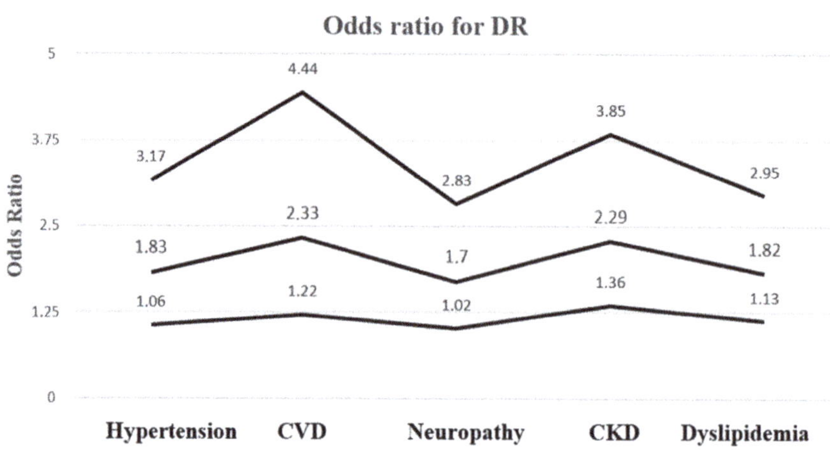

Figure 8. Odds ratio for DR development. CVD, cardiovascular disease; CKD, chronic kidney disease.

4. Discussion

This present study aimed to evaluate the main risk factors involved in the development and progression of DR among patients with T2DM. From all patients included in this study, 34.8% presented DR in different stages of severity. These results align with recent literature, which reports a median prevalence of this disease at 27.9% (range: 22–37%) among patients with type 2 diabetes [7].

An important fact to be noted regarding DR prevalence is outlined by a study conducted by Markle et al. that highlighted a current increase in DR prevalence among younger diabetic patients, while older ones exhibit a slight decrease in its occurrence [8]. Taking this recent research into consideration, and the fact that our study group was comprised mainly of elderly patients (median age 64 years old), results regarding prevalence could increase if the study group was extended to a younger category of T2DM patients.

Facing a global ageing population [9], the concept of multimorbidity has gained increasing interest among primary care physicians [10], especially regarding T2DM patients, as they are at a higher risk of presenting multiple co-occurring conditions [11]. In our study group, most of the patients presented more than one comorbidity alongside DM. Our focus was on observing the main systemic pathologies such as hypertension, CVD, CKD and dyslipidaemia, diseases that are known to be highly prevalent in the elderly population with a significant impact on diabetes-related ocular complications such as the vision-threatening DR. Regarding polyneuropathy, one of the most frequent chronic DM complications, we obtained a strong correlation between DR occurrence and the presence of polyneuropathy among T2DM patients as stated in current literature [2,12]. We found that the above mentioned pathologies (hypertension, CVD, polyneuropathy and dyslipidaemia) are highly prevalent among our general study group, but more importantly a high prevalence was observed regarding the subpopulation represented by patients with DR. Hypertension and CVD had one of the highest predictive values in our study regarding probability of DR occurrence, similarly to current literature data [13,14]. Identifying a positive correlation between polyneuropathy, dyslipidaemia and DR has been the purpose of multiple international studies [15,16], our results being superposable with current literature.

Regarding other ocular pathologies, we observed the presence of cataract or previous cataract surgery with IOL implant, IOP values and last but not least DME presence. Cataract is known to be more frequent among diabetic patients [17], with 10-year incidence of cataract surgery being 24.9% among this category of patients according to the Wisconsin Epidemiologic Study of Diabetic Retinopathy [18]. In our research, 20.2% of T2DM patients without DR and 21% of patients with DR presented cataract or previous cataract surgery. IOP values obtained in our group were within normal range with a median value of 15 mmHg in both patients with or without DR, still, positive correlations are known between higher IOP and presence of glaucoma among diabetic patients [19]. DME can virtually occur in any stage of DR, but remains more frequent among patients with PDR [20]. Population-based studies show a reported prevalence of DME of up to 12.8% [21], while our research obtained similar results, more precisely 18.1% prevalence among our studied population.

Our research population consisted of mainly overweight patients. BMI had a median value of 27 kg/m^2 [25; 30.8] across the entire study group, with a higher median value of 28.3 kg/m^2 [25.7; 31] among patients who also had DR. This is lower than the prevalence of overweight patients reported in the current literature for those with T2DM, which ranges from 31.2% to 67.8%, a condition known to be linked to DR progression [22,23]. These differences could be attributed to the fact that our study group mainly consisted of elderly patients with longer diabetes duration and poor glycaemic control, factors that could suggest subsequent weight loss due to uncontrolled DM and the presence of metabolic complications [23]. General DM management typically focuses on weight loss for overweight and obese patients; however, some precautions should be taken when applying these measures in the elderly diabetic population, as recent data suggest fewer benefits from extensive weight control in this age group [24].

Behavioural aspects like smoking, alcohol use or practicing physical activity are key factors in maintaining a healthy lifestyle in general population but more so in diabetic patients. Improving these negative patterns, diabetes incidence is reduced among the general population, while it significantly decreases the risk of complications, especially CVD among diabetics [25]. Our study has focused on smoking assessment, as it is considered one of the most avertible causes of death globally. Results were noted after patients self-report, illustrating that smoking was more prevalent in DR subpopulation (25.7%) than in the whole study group (19.5%), data that aligned with current literature [26]. In our research, we only considered active smokers, as nicotine intake contributes to impairment in insulin activity and has a subsequent negative effect on glycaemic control. However, data are inconclusive regarding a direct impact of smoking on the progression of DR [26,27].

Our research strengths consists of a relatively large study population that we consider accurately reflects health status among elderly T2DM patients in our country, but we also weigh the need to include a younger demographic group in further research, as early-onset T2DM patients seem to develop systemic complication earlier and more aggressively [28].

All patients included in this study were subjected to a complete fundus examination with prior pupil dilation in order to evaluate the presence of DR and DME. Still, this method remains slightly subjective and consequently can lead to underdiagnosis of the extend of retinal disease and presence of macular thickening [29]. We consider a more extended ophthalmologic evaluation of these patients is needed, utilising fundus photography, but more important optical coherence tomography (OCT). OCT and the more novel OCT-angiography offer high-resolution images of retinal structures and vasculature in order to properly identify diabetes related ophthalmic complications, aiding ophthalmologists in establishing a proper treatment protocol and a precise follow-up [30–32].

The not so new concept of empowerment, which according to WHO refers to a practice in which people gain control over their own actions regarding their health, has become prominent lately also among diabetic patients. This concept is considered to improve the patient–physician relationship, and ultimately determining patients to become more adherent to adequate medical conduct [33]. Nevertheless, in order to achieve an empowered status among diabetic population, more thorough patient education is due. Besides the strict management of the risk factors that has been the object of many studies, including the present one, patients should be more informed about possible DR symptoms like sudden or gradual vision loss, presence of floaters in the visual field, loss of central vision or impaired night vision. Lack of treatment adherence among diabetic patients is a very common issue; therefore, a more intensive patient education regarding their disease might overcome this barrier, ultimately improving their long-term quality of life [34].

5. Conclusions

The results obtained from our present research confirm current literature data which state that the most important risk factors regarding T2DM evolution and management involved in the occurrence of DR are represented by poor glycaemic control and longer DM duration, while the most impacting comorbidities are hypertension and CVD, CKD and dyslipidaemia. Early detection and management of systemic risk factors can avert this DM complication. However, the primary and fundamental strategy for preventing ocular complications in diabetic patients continues to be the maintenance of a tight glycaemic control.

Author Contributions: Conceptualization, A.I., S.P. and R.T.; methodology, R.T.; software, S.P.; validation, S.P. and R.T.; formal analysis, R.T.; investigation, M.P.; data curation, R.I.; writing—original draft preparation, A.I.; writing—review and editing, A.I. and S.P.; visualization, R.I.; supervision, R.T.; project administration, R.T.; funding acquisition, A.I. All authors have read and agreed to the published version of the manuscript.

Funding: This research received no external funding. We would like to acknowledge 'Victor Babes' University of Medicine and Farmacy, Timisoara, for their support in covering the publishing costs.

Institutional Review Board Statement: This study was conducted according to the Declaration of Helsinki (2013 version) and was approved by the Ethics Committee of the Emergency County Hospital "Pius Brinzeu" Timișoara, Romania (approval no. 467, approved on 20 May 2024).

Informed Consent Statement: Informed consent was obtained from all participants involved in the present study.

Data Availability Statement: All available data can be provided upon request to the corresponding author.

Conflicts of Interest: The authors declare no conflicts of interest. The funders had no role in study design, data collection, analysis or interpretation nor in writing or publishing the results of the current manuscript.

References

1. Sun, H.; Saeedi, P.; Karuranga, S.; Pinkepank, M.; Ogurtsova, K.; Duncan, B.B.; Stein, C.; Basit, A.; Chan, J.C.N.; Mbanya, J.C.; et al. IDF Diabetes Atlas: Global, Regional and Country-Level Diabetes Prevalence Estimates for 2021 and Projections for 2045. *Diabetes Res. Clin. Pract.* **2022**, *183*, 109119. [CrossRef] [PubMed]
2. Ting, D.S.W.; Cheung, G.C.M.; Wong, T.Y. Diabetic Retinopathy: Global Prevalence, Major Risk Factors, Screening Practices and Public Health Challenges: A Review. *Clin. Exper. Ophthalmol.* **2016**, *44*, 260–277. [CrossRef] [PubMed]
3. Teo, Z.L.; Tham, Y.-C.; Yu, M.; Chee, M.L.; Rim, T.H.; Cheung, N.; Bikbov, M.M.; Wang, Y.X.; Tang, Y.; Lu, Y.; et al. Global Prevalence of Diabetic Retinopathy and Projection of Burden through 2045. *Ophthalmology* **2021**, *128*, 1580–1591. [CrossRef] [PubMed]
4. Vujosevic, S.; Aldington, S.J.; Silva, P.; Hernández, C.; Scanlon, P.; Peto, T.; Simó, R. Screening for Diabetic Retinopathy: New Perspectives and Challenges. *Lancet Diabetes Endocrinol.* **2020**, *8*, 337–347. [CrossRef] [PubMed]
5. DCCT Research Group. Diabetes Control and Complications Trial (DCCT): Results of Feasibility Study. The DCCT Research Group. *Diabetes Care* **1987**, *10*, 1–19. [CrossRef] [PubMed]
6. UK Prospective Diabetes Study (UKPDS) Group. Intensive Blood-Glucose Control with Sulphonylureas or Insulin Compared with Conventional Treatment and Risk of Complications in Patients with Type 2 Diabetes (UKPDS 33). *Lancet* **1998**, *352*, 837–853. [CrossRef]
7. Ruta, L.M.; Magliano, D.J.; Lemesurier, R.; Taylor, H.R.; Zimmet, P.Z.; Shaw, J.E. Prevalence of Diabetic Retinopathy in Type 2 Diabetes in Developing and Developed Countries. *Diabet. Med.* **2013**, *30*, 387–398. [CrossRef] [PubMed]
8. Rein, D.B.; Wittenborn, J.S. Prevalence of Diabetic Retinopathy in Health Care Settings—An Early Warning Sign? *JAMA Ophthalmol.* **2024**, *142*, 607–608. [CrossRef]
9. Guseh, J.S. Aging of the World's Population. In *Encyclopedia of Family Studies*; Shehan, C.L., Ed.; Wiley: Hoboken, NJ, USA, 2015; pp. 1–5, ISBN 978-1-119-08562-1.
10. Nicholson, K.; Almirall, J.; Fortin, M. The Measurement of Multimorbidity. *Health Psychol.* **2019**, *38*, 783–790. [CrossRef]
11. Cicek, M.; Buckley, J.; Pearson-Stuttard, J.; Gregg, E.W. Characterizing Multimorbidity from Type 2 Diabetes: Insights from Clustering Approaches. *Endocrinol. Metab. Clin. N. Am.* **2021**, *50*, 531–558. [CrossRef] [PubMed]
12. Graue-Hernandez, E.O.; Rivera-De-La-Parra, D.; Hernandez-Jimenez, S.; Aguilar-Salinas, C.A.; Kershenobich-Stalnikowitz, D.; Jimenez-Corona, A. Prevalence and Associated Risk Factors of Diabetic Retinopathy and Macular Oedema in Patients Recently Diagnosed with Type 2 Diabetes. *BMJ Open Ophthalmol.* **2020**, *5*, e000304. [CrossRef] [PubMed]
13. Zhang, M.; Wu, J.; Wang, Y.; Wu, J.; Hu, W.; Jia, H.; Sun, X. Associations between Blood Pressure Levels and Diabetic Retinopathy in Patients with Diabetes Mellitus: A Population-Based Study. *Heliyon* **2023**, *9*, e16830. [CrossRef] [PubMed]
14. Li, L.; Gao, J.; Rao, X.; Liu, X. Relationship between Atherosclerotic Cardiovascular Disease and Diabetic Retinopathy in Patients with Type 2 Diabetes Mellitus. *Medicine* **2024**, *103*, e38051. [CrossRef] [PubMed]
15. Hafeez, M.; Achar, P.; Neeralagi, M.; Naik, G.T. Correlation between Diabetic Retinopathy and Diabetic Peripheral Neuropathy in Patients with Type II Diabetes Mellitus. *J. Pharm. Bioallied Sci.* **2022**, *14*, S658–S661. [CrossRef] [PubMed]
16. Chatziralli, I.P. The Role of Dyslipidemia Control in the Progression of Diabetic Retinopathy in Patients with Type 2 Diabetes Mellitus. *Diabetes Ther.* **2017**, *8*, 209–212. [CrossRef] [PubMed]
17. Kiziltoprak, H.; Tekin, K.; Inanc, M.; Goker, Y.S. Cataract in Diabetes Mellitus. *World J. Diabetes* **2019**, *10*, 140–153. [CrossRef] [PubMed]
18. Klein, B.E.; Klein, R.; Moss, S.E. Incidence of Cataract Surgery in the Wisconsin Epidemiologic Study of Diabetic Retinopathy. *Am. J. Ophthalmol.* **1995**, *119*, 295–300. [CrossRef] [PubMed]
19. Ojha, S.; Kukreja, P.; Verma, S. Association of Intraocular Pressure with Blood Sugar Levels in Patients of Type 2 Diabetes Mellitus and Control Group. *TNOA J. Ophthalmic Sci. Res.* **2022**, *60*, 294. [CrossRef]

20. Wong, T.Y.; Sun, J.; Kawasaki, R.; Ruamviboonsuk, P.; Gupta, N.; Lansingh, V.C.; Maia, M.; Mathenge, W.; Moreker, S.; Muqit, M.M.K.; et al. Guidelines on Diabetic Eye Care: The International Council of Ophthalmology Recommendations for Screening, Follow-up, Referral, and Treatment Based on Resource Settings. *Ophthalmology* **2018**, *125*, 1608–1622. [CrossRef] [PubMed]
21. Acan, D.; Calan, M.; Er, D.; Arkan, T.; Kocak, N.; Bayraktar, F.; Kaynak, S. The Prevalence and Systemic Risk Factors of Diabetic Macular Edema: A Cross-Sectional Study from Turkey. *BMC Ophthalmol.* **2018**, *18*, 91. [CrossRef]
22. Mugharbel, K.M.; Al-Mansouri, M.A. Prevalence of Obesity among Type 2 Diabetic Patients in Al-Khobar Primary Health Care Centers. *J. Family Community Med.* **2003**, *10*, 49–53. [CrossRef] [PubMed]
23. Li, W.; Gong, X.; Wang, W.; Xiong, K.; Meng, J.; Li, Y.; Wang, L.; Liang, X.; Jin, L.; Huang, W. Association of Different Kinds of Obesity with Diabetic Retinopathy in Patients with Type 2 Diabetes. *BMJ Open* **2022**, *12*, e056332. [CrossRef]
24. Zhou, Q.; Sun, J.; Wu, Z.; Wu, W.; Zhang, X.; Pan, Q.; Qi, H.; Yuan, H.; Shi, H.; Cao, S.; et al. The Older, the Less Potential Benefit for Type 2 Diabetes from Weight Control. *BMC Geriatr.* **2022**, *22*, 346. [CrossRef] [PubMed]
25. Galaviz, K.I.; Narayan, K.M.V.; Lobelo, F.; Weber, M.B. Lifestyle and the Prevention of Type 2 Diabetes: A Status Report. *Am. J. Lifestyle Med.* **2018**, *12*, 4–20. [CrossRef] [PubMed]
26. Durlach, V.; Vergès, B.; Al-Salameh, A.; Bahougne, T.; Benzerouk, F.; Berlin, I.; Clair, C.; Mansourati, J.; Rouland, A.; Thomas, D.; et al. Smoking and Diabetes Interplay: A Comprehensive Review and Joint Statement. *Diabetes Metab.* **2022**, *48*, 101370. [CrossRef] [PubMed]
27. Cai, X.; Chen, Y.; Yang, W.; Gao, X.; Han, X.; Ji, L. The Association of Smoking and Risk of Diabetic Retinopathy in Patients with Type 1 and Type 2 Diabetes: A Meta-Analysis. *Endocrine* **2018**, *62*, 299–306. [CrossRef] [PubMed]
28. Hillier, T.A.; Pedula, K.L. Complications in Young Adults with Early-Onset Type 2 Diabetes: Losing the Relative Protection of Youth. *Diabetes Care* **2003**, *26*, 2999–3005. [CrossRef] [PubMed]
29. Aljefri, S.; Al Adel, F. The Validity of Diabetic Retinopathy Screening Using Nonmydriatic Fundus Camera and Optical Coherence Tomography in Comparison to Clinical Examination. *Saudi J. Ophthalmol.* **2020**, *34*, 266–272. [CrossRef] [PubMed]
30. Zeppieri, M.; Marsili, S.; Enaholo, E.S.; Shuaibu, A.O.; Uwagboe, N.; Salati, C.; Spadea, L.; Musa, M. Optical Coherence Tomography (OCT): A Brief Look at the Uses and Technological Evolution of Ophthalmology. *Medicina* **2023**, *59*, 2114. [CrossRef] [PubMed]
31. Agarwal, D.; Gelman, R.; Prospero Ponce, C.; Stevenson, W.; Christoforidis, J.B. The Vitreomacular Interface in Diabetic Retinopathy. *J. Ophthalmol.* **2015**, *2015*, 392983. [CrossRef] [PubMed]
32. Hagag, A.; Gao, S.; Jia, Y.; Huang, D. Optical Coherence Tomography Angiography: Technical Principles and Clinical Applications in Ophthalmology. *Taiwan. J. Ophthalmol.* **2017**, *7*, 115. [CrossRef] [PubMed]
33. Tol, A.; Baghbanian, A.; Mohebbi, B.; Shojaeizadeh, D.; Azam, K.; Shahmirzadi, S.E.; Asfia, A. Empowerment Assessment and Influential Factors among Patients with Type 2 Diabetes. *J. Diabetes Metab. Disord.* **2013**, *12*, 6. [CrossRef] [PubMed]
34. Pourhabibi, N.; Mohebbi, B.; Sadeghi, R.; Shakibazadeh, E.; Sanjari, M.; Tol, A.; Yaseri, M. Determinants of Poor Treatment Adherence among Patients with Type 2 Diabetes and Limited Health Literacy: A Scoping Review. *J. Diabetes Res.* **2022**, *2022*, 2980250. [CrossRef] [PubMed]

biomedicines

MDPI

Review

Diabetes and Heart Failure: A Literature Review, Reflection and Outlook

Xiya Li [†], Xiaoyang Zhou [†] and Ling Gao [*]

Department of Endocrinology, Renmin Hospital, Wuhan University, Wuhan 430060, China; lxy958619764@outlook.com (X.L.); xiaoyangzh@whu.edu.cn (X.Z.)

* Correspondence: ling.gao@whu.edu.cn; Tel.: +86-15927469449; Fax: +86-(27)-88042292

† These authors contributed equally to this work.

Abstract: Heart failure (HF) is a complex clinical syndrome caused by structural or functional dysfunction of the ventricular filling or blood supply. Diabetes mellitus (DM) is an independent predictor of mortality for HF. The increase in prevalence, co-morbidity and hospitalization rates of both DM and HF has further fueled the possibility of overlapping disease pathology between the two. For decades, antidiabetic drugs that are known to definitively increase the risk of HF are the thiazolidinediones (TZDs) and saxagliptin in the dipeptidyl peptidase-4 (DPP-4) inhibitor, and insulin, which causes sodium and water retention, and whether metformin is effective or safe for HF is not clear. Notably, sodium-glucose transporter 2 (SGLT2) inhibitors and partial glucagon-like peptide-1 receptor agonists (GLP-1 RA) all achieved positive results for HF endpoints, with SGLT2 inhibitors in particular significantly reducing the composite endpoint of cardiovascular mortality and hospitalization for heart failure (HHF). Further understanding of the mutual pathophysiological mechanisms between HF and DM may facilitate the detection of novel therapeutic targets to improve the clinical outcome. This review focuses on the association between HF and DM, emphasizing the efficacy and safety of antidiabetic drugs and HF treatment. In addition, recent therapeutic advances in HF and the important mechanisms by which SGLT2 inhibitors/mineralocorticoid receptor antagonist (MRA)/vericiguat contribute to the benefits of HF are summarized.

Keywords: heart failure; diabetes; left ventricular ejection fraction; antidiabetic drugs; SGLT2 inhibitor; randomized controlled trial

1. Background

HF is a multifaceted clinical syndrome, associated with an impaired quality of life, frequent hospitalizations and increased mortality [1]. And DM is a major risk factor for HF, which, in turn, exacerbates the metabolic disturbances and complications of DM, with a worse prognosis for patients [2]. In the Framingham Heart Study, DM resulted in a nearly twofold increase in the risk of HF in men and a fourfold increase in women [3]. In terms of possible mechanisms, DM may cause myocardial ischemia through microcirculatory disturbances and macrovascular lesions and may directly adversely affect the myocardium [4]. Hyperglycemia, hyperinsulinemia and insulin resistance can lead to fatty acid overload in cardiomyocytes and lipid deposition in the epicardium, resulting in an altered cardiac structure and impaired myocardial energy metabolism [5,6]. Advanced glycosylation products (AGEs) are deposited in endothelial cells and cross-link with myocardial collagen, worsening inflammation and oxidative stress [7]. Following a notable increase in interest in the role of antidiabetic drugs for DM in HF, a number of outcome trials for antidiabetic drugs are being demonstrated. This review will summarize the pathophysiology of DM and HF interactions, as well as antidiabetic drugs and emerging pharmacological treatments for HF.

2. The Pathogenesis of Heart Failure and Its Treatment

HF is primarily characterized by myocardial remodeling due to increased mechanical stress, with alterations in neural, humoral, endocrine, inflammatory, immune and energy metabolism [8]. Hyperglycemia, insulin resistance and hyperinsulinemia are the main physiological disorders of DM contributing to functional and structural disorders of the cardiovascular system through multiple pathways, finally leading to various pathological conditions, such as myocardial infarction, myocardial hypertrophy, coronary artery disease, myocardial ischemia and hypertension, and, ultimately, leading to HF [8,9] (Figure 1). Numerous underlying risk factors of HF have been identified over the decades, including hypertension, diabetes, obesity, smoking, alcohol abuse, etc. [10] However, suboptimal primary prevention of HF persists, and the incidence of HF remains high compared to ischemic heart disease and stroke [11].

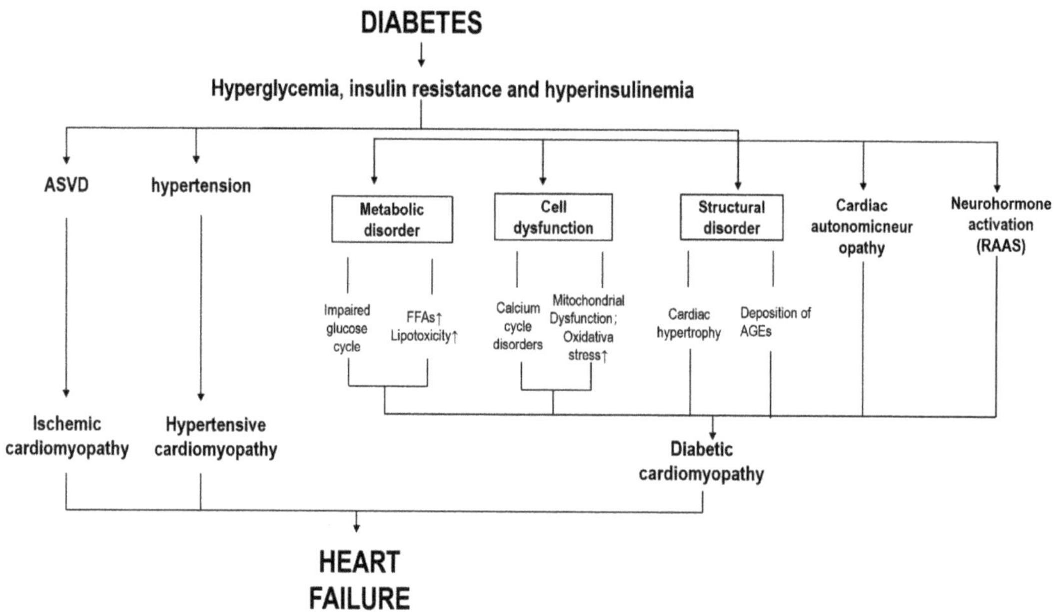

Figure 1. Pathophysiological mechanism of diabetic heart failure. Diabetic patients with hyperglycemia, insulin resistance, and hyperinsulinemia trigger vascular lesions, metabolic abnormalities, cellular dysfunction, and abnormal activation of the endocrine and nervous systems of the body, leading to ischemic heart disease, hypertensive heart disease, diabetic cardiomyopathy, and ultimately heart failure. ASVD, atherosclerotic vascular disease; FFAs, free fatty acids; AGEs, advanced glycosylation products; RAAS, renin–angiotensin–aldosterone system.

3. Different Pathogenesis of Two Traditional Types of Heart Failure

Based on the left ventricular ejection fraction (LVEF), HF has three types: heart failure with reduced ejection fraction (HFrEF; EF < 40%), heart failure with mid-range ejection fraction (HFmrEF; EF: 40–49%), and heart failure with preserved ejection fraction (HFpEF; EF $\geq$ 50%). However, clinical and epidemiologic data and experimental data focus more on HFrEF and HFpEF, and this review also focuses on the two (Table 1). HFrEF is usually preceded by acute or chronic myocardial cell loss due to ischemia, genetic mutations, myocarditis or valvular disease [12]. Additionally, HFrEF is often associated with neurohormonal activation, which can further exacerbate myocardial dysfunction and adverse remodeling. In contrast, the development of HFpEF is closely related to the presence of co-morbidities [13], including obesity, diabetes, anemia, hypertension, chronic obstructive pulmonary disease (COPD), etc. A landmark invasive study showed significant impaired active diastolic function and increased passive stiffness in patients with HFpEF [14] and even concomitant adverse remodeling and dysfunction of the atrial and vascular systems [15]. Chronic low-grade systemic inflammation results from the accumulation of metabolic risk factors, simultaneously leading to inflammation in HFpEF. However, the inflammatory response in HFrEF is mostly a consequence of myocardial cell injury [16]. In addition, older women are more likely to be affected by HFpEF. However, HFrEF is more prevalent in men due to their susceptibility to myocardial infarction [17]. Notably, though medical advances have led to the development of effective and specific treatments for HFrEF by targeting the neurohumoral axis, effective drugs to treat HFpEF are currently lacking [18].

Table 1. Difference in pathogenesis of HFpEF and HFrEF.

	HFpEF	HFrEF
Diagnostic criteria	① Symptoms/signs of HF; ② LVEF $\geq$ 50%; ③ Natriuretic peptide + (left ventricular hypertrophy, left atrial enlargement, cardiac diastolic dysfunction).	① Symptoms/signs of heart failure; ② LVEF < 40%.
Pathogenesis	Mostly associated with ischemic diseases, endothelial dysfunction at early stages and microvascular events more prevalent.	Altered left ventricular structure and function;Neurohormonal activation and endothelial dysfunction at all stages;
Co-morbidities	Obesity, diabetes, anemia, hypertension, chronic obstructive pulmonary disease, autoimmune disease and renal insufficiency.	Acute or chronic Cardiomyocyte loss due to prior ischemia, genetic mutation, myocarditis, or valvular disease;
Age and sex	Older women with obesity.	Men with coronary heart disease, valvular disease or uncontrolled hypertension.
Inflammation	Low-grade systemic inflammation.	Consequence of myocardial cell injury.
Treatment	Effective treatment is still lacking.	ACEIs, β-blockers, ARBs, MRAs, ARNI, If-channel blockers are recommended.

HF, heart failure; LVEF, left ventricular ejection fraction; HFrEF, heart failure with reduced ejection fraction; HFpEF, heart failure with preserved ejection fraction; ACEIs, Angiotensin-converting enzyme inhibitors; β-blockers, β-adrenergic blockers; ARBs, angiotensin receptor blockers; MRAs, mineralocorticoid receptor antagonists; ARNI, angiotensin receptor neprilysin inhibitors; If-channel, IF channel inhibitors.

4. Diabetes Increases the Risk of Heart Failure

HF affects approximately 64 million people worldwide [19,20]. Sadly, nearly half of all HF patients die within five years of diagnosis [21]. The prevalence of DM in patients with HF ranges from approximately 25% to 40% (vs. 10.5% in general population) [22]. DM and hypertension are independent risk factors for HF, and the co-existence of the two significantly increases the risk of HF and cardiomyopathy [23]. The Heart and Soul study followed 839 patients with stable coronary artery disease and no signs of HF at baseline, finding that the risk of developing HF was twice as high in diabetic compared to nondiabetic subjects [24]. A retrospective cohort study showed that the incidence of HF was 30.9/1000 person-years in diabetic participants, which was higher than the incidence of 12.4/1000 person-years in nondiabetic participants [25]. According to a Medicare study, the mortality for people with type 2 diabetes mellitus (T2DM) and HF was 32.7/1000 person-years, compared to 3.7/1000-years for normoglycemic HF patients [26]. While few studies directly compare the prevalence and incidence of DM in HFrEF and HFpEF patients, in a study of inpatients with HF, the prevalence of DM was approximately 40% in both HFrEF and HFpEF patients [27].

4.1. Mechanism of Heart Failure Due to Diabetes Mellitus

The pathophysiological mechanisms between DM and HF are complex and multifactorial. Hyperglycemia, insulin resistance and hyperinsulinemia all seem to provoke and perpetuate the progression of HF, though the exact mechanisms are unclear [28]. Excessive production and accumulation of AGEs in plasma and vascular tissues lead to arterial stiffness and reduced elasticity [29]. Meanwhile, AGE accumulation triggers the production of reactive oxygen species (ROS), leading to myocardial and microcirculatory inflammation, mitochondrial dysfunction and myocardial apoptosis. Additionally, chronic hyperglycemia and insulin resistance may cause direct damage to the myocardium, along with the associated metabolic abnormalities, promoting the development of atherosclerosis and vascular damage. Hyperglycemia contributes to disturbed energy metabolism, inappropriate lipid deposition in extra-adipose tissues (including epicardium) [30] and lipotoxicity, provoking cardiomyocyte damage and triggering myocardial stiffness and ischemia [31]. Eventually, HF leads to renin–angiotensin–aldosterone system (RAAS) and sympathetic nervous system activation. When coupled with the typical Western diet, obesity and fatty liver, HF aggravates insulin resistance, and thus begins a vicious cycle [32] (Figure 2).

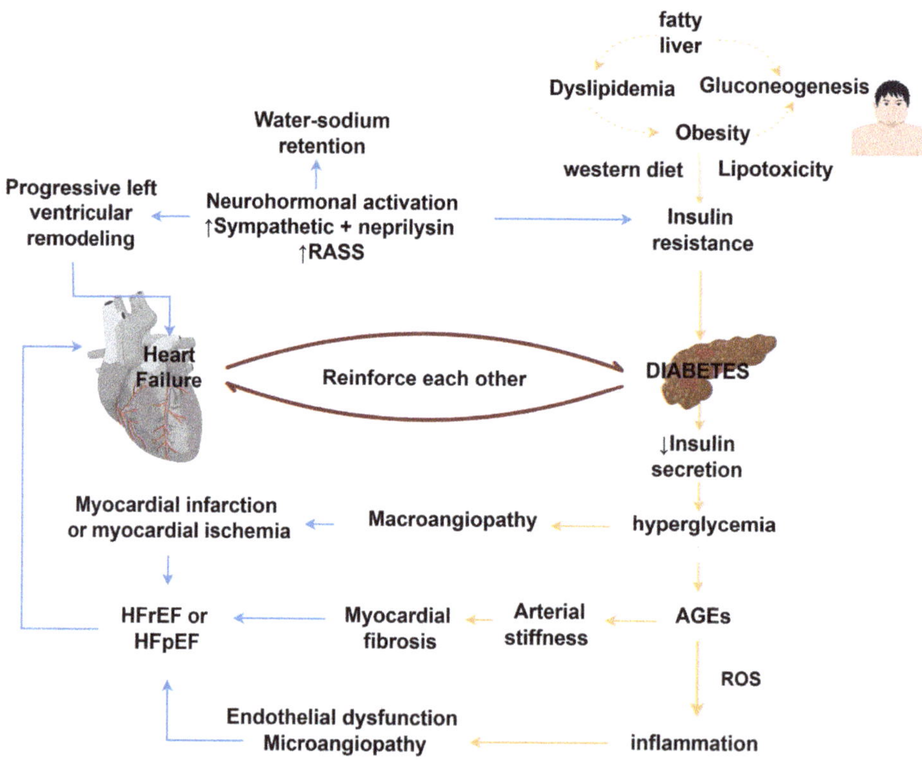

Figure 2. The pathological mechanism of interaction between heart failure and diabetes. Diabetes mellitus leads to hyperglycemia and insulin resistance, and the chronic hyperglycemic leads to chronic inflammation, endothelial and cardiomyocyte damage, promoting cardiac fibrosis, myocardial ischemia, cardiac remodeling, and further worsening heart failure. Heart failure leads to decreased cardiac output, sodium and water retention, activation of sympathetic nerves and the RASS system, which further reduces insulin secretion and exacerbates hyperglycemia, creating a vicious cycle. By Figdraw. RAAS, renin–angiotensin–aldosterone system; AGEs, advanced glycosylation products; ROS, reactive oxygen species; HFrEF, heart failure with reduced ejection fraction; HFpEF, heart failure with preserved ejection fraction.

4.2. Diabetes and Risk Factor Management

Many studies have attempted to predict HF through markers of DM or prevent it by intervening in the course of DM. The UKPDS findings suggest that the mean value of HemoglobinA1c (HbA1c) is a predictor of cardiovascular events [33], and an early 1% reduction in HbA1c increases the long-term survival benefit by threefold. In addition, inflammatory biomarkers (TNFR-1a, osteopontin), N-terminal pro-B-type natriuretic peptide (NT-proBNP) and angiopoietin may predict cardiac remodeling, inflammation and fibrosis in patients with HF and DM [34]. A cohort study based on the Swedish National Diabetes Registry database, where risk factors (HbA1c level, VLDL level, proteinuria, smoking, hypertension) were controlled, showed that the risk of death, myocardial infarction or stroke significantly decreased, while the excess risk of HHF remained and was only slightly reduced at HbA1c less than 53 mmol/L (equivalent to 7.0%) [9]. In terms of treatment, a meta-analysis of four studies, ACCORD, ADVANCE, UKPDS33 and VADT, showed that intensive glycemic control merely leads to a small but significant cardiovascular benefit in the short to medium term but not in all-cause mortality and cardiovascular mortality [9]. The failure of many clinical trials in the past may have been due to the fact that conventional antidiabetic drugs may have additional harmful effects on the heart [35]. However, nowadays, the therapeutic role of SGLT2 inhibitors in HF across the entire spectrum of ejection fraction has shown robust evidence of a clinical benefit [36].

4.3. Hypoglycemia and Heart Failure

T2DM and hypoglycemia are independent risk factors for MACE and mortality in HF patients [37]. Hypoglycemia induces acute cardiovascular events, accelerates chronic complications and increases all-cause mortality [38]. In terms of the mechanism, hypoglycemia triggers counter-regulatory defense reactions, activating the renin–angiotensin system, leading to cardiac arrhythmias and hemodynamic changes [39]. It also activates inflammatory responses, platelets, macrophages and coagulation factor VIII, causing endothelial dysfunction, coagulation abnormalities and promoting atherosclerosis [40]. Additionally, it directly harms the heart by affecting myocardial energy metabolism. Notably, rebound hyperglycemia amplifies inflammation, exacerbating endothelial dysfunction and thrombus activation [41]. Major trials, like ACCORD, ADVANCE, ORIGIN and VADT, link hypoglycemia to increased cardiovascular risk and mortality [39,42,43]. The SAVOR study associates increased HF hospitalization with severe hypoglycemia from sulfonylurea combinations [44]. While the DAPA-HF study reported zero major hypoglycemic events with dapagliflozin in HF patients [45], emphasis should be placed on medications associated with an increased risk of hypoglycemia, such as insulin and sulfonylureas.

5. Pharmacological Treatment of Heart Failure

Prior to 2010, many randomized controlled trials (RCTs) had been conducted in the field of chronic HF, establishing the classic golden triangle treatment model of angiotensin-converting enzyme inhibitor (ACEI)/angiotensin receptor blocker (ARB), beta-blocker (BB) and MRA. After 2019, many RCTs were carried out on new drugs for HF, such as angiotensin receptor-neprilysin inhibitor (ARNI), SGLT2 inhibitors, ivabradine (Iva), etc. PARADIGM-HF suggested that ARNI represented by Sacubitril valsartan is recommended as the drug of choice for the treatment of HFrEF patients [46]. Vericiguat is a soluble guanylate cyclase (sGC) stimulator, approved for use in patients with HFrEF in several countries in 2021 and 2022, reducing the risk of HHF or the need for emergency intravenous diuretic therapy [47]. Finerenone, a third-generation mineralocorticoid receptor antagonist, shows superior renal-cardio protection. Since its first approval in the United States in 2021, it has been unanimously recommended by many domestic and international authoritative guidelines [48]. A new quadruple, ARNI/ACEI/ ARB, SGLT2 inhibitors, β-blocker and MRA, was formed in 2021, shown to provide sustained benefits [49], such as reducing the risk of cardiovascular death or HHF by 62% through early application [36]. While evolving from the golden triangle to the new quadruple therapy, the studies conducted have focused on HFrEF, even if ARNI and SGLT2 inhibitors have shown promising results in treating HFpEF, primarily by reducing HHF. Notably, patients with cardiovascular diseases with low blood pressure and fast heart rates are subjected to various limitations in the use of drugs such as ARNI and β-blockers. However, SGLT2 inhibitors have looser requirements for blood pressure and cardiac function and are better tolerated and safer. SGLT2 inhibitors are being studied in large clinical trials as other promising options [50], though we are still waiting for drugs to significantly prolong survival in HFpEF patients.

6. Antidiabetic Drugs and Heart Failure

DM is an independent risk factor for HF, and, ideally, effective treatment for one should benefit the other without causing harm (Table 2).

Table 2. Summary of antidiabetic drug classes on heart failure [51–58].

	Class	Common Medications	Effects in Heart Failure	Clinical Practice Recommendations
Novel antidiabetic drugs	SGLT2 inhibitors	Dapagliflozin Empagliflozin	Beneficial	Symptomatic HFrEF patients are recommended regardless of DM.
	GLP-1 RA	Semaglutide	Beneficial	If SGLT2 inhibitors are contraindicated or not tolerated, consider GLP-1 RA. Recommended for HFpEF patients (BMI $\geq$ 30 kg/m^2, NYHA class II-IV, LVEF $\geq$ 45%).
	DPP-4i	Saxagliptin	• Saxagliptin harmful • Others potentially harmful	Saxagliptin is not recommended for T2DM with HF.
	GKA	Dorzagliatin	Potential cardiovascular benefits	Solid protection for CHD and HF, but more RCTs are needed.
Traditional antidiabetic drugs	Metformin	Metformin	Beneficial	Recommended for stable T2DM patients with normal renal function and chronic HF; not recommended for acute or decompensated HF patients.
	Glycosidase inhibitor	Acarbose	Beneficial	Second- or third-line medication. If digoxin is used to treat HF, avoid or discontinue acarbose.
	Glinides	Repaglinide	Neutral	Second- or third-line medication. Does not increase cardiovascular events in patients with T2DM.
	Sulfonylureas	Glimepiride	Potentially harmful	Sulfonylureas are not recommended for T2DM with HF.
	Insulin	Insulin	Potentially harmful	Rapid-acting and short-acting insulin analogs appears safer, with close monitoring for potential worsening of HF.
	TZDs	Pioglitazone	Harmful	TZDs are not recommended for T2DM with HF.

SGLT2i, sodium-glucose transporter 2 inhibitor; GLP-1 RA, glucagon-like peptide-1 receptor agonists; DPP-4i, dipeptidyl peptidase-4 inhibitor; GKA, glucokinase activator; TZDs, thiazolidinedions; HFrEF, heart failure with reduced ejection fraction; HFpEF, heart failure with preserved ejection fraction; DM, diabetes mellitus; HF, heart failure; CHD, coronary heart disease; NYHA, New York Heart Association; RCTs, randomized controlled studies.

However, some antidiabetic drugs have no significant effect on HF and may even act negatively. Conventional TZDs mainly activate peroxisome proliferator-activated receptors γ(PPARγ), but overactivation often leads to significant water and sodium retention [59]. The RECORD Study and PROactive Study revealed that TZDs significantly increase the risk of HF and mortality [60]. In contrast, chiglitazar sodium, a full agonist of PPAR, has not been associated with HF in studies and has lower incidences of edema, fractures and weight gain [61]. A meta-analysis of 115 trials showed that sulfonylureas were associated with increased mortality [62]. Retrospective studies suggest insulin is associated with worse outcomes in HF patients with T2DM, but RCTs have not shown that [63]. Currently, sulfonylureas and insulin are used as second- or third-line therapies in T2DM with HF, though their safety remains controversial [64]. The MeRIA study found that acarbose reduced the absolute risk of HF in T2DM patients by up to 45% [65]. The 2013 SAVOR-TIMI 53 study showed that saxagliptin, a DPP-4 inhibitor, was cardiovascular safe compared to placebo but increased the risk of HHF [66]. However, the EXAMINE trial found that cardiovascular outcomes were similar between the alogliptin and placebo groups [67]. Meta-analyses and animal studies have shown conflicting evidence on DPP-4 inhibitors.

Some other antidiabetic drugs, however, show a more favorable outcome. The use of metformin in T2DM patients with HF has been a long-standing concern due to the potential risk of lactic acidosis [68]. However, metformin has been proven to activate AMP-activated protein kinase (AMPK), reducing cardiomyocyte apoptosis and AGE formation, enhancing mitochondrial β-oxidation of FFAs and improving myocardial function [69]. Additionally, it modulates gut microbiome changes in HF patients, particularly affecting short-chain fatty acid-producing bacteria [56]. Meta-analyses have indicated that metformin reduces the risk of all-cause and cardiovascular death, and readmission for chronic HF in T2DM patients [70,71]. Since 2007, the American Diabetes Association has recommended metformin for HF patients with normal, stable renal function [72]. Glucokinase activator (GKA), dorzagliatin, rough allosteric modulation, fully activates GK by stabilizing its active conformation, thereby improving β-cell function, reducing insulin resistance and remodeling glycemic homeostasis in patients with T2DM [73,74]. The phase III expansion study of dorzagliatin showed an improvement in time in target range (TIR) for glucose from 59.9% at baseline to 83.7% at 46 weeks of dorzagliatin treatment [75]. And while a 6% reduction in major adverse cardiovascular event (MACE) risk for every 10% increase in TIR may provide support for the cardiovascular benefits of dorzagliatin, more prospective studies are needed [76]. GLP-1 RA may improve cardiovascular outcomes by reducing appetite and body weight through central nervous system actions, decreasing hepatic steatosis to lower triglyceride and LDL-C levels [51]. In HFpEF, GLP-1RA attenuated atrial enlargement and reduced epicardial fat storage; in HFrEF, GLP-1RA attenuated adverse left ventricular remodeling and cardiac inflammation while increasing AMPK activity [77]. Recently, in the STEP-HFpEF and STEP-HFpEF DM trials, Semaglutide was superior to placebo in improving HF-related symptoms and reducing body weight in obesity-associated HFpEF [78]. SGLT2 inhibitors were effective in lowering mean HbAlc, BMI, and systolic blood pressure, as well as reducing the risk of HHF [79]. However, concerns regarding the heightened risk of genitourinary (GU) infections, particularly urinary tract infections, remain a significant barrier to their wider adoption [80].

The Grading of Recommendations Assessment, Development and Evaluation (GRADE) method of summarizing and assessing the quality of evidence is used by more than 110 organizations worldwide and has advantages over any alternative [81]. Five factors may reduce the quality of evidence: risk of bias, inconsistency, inaccuracy, indirectness and publication bias [82]. These five factors will be assessed using using the online tool, GRADEproGPT. The quality of evidence will be categorized into the following four levels: high, moderate, low and very low. Of note, the SGLT2 inhibitor is recommended in several guidelines with a high strength and quality of evidence of A, both for HFrEF and HFpEF [83,84].

7. SGLT2 Inhibitors and Heart Failure

Landmark trials have demonstrated the efficacy of SGLT2 inhibitors through prospective evaluations (Table 3). The EMPEROR-Reduced and DAPA-HF trials showed that SGLT2 inhibitors benefit HFrEF by reducing HHF, cardiovascular death and slowing renal function decline in chronic kidney disease (CKD) patients [85,86]. The EMPEROR-Preserved and DELIVER trials showed that SGLT2 inhibitors significantly reduced cardiovascular death and HHF in HFpEF, and modestly improved symptoms measured by the Kansas City Cardiomyopathy Questionnaire (KCCQ) [85]. Real-world database studies have also validated the clinical benefits of SGLT2 inhibitors on cardiovascular events (Table 4).

Table 3. RCT: SGLT2i on HF.

Name	Method	Result	Conclusion
The DAPA-HF study [45]	N = 4744 Dapagliflozin 10 mg vs. placebo Follow-up of 18.2 years	Dapagliflozin can reduce the risk of cardiovascular death or HHF in HFrEF patients by 26% and the risk of all-cause mortality by 17%.	Dapagliflozin reduces the risk of ventricular arrhythmia, cardiac arrest, or sudden death in patients with HFrEF.
The EMPEROR-Reduced study [86]	N = 3730 Empagliflozin 10 mg vs. placebo Follow-up of 1.5 years	Empagliflozin reduced the primary outcome (first cardiovascular death or HF with or without CKD), as well as the secondary outcome (patients' first and recurrent hospitalizations for HF) and may slow the rate of decline in eGFR.	The use of empagliflozin in HFrEF patients is recommeded.
The DELIVER study [87]	N = 6263 Dapagliflozin 10 mg vs. placebo Follow-up of 2.3 years	Dapagliflozin significantly reduced the rate of cardiovascular deaths and HHF by 18%, regardless of left ventricular function.	Dapagliflozin reduce the risk of the primary composite endpoint.
The PRESERVED-HF study [88]	N = 324 Dapagliflozin 10 mg vs. placebo Follow-up of 12 weeks	Dapagliflozin significant benefit in symptoms, physical limitations and 6-min walk test with 12 weeks of dapagliflozin.	Within 12 weeks, dapagliflozin significantly improved symptoms and physical activity limitations in patients with HFpEF.
The CAMEO-DAPA study [89]	N = 38 NYHAII/III, LVEF > 50% and PCWP patients were randomly divided into the dapagliflozin group and placebo group. Follow-up of 24 weeks	Resting PCWP decreased by 3.5 mmHg (p = 0.029); Exercise PCWP decreased by 6.1 mmHg (p = 0.019)	Dapagliflozin offers potential benefits for HFpEF.
The EMPEROR-Preserved study [90]	N = 5988 Empagliflozin 10 mg vs. placebo, Follow-up of 26.2 months	Empagliflozin significantly improved cardiovascular death and HHF in patients with HFpEF, the treatment effect of empagliflozin was not affected by heart rate.	Empagliflozin significantly reduced the rate of cardiovascular death or HHF composite endpoint events compared to placebo, and independent of the presence of comorbid diabetes.
The EMPA-RESPONSE-AHF study [91]	N = 80 Empagliflozin 10 mg vs. placebo Follow-up of 60 days	Empagliflozin significantly reduced the composite endpoint events including worsening heart failure during hospitalization, HF rehospitalization, and death.	Empagliflozin is safe and well-tolerated in the treatment of acute decompensated HF.

Table 3. *Cont.*

Name	Method	Result	Conclusion
the EMPA-REG OUTCOME study [92]	N = 7020 Empagliflozin 10 mg vs. Empagliflozin 25 mg vs. placebo	Empagliflozin significantly reduced the risk of 3P-MACE in patients by up to 14% and the risk of cardiovascular death by up to 38% on top of standard therapy.	Treatment with empagliflozin (10 mg) significantly prolonged survival in patients of all ages.
The EMBRACE-HF study [91]	N = 65 Empagliflozin 10mg vs. placebo Follow-up of 12 weeks	The empagliflozin group significantly reduced mean pulmonary artery diastolic pressure at 8–12 weeks.	Empagliflozin significantly reduced pulmonary artery diastolic blood pressure.
The EMPULSE study [93]	N = 530 Empagliflozin 10 mg vs. placebo Follow-up of 90 days	Patients treated with empagliflozin were 36% more likely to achieve clinical benefit, and no treatment heterogeneity.	Patients hospitalized with acute HF were significantly more likely to have clinical benefit within 90 days with empagliflozin.
The EMPAG-HF study [94]	Empagliflozin 25 mg vs. placebo Follow-up on days 6–10 (at discharge) and after 30 days	Treatment of acute decompensated HF with empagliflozin does not result in additional renal injury.	Empagliflozin was safe and well tolerated.
The VERTIS CV study [95]	N = 8246 Ertugliflozin 5 mg vs. Ertugliflozin 15 mg vs. placebo Follow-up of 3.5 years	The risk of 3P-MACE was noninferior in the Ertugliflozin (5 and 10 mg) groups compared with the placebo group.	Ertugliflozin reduces the risk of first HF and all HF after enrollment, which is not influenced by the presence or absence of a history of HF at baseline or LVEF.
The CHIENT-HF study [96]	N = 476 HF Canagliflozin 100 mg vs. placebo	The benefit of canagliflozin in significantly improving patient symptom regardless of EF or T2DM.	Canagliflozin not only improves prognosis, but also significantly improves symptoms, function and quality of life.

HF, heart failure; HHF, hospitalization for heart failure; EF, ejection fraction; LVEF, left ventricular ejection fraction; NYHA, New York Heart Association; PCWP, pulmonary capillary wedge pressure; HFrEF, heart failure with reduced ejection fraction; HFpEF, heart failure with preserved ejection fraction; CKD, chronic kidney disease; T2DM, type 2 diabetes mellitus.

Table 4. Real world: SGLT2 inhibitor on HF [97–100].

Name	Populations Included	Method	Conclusion
CVD-REAL study	Patients treated with any SGLT-2i versus other antidiabetic drugs in 6 countries (USA, Norway, Denmark, Sweden, Germany and UK).	Using medical claims, hospital records and national registry data, HHF and mortality were estimated by country and aggregated to determine a weighted effect size.	Treatment with SGLT-2 inhibitor was associated with lower incidence of HHF and mortality, with no heterogeneity in outcomes between countries.
Scandinavian register based on cohort study	National registry data from Denmark, Norway, and Sweden including 19% of the population with a history of major cardiovascular disease and 6% with a history of HF.	83% were on dapagliflozin, 16% empagliflozin, and 1% canagliflozin, compared SGLT-2 inhibitor versus DPP-4is on heart failures hospitalization.	SGLT-2i reduced the risk of primary heart failure by 34%.

Table 4. *Cont.*

Name	Populations Included	Method	Conclusion
Real-world study in Taiwan	12,681 patients with T2DM who were new to SGLT2 inhibitors were included, of which 5812 were on dapagliflozin and 6869 were on empagliflozin.	Through analysis of multi-institutional electronic medical records (Chang Gung Research Database, Taiwan), the risk of cardiovascular events was compared and analyzed between the two groups.	In terms of risk of cardiovascular events, both risks were similar, but dapagliflozin was significantly better than empagliflozin in reducing HF.

HF, heart failure; HHF, hospitalization for HF; SGLT2, sodium-glucose transporter 2; T2DM, type 2 diabetes mellitus.

Possible Mechanism of SGLT2i for Heart Failure

SGLT2 inhibitors lower glucose by increasing urinary glucose excretion, but their cardiovascular benefits may be independent of their hypoglycemic effects [101]. Sustained cardiovascular benefits may occur through multiple mechanisms, such as diuresis, sodium excretion, improved ventricular remodeling and cardiac function, inhibition of sodium-hydrogen exchangers, improved myocardial energy metabolism, reduced sympathetic activity, anti-inflammatory, and antioxidant activities [102] (Figure 3). The EMPA-REG OUTCOME trial showed that about 50% of the cardiovascular benefit is due to elevated hematocrit. Notably, after dapagliflozin treatment in T2DM patients, Erythropoietin (EPO) levels still increased after 2 months, suggesting that elevated hematocrit is due to both diuretic-induced hemoconcentration and increased EPO [103]. In addition, SGLT2 inhibitors protect vascular endothelial cells by enhancing NO synthesis and preventing degradation [104,105], improving ventricular remodeling and cardiac function by decreasing epicardial fat [106]. Dapagliflozin directly inhibits Sodium Hydrogen Antiporter (NHE-1), reduces intracellular Na ion concentration, and decreases glucose dependence in favor of increasing fatty acid and ketone use, an improved fuel source that requires less oxygen for cardiomyocytes. Recent studies have found SGLT2 inhibitor increased heme oxygenase expression, reduced AGEs and increased antioxidant effects of ketogenicity to alleviate oxidative stress [107,108]. SGLT 2 inhibitors can decrease activation of the transcription factor nuclear factor-κB (NF-κB), also reducing the production of pro-inflammatory cytokines and chemokines [109]. Interestingly, SGLT2 inhibitors mediated the doubling of ketone levels more significantly in diabetic patients, blocking the NLPR 3 inflammasome [110]. Additional cardiac benefits may be mediated through weight loss, reduced insulin resistance, lower serum uric acid levels, etc. [111]. In conclusion, establishing the exact mechanism of benefit is key to understanding SGLT2 inhibitors and may also provide a richer pathway to fully understand the pathophysiology of HF and the potential therapeutic approaches.

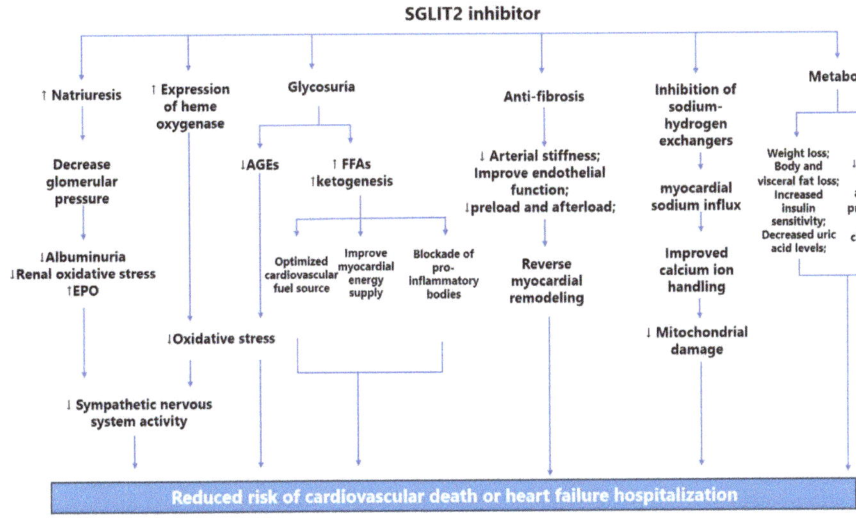

Figure 3. Potential mechanisms of clinical benefit of SGLT2 inhibitors. SGLT2 inhibitors exert beneficial effects on the cardiovascular system through a variety of mechanisms, including hypoglycemia, antihypertension, diuresis, weight loss, improvement of myocardial energy metabolism, reduction of oxidative stress and inflammation, protection of renal function, body weight reduction, and metabolic improvement. Recently, SGLT2 inhibitors have been found to have novel mechanisms of increased heme oxygenase expression, increased ketone bodies as a better fuel for the myocardium, and decreased epicardial fat, which together reduced risk of cardiovascular death or heart failure hospitalization. SGLT2, sodium-glucose transporter 2; EPO, erythropoietin; AGEs, advanced glycosylation products; FFAs, free fatty acids.

8. Finerenone—Non-Steroidal Mineralocorticoid Receptor Antagonists in Heart Failure

Non-aldosterone-mediated activation of the mineralocorticoid receptor (MR) promotes reactive oxygen species generation and mediates tissue inflammation and fibrosis, leading to myocardial hypertrophy, ventricular remodeling, glomerular hypertrophy and glomerulosclerosis, ultimately causing renal-cardiac adverse outcomes [112,113]. Specific MRA has become a major focus of research and development. Finerenone is the first novel non-steroidal MRA approved globally for treating T2D-related CKD [114]. It acts on multiple MR sites in the glomerulus, tubule and heart, binding specifically to Ala-773 and Ser-810 residues, leading to C-terminal ligand-dependent binding. Upon binding, helix 12 of the activation domain AF2 protrudes, forming an "inactive conformation" that fully inhibits co-regulatory factor recruitment [115,116]. Additionally, finerenone does not bind to glucocorticoid, androgen or progesterone receptors, making it more selective and providing direct anti-inflammatory and antifibrotic effects [117]. Furthermore, finerenone does not cross the blood–brain barrier, has a short half-life and allows for quicker correction of hyperkalemia, balancing efficacy and safety [118,119]. In two landmark phase III studies, FIDELIO-DKD and FIGARO-DKD, finerenone demonstrated significant renoprotective effects on top of RAAS inhibitor therapy at the maximum tolerable dose, reducing cardiovascular adverse events and proteinuria [120]. The European Society of Cardiology (ESC) gave finerenone the highest recommendation for cardiovascular disease in patients with acute and chronic HF and DM [121]. In contrast, recent subgroup analysis of the FIDELITY study showed that finerenone treatment benefit was not related to the presence or absence of SGLT2 inhibitor use [114]. However, there was an effect of better renal-cardiac benefit and lower hyperkalemia in the combination treatment group compared with the placebo group (10.3% and 2.7%, respectively) [122]. Notably, since both SGLT2 inhibitors and finerenone can cause a transient decrease in the estimated glomerular filtration rate (eGFR), sequential therapy is recommended for efficacy and safety [114]. The China Expert Consensus (2023) recommended applying finerenone with an interval of at least 2–4 weeks and to closely monitor eGFR fluctuations during treatment.

9. Vericiguat—A Novel Drug in HF Treatment

The 2021 ESC Heart Failure Guidelines included, for the first time, a new generation of sGC agonist vericiguat [123] (Figure 4). sGC is a key enzyme that promotes the production of cyclic guanosine monophosphate (cGMP) when nitric oxide NO binds to sGC, playing a vital role in the regulation of vascular tone, contractile function of the heart and remodeling of cardiac structure [47]. On the one hand, vericiguat improves sGC receptor sensitivity to NO by stabilizing the NO-sGC binding site, resulting in increased cGMP production in cardiomyocytes and vascular smooth muscle cells [124]. On the other hand, acting on the NO-independent binding site, it directly binds to the sGC receptor and further enhances the expression of cGMP [47]. The above dual mechanism repairs the NO-sGC-cGMP signaling pathway, improves endothelial and vascular function, and reduces ventricular remodeling and myocardial hypertrophy. The VICTORIA phase III study showed that vericiguat reduced the annual absolute risk (ARR) of the primary composite endpoint by 4.2%, with a number needed to treat (NNT) of 24, meaning one primary endpoint event is prevented per year for every 24 patients treated [125]. Continued vericiguat treatment led to significant improvements in LVEF, blood NT-proBNP levels and quality of life in patients [126]. Importantly, no adverse effects on blood pressure or renal function were observed, ensuring treatment safety [127]. Notably, for patients with worsening HFrEF, even with optimal treatment with quadruple dosing, there is still a higher risk of adverse clinical events and a higher risk of HHF [128]. Based on the results of the VICTORIA trial, vericiguat was approved for the treatment of symptomatic chronic HF with an ejection fraction <45% after a worsening event in HF due to its well-tolerated, safe and reduced rate of HHF [129].

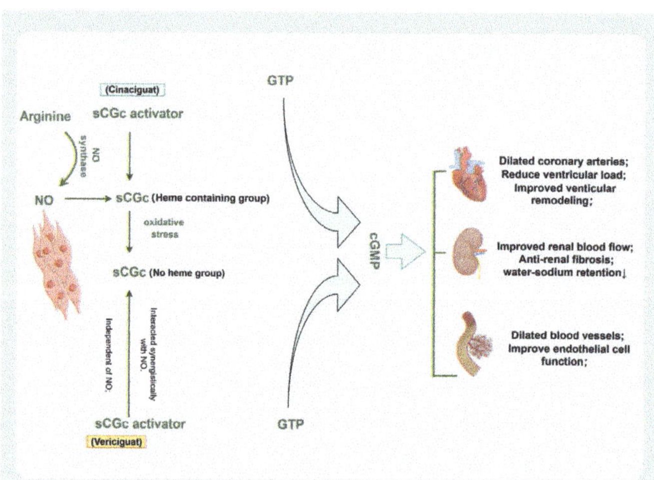

Figure 4. Mechanism of cardiorenal benefits of vericiguat. Vericiguat is the first sGC agonist that can directly stimulate sGC or synergize with endogenous NO to jointly increase intracellular levels of cGMP, leading to smooth muscle relaxation and vasodilation. By repairing damage to NO-sGC-cGMP, a cellular signaling pathway, the three major target organs, heart, blood vessels, and kidneys, are benefited. By Figdraw. SCG, soluble guanylate cyclase; NO, nitric oxide; cGMP, cyclic guanosine monophosphate; GTP, guanosine triphosphate.

10. The Reflection on Choosing the Research Endpoint in the SGLT2 Inhibitor HFpEF Test

The selection of clinical trial endpoints in ongoing studies of new drugs is fraught with challenges. Clinical trials have been a crucial tool for identifying primary endpoints since the 1960s, typically described in a non-stratified manner in the study protocol. However, when multiple primary endpoints are specified without comparing and adjusting for multiplicity, it is possible for researchers to erroneously conclude that a treatment is effective if just one of the endpoints meets a threshold of 0.05 [130]. For example, the EMPEROR-Preserved study, which used SGLT2 inhibitors as a composite endpoint for cardiovascular death or HHF, was arguably the first large HFpEF trial to meet the primary endpoint, but the improvement in this endpoint was primarily due to a reduction in HHF, with no significant differences observed in total or cardiovascular mortality, quality of life or NT-proBNP levels [131].

11. Future Directions in Heart Failure Research

RCTs include patients with HFrEF to improve statistical efficacy, ignoring the diverse and heterogeneous phenotypes of HF patients [132]. Future studies should focus on the characteristics of the HF spectrum, moving from analyses of large, heterogeneous groups with unspecified LVEF to more individualized [133], mechanistic studies with smaller, homogeneous groups. Additionally, benefits have been shown in patients with DM and/or HF, suggesting that evaluating their potential synergy with SGLT2 inhibitors is promising [51]. Recent cohort studies indicate that co-administering GLP-1 RA and SGLT2 inhibitors reduces the risk of MACE and serious renal events compared to using either drug alone [134]. The combination of an SGLT2 inhibitor and MRA will be evaluated in patients with cardiorenal disease in the MIRACLE and CONFIDENCE trials [135]. Moreover, SGLT2 inhibitors will be applied to address causative factors leading to HF and other cardiovascular diseases. Since atrial fibrillation is significantly associated with HFpEF, SGLT2 inhibitors have been shown to reduce atrial fibrillation events in a recent analysis of adverse event reports from RCTs [136]. Additionally, starting SGLT2 inhibitors in patients with T2DM and a history of percutaneous coronary intervention (PCI) was significantly associated with reduced risks of cardiorenal outcomes and mortality, regardless of the time since the last PCI [137]. Finally, ongoing trials (DAPA-MI and EMPACT-MI) are assessing the role of SGLT2 inhibitors after myocardial infarction [84].

12. Conclusions

HF and DM are mutual risk factors for each other. Long-term hyperglycemia can lead to autonomic neuropathy, microcirculatory dysfunction and metabolic and energy changes. Therefore, hypoglycemic therapy has been widely researched as an important potential target for HF. Encouragingly, many antidiabetic drugs applied to HF have achieved good efficacy, such as SGLT2 inhibitor and some GLP-1 RA. HFpEF accounts for nearly 50% of cases, with hospitalization and mortality rates comparable to HFrEF, and still lacks ideal treatment, while SGLT2 inhibitors have shown significant benefit in preventing hospitalization. The potential mechanisms of the SGLT2 inhibitor cannot be attributed solely to improvements in traditional risk factors (e.g., blood pressure, glucose, volume status and renal function), and an increasing amount of experimental evidence suggests an improvement in energy efficiency and a reduction in inflammation and oxidative stress and fibrosis, which can help to reduce adverse remodeling and diastolic dysfunction. These studies will provide important insights into the key pathways involved in the cardioprotective effects associated with SGLT2 inhibitor therapy. In addition, novel drugs such as vericiguat and finerenone have been documented in several clinical trials for very promising cardiovascular benefits in HF. Hopefully, as clinical evidence increases, they will become an additional powerful tool in the treatment of patients with HF. While this review comprehensively synthesizes the current literature on DM, HF and antidiabetic drugs for HF treatment, several limitations should be noted. The literature search may have been restricted by the timeframe, language biases and specific database reliance, potentially excluding relevant high-quality studies. Additionally, this review primarily aligns with authoritative guidelines, rather than autonomously applying the GRADE methodology to assess antidiabetic drug recommendations based on evidence quality and clinical context, and to indicate the recommendation strength clearly. Moreover, long-term safety data for some drugs remain unclear due to limited clinical trial follow-up. Future research should address these limitations.

Author Contributions: X.L. wrote the manuscript. X.Z. and L.G. participated in the writing and revised the manuscript. All authors have read and agreed to the published version of the manuscript.

Funding: This study was supported by the National Science Foundation of China (Project # 82270861 to L.G.), the Fundamental Research Funds for the Central Universities (Project # 2042020kf1079 to L.G.), the Planned international development Project of Wuhan University (Project # WHU-GJZDZX TS03 to L.G.), China UK joint training program for young scientists of Wuhan University.

Acknowledgments: The authors greatly appreciate Li Qiang for his help in searching the data.

Conflicts of Interest: The authors declare that the research was conducted in the absence of any commercial or financial relationships that could be construed as a potential conflict of interest. The authors declare no conflicts of interest.

References

1. Mudd, J.O.; Kass, D.A. Tackling Heart Failure in the Twenty-First Century. *Nature* **2008**, *451*, 919–928. [CrossRef] [PubMed]
2. From, A.M.; Leibson, C.L.; Bursi, F.; Redfield, M.M.; Weston, S.A.; Jacobsen, S.J.; Rodeheffer, R.J.; Roger, V.L. Diabetes in Heart Failure: Prevalence and Impact on Outcome in the Population. *Am. J. Med.* **2006**, *119*, 591–599. [CrossRef] [PubMed]
3. Kannel, W.B.; McGee, D.L. Diabetes and Cardiovascular Disease. The Framingham Study. *JAMA* **1979**, *241*, 2035–2038. [CrossRef] [PubMed]
4. Wei, M.; Gaskill, S.P.; Haffner, S.M.; Stern, M.P. Effects of Diabetes and Level of Glycemia on All-Cause and Cardiovascular Mortality. The San Antonio Heart Study. *Diabetes Care* **1998**, *21*, 1167–1172. [CrossRef] [PubMed]
5. Gambardella, J.; Lombardi, A.; Santulli, G. Metabolic Flexibility of Mitochondria Plays a Key Role in Balancing Glucose and Fatty Acid Metabolism in the Diabetic Heart. *Diabetes* **2020**, *69*, 2054–2057. [CrossRef] [PubMed]
6. Wisneski, J.A.; Gertz, E.W.; Neese, R.A.; Mayr, M. Myocardial Metabolism of Free Fatty Acids. Studies with 14C-Labeled Substrates in Humans. *J. Clin. Investig.* **1987**, *79*, 359–366. [CrossRef]
7. Goldin, A.; Beckman, J.A.; Schmidt, A.M.; Creager, M.A. Advanced Glycation End Products: Sparking the Development of Diabetic Vascular Injury. *Circulation* **2006**, *114*, 597–605. [CrossRef] [PubMed]
8. Pop-Busui, R.; Januzzi, J.L.; Bruemmer, D.; Butalia, S.; Green, J.B.; Horton, W.B.; Knight, C.; Levi, M.; Rasouli, N.; Richardson, C.R. Heart Failure: An Underappreciated Complication of Diabetes. A Consensus Report of the American Diabetes Association. *Diabetes Care* **2022**, *45*, 1670–1690. [CrossRef] [PubMed]
9. Rawshani, A.; Rawshani, A.; Franzén, S.; Sattar, N.; Eliasson, B.; Svensson, A.-M.; Zethelius, B.; Miftaraj, M.; McGuire, D.K.; Rosengren, A.; et al. Risk Factors, Mortality, and Cardiovascular Outcomes in Patients with Type 2 Diabetes. *N. Engl. J. Med.* **2018**, *379*, 633–644. [CrossRef]
10. Gebreegziabher, Y.; McCullough, P.A.; Bubb, C.; Loney-Hutchinson, L.; Makaryus, J.N.; Anand, N.; Divakaran, V.; Akhrass, P.; Alam, A.; von Gizycki, H.; et al. Admission Hyperglycemia and Length of Hospital Stay in Patients with Diabetes and Heart Failure: A Prospective Cohort Study. *Congest. Heart Fail.* **2008**, *14*, 117–120. [CrossRef]
11. Banerjee, A.; Pasea, L.; Chung, S.-C.; Direk, K.; Asselbergs, F.W.; Grobbee, D.E.; Kotecha, D.; Anker, S.D.; Dyszynski, T.; Tyl, B.; et al. A Population-Based Study of 92 Clinically Recognized Risk Factors for Heart Failure: Co-Occurrence, Prognosis and Preventive Potential. *Eur. J. Heart Fail.* **2022**, *24*, 466–480. [CrossRef]
12. Borlaug, B.A.; Melenovsky, V.; Russell, S.D.; Kessler, K.; Pacak, K.; Becker, L.C.; Kass, D.A. Impaired Chronotropic and Vasodilator Reserves Limit Exercise Capacity in Patients with Heart Failure and a Preserved Ejection Fraction. *Circulation* **2006**, *114*, 2138–2147. [CrossRef] [PubMed]
13. Ergatoudes, C.; Schaufelberger, M.; Andersson, B.; Pivodic, A.; Dahlström, U.; Fu, M. Non-Cardiac Comorbidities and Mortality in Patients with Heart Failure with Reduced vs. Preserved Ejection Fraction: A Study Using the Swedish Heart Failure Registry. *Clin. Res. Cardiol.* **2019**, *108*, 1025–1033. [CrossRef]
14. Zile, M.R.; Baicu, C.F.; Gaasch, W.H. Diastolic Heart Failure--Abnormalities in Active Relaxation and Passive Stiffness of the Left Ventricle. *N. Engl. J. Med.* **2004**, *350*, 1953–1959. [CrossRef] [PubMed]
15. Mishra, S.; Kass, D.A. Cellular and Molecular Pathobiology of Heart Failure with Preserved Ejection Fraction. *Nat. Rev. Cardiol.* **2021**, *18*, 400–423. [CrossRef] [PubMed]
16. Tsutsui, H.; Kinugawa, S.; Matsushima, S. Oxidative Stress and Heart Failure. *Am. J. Physiol. Heart Circ. Physiol.* **2011**, *301*, H2181–H2190. [CrossRef]

17. Ho, J.E.; Lyass, A.; Lee, D.S.; Vasan, R.S.; Kannel, W.B.; Larson, M.G.; Levy, D. Predictors of New-Onset Heart Failure: Differences in Preserved versus Reduced Ejection Fraction. *Circ. Heart Fail.* **2013**, *6*, 279–286. [CrossRef]
18. Kass, D.A.; Bronzwaer, J.G.F.; Paulus, W.J. What Mechanisms Underlie Diastolic Dysfunction in Heart Failure? *Circ. Res.* **2004**, *94*, 1533–1542. [CrossRef]
19. Dickstein, K.; Cohen-Solal, A.; Filippatos, G.; McMurray, J.J.V.; Ponikowski, P.; Poole-Wilson, P.A.; Strömberg, A.; van Veldhuisen, D.J.; Atar, D.; Hoes, A.W.; et al. ESC Guidelines for the Diagnosis and Treatment of Acute and Chronic Heart Failure 2008: The Task Force for the Diagnosis and Treatment of Acute and Chronic Heart Failure 2008 of the European Society of Cardiology. Developed in Collaboration with the Heart Failure Association of the ESC (HFA) and Endorsed by the European Society of Intensive Care Medicine (ESICM). *Eur. J. Heart Fail.* **2008**, *10*, 933–989. [CrossRef]
20. GBD 2016 Disease and Injury Incidence and Prevalence Collaborators. Global, Regional, and National Incidence, Prevalence, and Years Lived with Disability for 328 Diseases and Injuries for 195 Countries, 1990–2016: A Systematic Analysis for the Global Burden of Disease Study 2016. *Lancet* **2017**, *390*, 1211–1259. [CrossRef]
21. Writing Group Members; Mozaffarian, D.; Benjamin, E.J.; Go, A.S.; Arnett, D.K.; Blaha, M.J.; Cushman, M.; Das, S.R.; de Ferranti, S.; Després, J.-P.; et al. Heart Disease and Stroke Statistics-2016 Update: A Report From the American Heart Association. *Circulation* **2016**, *133*, e38–e360. [CrossRef] [PubMed]
22. Matsue, Y.; Suzuki, M.; Nakamura, R.; Abe, M.; Ono, M.; Yoshida, S.; Seya, M.; Iwatsuka, R.; Mizukami, A.; Setoguchi, M.; et al. Prevalence and Prognostic Implications of Pre-Diabetic State in Patients with Heart Failure. *Circ. J.* **2011**, *75*, 2833–2839. [CrossRef] [PubMed]
23. Bae, J.H.; Han, K.-D.; Ko, S.-H.; Yang, Y.S.; Choi, J.H.; Choi, K.M.; Kwon, H.-S.; Won, K.C. Diabetes Fact Sheet in Korea 2021. *Diabetes Metab. J.* **2022**, *46*, 417–426. [CrossRef]
24. van Melle, J.P.; Bot, M.; de Jonge, P.; de Boer, R.A.; van Veldhuisen, D.J.; Whooley, M.A. Diabetes, Glycemic Control, and New-Onset Heart Failure in Patients with Stable Coronary Artery Disease: Data from the Heart and Soul Study. *Diabetes Care* **2010**, *33*, 2084–2089. [CrossRef] [PubMed]
25. Nichols, G.A.; Gullion, C.M.; Koro, C.E.; Ephross, S.A.; Brown, J.B. The Incidence of Congestive Heart Failure in Type 2 Diabetes: An Update. *Diabetes Care* **2004**, *27*, 1879–1884. [CrossRef] [PubMed]
26. Bertoni, A.G.; Hundley, W.G.; Massing, M.W.; Bonds, D.E.; Burke, G.L.; Goff, D.C. Heart Failure Prevalence, Incidence, and Mortality in the Elderly with Diabetes. *Diabetes Care* **2004**, *27*, 699–703. [CrossRef] [PubMed]
27. Kristensen, S.L.; Jhund, P.S.; Lee, M.M.Y.; Køber, L.; Solomon, S.D.; Granger, C.B.; Yusuf, S.; Pfeffer, M.A.; Swedberg, K.; McMurray, J.J.V.; et al. Prevalence of Prediabetes and Undiagnosed Diabetes in Patients with HFpEF and HFrEF and Associated Clinical Outcomes. *Cardiovasc. Drugs Ther.* **2017**, *31*, 545–549. [CrossRef]
28. Zhong, P.; Peng, J. Sarcolipin Acts as a Bridge between Diabetes and Heart Failure. *ESC Heart Fail.* **2020**, *7*, 4488. [CrossRef]
29. Paradela-Dobarro, B.; Agra, R.M.; Álvarez, L.; Varela-Román, A.; García-Acuña, J.M.; González-Juanatey, J.R.; Álvarez, E.; García-Seara, F.J. The Different Roles for the Advanced Glycation End Products Axis in Heart Failure and Acute Coronary Syndrome Settings. *Nutr. Metab. Cardiovasc. Dis.* **2019**, *29*, 1050–1060. [CrossRef]
30. Ertunc, M.E.; Hotamisligil, G.S. Lipid Signaling and Lipotoxicity in Metaflammation: Indications for Metabolic Disease Pathogenesis and Treatment. *J. Lipid Res.* **2016**, *57*, 2099–2114. [CrossRef]
31. Glass, C.K.; Olefsky, J.M. Inflammation and Lipid Signaling in the Etiology of Insulin Resistance. *Cell Metab.* **2012**, *15*, 635–645. [CrossRef] [PubMed]
32. Braunwald, E. Diabetes, Heart Failure, and Renal Dysfunction: The Vicious Circles. *Prog. Cardiovasc. Dis.* **2019**, *62*, 298–302. [CrossRef] [PubMed]
33. Iribarren, C.; Karter, A.J.; Go, A.S.; Ferrara, A.; Liu, J.Y.; Sidney, S.; Selby, J.V. Glycemic Control and Heart Failure among Adult Patients with Diabetes. *Circulation* **2001**, *103*, 2668–2673. [CrossRef] [PubMed]
34. Ceriello, A.; Catrinoiu, D.; Chandramouli, C.; Cosentino, F.; Dombrowsky, A.C.; Itzhak, B.; Lalic, N.M.; Prattichizzo, F.; Schnell, O.; Seferović, P.M.; et al. Heart Failure in Type 2 Diabetes: Current Perspectives on Screening, Diagnosis and Management. *Cardiovasc. Diabetol.* **2021**, *20*, 218. [CrossRef]
35. Control Group; Turnbull, F.M.; Abraira, C.; Anderson, R.J.; Byington, R.P.; Chalmers, J.P.; Duckworth, W.C.; Evans, G.W.; Gerstein, H.C.; Holman, R.R.; et al. Intensive Glucose Control and Macrovascular Outcomes in Type 2 Diabetes. *Diabetologia* **2009**, *52*, 2288–2298. [CrossRef]
36. Turner, R.C.; Millns, H.; Neil, H.A.; Stratton, I.M.; Manley, S.E.; Matthews, D.R.; Holman, R.R. Risk Factors for Coronary Artery Disease in Non-Insulin Dependent Diabetes Mellitus: United Kingdom Prospective Diabetes Study (UKPDS: 23). *BMJ* **1998**, *316*, 823–828. [CrossRef] [PubMed]
37. Braunwald, E. SGLT2 Inhibitors: The Statins of the 21st Century. *Eur. Heart J.* **2022**, *43*, 1029–1030. [CrossRef]
38. Echouffo-Tcheugui, J.B.; Daya, N.; Lee, A.K.; Tang, O.; Ndumele, C.E.; Windham, B.G.; Shah, A.M.; Selvin, E. Severe Hypoglycemia, Cardiac Structure and Function, and Risk of Cardiovascular Events Among Older Adults With Diabetes. *Diabetes Care* **2021**, *44*, 248–254. [CrossRef]
39. Rezende, P.C.; Everett, B.M.; Brooks, M.M.; Vlachos, H.; Orchard, T.J.; Frye, R.L.; Bhatt, D.L.; Hlatky, M.A. Hypoglycemia and Elevated Troponin in Patients With Diabetes and Coronary Artery Disease. *J. Am. Coll. Cardiol.* **2018**, *72*, 1778–1786. [CrossRef]

40. ORIGIN Trial Investigators; Mellbin, L.G.; Rydén, L.; Riddle, M.C.; Probstfield, J.; Rosenstock, J.; Díaz, R.; Yusuf, S.; Gerstein, H.C. Does Hypoglycaemia Increase the Risk of Cardiovascular Events? A Report from the ORIGIN Trial. *Eur. Heart J.* **2013**, *34*, 3137–3144. [CrossRef]
41. Frier, B.M.; Schernthaner, G.; Heller, S.R. Hypoglycemia and Cardiovascular Risks. *Diabetes Care* **2011**, *34* (Suppl. S2), S132–S137. [CrossRef] [PubMed]
42. Desouza, C.; Salazar, H.; Cheong, B.; Murgo, J.; Fonseca, V. Association of Hypoglycemia and Cardiac Ischemia: A Study Based on Continuous Monitoring. *Diabetes Care* **2003**, *26*, 1485–1489. [CrossRef] [PubMed]
43. Zhou, J.J.; Koska, J.; Bahn, G.; Reaven, P. Fasting Glucose Variation Predicts Microvascular Risk in ACCORD and VADT. *J. Clin. Endocrinol. Metab.* **2021**, *106*, 1150–1162. [CrossRef] [PubMed]
44. Nuyujukian, D.S.; Koska, J.; Bahn, G.; Reaven, P.D.; Zhou, J.J. VADT Investigators Blood Pressure Variability and Risk of Heart Failure in ACCORD and the VADT. *Diabetes Care* **2020**, *43*, 1471–1478. [CrossRef] [PubMed]
45. Cahn, A.; Mosenzon, O.; Bhatt, D.L.; Leibowitz, G.; Yanuv, I.; Rozenberg, A.; Iqbal, N.; Hirshberg, B.; Stahre, C.; Im, K.; et al. Hypoglycaemia Manifestations and Recurrent Events: Lessons from the SAVOR-TIMI 53 Outcome Study. *Diabetes Obes. Metab.* **2017**, *19*, 1045–1050. [CrossRef] [PubMed]
46. McMurray, J.J.V.; DeMets, D.L.; Inzucchi, S.E.; Køber, L.; Kosiborod, M.N.; Langkilde, A.M.; Martinez, F.A.; Bengtsson, O.; Ponikowski, P.; Sabatine, M.S.; et al. A Trial to Evaluate the Effect of the Sodium-Glucose Co-Transporter 2 Inhibitor Dapagliflozin on Morbidity and Mortality in Patients with Heart Failure and Reduced Left Ventricular Ejection Fraction (DAPA-HF). *Eur. J. Heart Fail.* **2019**, *21*, 665–675. [CrossRef]
47. Ruilope, L.M.; Dukat, A.; Böhm, M.; Lacourcière, Y.; Gong, J.; Lefkowitz, M.P. Blood-Pressure Reduction with LCZ696, a Novel Dual-Acting Inhibitor of the Angiotensin II Receptor and Neprilysin: A Randomised, Double-Blind, Placebo-Controlled, Active Comparator Study. *Lancet* **2010**, *375*, 1255–1266. [CrossRef]
48. Hulot, J.-S.; Trochu, J.-N.; Donal, E.; Galinier, M.; Logeart, D.; De Groote, P.; Juillière, Y. Vericiguat for the Treatment of Heart Failure: Mechanism of Action and Pharmacological Properties Compared with Other Emerging Therapeutic Options. *Expert Opin. Pharmacother.* **2021**, *22*, 1847–1855. [CrossRef]
49. Agarwal, R.; Filippatos, G.; Pitt, B.; Anker, S.D.; Rossing, P.; Joseph, A.; Kolkhof, P.; Nowack, C.; Gebel, M.; Ruilope, L.M.; et al. Cardiovascular and Kidney Outcomes with Finerenone in Patients with Type 2 Diabetes and Chronic Kidney Disease: The FIDELITY Pooled Analysis. *Eur. Heart J.* **2022**, *43*, 474–484. [CrossRef]
50. Butler, J.; Zannad, F.; Filippatos, G.; Anker, S.D.; Packer, M. Totality of Evidence in Trials of Sodium-Glucose Co-Transporter-2 Inhibitors in the Patients with Heart Failure with Reduced Ejection Fraction: Implications for Clinical Practice. *Eur. Heart J.* **2020**, *41*, 3398–3401. [CrossRef]
51. Ilieșiu, A.M.; Hodorogea, A.S. Treatment of Heart Failure with Preserved Ejection Fraction. *Adv. Exp. Med. Biol.* **2018**, *1067*, 67–87. [CrossRef] [PubMed]
52. Scheen, A.J. GLP-1 Receptor Agonists and Heart Failure in Diabetes. *Diabetes Metab.* **2017**, *43* (Suppl. S1), 2S13–12S19. [CrossRef] [PubMed]
53. Li, L.; Li, S.; Liu, J.; Deng, K.; Busse, J.W.; Vandvik, P.O.; Wong, E.; Sohani, Z.N.; Bala, M.M.; Rios, L.P.; et al. Glucagon-like Peptide-1 Receptor Agonists and Heart Failure in Type 2 Diabetes: Systematic Review and Meta-Analysis of Randomized and Observational Studies. *BMC Cardiovasc. Disord.* **2016**, *16*, 91. [CrossRef] [PubMed]
54. Staszewsky, L.; Baviera, M.; Tettamanti, M.; Colacioppo, P.; Robusto, F.; D'Ettorre, A.; Lepore, V.; Fortino, I.; Bisceglia, L.; Attolini, E.; et al. Insulin Treatment in Patients with Diabetes Mellitus and Heart Failure in the Era of New Antidiabetic Medications. *BMJ Open Diabetes Res. Care* **2022**, *10*, e002708. [CrossRef]
55. Arnold, S.V.; Echouffo-Tcheugui, J.B.; Lam, C.S.P.; Inzucchi, S.E.; Tang, F.; McGuire, D.K.; Goyal, A.; Maddox, T.M.; Sperling, L.S.; Fonarow, G.C.; et al. Patterns of Glucose-Lowering Medication Use in Patients with Type 2 Diabetes and Heart Failure. Insights from the Diabetes Collaborative Registry (DCR). *Am. Heart J.* **2018**, *203*, 25–29. [CrossRef] [PubMed]
56. Keller, D.M.; Ahmed, N.; Tariq, H.; Walgamage, M.; Walgamage, T.; Mohammed, A.; Chou, J.T.-T.; Kałużna-Oleksy, M.; Lesiak, M.; Straburzyńska-Migaj, E. SGLT2 Inhibitors in Type 2 Diabetes Mellitus and Heart Failure-A Concise Review. *J. Clin. Med.* **2022**, *11*, 1470. [CrossRef] [PubMed]
57. Schernthaner, G.; Brand, K.; Bailey, C.J. Metformin and the Heart: Update on Mechanisms of Cardiovascular Protection with Special Reference to Comorbid Type 2 Diabetes and Heart Failure. *Metab. Clin. Exp.* **2022**, *130*, 155160. [CrossRef]
58. Weir, D.L.; McAlister, F.A.; Senthilselvan, A.; Minhas-Sandhu, J.K.; Eurich, D.T. Sitagliptin Use in Patients with Diabetes and Heart Failure: A Population-Based Retrospective Cohort Study. *JACC. Heart Fail.* **2014**, *2*, 573–582. [CrossRef]
59. Eurich, D.T.; McAlister, F.A.; Blackburn, D.F.; Majumdar, S.R.; Tsuyuki, R.T.; Varney, J.; Johnson, J.A. Benefits and Harms of Antidiabetic Agents in Patients with Diabetes and Heart Failure: Systematic Review. *BMJ (Clin. Res. Ed.)* **2007**, *335*, 497. [CrossRef]
60. He, B.K.; Ning, Z.Q.; Li, Z.B.; Shan, S.; Pan, D.S.; Ko, B.C.B.; Li, P.P.; Shen, Z.F.; Dou, G.F.; Zhang, B.L.; et al. In Vitro and In Vivo Characterizations of Chiglitazar, a Newly Identified PPAR Pan-Agonist. *PPAR Res.* **2012**, *2012*, 546548. [CrossRef]
61. Rohatgi, A.; McGuire, D.K. Effects of the Thiazolidinedione Medications on Micro- and Macrovascular Complications in Patients with Diabetes—Update 2008. *Cardiovasc. Drugs Ther.* **2008**, *22*, 233–240. [CrossRef] [PubMed]
62. Norris, S.L.; Carson, S.; Roberts, C. Comparative Effectiveness of Pioglitazone and Rosiglitazone in Type 2 Diabetes, Prediabetes, and the Metabolic Syndrome: A Meta-Analysis. *Curr. Diabetes Rev.* **2007**, *3*, 127–140. [CrossRef] [PubMed]

63. Lincoff, A.M.; Wolski, K.; Nicholls, S.J.; Nissen, S.E. Pioglitazone and Risk of Cardiovascular Events in Patients with Type 2 Diabetes Mellitus: A Meta-Analysis of Randomized Trials. *JAMA* **2007**, *298*, 1180–1188. [CrossRef] [PubMed]
64. Avogaro, A.; Fadini, G.P. Insulin Treatment in Patients with Diabetes and Heart Failure: Defendant on the Stand. *Eur. J. Heart Fail.* **2018**, *20*, 896–897. [CrossRef] [PubMed]
65. Clawson, R.; Weidman-Evans, E.; Fort, A. Which Drug Is Best for a Patient with Type 2 Diabetes and Heart Failure? *JAAPA Off. J. Am. Acad. Physician Assist.* **2021**, *34*, 49–52. [CrossRef] [PubMed]
66. Hanefeld, M.; Schaper, F. Acarbose: Oral Anti-Diabetes Drug with Additional Cardiovascular Benefits. *Expert Rev. Cardiovasc. Ther.* **2008**, *6*, 153–163. [CrossRef] [PubMed]
67. Scirica, B.M.; Bhatt, D.L.; Braunwald, E.; Steg, P.G.; Davidson, J.; Hirshberg, B.; Ohman, P.; Frederich, R.; Wiviott, S.D.; Hoffman, E.B.; et al. Saxagliptin and Cardiovascular Outcomes in Patients with Type 2 Diabetes Mellitus. *N. Engl. J. Med.* **2013**, *369*, 1317–1326. [CrossRef] [PubMed]
68. Ferreira, J.P.; Mehta, C.; Sharma, A.; Nissen, S.E.; Rossignol, P.; Zannad, F. Alogliptin after Acute Coronary Syndrome in Patients with Type 2 Diabetes: A Renal Function Stratified Analysis of the EXAMINE Trial. *BMC Med.* **2020**, *18*, 165. [CrossRef] [PubMed]
69. Khan, M.S.; Solomon, N.; DeVore, A.D.; Sharma, A.; Felker, G.M.; Hernandez, A.F.; Heidenreich, P.A.; Matsouaka, R.A.; Green, J.B.; Butler, J.; et al. Clinical Outcomes With Metformin and Sulfonylurea Therapies Among Patients With Heart Failure and Diabetes. *JACC Heart Fail.* **2022**, *10*, 198–210. [CrossRef]
70. Larsen, A.H.; Jessen, N.; Nørrelund, H.; Tolbod, L.P.; Harms, H.J.; Feddersen, S.; Nielsen, F.; Brøsen, K.; Hansson, N.H.; Frøkiaer, J.; et al. A Randomised, Double-Blind, Placebo-Controlled Trial of Metformin on Myocardial Efficiency in Insulin-Resistant Chronic Heart Failure Patients without Diabetes. *Eur. J. Heart Fail.* **2020**, *22*, 1628–1637. [CrossRef]
71. Anabtawi, A.; Miles, J.M. Metformin: Nonglycemic effects and potential novel indications. *Endocr. Pr.* **2016**, *22*, 999–1007. [CrossRef] [PubMed]
72. Aguilar, D.; Chan, W.; Bozkurt, B.; Ramasubbu, K.; Deswal, A. Metformin Use and Mortality in Ambulatory Patients with Diabetes and Heart Failure. *Circ. Heart Fail.* **2011**, *4*, 53–58. [CrossRef] [PubMed]
73. American Diabetes Association 5. Lifestyle Management: Standards of Medical Care in Diabetes-2019. *Diabetes Care* **2019**, *42*, S46–S60. [CrossRef] [PubMed]
74. Agius, L. Glucokinase and Molecular Aspects of Liver Glycogen Metabolism. *Biochem. J.* **2008**, *414*, 1–18. [CrossRef] [PubMed]
75. Lenzen, S. A Fresh View of Glycolysis and Glucokinase Regulation: History and Current Status. *J. Biol. Chem.* **2014**, *289*, 12189–12194. [CrossRef] [PubMed]
76. Zeng, J.; Gan, S.; Mi, N.; Liu, Y.; Su, X.; Zhang, W.; Zhang, J.; Yu, F.; Dong, X.; Han, M.; et al. Diabetes Remission in Drug-Naïve Patients with Type 2 Diabetes after Dorzagliatin Treatment: A Prospective Cohort Study. *Diabetes Obes. Metab.* **2023**, *25*, 2878–2887. [CrossRef] [PubMed]
77. Virdi, N.; Poon, Y.; Abaniel, R.; Bergenstal, R.M. Prevalence, Cost, and Burden of Diabetic Ketoacidosis. *Diabetes Technol. Ther.* **2023**, *25*, S75–S84. [CrossRef] [PubMed]
78. Ussher, J.R.; Drucker, D.J. Glucagon-like Peptide 1 Receptor Agonists: Cardiovascular Benefits and Mechanisms of Action. *Nat. Rev. Cardiol.* **2023**, *20*, 463–474. [CrossRef] [PubMed]
79. Butler, J.; Shah, S.J.; Petrie, M.C.; Borlaug, B.A.; Abildstrøm, S.Z.; Davies, M.J.; Hovingh, G.K.; Kitzman, D.W.; Møller, D.V.; Verma, S.; et al. Semaglutide versus Placebo in People with Obesity-Related Heart Failure with Preserved Ejection Fraction: A Pooled Analysis of the STEP-HFpEF and STEP-HFpEF DM Randomised Trials. *Lancet* **2024**, *403*, 1635–1648. [CrossRef]
80. Bidulka, P.; Lugo-Palacios, D.G.; Carroll, O.; O'Neill, S.; Adler, A.I.; Basu, A.; Silverwood, R.J.; Bartlett, J.W.; Nitsch, D.; Charlton, P.; et al. Comparative Effectiveness of Second Line Oral Antidiabetic Treatments among People with Type 2 Diabetes Mellitus: Emulation of a Target Trial Using Routinely Collected Health Data. *BMJ (Clin. Res. Ed.)* **2024**, *385*, e077097. [CrossRef]
81. Kittipibul, V.; Cox, Z.L.; Chesdachai, S.; Fiuzat, M.; Lindenfeld, J.; Mentz, R.J. Genitourinary Tract Infections in Patients Taking SGLT2 Inhibitors: JACC Review Topic of the Week. *J. Am. Coll. Cardiol.* **2024**, *83*, 1568–1578. [CrossRef] [PubMed]
82. Goldet, G.; Howick, J. Understanding GRADE: An Introduction. *J. Evid. Based Med.* **2013**, *6*, 50–54. [CrossRef] [PubMed]
83. Cosentino, F.; Grant, P.J.; Aboyans, V.; Bailey, C.J.; Ceriello, A.; Delgado, V.; Federici, M.; Filippatos, G.; Grobbee, D.E.; Hansen, T.B.; et al. 2019 ESC Guidelines on Diabetes, Pre-Diabetes, and Cardiovascular Diseases Developed in Collaboration with the EASD. *Eur. Heart J.* **2020**, *41*, 255–323. [CrossRef] [PubMed]
84. Packer, M.; Anker, S.D.; Butler, J.; Filippatos, G.; Pocock, S.J.; Carson, P.; Januzzi, J.; Verma, S.; Tsutsui, H.; Brueckmann, M.; et al. Cardiovascular and Renal Outcomes with Empagliflozin in Heart Failure. *N. Engl. J. Med.* **2020**, *383*, 1413–1424. [CrossRef] [PubMed]
85. Guyatt, G.H.; Oxman, A.D.; Vist, G.E.; Kunz, R.; Falck-Ytter, Y.; Alonso-Coello, P.; Schünemann, H.J.; GRADE Working Group. GRADE: An Emerging Consensus on Rating Quality of Evidence and Strength of Recommendations. *BMJ* **2008**, *336*, 924–926. [CrossRef] [PubMed]
86. Caparrotta, T.M.; Blackbourn, L.A.K.; McGurnaghan, S.J.; Chalmers, J.; Lindsay, R.; McCrimmon, R.; McKnight, J.; Wild, S.; Petrie, J.R.; Philip, S.; et al. Prescribing Paradigm Shift? Applying the 2019 European Society of Cardiology-Led Guidelines on Diabetes, Prediabetes, and Cardiovascular Disease to Assess Eligibility for Sodium-Glucose Cotransporter 2 Inhibitors or Glucagon-Like Peptide 1 Receptor Agonists as First-Line Monotherapy (or Add-on to Metformin Monotherapy) in Type 2 Diabetes in Scotland. *Diabetes Care* **2020**, *43*, 2034–2041. [CrossRef]

87. Greene, S.J.; Butler, J. Primary Prevention of Heart Failure in Patients With Type 2 Diabetes Mellitus. *Circulation* **2019**, *139*, 152–154. [CrossRef] [PubMed]
88. Zannad, F.; Ferreira, J.P.; Pocock, S.J.; Zeller, C.; Anker, S.D.; Butler, J.; Filippatos, G.; Hauske, S.J.; Brueckmann, M.; Pfarr, E.; et al. Cardiac and Kidney Benefits of Empagliflozin in Heart Failure Across the Spectrum of Kidney Function: Insights From EMPEROR-Reduced. *Circulation* **2021**, *143*, 310–321. [CrossRef] [PubMed]
89. Solomon, S.D.; McMurray, J.J.V.; Claggett, B.; de Boer, R.A.; DeMets, D.; Hernandez, A.F.; Inzucchi, S.E.; Kosiborod, M.N.; Lam, C.S.P.; Martinez, F.; et al. Dapagliflozin in Heart Failure with Mildly Reduced or Preserved Ejection Fraction. *N. Engl. J. Med.* **2022**, *387*, 1089–1098. [CrossRef]
90. Nassif, M.E.; Windsor, S.L.; Borlaug, B.A.; Kitzman, D.W.; Shah, S.J.; Tang, F.; Khariton, Y.; Malik, A.O.; Khumri, T.; Umpierrez, G.; et al. The SGLT2 Inhibitor Dapagliflozin in Heart Failure with Preserved Ejection Fraction: A Multicenter Randomized Trial. *Nat. Med.* **2021**, *27*, 1954–1960. [CrossRef]
91. Borlaug, B.A.; Reddy, Y.N.V.; Braun, A.; Sorimachi, H.; Omar, M.; Popovic, D.; Alogna, A.; Jensen, M.D.; Carter, R. Cardiac and Metabolic Effects of Dapagliflozin in Heart Failure With Preserved Ejection Fraction: The CAMEO-DAPA Trial. *Circulation* **2023**, *148*, 834–844. [CrossRef] [PubMed]
92. Kalluri, S.R.; Bhutta, T.H.; Hannoodee, H.; Al Khalili, M.; Theik, N.W.Y.; Raji, O.E.; Shenwai, P.; Shah, R.; Khan, S. Do SGLT2 Inhibitors Improve Cardio-Renal Outcomes in Patients With Type II Diabetes Mellitus: A Systematic Review. *Cureus* **2021**, *13*, e17668. [CrossRef] [PubMed]
93. Damman, K.; Beusekamp, J.C.; Boorsma, E.M.; Swart, H.P.; Smilde, T.D.J.; Elvan, A.; van Eck, J.W.M.; Heerspink, H.J.L.; Voors, A.A. Randomized, Double-Blind, Placebo-Controlled, Multicentre Pilot Study on the Effects of Empagliflozin on Clinical Outcomes in Patients with Acute Decompensated Heart Failure (EMPA-RESPONSE-AHF). *Eur. J. Heart Fail.* **2020**, *22*, 713–722. [CrossRef] [PubMed]
94. Claggett, B.; Lachin, J.M.; Hantel, S.; Fitchett, D.; Inzucchi, S.E.; Woerle, H.J.; George, J.T.; Zinman, B. Long-Term Benefit of Empagliflozin on Life Expectancy in Patients With Type 2 Diabetes Mellitus and Established Cardiovascular Disease. *Circulation* **2018**, *138*, 1599–1601. [CrossRef] [PubMed]
95. Voors, A.A.; Angermann, C.E.; Teerlink, J.R.; Collins, S.P.; Kosiborod, M.; Biegus, J.; Ferreira, J.P.; Nassif, M.E.; Psotka, M.A.; Tromp, J.; et al. The SGLT2 Inhibitor Empagliflozin in Patients Hospitalized for Acute Heart Failure: A Multinational Randomized Trial. *Nat. Med.* **2022**, *28*, 568–574. [CrossRef] [PubMed]
96. Schulze, P.C.; Bogoviku, J.; Westphal, J.; Aftanski, P.; Haertel, F.; Grund, S.; von Haehling, S.; Schumacher, U.; Möbius-Winkler, S.; Busch, M. Effects of Early Empagliflozin Initiation on Diuresis and Kidney Function in Patients With Acute Decompensated Heart Failure (EMPAG-HF). *Circulation* **2022**, *146*, 289–298. [CrossRef] [PubMed]
97. Cosentino, F.; Cannon, C.P.; Cherney, D.Z.I.; Masiukiewicz, U.; Pratley, R.; Dagogo-Jack, S.; Frederich, R.; Charbonnel, B.; Mancuso, J.; Shih, W.J.; et al. Efficacy of Ertugliflozin on Heart Failure-Related Events in Patients With Type 2 Diabetes Mellitus and Established Atherosclerotic Cardiovascular Disease: Results of the VERTIS CV Trial. *Circulation* **2020**, *142*, 2205–2215. [CrossRef] [PubMed]
98. Spertus, J.A.; Birmingham, M.C.; Nassif, M.; Damaraju, C.V.; Abbate, A.; Butler, J.; Lanfear, D.E.; Lingvay, I.; Kosiborod, M.N.; Januzzi, J.L. The SGLT2 Inhibitor Canagliflozin in Heart Failure: The CHIEF-HF Remote, Patient-Centered Randomized Trial. *Nat. Med.* **2022**, *28*, 809–813. [CrossRef]
99. Shao, S.-C.; Chang, K.-C.; Hung, M.-J.; Yang, N.-I.; Chan, Y.-Y.; Chen, H.-Y.; Kao Yang, Y.-H.; Lai, E.C.-C. Comparative Risk Evaluation for Cardiovascular Events Associated with Dapagliflozin vs. Empagliflozin in Real-World Type 2 Diabetes Patients: A Multi-Institutional Cohort Study. *Cardiovasc. Diabetol.* **2019**, *18*, 120. [CrossRef]
100. Kosiborod, M.; Cavender, M.A.; Fu, A.Z.; Wilding, J.P.; Khunti, K.; Holl, R.W.; Norhammar, A.; Birkeland, K.I.; Jørgensen, M.E.; Thuresson, M.; et al. Lower Risk of Heart Failure and Death in Patients Initiated on Sodium-Glucose Cotransporter-2 Inhibitors Versus Other Glucose-Lowering Drugs: The CVD-REAL Study (Comparative Effectiveness of Cardiovascular Outcomes in New Users of Sodium-Glucose Cotransporter-2 Inhibitors). *Circulation* **2017**, *136*, 249–259. [CrossRef]
101. Kosiborod, M.; Lam, C.S.P.; Kohsaka, S.; Kim, D.J.; Karasik, A.; Shaw, J.; Tangri, N.; Goh, S.-Y.; Thuresson, M.; Chen, H.; et al. Cardiovascular Events Associated With SGLT-2 Inhibitors Versus Other Glucose-Lowering Drugs: The CVD-REAL 2 Study. *J. Am. Coll. Cardiol.* **2018**, *71*, 2628–2639. [CrossRef] [PubMed]
102. Pasternak, B.; Ueda, P.; Eliasson, B.; Svensson, A.-M.; Franzén, S.; Gudbjörnsdottir, S.; Hveem, K.; Jonasson, C.; Wintzell, V.; Melbye, M.; et al. Use of Sodium Glucose Cotransporter 2 Inhibitors and Risk of Major Cardiovascular Events and Heart Failure: Scandinavian Register Based Cohort Study. *BMJ (Clin. Res. Ed.)* **2019**, *366*, l4772. [CrossRef] [PubMed]
103. McHugh, K.; DeVore, A.D.; Wu, J.; Matsouaka, R.A.; Fonarow, G.C.; Heidenreich, P.A.; Yancy, C.W.; Green, J.B.; Altman, N.; Hernandez, A.F. Heart Failure With Preserved Ejection Fraction and Diabetes: JACC State-of-the-Art Review. *J. Am. Coll. Cardiol.* **2019**, *73*, 602–611. [CrossRef] [PubMed]
104. Liu, Y.; Wu, M.; Xu, B.; Kang, L. Empagliflozin Alleviates Atherosclerosis Progression by Inhibiting Inflammation and Sympathetic Activity in a Normoglycemic Mouse Model. *J. Inflamm. Res.* **2021**, *14*, 2277–2287. [CrossRef] [PubMed]
105. Heyman, S.N.; Armaly, Z.; Hamo-Giladi, D.B.; Abassi, Z. Novel Perspectives Regarding the Physiologic Mechanisms by Which Gliflozins Induce Reticulocytosis and Erythrocytosis. *Am. J. Physiol. Endocrinol. Metab.* **2023**, *325*, E621–E623. [CrossRef] [PubMed]

106. Zhang, N.; Feng, B.; Ma, X.; Sun, K.; Xu, G.; Zhou, Y. Dapagliflozin Improves Left Ventricular Remodeling and Aorta Sympathetic Tone in a Pig Model of Heart Failure with Preserved Ejection Fraction. *Cardiovasc. Diabetol.* **2019**, *18*, 107. [CrossRef] [PubMed]
107. Uthman, L.; Homayr, A.; Juni, R.P.; Spin, E.L.; Kerindongo, R.; Boomsma, M.; Hollmann, M.W.; Preckel, B.; Koolwijk, P.; van Hinsbergh, V.W.; et al. Empagliflozin and Dapagliflozin Reduce ROS Generation and Restore NO Bioavailability in Tumor Necrosis Factor α-Stimulated Human Coronary Arterial Endothelial Cells. *Cell. Physiol. Biochem. Int. J. Exp. Cell. Physiol. Biochem. Pharmacol.* **2019**, *53*, 865–886. [CrossRef]
108. Sato, T.; Aizawa, Y.; Yuasa, S.; Kishi, S.; Fuse, K.; Fujita, S.; Ikeda, Y.; Kitazawa, H.; Takahashi, M.; Sato, M.; et al. The Effect of Dapagliflozin Treatment on Epicardial Adipose Tissue Volume. *Cardiovasc. Diabetol.* **2018**, *17*, 6. [CrossRef] [PubMed]
109. Zhou, H.; Wang, S.; Zhu, P.; Hu, S.; Chen, Y.; Ren, J. Empagliflozin Rescues Diabetic Myocardial Microvascular Injury via AMPK-Mediated Inhibition of Mitochondrial Fission. *Redox Biol.* **2018**, *15*, 335–346. [CrossRef]
110. Pabel, S.; Hamdani, N.; Singh, J.; Sossalla, S. Potential Mechanisms of SGLT2 Inhibitors for the Treatment of Heart Failure With Preserved Ejection Fraction. *Front. Physiol.* **2021**, *12*, 752370. [CrossRef]
111. Bonora, B.M.; Avogaro, A.; Fadini, G.P. Extraglycemic Effects of SGLT2 Inhibitors: A Review of the Evidence. *Diabetes Metab. Syndr. Obes. Targets Ther.* **2020**, *13*, 161–174. [CrossRef] [PubMed]
112. Swanson, K.V.; Deng, M.; Ting, J.P.-Y. The NLRP3 Inflammasome: Molecular Activation and Regulation to Therapeutics. *Nat. Rev. Immunol.* **2019**, *19*, 477–489. [CrossRef]
113. Yaribeygi, H.; Sathyapalan, T.; Maleki, M.; Jamialahmadi, T.; Sahebkar, A. Molecular Mechanisms by Which SGLT2 Inhibitors Can Induce Insulin Sensitivity in Diabetic Milieu: A Mechanistic Review. *Life Sci.* **2020**, *240*, 117090. [CrossRef] [PubMed]
114. González-Juanatey, J.R.; Górriz, J.L.; Ortiz, A.; Valle, A.; Soler, M.J.; Facila, L. Cardiorenal Benefits of Finerenone: Protecting Kidney and Heart. *Ann. Med.* **2023**, *55*, 502–513. [CrossRef]
115. Kolkhof, P.; Joseph, A.; Kintscher, U. Nonsteroidal Mineralocorticoid Receptor Antagonism for Cardiovascular and Renal Disorders—New Perspectives for Combination Therapy. *Pharmacol. Res.* **2021**, *172*, 105859. [CrossRef] [PubMed]
116. Rossing, P.; Anker, S.D.; Filippatos, G.; Pitt, B.; Ruilope, L.M.; Birkenfeld, A.L.; McGill, J.B.; Rosas, S.E.; Joseph, A.; Gebel, M.; et al. Finerenone in Patients With Chronic Kidney Disease and Type 2 Diabetes by Sodium-Glucose Cotransporter 2 Inhibitor Treatment: The FIDELITY Analysis. *Diabetes Care* **2022**, *45*, 2991–2998. [CrossRef] [PubMed]
117. Marzolla, V.; Infante, M.; Armani, A.; Rizzo, M.; Caprio, M. Efficacy and Safety of Finerenone for Treatment of Diabetic Kidney Disease: Current Knowledge and Future Perspective. *Expert Opin. Drug Saf.* **2022**, *21*, 1161–1170. [CrossRef]
118. Yang, P.; Huang, T.; Xu, G. The Novel Mineralocorticoid Receptor Antagonist Finerenone in Diabetic Kidney Disease: Progress and Challenges. *Metabolism* **2016**, *65*, 1342–1349. [CrossRef] [PubMed]
119. Pandey, A.K.; Bhatt, D.L.; Cosentino, F.; Marx, N.; Rotstein, O.; Pitt, B.; Pandey, A.; Butler, J.; Verma, S. Non-Steroidal Mineralocorticoid Receptor Antagonists in Cardiorenal Disease. *Eur. Heart J.* **2022**, *43*, 2931–2945. [CrossRef]
120. Bakris, G.L.; Agarwal, R.; Anker, S.D.; Pitt, B.; Ruilope, L.M.; Rossing, P.; Kolkhof, P.; Nowack, C.; Schloemer, P.; Joseph, A.; et al. Effect of Finerenone on Chronic Kidney Disease Outcomes in Type 2 Diabetes. *N. Engl. J. Med.* **2020**, *383*, 2219–2229. [CrossRef]
121. Pitt, B.; Filippatos, G.; Agarwal, R.; Anker, S.D.; Bakris, G.L.; Rossing, P.; Joseph, A.; Kolkhof, P.; Nowack, C.; Schloemer, P.; et al. Cardiovascular Events with Finerenone in Kidney Disease and Type 2 Diabetes. *N. Engl. J. Med.* **2021**, *385*, 2252–2263. [CrossRef] [PubMed]
122. Agarwal, R.; Joseph, A.; Anker, S.D.; Filippatos, G.; Rossing, P.; Ruilope, L.M.; Pitt, B.; Kolkhof, P.; Scott, C.; Lawatscheck, R.; et al. Hyperkalemia Risk with Finerenone: Results from the FIDELIO-DKD Trial. *J. Am. Soc. Nephrol.* **2022**, *33*, 225–237. [CrossRef]
123. Bauersachs, J.; Soltani, S. Heart failure: Update of the ESC 2023 guidelines. *Herz* **2024**, *49*, 19–21. [CrossRef] [PubMed]
124. Rossing, P.; Burgess, E.; Agarwal, R.; Anker, S.D.; Filippatos, G.; Pitt, B.; Ruilope, L.M.; Gillard, P.; MacIsaac, R.J.; Wainstein, J.; et al. Finerenone in Patients With Chronic Kidney Disease and Type 2 Diabetes According to Baseline HbA1c and Insulin Use: An Analysis From the FIDELIO-DKD Study. *Diabetes Care* **2022**, *45*, 888–897. [CrossRef] [PubMed]
125. McDonagh, T.A.; Metra, M.; Adamo, M.; Gardner, R.S.; Baumbach, A.; Böhm, M.; Burri, H.; Butler, J.; Čelutkienė, J.; Chioncel, O. 2021 ESC Guidelines for the Diagnosis and Treatment of Acute and Chronic Heart Failure: Developed by the Task Force for the Diagnosis and Treatment of Acute and Chronic Heart Failure of the European Society of Cardiology (ESC). With the Special Contribution of the Heart Failure Association (HFA) of the ESC. *Eur. J. Heart Fail.* **2022**, *24*, 4–131. [CrossRef] [PubMed]
126. Blanton, R.M. cGMP Signaling and Modulation in Heart Failure. *J. Cardiovasc. Pharmacol.* **2020**, *75*, 385–398. [CrossRef] [PubMed]
127. Armstrong, P.W.; Pieske, B.; Anstrom, K.J.; Ezekowitz, J.; Hernandez, A.F.; Butler, J.; Lam, C.S.P.; Ponikowski, P.; Voors, A.A.; Jia, G.; et al. Vericiguat in Patients with Heart Failure and Reduced Ejection Fraction. *N. Engl. J. Med.* **2020**, *382*, 1883–1893. [CrossRef] [PubMed]
128. Coats, A.J.S.; Tolppanen, H. Drug Treatment of Heart Failure with Reduced Ejection Fraction: Defining the Role of Vericiguat. *Drugs* **2021**, *81*, 1599–1604. [CrossRef] [PubMed]
129. Follmann, M.; Ackerstaff, J.; Redlich, G.; Wunder, F.; Lang, D.; Kern, A.; Fey, P.; Griebenow, N.; Kroh, W.; Becker-Pelster, E.-M.; et al. Discovery of the Soluble Guanylate Cyclase Stimulator Vericiguat (BAY 1021189) for the Treatment of Chronic Heart Failure. *J. Med. Chem.* **2017**, *60*, 5146–5161. [CrossRef]
130. Voors, A.A.; Mulder, H.; Reyes, E.; Cowie, M.R.; Lassus, J.; Hernandez, A.F.; Ezekowitz, J.A.; Butler, J.; O'Connor, C.M.; Koglin, J.; et al. Renal Function and the Effects of Vericiguat in Patients with Worsening Heart Failure with Reduced Ejection Fraction: Insights from the VICTORIA (Vericiguat Global Study in Subjects with HFrEF) Trial. *Eur. J. Heart Fail.* **2021**, *23*, 1313–1321. [CrossRef]

131. Greene, S.J.; Bauersachs, J.; Brugts, J.J.; Ezekowitz, J.A.; Filippatos, G.; Gustafsson, F.; Lam, C.S.P.; Lund, L.H.; Mentz, R.J.; Pieske, B.; et al. Management of Worsening Heart Failure With Reduced Ejection Fraction: JACC Focus Seminar 3/3. *J. Am. Coll. Cardiol.* **2023**, *82*, 559–571. [CrossRef] [PubMed]
132. Butler, J.; Packer, M.; Greene, S.J.; Fiuzat, M.; Anker, S.D.; Anstrom, K.J.; Carson, P.E.; Cooper, L.B.; Fonarow, G.C.; Hernandez, A.F.; et al. Heart Failure End Points in Cardiovascular Outcome Trials of Sodium Glucose Cotransporter 2 Inhibitors in Patients With Type 2 Diabetes Mellitus: A Critical Evaluation of Clinical and Regulatory Issues. *Circulation* **2019**, *140*, 2108–2118. [CrossRef] [PubMed]
133. Fu, S.; Litwin, S.E.; Tedford, R.J. Lessons from SGLT-2 Inhibitors: Rethinking Endpoints for Heart Failure Studies. *Nat. Med.* **2021**, *27*, 1872–1873. [CrossRef] [PubMed]
134. Greene, S.J.; Vaduganathan, M.; Khan, M.S.; Bakris, G.L.; Weir, M.R.; Seltzer, J.H.; Sattar, N.; McGuire, D.K.; Januzzi, J.L.; Stockbridge, N.; et al. Prevalent and Incident Heart Failure in Cardiovascular Outcome Trials of Patients With Type 2 Diabetes. *J. Am. Coll. Cardiol.* **2018**, *71*, 1379–1390. [CrossRef]
135. Triposkiadis, F.; Butler, J.; Abboud, F.M.; Armstrong, P.W.; Adamopoulos, S.; Atherton, J.J.; Backs, J.; Bauersachs, J.; Burkhoff, D.; Bonow, R.O.; et al. The Continuous Heart Failure Spectrum: Moving beyond an Ejection Fraction Classification. *Eur. Heart J.* **2019**, *40*, 2155–2163. [CrossRef] [PubMed]
136. Simms-Williams, N.; Treves, N.; Yin, H.; Lu, S.; Yu, O.; Pradhan, R.; Renoux, C.; Suissa, S.; Azoulay, L. Effect of Combination Treatment with Glucagon-like Peptide-1 Receptor Agonists and Sodium-Glucose Cotransporter-2 Inhibitors on Incidence of Cardiovascular and Serious Renal Events: Population Based Cohort Study. *BMJ (Clin. Res. Ed.)* **2024**, *385*, e078242. [CrossRef]
137. Green, J.B.; Mottl, A.K.; Bakris, G.; Heerspink, H.J.L.; Mann, J.F.E.; McGill, J.B.; Nangaku, M.; Rossing, P.; Scott, C.; Gay, A.; et al. Design of the COmbinatioN Effect of FInerenone anD EmpagliflloziN in Participants with Chronic Kidney Disease and Type 2 Diabetes Using a UACR Endpoint Study (CONFIDENCE). *Nephrol. Dial. Transplant. Off. Publ. Eur. Dial. Transpl. Assoc. Eur. Ren. Assoc.* **2023**, *38*, 894–903. [CrossRef]

biomedicines

MDPI

Review

Unraveling the Cardiac Matrix: From Diabetes to Heart Failure, Exploring Pathways and Potential Medications

Bogdan-Sorin Tudurachi [1,2], Larisa Anghel [1,2,*], Andreea Tudurachi [2], Radu Andy Sascău [1,2], Răzvan-Liviu Zanfirescu [2,3] and Cristian Stătescu [1,2]

1 Internal Medicine Department, "Grigore T. Popa" University of Medicine and Pharmacy, 700503 Iasi, Romania; bogdan-sorin.tudurachi@d.umfiasi.ro (B.-S.T.); radu.sascau@umfiasi.ro (R.A.S.); cristian.statescu@umfiasi.ro (C.S.)

2 Cardiology Department, Cardiovascular Diseases Institute "Prof. Dr. George I. M. Georgescu", 700503 Iasi, Romania; leonteandreea32@gmail.com (A.T.); zanfirescu_razvan-liviu@d.umfiasi.ro (R.-L.Z.)

3 Physiology Department, "Grigore T. Popa" University of Medicine and Pharmacy, 700503 Iasi, Romania

* Correspondence: larisa.anghel@umfiasi.ro; Tel.: +40-0232-211834

Abstract: Myocardial infarction (MI) often leads to heart failure (HF) through acute or chronic maladaptive remodeling processes. This establishes coronary artery disease (CAD) and HF as significant contributors to cardiovascular illness and death. Therefore, treatment strategies for patients with CAD primarily focus on preventing MI and lessening the impact of HF after an MI event. Myocardial fibrosis, characterized by abnormal extracellular matrix (ECM) deposition, is central to cardiac remodeling. Understanding these processes is key to identifying new treatment targets. Recent studies highlight SGLT2 inhibitors (SGLT2i) and GLP-1 receptor agonists (GLP1-RAs) as favorable options in managing type 2 diabetes due to their low hypoglycemic risk and cardiovascular benefits. This review explores inflammation's role in cardiac fibrosis and evaluates emerging anti-diabetic medications' effectiveness, such as SGLT2i, GLP1-RAs, and dipeptidyl peptidase-4 inhibitors (DPP4i), in preventing fibrosis in patients with diabetes post-acute MI. Recent studies were analyzed to identify effective medications in reducing fibrosis risk in these patients. By addressing these areas, we can advance our understanding of the potential benefits of anti-diabetic medications in reducing cardiac fibrosis post-MI and improve patient outcomes in individuals with diabetes at risk of HF.

Keywords: diabetes; myocardial infarction; heart failure; myocardial fibrosis; SGLT2 inhibitors; GLP-1 agonist; dipeptidyl peptidase-4 inhibitors

1. Introduction

The cardiac muscle, comprising cardiomyocytes, capillaries, and ECM rich in collagen fibers, constitutes the fundamental elements crucial for efficient contraction. Left ventricular (LV) remodeling, an adaptive response to mechanical, neurohormonal, and genetic stimuli, orchestrates alterations in ventricular dimension, shape, and function. While physiological cardiomyocyte proliferation in scenarios like pregnancy signifies a reversible process facilitated by augmented microcirculatory perfusion, pathological remodeling after cardiac events such as MI poses a substantial risk for HF [1]. HF, a complex syndrome stemming from structural and functional aberrations within the heart, manifests pathologically through interstitial fibrosis, chamber remodeling, and diminished ventricular compliance [2]. Diabetes mellitus (DM) emerges as an independent risk factor for HF, with diabetic cardiomyopathy representing a significant complication fueled by metabolic perturbations including glucose and lipotoxicity, insulin resistance, endothelial dysfunction, and microvascular impairment, alongside ischemic heart disease sequelae, involving multifaceted pathophysiological pathways [3]. Type 2 diabetes mellitus (T2DM) assumes a pivotal role in cardiovascular (CV) pathology, directly intertwining with diabetic cardiomyopathy and exacerbating CV risk factors, thus amplifying susceptibility to CAD. CAD-induced MI and ischemia/reperfusion injuries frequently instigate HF via acute or chronic maladaptive remodeling processes, establishing CAD and HF as principal contributors to CV morbidity and mortality. Consequently, therapeutic strategies for patients with CAD focus on averting MI occurrence and mitigating HF burden post-MI [4,5].

Traditionally, T2DM management commenced with insulin therapy; however, the evolution of oral anti-diabetic agents revolutionized glycemic control. Nonetheless, concerns regarding the CV safety profile of certain anti-diabetic drugs prompted extensive research aimed at elucidating their CV risk. Notably, studies unveiled two drug classes, SGLT2i and GLP1-RAs, which not only demonstrated CV safety but also exhibited remarkable reductions in major adverse CV events, including CV mortality, thereby positioning them as favorable options in T2DM management due to their low hypoglycemic risk and beneficial cardiovascular effects (CV benefits) [6]. Fibrosis, a chronic pathological process characterized by aberrant ECM deposition, serves as a hallmark feature across various cardiac pathologies, reflecting both reparative and maladaptive responses to injury. While initially pivotal for wound healing and tissue repair, persistent ECM accumulation engenders structural distortion and functional impairment within the heart. Myocardial fibrosis encompasses both interstitial and replacement forms, driven by diverse cellular and paracrine mechanisms involving inflammatory mediators, growth factors, and collagen-modulating enzymes such as matrix metalloproteinases (MMPs). Dysregulated collagen turnover precipitates myocardial fibrosis progression, further underscoring its pivotal role in cardiac remodeling [7].

Understanding key pathophysiological processes holds paramount importance for identifying novel therapeutic targets and leveraging diagnostic and prognostic modalities, including biomarkers and imaging techniques, to tailor medical interventions, thereby enhancing patient outcomes and clinical management strategies (Figure 1).

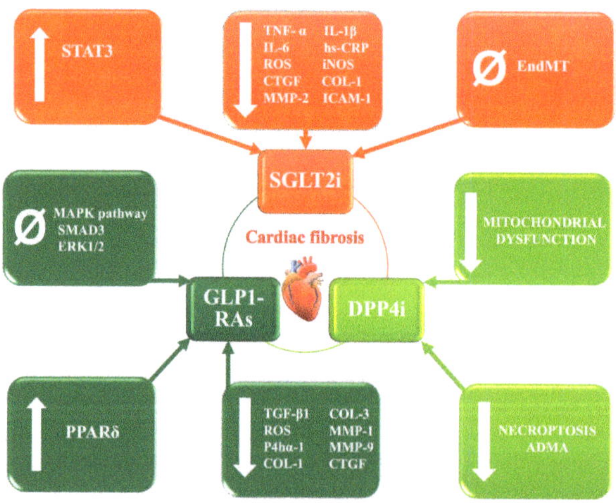

Figure 1. Pathways and potential medications related to cardiac fibrosis. ↑ = increase; ↓ = decrease; ∅ = inhibit; STAT3 = signal transducer and activator of transcription 3; TNF-α = tumor necrosis factor-α; IL-1β = interleukin-1β; IL-6 = interleukin-6; hs-CRP = high sensitivity c-reactive protein; COL-1 = type 1 collagen; COL-3 = type 3 collagen; MMP-1 = matrix metalloproteinase 1; MMP-2 = matrix metalloproteinase 2; MMP-9 = matrix metalloproteinase 9; PPARα = peroxisome proliferator-activated receptor alpha; DPP4i = dipeptidyl peptidase-4 inhibitor; SGLT2i = sodium-glucose cotransporter 2 inhibitors; GLP-1RAs = glucagon-like peptide-1 receptor agonists; CTGF = connective tissue growth factor; iNOS = inducible form of nitric oxide synthase; ROS = reactive oxygen species; ICAM-1 = intercellular adhesion molecule 1; MAPK = mitogen-activated protein kinase; ERK1/2 = extracellular signal-regulated kinase 1/2; EndMT = endothelial-to-mesenchymal transition; TGF- β1 = transforming growth factor-β; P4hα-1 = prolyl 4-hydroxylase subunit alpha 1; and ADMA = asymmetric dimethylarginine.

2. Materials and Methods

Myocardial fibrosis, often a leading cause of sudden cardiac death, occurs due to an accumulation of ECM, sometimes called interstitial myocardial enlargement. Myocardial ischemia/reperfusion (MI/R) injury damages cardiomyocytes, triggering fibroblast activation and fibrosis formation. In MI, "interstitial fibrosis" emerges as collagen-based scars that replace necrotic cardiac cells from ischemia. Another aspect, "perivascular fibrosis", involves the thickening of microvascular adventitia. While dilated cardiomyopathy (DCM) does not typically result in immediate cardiomyocyte loss, abnormal metabolism can lead to their atypical demise, causing "replacement fibrosis" that worsens DCM. Although there is an established connection between cardiac fibrosis and acute myocardial infarction (AMI) as well as diabetes, the current research on the correlation between emerging anti-diabetic medications and this phenomenon is insufficient. Therefore, the present study aims to examine the inflammation role in cardiac fibrosis and the efficacy of drugs like SGLT2i, GLP-1RAs, or DPP4i in preventing fibrosis in patients with diabetes following acute MI [2,8,9]. We conducted a narrative review incorporating contemporary studies from the last five years, published in MEDLINE, PubMed, and EMBASE databases, with the goal to identify effective medications in reducing fibrosis risk in these patients.

3. Collagen Synthesis

3.1. C-Terminal Propeptide of Procollagen Type I

The C-Terminal Propeptide of Procollagen Type I (PICP) is released into the bloodstream when procollagen type I carboxy-terminal proteinase cleaves it from the protein to produce fibril-forming collagen type I. In individuals without liver cirrhosis, PICP serves as a marker of collagen type I production and is metabolized by the liver [10]. Elevated levels of PICP have been observed in the blood of patients with heart failure and hypertension, correlating with myocardial thickening and impaired heart relaxation in those with arterial hypertension [11]. Prior to receiving medication therapy, hypertensive individuals have notably higher levels of PICP in their bloodstreams [12]. Currently, there is no evidence indicating a relationship between PICP levels and the progression towards heart failure in individuals experiencing acute ischemic events who also have diabetes.

3.2. Procollagen Type I N-Terminal Propeptide

The Procollagen type I N-Terminal Propeptide (PINP), indicative of collagen type I production, is generated through the conversion of collagen type I. Unlike PICP, PINP is characterized by its delayed release. In a case–control study, it was revealed that patients with HF had significantly higher baseline serum PINP levels compared to controls. Furthermore, another study observed a notable increase in plasma PINP levels in the MI group compared to the normal control group in rats with ischemic cardiomyopathy [13,14].

3.3. Procollagen Type III Amino-Terminal Propeptide

Procollagen Type III Amino-Terminal Propeptide (PIIINP) is released into the bloodstream as a result of increased collagen type III production during cardiac fibrosis, and it plays a crucial role in myocardial elasticity. A study on DCM revealed that patients with idiopathic or ischemic DCM exhibited higher baseline blood PIIINP levels compared to healthy individuals. Additionally, in rats with a MI model, the reduction in fibrosis attributed to tanshinone IIA was associated with a decrease in serum PIIINP levels [7,15]. Osokina et al. demonstrated that the risk of cardiac fibrosis increases when PIIINP levels reach or exceed 381.4 ng/mL on the 12th day after ST-segment elevation myocardial infarction (STEMI) with maintained left ventricular ejection fraction (LVEF). Monitoring PIIINP levels during hospitalization may aid in identifying individuals at high risk of cardiac fibrosis one year after STEMI with normal LVEF [16].

4. Collagen Degradation

4.1. C-Terminal Telopeptide of Collagen Type I

As a marker of collagen turnover and a potential indicator for the early detection of adverse remodeling, C-terminal telopeptide, also referred to as beta-CTx, is a fragment of Type I collagen released into circulation following its breakdown. According to Zelniker et al., in individuals with non-ST-elevation acute coronary syndrome (NSTEMI), beta-CTx levels were associated with both HF and CV mortality [17]. Manhenke et al. suggested that, in patients experiencing AMI, plasma beta-CTx served as an independent predictor of CV death, with levels rising in those who died from any cause [18].

4.2. Matrix Metalloproteinases

The extracellular matrix is viewed as a dynamic and vital framework essential for cardiac healing processes. MMPs are zinc ion-dependent proteases responsible for collagen and proteoglycan breakdown, playing a critical role in atherosclerosis progression. MMPs also play a pivotal role in post-AMI cardiac remodeling and the development of associated complications, with the myocardium expressing numerous MMPs [19,20]. Research suggests that matrix metalloproteinase 28 (MMP-28) is associated with CV events and mortality both during hospitalization and within 30 days after discharge, serving as a potential predictor of short-term prognosis for individuals with MI [21]. Recent studies have shown that young patients experiencing STEMI exhibit significantly elevated levels of matrix metalloproteinase 3 (MMP-3), matrix metalloproteinase 9 (MMP-9), and tissue inhibitors of metalloproteinase (TIMP) compared to healthy individuals. Those experiencing Major Adverse Cardiovascular Events (MACEs), particularly HF hospitalizations, demonstrate markedly increased levels of MMP-9, suggesting its involvement in cardiac remodeling and its impact on LV function [22]. Furthermore, elevated MMP-9 levels have been associated with a notable increase in CV mortality over a two-year period, with patients with advanced HF being more prevalent in the high MMP-9 group during the monitoring period [23].

Watson et al. propose that the minor allele of genetic variation rs3918242 in the promoter region of the MMP-9 gene may be linked to hypertension and/or MI. Patients with diabetes patients carrying the minor T allele of rs3918242 showed a higher likelihood of experiencing MI, reduced ejection fraction (EF), and increased progression of LV systolic dysfunction over a 3.5-year follow-up period, indicating an elevated risk for developing HF [24].

4.3. Tissue Inhibitors of Metalloproteinases

TIMPs constitute a subgroup of small glycoproteins synthesized and released by fibroblasts, epithelial cells, and endothelial cells, prevalent in various tissues. They play a role in initiating the conversion of fibroblasts into myofibroblasts at sites of tissue damage and regulate the enzymatic activity of MMPs by inhibiting the activation of latent MMPs. Thus, maintaining an appropriate balance between MMPs and TIMP production is critical for the reconstruction of the extracellular matrix in cardiac tissues. Four types of TIMPs have been identified to be associated with myocardial fibrosis [7].

A retrospective cohort study has indicated that blood levels of tissue inhibitors of metalloproteinase 3 (TIMP-3), CA125, and NT-proBNP can predict ventricular remodeling in patients with HF following AMI. These three markers demonstrated excellent specificity and moderate sensitivity. Early detection of serum TIMP-3, CA125, and NT-proBNP levels may enhance the accuracy of predicting cardiac remodeling and facilitate early detection and management of HF post-AMI [25].

Clinical investigations have shown that MMP and TIMP levels during the acute phase may predict the development of HF or CV events within a 30-day follow-up period in patients with AMI who did not receive reperfusion treatment. Specifically, plasma levels of tissue inhibitors of metalloproteinase 1 (TIMP1) and the matrix metalloproteinase 2 (MMP2)/TIMP1 ratio can indicate the likelihood of HF and CV events. The matrix metalloproteinase 8 (MMP8)/TIMP1 ratio has shown predictive utility for the risk of CV-related events [26].

5. Collagen Metabolism

5.1. *Transforming Growth Factor-B and SMADS*

Transforming growth factor-β (TGF-β) is a crucial cytokine involved in promoting fibrosis within the heart muscle. It regulates the fibroblast growth, differentiation, migration, and synthesis of the ECM. The mammalian TGF-β subfamily comprises three isoforms (TGF-β1, 2, and 3) that bind to identical receptors and target similar cellular substrates. However, they exhibit distinct regulatory patterns and different affinities for their receptors and co-receptors, suggesting unique functions in fibrotic disease development [2].

TGF-β induces fibrosis in cardiac fibroblasts by activating the Smad3, PI3K/Akt, and mitogen-activated protein kinase (MAPK) signaling pathways as a cytokine upstream of the oxidized low-density-lipoprotein receptor (LOX) [7]. Following MI, there is a significant increase in TGF-β1 expression, which may interact with the renin–angiotensin system to promote heart remodeling. TGF-β1 stimulates the activation of fetal genes in myocardial cells and induces fibroblasts in the heart to produce ECM proteins.

Research by Zhang et al. investigated the effects of TGF-β1 therapy on myocardial cell death in rats with MI. AMI was induced in rats by occluding the left anterior descending coronary artery. Both the model and control groups were assessed for mRNA and protein expression levels of TGF-β1 in myocardial cells. AMI rats exhibited significantly higher levels of TGF-β1 mRNA and protein expression compared to the control group. The study suggested that the TGF-β1/MAPK signaling pathway was activated in myocardial cells during AMI, and administration of TGF-β1 was shown to attenuate myocardial cell death in AMI rats [27].

TGF-β transmits signals through intracellular effector proteins called Smads, as well as through Smad-independent pathways. In vivo research indicates that Smad3 signaling plays a crucial role in activating reparative fibroblasts after MI, leading to ECM protein synthesis and integrin transcription, which contribute to scar formation. Collagen levels decreased in the infarcted hearts of Smad3-deficient animals 7 days post-reperfusion, with reduced collagen deposition in the non-infarcted, remodeling myocardium. Smad3 signaling in myofibroblasts within the infarcted area inhibits cell proliferation, resulting in organized clusters of activated myofibroblasts and maintaining structural integrity through integrin and reactive oxygen species (ROS)-mediated pathways [2,7,28]. Disruption of the Smad gene appears to attenuate the remodeling process.

5.2. *Corin*

Corin, a transmembrane serine protease of type II, is predominantly found in atrial cardiomyocytes. It is a complex protein comprising a transmembrane domain near the N terminus, two frizzled-like domains, eight low-density lipoprotein (LDL) receptor repeats, a scavenger receptor-like domain, and a trypsin-like protease domain at the C terminus. Corin plays a crucial role in converting pro-atrial natriuretic peptide (pro-ANP) into its active form, ANP. Numerous studies have indicated that circulating corin levels have predictive value regarding various CV outcomes in individuals with AMI, chronic HF, and acute stroke [29–32]. However, preliminary findings from a small study suggest that serum levels of PCSK6 and corin are not independent predictors of CV outcomes in patients undergoing coronary angiography. Nonetheless, elevated blood PCSK6 levels in patients with non-chronic kidney disease (CKD) may indicate a higher risk of CV events [32]. To elucidate the critical genes and pathways involved in abnormal myocardial remodeling following prolonged ischemia, a study utilized a rhesus monkey model of MI. It revealed that cardiac remodeling may be aggravated by an imbalance in the expression of corin and natriuretic peptide A/natriuretic peptide B [33].

6. Inflammatory Factors

6.1. Galectin-3

The lectin family includes Galectin-3 (Gal-3), which has been associated with myocardial fibrosis, acute CV events, autoimmune diseases, and various inflammatory conditions. Animal models and a limited number of human samples have demonstrated its significant role in tissue healing following AMI. Gal-3 is primarily produced by activated macrophages and injured cardiomyocytes, highlighting its critical involvement in myocardial fibrosis. Elevated Gal-3 expression has a strong correlation with the onset and progression of CV disorders, making it closely linked to the adverse remodeling of the heart and MACEs [34]. MACE remains the leading cause of morbidity and mortality in patients with AMI, and several studies suggest that Gal-3 plays a significant role in predicting adverse events post-AMI [34–39]. According to research by Grandin E. and colleagues, patients with elevated levels of both BNP and Gal-3 have the highest likelihood of developing HF, suggesting that Gal-3 may provide additional value in assessing HF risk after acute coronary syndrome (ACS) [40].

Increased levels of fibrosis and indicators of ECM remodeling, such as collagen, fibronectin, TGF-β, fibroblast proliferation, alpha smooth muscle actin (αSMA), and MMPs, have been associated with peak levels of Gal-3 in the ischemic region [41,42]. In addition to promoting ECM remodeling, Gal-3 may facilitate neutrophil adhesion and recruitment to the injured heart. While recent research suggests that neutrophils contribute to healing and the temporal progression of MI, their involvement is typically limited to the first week post-AMI. Neutrophils can alter their phenotype during the healing process, transitioning from a pro-inflammatory to an anti-inflammatory profile and contributing to scar formation [43–45].

In a rat model of MI, the inhibition of Gal-3 led to decreased collagen synthesis and reduced myocardial fibrosis [46]. Additionally, through its dual roles as a chemotactic factor for macrophage recruitment and a regulator of their polarization towards the reparative M2 phenotype, Gal-3 plays a multifaceted role in post-infarction wound healing. Gal-3′s dual function is crucial for coordinating the immune response and tissue repair mechanisms after myocardial infarction, ultimately aiding in the recovery of heart tissue [41,47]. Animals with Gal-3 knockdown and pharmacologic suppression of Galectin exhibited decreased fibrosis, apoptosis, inflammation, and infarct size [48,49].

Gal-3 is intricately linked to inflammation, fibrosis, remodeling, and dysfunction in CV pathophysiology. Its significant involvement in cardiac remodeling underscores the importance of understanding its role in cardiac function. Understanding how Gal-3 operates in the heart holds promise for therapeutic interventions aimed at reducing HF.

6.2. Tumor Necrosis Factor-α and Interleukins

Macrophages and monocytes can generate and release numerous pro-inflammatory mediators, including interleukin-1β (IL-1β), interleukin-4 (IL-4), interleukin-6 (IL-6), and tumor necrosis factor-α (TNF-α). These inflammatory factors collectively form a complex regulatory network that promotes fibrotic degenerative processes and the activation of myofibroblasts [50]. Kang et al. demonstrated elevated concentrations of TNF-α, IL-6, and IL-1β, as well as increased expression of collagen I and III mRNAs compared to normal controls, suggesting a correlation between fibrosis and inflammation [51]. Fang et al. conducted a cross-sectional study on hypertrophic cardiomyopathy (HCM) and observed a positive correlation between plasma levels of IL-4, IL-6, and interleukin-10 (IL-10) with both diffuse and localized myocardial fibrosis [52].

TGF-β plays a critical role in transitioning from inflammation to fibrosis by inhibiting inflammation and promoting ECM deposition. Studies have shown that mice lacking TGF-β in their heart muscle exhibit reduced cardiac fibrosis and increased survival rates [53–55]. The IL-6 trans-signaling cascade has been implicated in cardiac fibrosis induced by aldosterone. Conversely, blocking IL-6 has shown beneficial effects by reducing inflammation and fibrosis in mice subjected to high salt intake after nephrectomy [56,57]. Interleukin-33 (IL-33) has been associated with pro-fibrotic signaling in rats with MI and in individuals diagnosed with HF. IL-4 has been identified as a contributor to heart fibrosis, as it stimulates pro-fibrotic activity in macrophages [58–60].

6.3. MicroRNA

The development of fibrosis in patients with diabetes or post-AMI may be attributed to pathophysiological processes, which may include the dysfunction of microRNA (miRNA, miR). These are tiny, single-stranded, non-coding RNAs that control gene expression after the transcription process. miRNAs have widespread expression in both the nucleus and cytoplasm. Nevertheless, miRNAs may still be detected in the bloodstream. They have a significant impact on several biological processes such as cell growth, specialization, programmed cell death, and metabolism by either inhibiting or promoting the expression of genes. Due to their stable expression in blood, miRNAs have the potential to serve as biomarkers for diagnosing, predicting outcomes, and developing new treatment approaches for cardiovascular disease [61–63].

In individuals with diabetes, there is an abnormal regulation of miRNA expression in the serum or plasma. Each miRNA has one or many targets that play a role in the development of diabetic fibrosis in the heart. Each gene might potentially be associated with one or many miRNAs, which can then inhibit its expression. Cardiac fibroblasts, endothelial cells, and cardiomyocytes have a role in the development of cardiac fibrosis. Every microRNA has a distinct target in certain cells, but many microRNAs have several targets in diverse cells. Mimicking of microRNAs inhibits the production of molecules of interest. Research indicates that cardiac fibrosis may include the activation of many crucial signaling pathways to enhance the production of pro-fibrotic molecules or hinder the production of anti-fibrotic molecules at the levels of gene expression and protein synthesis. miRNAs selectively target these molecules to exert an influence on the development of cardiac fibrosis in the diabetic heart or after a MI [64]. Several miRNAs have a function in reducing fibrosis in the diabetic heart affected by cardiac fibrosis. Those are represented by miR-15a/b, miR-18a-5p, miR-20a-5p, miR-26b-5p, miR-29, miR-133a, miR-141, miR-146a, miR-200b, miR-203, miR-222, and miR-551b-5p. Increased production of these miRNAs with anti-fibrotic properties inhibits the development of cardiac fibrosis in vivo and decreases the levels of molecules that promote fibrosis [65–76].

In addition, some miRNAs are increased in expression in the presence of high blood sugar levels. Typically, their specific objectives are genes or proteins that are suppressed in the heart of individuals with diabetes or in cells that are exposed to high levels of glucose. Myocardial fibrosis and heightened production of pro-fibrotic molecules are a consequence of overproduction of these miRNAs (miR-21–5p, miR-21–3p, miR-150–5p, miR-155, miR-221–3p, miR-223, miR-451). Antagomirs of these molecules, which are modified antisense oligonucleotides designed to target certain mature miRNA sequences, have been shown to provide cardiac protection and decrease cardiac fibrosis [77–87].

Following a MI, it has been proposed that miRNAs target many important fibrogenic pathways, including TGF-b/Smad, PTEN/Akt, angiotensin II/MAPK, or PIGF/VEGF-A. A full understanding of the function of miRNAs in fibrotic circumstances is hindered by the intricate nature of their activities in many cell types, as well as the extensive array of their molecular targets. Research findings indicate that certain miRNAs, such as miR-1, miR-19b, and miR-590-3p, could have a role in suppressing cardiac fibrosis by inhibiting the pathways triggered by fibrogenic growth factors or matricellular proteins [88–90]. The suppression of miR-34a and miR-1955 inhibits the pro-fibrogenic effects of TGF-β1 or those caused by angiotensin II in cardiac fibroblasts [91,92]. On the other hand, it has been proposed that miR-21, miR-92a, miR-195, miR-200a-3p, miR-125b, miR-34a, miR-146b-5p and miR-144-3p have fibrogenic effects [91,93–101].

The primary goal of miRNA-based therapeutics post-MI is to reinstate miRNA expression levels. According to the findings, administering a miR-21 mimic to mice with cardiac macrophages changed their condition from one that promotes inflammation to one that reduces inflammatory processes. This alteration led to an increase in angiogenesis, a decrease in apoptosis, and abnormal restructuring in the infarct-affected region [102]. Cardiomyocyte apoptosis is closely associated with the suppression of a particular gene known as protein phosphatase 1 regulatory subunit 10 or PNUTS. A microRNA known as miR-34a controls the expression of this gene. In mice, PNUTS improves function recovery following a heart attack [103]. Other therapeutic targets for miRNAs and exosomal miRNAs in MI are represented by miR-210, miR-15, exosomal miR-4943p, and miR-132 [104–107].

Future research should focus on identifying miRNAs as biomarkers and therapeutic targets that are common to various components of the metabolic illness group or ischemic disease.

7. Insulin Resistance and Hyperinsulinemia

Diabetic cardiomyopathy (DC) is a critical complication of DM marked by structural and functional impairments in the heart muscle, occurring without typical cardiovascular issues like coronary artery disease or valve disorders. It primarily develops due to prolonged high levels of hemoglobin A1c (HbA1c), a long duration of diabetes, and older age [108,109].

The etiology of DC is complex, involving multiple cellular and molecular factors that contribute to heart dysfunction. These include the overproduction of advanced glycation end-products (AGEs), activation of the hexosamine biosynthetic pathway, lipotoxicity, mitochondrial dysfunction, increased oxidative stress, and activation of the renin–angiotensin system and calcium homeostasis. These processes compound the effects of hyperglycemia, hyperinsulinemia, and insulin resistance, exacerbating the structural and functional decline of the heart in individuals with diabetes [110].

Prolonged high blood sugar levels in individuals with diabetes lead to increased insulin resistance and higher insulin levels, causing the death of heart muscle cells and the formation of scar tissue in the heart. This condition also impairs glucose processing, reduces glucose clearance, and increases gluconeogenesis. In diabetic cardiomyopathy, the diminished functionality of glucose transporters GLUT1 and GLUT4 in cardiac cells further disrupts glucose absorption and metabolism, which normally meets only 30% to 40% of the energy requirements for heart functions through glycolysis [111,112]. There is also an intense proliferation of cardiac fibroblasts, key players in initiating cardiac fibrosis, and an increase in ECM synthesis. AGEs, formed from prolonged glucose exposure, bind to receptors on heart cells, triggering collagen production and other ECM proteins through pathways like TGFβ, ultimately exacerbating cardiac dysfunction through fibrosis. Furthermore, the AGEs-RAGE signaling pathway activates inflammatory responses and promotes interstitial fibrosis, while lipid-related metabolic changes further impair cardiac function by promoting cardiomyocyte death and reducing myocardial energy efficiency [113–115].

Oxidative stress plays a pivotal role in the development and progression of DC, primarily through the increased production of ROS and a reduction in antioxidant defenses such as glutathione peroxidase and superoxide dismutase, leading to heart fibrosis and mitochondrial damage. These oxidative changes impair mitochondrial function and calcium handling within cells, further reducing cardiac efficiency. Additionally, persistent ROS activity activates the TGFβ1/Smad3 signaling pathway, which enhances fibrotic changes in the heart by upregulating fibrotic markers and promoting the growth of cardiac fibroblasts, contributing significantly to the structural and functional decline observed in DC [116,117].

In individuals with diabetes, the chronic activation of the renin–angiotensin–aldosterone (RAS) pathway leads to the increased levels of angiotensin II (AT-II), which promotes left ventricular hypertrophy, vasoconstriction, cardiac dysfunction through fibrosis, oxidative stress, and cardiomyocyte death. This activation, further enhanced by elevated glucose, AGEs, and ROS, results in increased collagen production and decreased breakdown, contributing to the progression of cardiac fibrosis in DC [110,118].

In DM, identified as an inflammatory condition, the activation of pro-inflammatory genes and proteins, particularly through nuclear factor-KB (NF-kB), plays a crucial role in cardiac damage. NF-kB promotes the expression of pro-inflammatory cytokines and the NLRP3 inflammasome in the heart, leading to a self-perpetuating cycle of inflammation exacerbated by elevated ROS and the pro-inflammatory activation of monocytes/macrophages [119–121].

Inflammation, oxidative stress, activated RAS, compromised mitochondrial function, and disrupted calcium handling drive the structural and functional deterioration observed in DC.

8. Novel Drugs and Their Anti-Fibrotic Role

8.1. SGLT2 Inhibitors

SGLT2i works by enhancing glucose excretion in urine, primarily through inhibiting SGLT2, thereby reducing the renal threshold value of glucose and decreasing the reabsorption of filtered glucose. However, the benefits observed in HF associated with SGLT2i are unlikely to be solely attributed to glucose lowering. Rather, the advantages for CV and renal health have been linked to various mechanisms including hemodynamic effects, anti-inflammatory properties, anti-fibrotic effects, antioxidant actions, reno-protective effects, attenuation of glucotoxicity, reduction in uric acid levels, modification of the neurohumoral system, and cardiac metabolism [6,122–124]. While the CV benefits of SGLT2i are evident, the precise mechanisms underlying these effects are not fully understood.

SGLT2i plays a significant role in managing blood glucose levels by specifically targeting the SGLT2 transporter in the proximal renal tubules, leading to decreased glucose reabsorption and increased glucose excretion in the urine. This mechanism effectively reduces blood glucose concentrations independent of insulin pathways, thereby not triggering insulin release or causing hypoglycemia. Consequently, this reduction in circulating glucose helps to improve insulin sensitivity in muscle tissues and enhances β-cell function, contributing to the management of insulin resistance in patients with diabetes [125–129].

ACS is characterized by coronary artery obstruction, leading to myocardial ischemic damage, which can have life-threatening consequences. Immediate treatment is provided to restore oxygenation to the affected tissue, and patients are often prescribed secondary preventive medications to reduce the risk of future ACS events. Despite consistent prescription practices over the years, there is potential to include SGLT2i in this regimen due to their demonstrated CV benefits. Clinical research on the impact of SGLT2i on CV health in patients after MI has yielded conflicting results, with most trials focusing on MACEs rather than the underlying cellular processes including inflammation, cardiac metabolism, or cardiac fibrosis.

Inflammation plays a central role in myocardial fibrosis development, involving various inflammatory factors. However, it remains uncertain whether SGLT2i influences the inflammatory response and whether they can impede myocardial fibrosis progression by targeting inflammation. Wang et al. found that dapagliflozin effectively reduced levels of TNF-α, IL-1β, IL-6, and hs-CRP in patients with diabetes and HF, leading to a gradual decline in inflammation and alleviation of myocardial fibrosis [130]. Dapagliflozin also reduced cardiac fibrosis in T2DM rats by inhibiting endothelial-to-mesenchymal transition (EndMT) and fibroblast activation via AMPKα activation, which suppressed the TGF-β/Smad signaling pathway [131]. Dapagliflozin decreased oxidative stress in the heart and prevented the production of inflammatory substances, thereby inhibiting myocardial enlargement and scar tissue formation [132–134]. Additionally, via raising AMPK phosphorylation, it inhibits high glucose-induced endothelial cell dysfunction [135]. A recent clinical trial has shown the efficacy of dapagliflozin in improving glycemic fluctuations and reducing oxidative stress in individuals with T2DM [136]. Recent investigations have shown that dapagliflozin provides protection against myocardial ischemia/reperfusion injury (IRI) via restricting the activation of the NLRP3 inflammasome [137].

In mouse models, empagliflozin was found to reduce myocardial infarct size and preserve myocardial function after ischemia/reperfusion injury by regulating inflammatory responses and redox signaling in the ischemic myocardium [138,139]. Empagliflozin also reduced cardiomyocyte hypertrophy, interstitial fibrosis, and oxidative stress in non-diabetic rat models of HF [140,141]. However, long-term empagliflozin administration did not significantly improve LV function, shape, adiposity, or diffuse fibrosis in individuals with T2DM [142]. Similarly, no significant difference in mortality was observed between patients with diabetes receiving low-dose empagliflozin after percutaneous coronary intervention (PCI) for ACS and the placebo group [143]. Nonetheless, empagliflozin treatment improved heart function in mice with diabetes after infarction, particularly diastolic function, suggesting potential benefits in diabetic cardiomyopathy [144]. Nrf2 has a crucial role as a transcription factor in regulating the expression of genes that are involved in antioxidant and cytoprotective functions. Empagliflozin enhances Nrf2 expression and facilitates its nuclear translocation, therefore mitigating heart dysfunction in db/db mice with diabetes via the amelioration of oxidative stress and mitochondrial dysfunction [145,146].

Furthermore, SGLT2i such as dapagliflozin, canagliflozin, and empagliflozin have been shown to have anti-inflammatory effects by reducing the production of the NLRP3 inflammasome, IL-1β, IL-6, TNF-α, and LV ECM remodeling in diabetes animal models [137,147–151]. In the same line, Hodrea, J. et al. demonstrated that dapagliflozin effectively decreased the levels of IL-1β, IL-6, and TNF-α in the LV of rats with type 1 diabetes mellitus (T1DM), indicating its potential as an anti-inflammatory agent [149]. Empagliflozin attenuates TGF-β1-induced fibroblast activation and decreases pro-fibrotic markers such as type I collagen (COL-1), connective tissue growth factor (CTGF), and MMP-2 [152]. Additionally, it has been shown to alleviate cardiac fibrosis by downregulating the TGF-β/Smad pathway, triggering Nrf2/ARE signaling, and lowering the concentrations of Smad1, Smad2, and Smad3 in the heart tissue of mice with diabetes [146].

According to recent research, SGLT2i may have a role in LV remodeling in individuals with diabetes. Following this therapy, individuals with T2DM with or without CAD showed a decrease in LV mass measured by cardiac MRI, as stated by two randomized trials [153,154]. Recent results indicate that the treatment of SGLT2i to individuals with diabetes resulted in a decrease in blood hs-CRP levels and an improvement in endothelial function. In contrast, the EMBLEM study found that a 24-week therapy with empagliflozin did not lead to any improvement in endothelial dysfunction in patients with preexisting cardiovascular disease and T2DM [155–158]. Collectively, these findings suggest that SGLT2i may have potential therapeutic effects beyond glucose lowering, particularly in mitigating inflammation and fibrosis in CV diseases.

8.2. Glucagon-like Peptide-1 Receptor Agonists

Glucagon-like peptide-1 (GLP-1) is a hormone naturally produced and released by endocrine L-cells in the small intestine upon food ingestion. It binds to specific GLP-1 receptors in the pancreas, stimulating insulin release in a glucose dependent manner. Despite its widespread presence in various organs, natural GLP-1 has a short half-life due to rapid breakdown by dipeptidyl peptidase-4 (DPP-4) [159–161].

Incretin hormones significantly influence insulin production post-meal, accounting for 50–70% of total insulin release, but their effect is reduced in patients with T2DM due to various factors. These hormones, particularly GLP-1, enhance insulin secretion, delay stomach emptying, and suppress glucagon release, helping regulate postprandial blood glucose levels. To augment the actions of GLP-1, two therapeutic strategies are employed and are as follows: GLP-1RAs, which resist the degradation by DPP-4 enzyme and thus prolong receptor activation, and DPP-4 inhibitors, which extend the life of endogenous incretin hormones. GLP-1RAs improve glucose-dependent insulin release, reduce glucagon secretion, enhance insulin sensitivity, and have additional benefits on appetite suppression, cardiovascular protection, renal sodium excretion, and metabolic functions in adipose and muscle tissues. The efficacy of GLP-1RAs varies with their duration of action; long-acting forms are particularly effective in controlling both postprandial and fasting glucose levels, demonstrating significant improvements in glycemic control in patients with T2DM [162–165].

Studies have shown that GLP-1RAs can modulate ECM homeostasis by inhibiting the mitogen-activated protein kinase (MAPK) pathway and BATF/JUN heterodimer formation. They also downregulate the pro-fibrotic factor TGF-β1, suppressing SMAD3 and extracellular signal-regulated kinase 1/2 (ERK1/2) signaling while enhancing WNT/β-catenin signaling and other pathways, thus reducing extracellular matrix protein deposition and delaying fibrosis [166–168].

GLP-1RAs ameliorate diabetes-related cardiac fibrosis by stimulating PPARδ expression. Additionally, GLP-1 attenuates high glucose-induced ROS production in cardiomyocytes through an AMPK/mTORC1/p70S6K-dependent mechanism [169,170]. In vitro, semaglutide suppressed cardiomyocyte apoptosis produced by ischemia/reperfusion (I/R) via activating the PKG/PKCε/ERK1/2 pathway [171]. It also might potentially be a beneficial treatment target for preventing diabetic cardiomyopathy by modifying integrin-linked kinase (ILK)-associated TGF-β/SMAD signaling pathways [172].

Research has shown that GLP-1 analogs, such as liraglutide, may prevent myocardial damage by activating the Sirt1/AMPK signaling pathways to suppress cellular pyroptosis in diabetic cardiac tissues and by lowering the expression of fibrotic markers [173,174]. Moreover, treatment with liraglutide limits infarct size, expansion, and cardiac rupture in the normal and diabetic heart by activating prosurvival kinases and cytoprotective genes in the heart in a preclinical murine model of experimental ischemia following coronary artery obstruction. In mouse cardiomyocytes cultivated in vitro, it also raises cAMP and lowers apoptosis [175].

GLP-1 analog exendin-4 has been found to suppress fibrosis and PPARα-mediated lipid accumulation via the protein kinase A/Rho-associated protein kinase (PKA/ROCK) pathway [176]. Recent studies in vitro have shown that exendin-4 effectively reduces the formation of intracellular and mitochondrial ROS, prevents apoptosis, and improves mitochondrial membrane potential impairment. Additionally, it activates genes associated with mitochondrial functions and dynamics via the cAMP/Epac/PI3K/Akt pathway. By encouraging the nuclear translocation of TFEB, it restores autophagic flux. It also protects endothelial function by upregulating the expression of HDL scavenger receptor class BI via the AMPK/FoxO1 pathway and eNOS activation. Lastly, it decreases the size of infarcts and maintains cardiac function by having anti-apoptotic and antioxidative properties [177–179]. Research have demonstrated the cardioprotective benefits of exendin-4 in rats with diabetes. This is due to its capacity to enhance mitochondrial activities by targeting inflammatory and autophagy processes and suppressing cardiomyocyte pyroptosis via the AMPK-TXNIP pathway [180,181]. In mice models, after MI, the positive impacts of exendin-4 on cardiac remodeling may be achieved via activating the eNOS/cGMP/PKG pathway, β-arrestin-2, and protein phosphatase 2A and suppressing β-catenin, collagen I, collagen III, transforming growth factor-β1, and PI3K/AKT signaling pathway [181–184].

Modified mesenchymal stem cells engineered to secrete a fusion protein have demonstrated positive effects on cardiac recovery post infarction by reducing TGF-β expression and influencing extracellular matrix protein deposition. GLP-1RAs inhibit cardiac remodeling in rats after AMI by modulating various signaling pathways [182,185]. In murine models, liraglutide reduces cardiac fibrosis and enhances capillary density, potentially improving heart function [186,187].

Clinical studies have also shown the anti-fibrotic effects of GLP-1RAs. Reduced GLP-1 levels in plasma have been associated with atheroma instability and cardiac fibrosis in non-diabetic patients with ACS [188]. Initiating GLP-1RAs therapy shortly after a first AMI in patients with diabetes has been linked to a reduced risk of significant CV events [189]. Long-term treatment with GLP-1RAs and/or SGLT-2i positively impacts the clinical prognosis of patients with diabetes that are hospitalized with AMI [190,191].

However, conflicting results exist in clinical trials regarding the impact of GLP-1RAs on myocardial remodeling. While some studies show potential benefits, others reveal no significant effects on cardiac function or fibrosis parameters [192,193]. Nonetheless, retrospective studies suggest a reduced risk of CV events and mortality in patients with diabetes treated with GLP-1RAs [194].

In summary, the potential anti-fibrotic effects of GLP-1RAs offer promising avenues for clinical treatment by inhibiting epithelial–endothelial transformation, suppressing inflammatory responses, and reducing oxidative stress damage while controlling blood glucose levels.

8.3. Dipeptidyl Peptidase-4 Inhibitors

DPP4i are small, orally administered compounds that specifically interact with the catalytic site of DPP4 without affecting its other known activities, such as its immunomodulatory effects. DPP-4 is a serine protease primarily responsible for deactivating the GLP-1 and GIP generated in the intestines. The efficacy of DPP4i as anti-diabetic agents is closely tied to their ability to inhibit DPP4 enzyme activity, thus leading to a prolongation of the lifespan of incretin hormones and an improvement in insulin production, which is reliant on glucose levels. By prolonging the half-life of GLP-1, increasing insulin levels, and lowering blood glucose levels, DPP4i offer therapeutic benefits [195,196]. Contrary to the anti-diabetic medications stated above, DPP-4 inhibitors do not impact insulin sensitivity or secretion [197–200].

A meta-analysis has shown that DPP-4 inhibitors may effectively reduce low-grade inflammation in individuals with T2DM by decreasing levels of C-reactive protein (CRP), TNF-α, IL-6, and IL-1β [201]. Recent studies on diabetic animal models, such as db/db mice, have demonstrated the cardioprotective effects of DPP4 inhibitors like evogliptin. These inhibitors mitigate the primary drivers of diabetic cardiomyopathy, including cardiac hypertrophy, fibrosis, and systolic and diastolic dysfunction. Evogliptin has been shown to reduce mitochondrial dysfunction and lipotoxicity by reducing myocardial fat formation or modulating transcription factors [202]. Additionally, gemigliptin was also shown to reduce cardiomyocyte cross-sectional areas and interstitial and perivascular fibrosis [203]. In rats with HF, monotherapy with DPP4i like valsartan and vildagliptin has been found to decrease LV hypertrophy, alleviate cardiac interstitial fibrosis, and improve systolic and diastolic performance [204].

Studies by Wójcicka et al. investigated whether incretin drugs like exenatide and sitagliptin exert heart-protective and anti-fibrotic effects through their influence on asymmetric dimethylarginine (ADMA) metabolism. Both drugs reduced cardiac fibrosis and immune response around blood vessels. In metabolic syndrome, sitagliptin and exenatide positively impacted cardiac fibrotic remodeling and circulating levels of endogenous NOS inhibitors, such as ADMA, which inhibit NO production, essential for maintaining healthy blood vessels [205]. Additionally, DPP4i have been found to have antifibrotic effects by blocking the interaction between membrane-bound DPP-4, integrin, and the caveolin complex [206].

Linagliptin improved systolic and diastolic blood pressure and cardiac function while reducing cardiac fibrosis in animal models. It also ameliorated structural disruptions in the heart induced by diabetic conditions [207]. In db/db mice with MI, it targeted the NLRP3/ASC inflammasome, increasing EF and lowering IL-1β and IL-6 levels [208].

Sitagliptin treatment effectively hindered cardiac fibrosis development and alleviated cardiac hypertrophy [209]. It also mitigates heart dysfunction and unfavorable remodeling after AMI in diabetic animal models [210]. Additionally, it reduced the severity of diabetic cardiomyopathy by suppressing the JAK/STAT signaling pathway and decreasing TGF-β1 protein levels, therefore avoiding myocardial remodeling [211,212].

Alogliptin reduced interstitial fibrosis and decreased mitochondrial ROS generation, preventing the mitochondrial depolarization of membranes and swelling in rabbits with diabetes [213,214]. Interestingly, adding saxagliptin to dapagliflozinin may have reduced the degree of activation of the NLRP3/ASC inflammasome. Higher myocardial lipid deposits, oxidative stress, and apoptosis were all reduced by saxagliptin [150,176].

Despite several CV outcome trials evaluating the efficacy and safety of new glucose-lowering drugs for CV outcomes, there is limited research on their correlation with the reduction in cardiac fibrosis risk in patients with diabetes and ACS.

8.4. Neprilysin Inhibitor

Neutral endopeptidase, also known as neprilysin (NEP), breaks down natriuretic peptides (NPs) by hydrolysis. Neprilysin inhibitors (NEPis) have been discovered to elevate the concentration of defensive natriuretic peptides (NPs), hence enhancing their ability to defend against diabetic consequences. Nevertheless, NEPi alone proved inadequate in addressing cardiovascular disorders as mandated by conventional pharmacology, prompting the development of dual-acting inhibitors that target both neprilysin and the pressor arm (Ang II/ACE/AT1R) of the RAS. Recent human trials have shown that the dual angiotensin receptor–neprilysin inhibitor (ARNi) has been effective in enhancing glycemic control and insulin sensitivity in persons with T2DM and/or obesity. Additionally, preclinical research has also shown that inhibiting neprilysin, either on its own or in conjunction with renin–angiotensin system blockers, has positive effects on glucose regulation [215–217].

Studies have shown that ARNIs enhance glucose homeostasis, glucose management, and insulin sensitivity in individuals with T2DM [215]. Evidence from human research substantiates the efficacy of neprilysin inhibitors for both preventing and treating type 2 diabetes. The PARADIGM-HF study shown that administering the ARNi over a duration of 3 years led to a more significant decrease in HbA1c levels and a reduced number of patients needing to start oral glucose-lowering medicines or insulin therapy, in comparison to using just an ACE inhibitor. In an additional investigation, switching the therapy from either an ACE inhibitor or ARB to ARNi for a duration of 3 months led to a drop in serum neprilysin activity. This decrease was shown to be linked to lower levels of fructosamine, a marker used to measure protein glycation. The results of this study, along with a previous publication, indicated that ARNi may have positive effects on glycemic management by partially raising the levels of GLP-1 in the bloodstream [218,219].

In streptozotocin (STZ)-induced mice with diabetes and HF and a decreased EF, LCZ696, the initial member of ARNi, has been shown to enhance cardiac functions and mitigate fibrosis by inhibiting TGF-ß [220]. According to research by Qing et al., mice with diabetes treated with LCZ696 had better cardiac function and ventricular remodeling than mice with diabetes that were left untreated. Additionally, LCZ696 reduced oxidative stress in vitro and in vivo. Finally, via lowering oxidative stress, apoptosis, and cardiac inflammation, LCZ696 ameliorated diabetic cardiomyopathy [221].

Researchers have created and tested omapatrilat, the most researched vasopeptidase inhibitor, against heart diseases associated with diabetes. Compared to ACEi, this medication had greater cardioprotective potential in spontaneously diabetic rats because it controlled systolic blood pressure, improved diastolic function, and decreased heart hypertrophy [222]. By restoring RAS and NPS activities, raising cGMP, and suppressing inflammatory, profibrotic, and apoptotic signaling, a recent study demonstrated the cardioprotective efficacy of NEPi and ACE2 activator combination treatment, which was successful in preventing DC [223].

In conclusion, not many studies have been conducted to determine how neprylisin inhibitors affect DC. Additional research is required to investigate the possible processes that underlie its effects, since this might serve as the foundation for a novel treatment approach for it.

8.5. Sarcoplasmic/Endoplasmic Reticulum Calcium ATPase

The pathological and molecular processes that underlie diabetes include irregularities in the control of calcium homeostasis within cardiomyocytes, which subsequently modifies the ventricular excitation–contraction coupling. A dysregulation of Ca2+ cycling in the diabetic heart involves a decrease in sarcoplasmic/endoplasmic reticulum calcium ATPase (SERCA) activity, which may also be accompanied by a drop in SERCA protein expression. Multiple preclinical and clinical experiments have shown that maintaining proper management of blood sugar levels is ineffective in slowing the course of diabetic cardiomyopathy, particularly in the intermediate and advanced phases. Thus, individuals with diabetic cardiomyopathy may continue to experience hyperglycemic stress despite the careful management of blood glucose levels. The etiology of DC is mostly investigated utilizing tiny molecular probes that have strong effectiveness against it. As a result, SERCA could be a target molecule for pharmacological intervention targeted at improving the mechanical performance and energy efficiency of the diabetic heart, which is characterized by a malfunctioning SR Ca2+ loading [224].

Recent research has shown that SJ-12, a new curcumin derivative, has therapeutic efficacy in STZ-induced diabetic cardiomiopathy. Furthermore, SJ-12 administration may reduce the fibrotic response. SJ-12 functions as an anti-fibrosis agent by specifically targeting the OGT-regulated O-GlcNAc-Sp1/SERCA2a/calcium signaling pathway [225].

A significant buildup of collagen and ECM proteins, linked to higher death rates, defines cardiac fibrosis. Recent findings suggest that the deregulation of SERCA2a and inappropriate handling of Ca2+ cause cardiac fibrosis. An imbalance in Ca2+ levels, on the other hand, can cause problems with energy metabolism, which in turn speeds up the development of cardiac fibrosis by making more matrix proteins. Conventional autophagy is responsible for breaking down and reusing cellular components, which helps to sustain cellular energy production. Excessive or inadequate autophagy may have a detrimental effect on the viability of cardiomyocytes, leading to a deterioration in both the structure and function of the heart. Latest research has shown that inhibiting the expression of SERCA might serve as a trigger for endoplasmic reticulum (ER) stress, which in turn leads to excessive autophagy and eventually results in cardiac fibrosis [226–228].

Most of the studies have mostly focused on the function of SERCA as the calcium pump responsible for transporting calcium from the cytosol to the SR lumen, working against the concentration gradient. However, there is little information about its involvement in cardiac fibrosis in patients with diabetes.

In Table 1, the main studies evaluating the antifibrotic effects of hypoglycemic medication are depicted.

Table 1. The main antifibrotic effect of novel medication.

Novel Medication	Antifibrotic Effect
SGLT2i	• Reduces the levels of TNF- α, IL-1β, IL-6, and hs-CRP in patients with HF and diabetes [130]. • Reduces cardiac fibrosis in rats with T2DM by inhibiting EndMT and fibroblast activation [131]. • Decreases oxidative stress and prevents the production of TNF-α, IL-1β, IL-6, and MCP-1 [132–134]. • Increases the phosphorylation and expression of STAT3 while reducing the expression of myocardial IL-6 and iNOS [138]. • Increases the activation of M2 macrophages, leading to a reduction in cardiac fibrosis at a molecular level [139]. • Decreases the production of the NLRP3 inflammasome, IL-1β, IL-6, and TNF-α [137,147,148]. • Attenuates TFG-β1-induced fibroblast activation and decreases COL-1, connective tissue growth factor, and MMP-2 [152]. • Alleviates cardiac fibrosis by downregulating the TGF-β/Smad pathway, triggering Nrf2/ARE signaling, and lowering the concentrations of Smad1, Smad2, and Smad3 in the heart tissue of mice with diabetes [146]. • Effectively decreases the levels of IL-1β, IL-6, and TNF-α in the LV of rats with T1DM [149]. • Enhances Nrf2 expression and facilitates its nuclear translocation, ameliorating oxidative stress and mitochondrial dysfunction [145].
GLP-1RAs	• By stimulating the expression of PPARδ, GLP-1RAs ameliorate diabetes-related cardiac fibrosis in a diabetic cardiomyopathy model [169]. • Decrease high glucose-induced ROS production in cardiomyocytes via a mechanism that is reliant on AMPK/mTORC1/p70S6K [170]. • Lower the expressions of P4hα-1, COL-1, COL-3, MMP-1, and MMP-9 [173]. • Suppress fibrosis and PPARα-mediated lipid accumulation and toxicity controlled by the PKA/ROCK pathway [176]. • Reduce cardiac remodeling in rats after AMI by inhibiting the activation of β-arrestin-2, PP2A, and GSK3β [182,185]. • Suppress the production of CTGF in both the infarcted and non-infarcted regions of mice after a heart attack by stimulating cAMP and decreasing the migration of collagen fibers from the infarcted region to the non-infarcted region [186,187]. • Suppress cardiomyocyte apoptosis produced by ischemia/reperfusion (I/R) via activating the PKG/PKCε/ERK1/2 pathway [171]. • Prevent myocardial damage by activating the Sirt1/AMPK signaling pathways to suppress cellular pyroptosis in diabetic cardiac tissues [173,174]. • Effectively reduce the formation of intracellular and mitochondrial ROS, prevent apoptosis, and improve mitochondrial membrane potential impairment [177–179]. • Activate genes associated with mitochondrial functions and dynamics via the cAMP/Epac/PI3K/Akt pathway [177–179]. • Enhance mitochondrial activities by targeting inflammatory and autophagy processes and suppressing cardiomyocyte pyroptosis via the AMPK-TXNIP pathway [180,181].
DPP4i	• Decreases LV hypertrophy, relieves cardiac interstitial fibrosis, and enhances systolic and diastolic performance [204]. • Decreases the amount of fibrosis around blood vessels and has positive impact on cardiac fibrotic remodeling and the circulating level of endogenous NOS inhibitors [205]. • Exhibits antifibrotic effects by blocking the interaction between membrane-bound DPP-4, integrin, and the caveolin complex [206]. • Linagliptin exhibits improvements by reducing disruptions in myocardial fiber, mitochondria, and sarcomere, along with the necroptosis [207]. • Sitagliptin treatment effectively hinders the development of cardiac fibrosis and alleviates cardiac hypertrophy [209]. • Reduces the severity of diabetic cardiomyopathy by suppressing the JAK/STAT signaling pathway and decreasing TGF-β1 protein levels, therefore avoiding myocardial remodeling [211,212].
ARNi	• Enhances cardiac functions and mitigates fibrosis by inhibiting TGF-ß [220]

HF = heart failure; LV = left ventricle; TNF-α = tumor necrosis factor-α; IL-1β = interleukin-1β; IL-6 = interleukin-6; hs-CRP = high sensitivity c-reactive protein; COL-1 = type 1 collagen; COL-3 = type 3 collagen; MMP-1 = matrix metalloproteinase 1; MMP-2 = matrix metalloproteinase 2; MMP-9 = matrix metalloproteinase 9; PPARα = peroxisome proliferator-activated receptor alpha; PKA/ROCK = protein kinase A/Rho-associated protein kinase; PP2A = protein phosphatase 2; DPP4 = dipeptidyl peptidase-4; DPP4i = dipeptidyl peptidase-4 inhibitor; SGLT2i = sodium-glucose cotransporter 2 inhibitors; GLP-1RAs = glucagon-like peptide-1 receptor agonists; CTGF = connective tissue growth factor; cAMP = cyclic adenosine monophosphate; GSK3β = glycogen synthase kinase 3 beta; STAT3 = signal transducer and activator of transcription 3; iNOS = inducible form of nitric oxide synthase; P4hα-1 = prolyl 4-hydroxylase subunit alpha 1; EndMT = endothelial-to-mesenchymal transition; ARNi = angiotensin receptor–neprilysin inhibitor; and T1DM = type 1 diabetes mellitus.

9. Limitations and Future Directions

While this research offers valuable insights, it is important to acknowledge certain limitations that may affect the interpretation and generalization of findings. Firstly, many studies assessing the effectiveness of anti-diabetic medications in reducing fibrosis risk post-MI have relatively short follow-up periods, limiting our understanding of their long-term effects. Secondly, variability in patient characteristics, such as age, comorbidities, and medication history, across different studies may affect the generalizability of findings. Finally, while some studies demonstrate the efficacy of anti-diabetic medications in reducing fibrosis, the exact mechanisms underlying these effects remain incompletely understood.

Thus, we recognize the need for future research to focus on addressing these limitations, exploring new directions, and contributing to advancing our knowledge in the field. Further research is needed to elucidate the precise mechanisms through which anti-diabetic medications exert their anti-fibrotic effects post-MI, potentially uncovering novel therapeutic targets. Longitudinal studies with extended follow-up periods are necessary to assess the sustained efficacy and safety of anti-diabetic medications in reducing fibrosis and improving CV outcomes. Investigating the potential synergistic effects of combining anti-diabetic medications with other therapeutic agents targeting different pathways involved in fibrosis could lead to enhanced treatment efficacy. In conclusion, future research should focus on elucidating the underlying mechanisms of action of these medications, conducting longitudinal studies with extended follow-up periods, and exploring personalized medicine approaches and combination therapies.

10. Conclusions

In conclusion, myocardial fibrosis is a critical contributor to adverse cardiac remodeling following AMI, particularly in patients with DM. Emerging evidence suggests that anti-diabetic medications, such as SGLT2i, GLP-1RAs, and DPP4i, may hold promise in attenuating fibrosis and improving CV outcomes in this patient population. Overall, the identification of effective anti-fibrotic strategies in patients with diabetes post-MI holds significant clinical implications for improving CV outcomes and reducing the burden of heart failure. Continued research efforts in this area are essential for advancing our understanding and refining treatment strategies to optimize patient care.

Author Contributions: Conceptualization, L.A. and A.T.; methodology, L.A.; software, A.T. and B.-S.T.; validation, L.A., R.A.S. and C.S.; formal analysis, L.A., C.S., R.-L.Z. and B.-S.T.; investigation, A.T. and B.-S.T., data curation, L.A., A.T. and B.-S.T.; writing—original draft preparation, L.A., A.T., R.-L.Z. and B.-S.T.; writing—review and editing, L.A., A.T. and B.-S.T.; supervision, R.A.S. and C.S. All authors have read and agreed to the published version of the manuscript.

Funding: This research received no external funding.

Institutional Review Board Statement: Not applicable.

Informed Consent Statement: Not applicable.

Conflicts of Interest: The authors declare no conflicts of interest.

References

1. Frantz, S.; Hundertmark, M.J.; Schulz-Menger, J.; Bengel, F.M.; Bauersachs, J. Left ventricular remodelling post-myocardial infarction: Pathophysiology, imaging, and novel therapies. *Eur. Heart J.* **2022**, *43*, 2549–2561. [CrossRef] [PubMed]
2. Frangogiannis, N.G. Cardiac fibrosis. *Cardiovasc. Res.* **2021**, *117*, 1450–1488. [CrossRef] [PubMed]
3. Nakamura, K.; Miyoshi, T.; Yoshida, M.; Akagi, S.; Saito, Y.; Ejiri, K.; Matsuo, N.; Ichikawa, K.; Iwasaki, K.; Naito, T.; et al. Pathophysiology and Treatment of Diabetic Cardiomyopathy and Heart Failure in Patients with Diabetes Mellitus. *Int. J. Mol. Sci.* **2022**, *23*, 3587. [CrossRef] [PubMed]
4. Preis, S.R.; Pencina, M.J.; Hwang, S.J.; D'Agostino, R.B., Sr.; Savage, P.J.; Levy, D.; Fox, C.S. Trends in cardiovascular disease risk factors in individuals with and without diabetes mellitus in the Framingham Heart Study. *Circulation* **2009**, *120*, 212–220. [CrossRef] [PubMed]
5. Matheus, A.S.; Tannus, L.R.; Cobas, R.A.; Palma, C.C.; Negrato, C.A.; Gomes, M.B. Impact of diabetes on cardiovascular disease: An update. *Int. J. Hypertens.* **2013**, *2013*, 653789. [CrossRef] [PubMed]

6. Davies, M.J.; Aroda, V.R.; Collins, B.S.; Gabbay, R.A.; Green, J.; Maruthur, N.M.; Rosas, S.E.; Del Prato, S.; Mathieu, C.; Mingrone, G.; et al. Management of Hyperglycemia in Type 2 Diabetes, 2022. A Consensus Report by the American Diabetes Association (ADA) and the European Association for the Study of Diabetes (EASD). *Diabetes Care* **2022**, *45*, 2753–2786. [CrossRef] [PubMed]
7. Ding, Y.; Wang, Y.; Zhang, W.; Jia, Q.; Wang, X.; Li, Y.; Lv, S.; Zhang, J. Roles of Biomarkers in Myocardial Fibrosis. *Aging Dis.* **2020**, *11*, 1157–1174. [CrossRef] [PubMed]
8. Frangogiannis, N.G. Cardiac fibrosis: Cell biological mechanisms, molecular pathways and therapeutic opportunities. *Mol. Aspects Med.* **2019**, *65*, 70–99. [CrossRef]
9. Ma, T.; Huang, X.; Zheng, H.; Huang, G.; Li, W.; Liu, X.; Liang, J.; Cao, Y.; Hu, Y.; Huang, Y. SFRP2 Improves Mitochondrial Dynamics and Mitochondrial Biogenesis, Oxidative Stress, and Apoptosis in Diabetic Cardiomyopathy. *Oxidative Med. Cell Longev.* **2021**, *2021*, 9265016. [CrossRef]
10. Salib, M.; Girerd, N.; Simon, A.; Kearney-Schwartz, A.; Duarte, K.; Leroy, C.; Rossignol, P.; Benetos, A.; Frimat, L.; Girerd, S. Levels of Procollagen Type I C-Terminal Pro-Peptide and Galectin-3, Arterial Stiffness Measured By Pulse Wave Velocity, and Cardiovascular Morbidity and Mortality in 44 Patients 2 Years After Kidney Transplantation. *Ann. Transplant.* **2023**, *28*, e938137. [CrossRef]
11. Ponikowska, B.; Iwanek, G.; Zdanowicz, A.; Urban, S.; Zymlinski, R.; Ponikowski, P.; Biegus, J. Biomarkers of Myocardial Injury and Remodeling in Heart Failure. *J. Pers. Med.* **2022**, *12*, 799. [CrossRef] [PubMed]
12. Ferreira, J.P.; Rossignol, P.; Pizard, A.; Machu, J.L.; Collier, T.; Girerd, N.; Huby, A.C.; Gonzalez, A.; Diez, J.; Lopez, B.; et al. Potential spironolactone effects on collagen metabolism biomarkers in patients with uncontrolled blood pressure. *Heart* **2019**, *105*, 307–314. [CrossRef] [PubMed]
13. Zile, M.R.; O'Meara, E.; Claggett, B.; Prescott, M.F.; Solomon, S.D.; Swedberg, K.; Packer, M.; McMurray, J.J.V.; Shi, V.; Lefkowitz, M.; et al. Effects of Sacubitril/Valsartan on Biomarkers of Extracellular Matrix Regulation in Patients With HFrEF. *J. Am. Coll. Cardiol.* **2019**, *73*, 795–806. [CrossRef] [PubMed]
14. Zhang, B.; Li, X.; Chen, C.; Jiang, W.; Lu, D.; Liu, Q.; Wang, K.; Yan, Y.; Jiang, Z.; Geng, J.; et al. Renal Denervation Effects on Myocardial Fibrosis and Ventricular Arrhythmias in Rats with Ischemic Cardiomyopathy. *Cell Physiol. Biochem.* **2018**, *46*, 2471–2479. [CrossRef] [PubMed]
15. Santanasto, A.J.; Cvejkus, R.K.; Wojczynski, M.K.; Marron, M.M.; Schupf, N.; Christensen, K.; Thyagarajan, B.; Zmuda, J.M. Circulating Procollagen Type III N-Terminal Peptide and Physical Function in Adults from the Long Life Family Study. *J. Gerontol. A Biol. Sci. Med. Sci.* **2021**, *76*, 1273–1279. [CrossRef] [PubMed]
16. Osokina, A.; Karetnikova, V.; Polikutina, O.; Ivanova, A.; Gruzdeva, O.; Dyleva, Y.; Kokov, A.; Brel, N.; Pecherina, T.; Barbarash, O. Prognostic potential of cardiac structural and functional parameters and N-terminal propeptide of type III procollagen in predicting cardiac fibrosis one year after myocardial infarction with preserved left ventricular ejection fraction. *Aging* **2021**, *13*, 194–203. [CrossRef] [PubMed]
17. Zelniker, T.A.; Jarolim, P.; Scirica, B.M.; Braunwald, E.; Park, J.G.; Das, S.; Sabatine, M.S.; Morrow, D.A. Biomarker of Collagen Turnover (C-Terminal Telopeptide) and Prognosis in Patients With Non- ST -Elevation Acute Coronary Syndromes. *J. Am. Heart Assoc.* **2019**, *8*, e011444. [CrossRef] [PubMed]
18. Manhenke, C.; Orn, S.; Squire, I.; Radauceanu, A.; Alla, F.; Zannad, F.; Dickstein, K. The prognostic value of circulating markers of collagen turnover after acute myocardial infarction. *Int. J. Cardiol.* **2011**, *150*, 277–282. [CrossRef] [PubMed]
19. Owolabi, U.S.; Amraotkar, A.R.; Coulter, A.R.; Singam, N.S.V.; Aladili, B.N.; Singh, A.; Trainor, P.J.; Mitra, R.; DeFilippis, A.P. Change in matrix metalloproteinase 2, 3, and 9 levels at the time of and after acute atherothrombotic myocardial infarction. *J. Thromb. Thrombolysis* **2020**, *49*, 235–244. [CrossRef]
20. Myasoedova, V.A.; Chistiakov, D.A.; Grechko, A.V.; Orekhov, A.N. Matrix metalloproteinases in pro-atherosclerotic arterial remodeling. *J. Mol. Cell Cardiol.* **2018**, *123*, 159–167. [CrossRef]
21. Zhou, K.; Li, Y.; Xu, Y.; Guo, R. Circulating Matrix Metalloproteinase-28 Levels Are Related to GRACE Scores and Short-Term Outcomes in Patients with Acute Myocardial Infarction. *Biomed. Res. Int.* **2020**, *2020*, 9206703. [CrossRef] [PubMed]
22. Basia, D.; Gupta, M.D.; Kunal, S.; Muheeb, G.; Girish, M.P.; Bansal, A.; Batra, V.; Yusuf, J.; Mukhopadhyay, S.; Tyagi, S.; et al. Matrix metalloproteinases and their gene polymorphism in young ST-segment elevation myocardial infarction. *Indian Heart J.* **2022**, *74*, 519–523. [CrossRef] [PubMed]
23. Somuncu, M.U.; Pusuroglu, H.; Karakurt, H.; Bolat, I.; Karakurt, S.T.; Demir, A.R.; Isiksacan, N.; Akgul, O.; Surgit, O. The prognostic value of elevated matrix metalloproteinase-9 in patients undergoing primary percutaneous coronary intervention for ST-elevation myocardial infarction: A two-year prospective study. *Rev. Port. Cardiol.* **2020**, *39*, 267–276. [CrossRef] [PubMed]
24. Watson, C.; Spiers, J.P.; Waterstone, M.; Russell-Hallinan, A.; Gallagher, J.; McDonald, K.; Ryan, C.; Gilmer, J.; Ledwidge, M. Investigation of association of genetic variant rs3918242 of matrix metalloproteinase-9 with hypertension, myocardial infarction and progression of ventricular dysfunction in Irish Caucasian patients with diabetes: A report from the STOP-HF follow-up programme. *BMC Cardiovasc. Disord.* **2021**, *21*, 87. [CrossRef] [PubMed]
25. Xie, Y.T.; Dang, Y.; Zhang, F.F.; Zhang, Q.H.; Wu, H.B.; Liu, G. Combination of serum TIMP-3, CA125, and NT-proBNP in predicting ventricular remodeling in patients with heart failure following acute myocardial infarction. *Cardiovasc. Diagn. Ther.* **2020**, *10*, 1184–1191. [CrossRef] [PubMed]

26. Pang, H.F.; Gao, Y.; Liu, J.M.; Lu, J.P.; Wang, Y.P.; Wang, S.M.; Hou, L.B.; Tian, A.X.; Gao, Y. Prognostic value of tissue inhibitor of metalloproteinase-matrix metalloproteinase biomarkers at 30 days in patients with acute myocardial infarction without reperfusion therapy. *Chin. Med. J.* **2020**, *134*, 481–483. [CrossRef] [PubMed]
27. Zhang, X.G.; Wei, Y.; Jiang, J.; Wang, L.; Liang, H.Y.; Lei, C.B. Effect of TGF-beta1 on myocardial cell apoptosis in rats with acute myocardial infarction via MAPK signaling pathway. *Eur. Rev. Med. Pharmacol. Sci.* **2020**, *24*, 1350–1356. [CrossRef] [PubMed]
28. Kong, P.; Shinde, A.V.; Su, Y.; Russo, I.; Chen, B.; Saxena, A.; Conway, S.J.; Graff, J.M.; Frangogiannis, N.G. Opposing Actions of Fibroblast and Cardiomyocyte Smad3 Signaling in the Infarcted Myocardium. *Circulation* **2018**, *137*, 707–724. [CrossRef] [PubMed]
29. Zhou, X.; Chen, J.; Zhang, Q.; Shao, J.; Du, K.; Xu, X.; Kong, Y. Prognostic Value of Plasma Soluble Corin in Patients With Acute Myocardial Infarction. *J. Am. Coll. Cardiol.* **2016**, *67*, 2008–2014. [CrossRef]
30. Zhou, X.; Chen, J.C.; Liu, Y.; Yang, H.; Du, K.; Kong, Y.; Xu, X.H. Plasma Corin as a Predictor of Cardiovascular Events in Patients With Chronic Heart Failure. *JACC Heart Fail.* **2016**, *4*, 664–669. [CrossRef]
31. Hu, W.; Chen, S.; Song, Y.; Zhu, F.; Shi, J.; Han, X.; Zhou, D.; Zhi, Z.; Zhang, F.; Shen, Y.; et al. Serum Soluble Corin Deficiency Predicts Major Disability within 3 Months after Acute Stroke. *PLoS ONE* **2016**, *11*, e0163731. [CrossRef] [PubMed]
32. Yang, S.F.; Chou, R.H.; Lin, S.J.; Li, S.Y.; Huang, P.H. Serum PCSK6 and corin levels are not associated with cardiovascular outcomes in patients undergoing coronary angiography. *PLoS ONE* **2019**, *14*, e0226129. [CrossRef] [PubMed]
33. Liu, X.; Zhang, J.; Li, P.; Han, P.; Kang, Y.J.; Zhang, W. Gene expression patterns and related pathways in the hearts of rhesus monkeys subjected to prolonged myocardial ischemia. *Exp. Biol. Med.* **2023**, *248*, 350–360. [CrossRef] [PubMed]
34. Vucic, R.M.; Andrejic, O.M.; Stokanovic, D.; Stoimenov, T.J.; McClements, L.; Nikolic, V.N.; Sreckovic, M.; Veselinovic, M.; Aleksandric, S.; Popadic, V.; et al. Galectin-3 as a Prognostic Biomarker in Patients with First Acute Myocardial Infarction without Heart Failure. *Diagnostics* **2023**, *13*, 3348. [CrossRef] [PubMed]
35. Li, M.; Guo, K.; Huang, X.; Feng, L.; Yuan, Y.; Li, J.; Lao, Y.; Guo, Z. Association Between Serum Galectin-3 Levels and Coronary Stenosis Severity in Patients With Coronary Artery Disease. *Front. Cardiovasc. Med.* **2022**, *9*, 818162. [CrossRef] [PubMed]
36. Kokturk, U.; Pusuroglu, H.; Somuncu, M.U.; Akgul, O.; Uygur, B.; Ozyilmaz, S.; Isiksacan, N.; Surgit, O.; Yildirim, A. Short and Long-Term Prognostic Significance of Galectin-3 in Patients with ST-Elevation Myocardial Infarction Undergoing Primary Percutaneous Coronary Intervention. *Angiology* **2023**, *74*, 889–896. [CrossRef] [PubMed]
37. Wang, Q.; Huai, W.; Ye, X.; Pan, Y.; Yang, X.; Chen, M.; Ma, Q.B.; Gao, Y.; Zhang, Y. Circulating plasma galectin-3 predicts new-onset atrial fibrillation in patients after acute myocardial infarction during hospitalization. *BMC Cardiovasc. Disord.* **2022**, *22*, 392. [CrossRef] [PubMed]
38. Erdogan, O.; Karaayvaz, E.; Erdogan, T.; Panc, C.; Sarikaya, R.; Oncul, A.; Bilge, A.K. A new biomarker that predicts ventricular arrhythmia in patients with ischemic dilated cardiomyopathy: Galectin-3. *Rev. Port. Cardiol.* **2021**, *40*, 829–835. [CrossRef] [PubMed]
39. Obeid, S.; Yousif, N.; Davies, A.; Loretz, R.; Saleh, L.; Niederseer, D.; Noor, H.A.; Amin, H.; Mach, F.; Gencer, B.; et al. Prognostic role of plasma galectin-3 levels in acute coronary syndrome. *Eur. Heart J. Acute Cardiovasc. Care* **2020**, *9*, 869–878. [CrossRef]
40. Grandin, E.W.; Jarolim, P.; Murphy, S.A.; Ritterova, L.; Cannon, C.P.; Braunwald, E.; Morrow, D.A. Galectin-3 and the development of heart failure after acute coronary syndrome: Pilot experience from PROVE IT-TIMI 22. *Clin. Chem.* **2012**, *58*, 267–273. [CrossRef]
41. Cassaglia, P.; Penas, F.; Betazza, C.; Fontana Estevez, F.; Miksztowicz, V.; Martinez Naya, N.; Llamosas, M.C.; Noli Truant, S.; Wilensky, L.; Volberg, V.; et al. Genetic Deletion of Galectin-3 Alters the Temporal Evolution of Macrophage Infiltration and Healing Affecting the Cardiac Remodeling and Function after Myocardial Infarction in Mice. *Am. J. Pathol.* **2020**, *190*, 1789–1800. [CrossRef] [PubMed]
42. Frangogiannis, N.G. Targeting galectin-3 in myocardial infarction: A unique opportunity for biomarker-guided therapy. *Cardiovasc. Res.* **2023**, *119*, 2495–2496. [CrossRef] [PubMed]
43. Daseke, M.J., 2nd; Valerio, F.M.; Kalusche, W.J.; Ma, Y.; DeLeon-Pennell, K.Y.; Lindsey, M.L. Neutrophil proteome shifts over the myocardial infarction time continuum. *Basic Res. Cardiol.* **2019**, *114*, 37. [CrossRef] [PubMed]
44. Daseke, M.J., 2nd; Chalise, U.; Becirovic-Agic, M.; Salomon, J.D.; Cook, L.M.; Case, A.J.; Lindsey, M.L. Neutrophil signaling during myocardial infarction wound repair. *Cell Signal* **2021**, *77*, 109816. [CrossRef] [PubMed]
45. Ma, Y. Role of Neutrophils in Cardiac Injury and Repair Following Myocardial Infarction. *Cells* **2021**, *10*, 1676. [CrossRef] [PubMed]
46. Li, W.; Jin, Q.; Zhang, L.; He, S.; Song, Y.; Xu, L.; Deng, C.; Wang, L.; Qin, X.; Xie, M. Ultrasonic Microbubble Cavitation Deliver Gal-3 shRNA to Inhibit Myocardial Fibrosis after Myocardial Infarction. *Pharmaceutics* **2023**, *15*, 729. [CrossRef] [PubMed]
47. Kubota, A.; Frangogiannis, N.G. Macrophages in myocardial infarction. *Am. J. Physiol. Cell Physiol.* **2022**, *323*, C1304–C1324. [CrossRef] [PubMed]
48. Mo, D.; Tian, W.; Zhang, H.N.; Feng, Y.D.; Sun, Y.; Quan, W.; Hao, X.W.; Wang, X.Y.; Liu, X.X.; Li, C.; et al. Cardioprotective effects of galectin-3 inhibition against ischemia/reperfusion injury. *Eur. J. Pharmacol.* **2019**, *863*, 172701. [CrossRef] [PubMed]
49. Zhang, M.; Cheng, K.; Chen, H.; Tu, J.; Shen, Y.; Pang, L.; Wu, W. Galectin-3 knock down inhibits cardiac ischemia-reperfusion injury through interacting with bcl-2 and modulating cell apoptosis. *Arch. Biochem. Biophys.* **2020**, *694*, 108602. [CrossRef]
50. Kong, P.; Christia, P.; Frangogiannis, N.G. The pathogenesis of cardiac fibrosis. *Cell Mol. Life Sci.* **2014**, *71*, 549–574. [CrossRef]
51. Kang, P.; Wang, J.; Fang, D.; Fang, T.; Yu, Y.; Zhang, W.; Shen, L.; Li, Z.; Wang, H.; Ye, H.; et al. Activation of ALDH2 attenuates high glucose induced rat cardiomyocyte fibrosis and necroptosis. *Free Radic. Biol. Med.* **2020**, *146*, 198–210. [CrossRef]

52. Fang, L.; Ellims, A.H.; Beale, A.L.; Taylor, A.J.; Murphy, A.; Dart, A.M. Systemic inflammation is associated with myocardial fibrosis, diastolic dysfunction, and cardiac hypertrophy in patients with hypertrophic cardiomyopathy. *Am. J. Transl. Res.* **2017**, *9*, 5063–5073.
53. Bhandary, B.; Meng, Q.; James, J.; Osinska, H.; Gulick, J.; Valiente-Alandi, I.; Sargent, M.A.; Bhuiyan, M.S.; Blaxall, B.C.; Molkentin, J.D.; et al. Cardiac Fibrosis in Proteotoxic Cardiac Disease is Dependent Upon Myofibroblast TGF -beta Signaling. *J. Am. Heart Assoc.* **2018**, *7*, e010013. [CrossRef]
54. Yao, Y.; Hu, C.; Song, Q.; Li, Y.; Da, X.; Yu, Y.; Li, H.; Clark, I.M.; Chen, Q.; Wang, Q.K. ADAMTS16 activates latent TGF-beta, accentuating fibrosis and dysfunction of the pressure-overloaded heart. *Cardiovasc. Res.* **2020**, *116*, 956–969. [CrossRef] [PubMed]
55. Dzialo, E.; Czepiel, M.; Tkacz, K.; Siedlar, M.; Kania, G.; Blyszczuk, P. WNT/beta-Catenin Signaling Promotes TGF-beta-Mediated Activation of Human Cardiac Fibroblasts by Enhancing IL-11 Production. *Int. J. Mol. Sci.* **2021**, *22*, 10072. [CrossRef] [PubMed]
56. Chou, C.H.; Hung, C.S.; Liao, C.W.; Wei, L.H.; Chen, C.W.; Shun, C.T.; Wen, W.F.; Wan, C.H.; Wu, X.M.; Chang, Y.Y.; et al. IL-6 trans-signalling contributes to aldosterone-induced cardiac fibrosis. *Cardiovasc. Res.* **2018**, *114*, 690–702. [CrossRef]
57. Tanaka, H.; Sun, T.; Kinashi, H.; Kamiya, K.; Yamaguchi, M.; Nobata, H.; Sakata, F.; Kim, H.; Mizuno, M.; Kunoki, S.; et al. Interleukin-6 blockade reduces salt-induced cardiac inflammation and fibrosis in subtotal nephrectomized mice. *Am. J. Physiol. Renal Physiol.* **2022**, *323*, F654–F665. [CrossRef] [PubMed]
58. Tseng, C.C.S.; Huibers, M.M.H.; van Kuik, J.; de Weger, R.A.; Vink, A.; de Jonge, N. The Interleukin-33/ST2 Pathway Is Expressed in the Failing Human Heart and Associated with Pro-fibrotic Remodeling of the Myocardium. *J. Cardiovasc. Transl. Res.* **2018**, *11*, 15–21. [CrossRef]
59. Zhong, C.; Min, K.; Zhao, Z.; Zhang, C.; Gao, E.; Huang, Y.; Zhang, X.; Baldini, M.; Roy, R.; Yang, X.; et al. MAP Kinase Phosphatase-5 Deficiency Protects Against Pressure Overload-Induced Cardiac Fibrosis. *Front. Immunol.* **2021**, *12*, 790511. [CrossRef]
60. Mia, M.M.; Cibi, D.M.; Ghani, S.; Singh, A.; Tee, N.; Sivakumar, V.; Bogireddi, H.; Cook, S.A.; Mao, J.; Singh, M.K. Loss of Yap/Taz in cardiac fibroblasts attenuates adverse remodelling and improves cardiac function. *Cardiovasc. Res.* **2022**, *118*, 1785–1804. [CrossRef]
61. Pordzik, J.; Jakubik, D.; Jarosz-Popek, J.; Wicik, Z.; Eyileten, C.; De Rosa, S.; Indolfi, C.; Siller-Matula, J.M.; Czajka, P.; Postula, M. Significance of circulating microRNAs in diabetes mellitus type 2 and platelet reactivity: Bioinformatic analysis and review. *Cardiovasc. Diabetol.* **2019**, *18*, 113. [CrossRef]
62. Zhao, Y.; Du, D.; Chen, S.; Chen, Z.; Zhao, J. New Insights into the Functions of MicroRNAs in Cardiac Fibrosis: From Mechanisms to Therapeutic Strategies. *Genes* **2022**, *13*, 1390. [CrossRef]
63. Guo, R.; Nair, S. Role of microRNA in diabetic cardiomyopathy: From mechanism to intervention. *Biochim. Biophys. Acta Mol. Basis Dis.* **2017**, *1863*, 2070–2077. [CrossRef]
64. Jin, Z.Q. MicroRNA targets and biomarker validation for diabetes-associated cardiac fibrosis. *Pharmacol. Res.* **2021**, *174*, 105941. [CrossRef]
65. Rawal, S.; Munasinghe, P.E.; Nagesh, P.T.; Lew, J.K.S.; Jones, G.T.; Williams, M.J.A.; Davis, P.; Bunton, D.; Galvin, I.F.; Manning, P.; et al. Down-regulation of miR-15a/b accelerates fibrotic remodelling in the Type 2 diabetic human and mouse heart. *Clin. Sci.* **2017**, *131*, 847–863. [CrossRef]
66. Geng, H.; Guan, J. MiR-18a-5p inhibits endothelial-mesenchymal transition and cardiac fibrosis through the Notch2 pathway. *Biochem. Biophys. Res. Commun.* **2017**, *491*, 329–336. [CrossRef]
67. Liu, X.; Guo, B.; Zhang, W.; Ma, B.; Li, Y. MiR-20a-5p overexpression prevented diabetic cardiomyopathy via inhibition of cardiomyocyte apoptosis, hypertrophy, fibrosis and JNK/NF-kappaB signalling pathway. *J. Biochem.* **2021**, *170*, 349–362. [CrossRef]
68. Tang, C.M.; Zhang, M.; Huang, L.; Hu, Z.Q.; Zhu, J.N.; Xiao, Z.; Zhang, Z.; Lin, Q.X.; Zheng, X.L.; Yang, M.; et al. CircRNA_000203 enhances the expression of fibrosis-associated genes by derepressing targets of miR-26b-5p, Col1a2 and CTGF, in cardiac fibroblasts. *Sci. Rep.* **2017**, *7*, 40342. [CrossRef]
69. Zhang, Y.; Wang, J.H.; Zhang, Y.Y.; Wang, Y.Z.; Wang, J.; Zhao, Y.; Jin, X.X.; Xue, G.L.; Li, P.H.; Sun, Y.L.; et al. Deletion of interleukin-6 alleviated interstitial fibrosis in streptozotocin-induced diabetic cardiomyopathy of mice through affecting TGFbeta1 and miR-29 pathways. *Sci. Rep.* **2016**, *6*, 23010. [CrossRef] [PubMed]
70. Chen, S.; Puthanveetil, P.; Feng, B.; Matkovich, S.J.; Dorn, G.W., 2nd; Chakrabarti, S. Cardiac miR-133a overexpression prevents early cardiac fibrosis in diabetes. *J. Cell Mol. Med.* **2014**, *18*, 415–421. [CrossRef] [PubMed]
71. Che, H.; Wang, Y.; Li, H.; Li, Y.; Sahil, A.; Lv, J.; Liu, Y.; Yang, Z.; Dong, R.; Xue, H.; et al. Melatonin alleviates cardiac fibrosis via inhibiting lncRNA MALAT1/miR-141-mediated NLRP3 inflammasome and TGF-beta1/Smads signaling in diabetic cardiomyopathy. *FASEB J.* **2020**, *34*, 5282–5298. [CrossRef] [PubMed]
72. Feng, B.; Chen, S.; Gordon, A.D.; Chakrabarti, S. miR-146a mediates inflammatory changes and fibrosis in the heart in diabetes. *J. Mol. Cell Cardiol.* **2017**, *105*, 70–76. [CrossRef] [PubMed]
73. Feng, B.; Cao, Y.; Chen, S.; Chu, X.; Chu, Y.; Chakrabarti, S. miR-200b Mediates Endothelial-to-Mesenchymal Transition in Diabetic Cardiomyopathy. *Diabetes* **2016**, *65*, 768–779. [CrossRef] [PubMed]
74. Yang, X.; Li, X.; Lin, Q.; Xu, Q. Up-regulation of microRNA-203 inhibits myocardial fibrosis and oxidative stress in mice with diabetic cardiomyopathy through the inhibition of PI3K/Akt signaling pathway via PIK3CA. *Gene* **2019**, *715*, 143995. [CrossRef] [PubMed]

75. Wang, Z.; Wang, Z.; Gao, L.; Xiao, L.; Yao, R.; Du, B.; Li, Y.; Wu, L.; Liang, C.; Huang, Z.; et al. miR-222 inhibits cardiac fibrosis in diabetic mice heart via regulating Wnt/beta-catenin-mediated endothelium to mesenchymal transition. *J. Cell Physiol.* **2020**, *235*, 2149–2160. [CrossRef] [PubMed]
76. Feng, Y.; Xu, W.; Zhang, W.; Wang, W.; Liu, T.; Zhou, X. LncRNA DCRF regulates cardiomyocyte autophagy by targeting miR-551b-5p in diabetic cardiomyopathy. *Theranostics* **2019**, *9*, 4558–4566. [CrossRef] [PubMed]
77. Li, Q.; Yao, Y.; Shi, S.; Zhou, M.; Zhou, Y.; Wang, M.; Chiu, J.J.; Huang, Z.; Zhang, W.; Liu, M.; et al. Inhibition of miR-21 alleviated cardiac perivascular fibrosis via repressing EndMT in T1DM. *J. Cell Mol. Med.* **2020**, *24*, 910–920. [CrossRef] [PubMed]
78. Liu, S.; Li, W.; Xu, M.; Huang, H.; Wang, J.; Chen, X. Micro-RNA 21Targets dual specific phosphatase 8 to promote collagen synthesis in high glucose-treated primary cardiac fibroblasts. *Can. J. Cardiol.* **2014**, *30*, 1689–1699. [CrossRef] [PubMed]
79. Li, X.; Meng, C.; Han, F.; Yang, J.; Wang, J.; Zhu, Y.; Cui, X.; Zuo, M.; Xu, J.; Chang, B. Vildagliptin Attenuates Myocardial Dysfunction and Restores Autophagy via miR-21/SPRY1/ERK in Diabetic Mice Heart. *Front. Pharmacol.* **2021**, *12*, 634365. [CrossRef]
80. Shi, P.; Zhao, X.D.; Shi, K.H.; Ding, X.S.; Tao, H. MiR-21-3p triggers cardiac fibroblasts pyroptosis in diabetic cardiac fibrosis via inhibiting androgen receptor. *Exp. Cell Res.* **2021**, *399*, 112464. [CrossRef]
81. Che, H.; Wang, Y.; Li, Y.; Lv, J.; Li, H.; Liu, Y.; Dong, R.; Sun, Y.; Xu, X.; Zhao, J.; et al. Inhibition of microRNA-150-5p alleviates cardiac inflammation and fibrosis via targeting Smad7 in high glucose-treated cardiac fibroblasts. *J. Cell Physiol.* **2020**, *235*, 7769–7779. [CrossRef] [PubMed]
82. Wang, J.; He, W.; Xu, X.; Guo, L.; Zhang, Y.; Han, S.; Shen, D. The mechanism of TGF-beta/miR-155/c-Ski regulates endothelial-mesenchymal transition in human coronary artery endothelial cells. *Biosci. Rep.* **2017**, *37*, BSR20160603. [CrossRef] [PubMed]
83. Zhang, D.; Cui, Y.; Li, B.; Luo, X.; Li, B.; Tang, Y. miR-155 regulates high glucose-induced cardiac fibrosis via the TGF-beta signaling pathway. *Mol. Biosyst.* **2016**, *13*, 215–224. [CrossRef]
84. Chen, D.; Zhang, M. GAS5 regulates diabetic cardiomyopathy via miR-221-3p/p27 axis-associated autophagy. *Mol. Med. Rep.* **2021**, *23*, 135. [CrossRef]
85. Xu, D.; Zhang, X.; Chen, X.; Yang, S.; Chen, H. Inhibition of miR-223 attenuates the NLRP3 inflammasome activation, fibrosis, and apoptosis in diabetic cardiomyopathy. *Life Sci.* **2020**, *256*, 117980. [CrossRef] [PubMed]
86. Liu, X.; Xu, Y.; Deng, Y.; Li, H. MicroRNA-223 Regulates Cardiac Fibrosis After Myocardial Infarction by Targeting RASA1. *Cell Physiol. Biochem.* **2018**, *46*, 1439–1454. [CrossRef] [PubMed]
87. Liang, C.; Gao, L.; Liu, Y.; Liu, Y.; Yao, R.; Li, Y.; Xiao, L.; Wu, L.; Du, B.; Huang, Z.; et al. MiR-451 antagonist protects against cardiac fibrosis in streptozotocin-induced diabetic mouse heart. *Life Sci.* **2019**, *224*, 12–22. [CrossRef]
88. Valkov, N.; King, M.E.; Moeller, J.; Liu, H.; Li, X.; Zhang, P. MicroRNA-1-Mediated Inhibition of Cardiac Fibroblast Proliferation Through Targeting Cyclin D2 and CDK6. *Front. Cardiovasc. Med.* **2019**, *6*, 65. [CrossRef]
89. Zhong, C.; Wang, K.; Liu, Y.; Lv, D.; Zheng, B.; Zhou, Q.; Sun, Q.; Chen, P.; Ding, S.; Xu, Y.; et al. miR-19b controls cardiac fibroblast proliferation and migration. *J. Cell Mol. Med.* **2016**, *20*, 1191–1197. [CrossRef]
90. Yuan, X.; Pan, J.; Wen, L.; Gong, B.; Li, J.; Gao, H.; Tan, W.; Liang, S.; Zhang, H.; Wang, X. MiR-590-3p regulates proliferation, migration and collagen synthesis of cardiac fibroblast by targeting ZEB1. *J. Cell Mol. Med.* **2020**, *24*, 227–237. [CrossRef]
91. Huang, Y.; Qi, Y.; Du, J.Q.; Zhang, D.F. MicroRNA-34a regulates cardiac fibrosis after myocardial infarction by targeting Smad4. *Expert. Opin. Ther. Targets* **2014**, *18*, 1355–1365. [CrossRef]
92. Wei, Y.; Yan, X.; Yan, L.; Hu, F.; Ma, W.; Wang, Y.; Lu, S.; Zeng, Q.; Wang, Z. Inhibition of microRNA-155 ameliorates cardiac fibrosis in the process of angiotensin II-induced cardiac remodeling. *Mol. Med. Rep.* **2017**, *16*, 7287–7296. [CrossRef]
93. Yuan, X.; Pan, J.; Wen, L.; Gong, B.; Li, J.; Gao, H.; Tan, W.; Liang, S.; Zhang, H.; Wang, X. MiR-144-3p Enhances Cardiac Fibrosis After Myocardial Infarction by Targeting PTEN. *Front. Cell Dev. Biol.* **2019**, *7*, 249. [CrossRef]
94. Zhou, X.L.; Xu, H.; Liu, Z.B.; Wu, Q.C.; Zhu, R.R.; Liu, J.C. miR-21 promotes cardiac fibroblast-to-myofibroblast transformation and myocardial fibrosis by targeting Jagged1. *J. Cell Mol. Med.* **2018**, *22*, 3816–3824. [CrossRef]
95. Surina, S.; Fontanella, R.A.; Scisciola, L.; Marfella, R.; Paolisso, G.; Barbieri, M. miR-21 in Human Cardiomyopathies. *Front. Cardiovasc. Med.* **2021**, *8*, 767064. [CrossRef]
96. Wang, X.; Morelli, M.B.; Matarese, A.; Sardu, C.; Santulli, G. Cardiomyocyte-derived exosomal microRNA-92a mediates post-ischemic myofibroblast activation both in vitro and ex vivo. *ESC Heart Fail.* **2020**, *7*, 284–288. [CrossRef]
97. Morelli, M.B.; Shu, J.; Sardu, C.; Matarese, A.; Santulli, G. Cardiosomal microRNAs Are Essential in Post-Infarction Myofibroblast Phenoconversion. *Int. J. Mol. Sci.* **2019**, *21*, 201. [CrossRef]
98. Ranjan, P.; Kumari, R.; Goswami, S.K.; Li, J.; Pal, H.; Suleiman, Z.; Cheng, Z.; Krishnamurthy, P.; Kishore, R.; Verma, S.K. Myofibroblast-Derived Exosome Induce Cardiac Endothelial Cell Dysfunction. *Front. Cardiovasc. Med.* **2021**, *8*, 676267. [CrossRef]
99. Jazbutyte, V.; Fiedler, J.; Kneitz, S.; Galuppo, P.; Just, A.; Holzmann, A.; Bauersachs, J.; Thum, T. MicroRNA-22 increases senescence and activates cardiac fibroblasts in the aging heart. *Age* **2013**, *35*, 747–762. [CrossRef] [PubMed]
100. Nagpal, V.; Rai, R.; Place, A.T.; Murphy, S.B.; Verma, S.K.; Ghosh, A.K.; Vaughan, D.E. MiR-125b Is Critical for Fibroblast-to-Myofibroblast Transition and Cardiac Fibrosis. *Circulation* **2016**, *133*, 291–301. [CrossRef] [PubMed]
101. Liao, Y.; Li, H.; Cao, H.; Dong, Y.; Gao, L.; Liu, Z.; Ge, J.; Zhu, H. Therapeutic silencing miR-146b-5p improves cardiac remodeling in a porcine model of myocardial infarction by modulating the wound reparative phenotype. *Protein Cell* **2021**, *12*, 194–212. [CrossRef] [PubMed]

102. Mohammed, O.A.; Alghamdi, M.; Alfaifi, J.; Alamri, M.M.S.; Al-Shahrani, A.M.; Alharthi, M.H.; Alshahrani, A.M.; Alhalafi, A.H.; Adam, M.I.E.; Bahashwan, E.; et al. The emerging role of miRNAs in myocardial infarction: From molecular signatures to therapeutic targets. *Pathol. Res. Pract.* **2024**, *253*, 155087. [CrossRef] [PubMed]
103. Boon, R.A.; Iekushi, K.; Lechner, S.; Seeger, T.; Fischer, A.; Heydt, S.; Kaluza, D.; Treguer, K.; Carmona, G.; Bonauer, A.; et al. MicroRNA-34a regulates cardiac ageing and function. *Nature* **2013**, *495*, 107–110. [CrossRef] [PubMed]
104. Song, R.; Dasgupta, C.; Mulder, C.; Zhang, L. MicroRNA-210 Controls Mitochondrial Metabolism and Protects Heart Function in Myocardial Infarction. *Circulation* **2022**, *145*, 1140–1153. [CrossRef] [PubMed]
105. Yang, Y.; Ding, S.; Xu, G.; Chen, F.; Ding, F. MicroRNA-15a inhibition protects against hypoxia/reoxygenation-induced apoptosis of cardiomyocytes by targeting mothers against decapentaplegic homolog 7. *Mol. Med. Rep.* **2017**, *15*, 3699–3705. [CrossRef] [PubMed]
106. Taubel, J.; Hauke, W.; Rump, S.; Viereck, J.; Batkai, S.; Poetzsch, J.; Rode, L.; Weigt, H.; Genschel, C.; Lorch, U.; et al. Novel antisense therapy targeting microRNA-132 in patients with heart failure: Results of a first-in-human Phase 1b randomized, double-blind, placebo-controlled study. *Eur. Heart J.* **2021**, *42*, 178–188. [CrossRef] [PubMed]
107. Liu, H.; Zhang, Y.; Yuan, J.; Gao, W.; Zhong, X.; Yao, K.; Lin, L.; Ge, J. Dendritic cell-derived exosomal miR-494-3p promotes angiogenesis following myocardial infarction. *Int. J. Mol. Med.* **2021**, *47*, 315–325. [CrossRef] [PubMed]
108. Seferovic, P.M.; Petrie, M.C.; Filippatos, G.S.; Anker, S.D.; Rosano, G.; Bauersachs, J.; Paulus, W.J.; Komajda, M.; Cosentino, F.; de Boer, R.A.; et al. Type 2 diabetes mellitus and heart failure: A position statement from the Heart Failure Association of the European Society of Cardiology. *Eur. J. Heart Fail.* **2018**, *20*, 853–872. [CrossRef]
109. Lee, M.M.Y.; McMurray, J.J.V.; Lorenzo-Almoros, A.; Kristensen, S.L.; Sattar, N.; Jhund, P.S.; Petrie, M.C. Diabetic cardiomyopathy. *Heart* **2019**, *105*, 337–345. [CrossRef]
110. Zamora, M.; Villena, J.A. Contribution of Impaired Insulin Signaling to the Pathogenesis of Diabetic Cardiomyopathy. *Int. J. Mol. Sci.* **2019**, *20*, 2833. [CrossRef]
111. Fazakerley, D.J.; Lawrence, S.P.; Lizunov, V.A.; Cushman, S.W.; Holman, G.D. A common trafficking route for GLUT4 in cardiomyocytes in response to insulin, contraction and energy-status signalling. *J. Cell Sci.* **2009**, *122*, 727–734. [CrossRef] [PubMed]
112. Huo, J.L.; Feng, Q.; Pan, S.; Fu, W.J.; Liu, Z.; Liu, Z. Diabetic cardiomyopathy: Early diagnostic biomarkers, pathogenetic mechanisms, and therapeutic interventions. *Cell Death Discov.* **2023**, *9*, 256. [CrossRef] [PubMed]
113. Xiong, J.; Dong, X.; Li, S.; Jiang, F.; Chen, J.; Yu, S.; Dong, B.; Su, Q. Effects of (Pro)renin Receptor on Diabetic Cardiomyopathy Pathological Processes in Rats via the PRR-AMPK-YAP Pathway. *Front. Physiol.* **2021**, *12*, 657378. [CrossRef] [PubMed]
114. Bodiga, V.L.; Eda, S.R.; Bodiga, S. Advanced glycation end products: Role in pathology of diabetic cardiomyopathy. *Heart Fail. Rev.* **2014**, *19*, 49–63. [CrossRef] [PubMed]
115. Jia, G.; DeMarco, V.G.; Sowers, J.R. Insulin resistance and hyperinsulinaemia in diabetic cardiomyopathy. *Nat. Rev. Endocrinol.* **2016**, *12*, 144–153. [CrossRef] [PubMed]
116. Biernacka, A.; Cavalera, M.; Wang, J.; Russo, I.; Shinde, A.; Kong, P.; Gonzalez-Quesada, C.; Rai, V.; Dobaczewski, M.; Lee, D.W.; et al. Smad3 Signaling Promotes Fibrosis While Preserving Cardiac and Aortic Geometry in Obese Diabetic Mice. *Circ. Heart Fail.* **2015**, *8*, 788–798. [CrossRef] [PubMed]
117. Wilson, A.J.; Gill, E.K.; Abudalo, R.A.; Edgar, K.S.; Watson, C.J.; Grieve, D.J. Reactive oxygen species signalling in the diabetic heart: Emerging prospect for therapeutic targeting. *Heart* **2018**, *104*, 293–299. [CrossRef] [PubMed]
118. Zhang, Y.C.; Mou, Y.L.; Xie, Y.Y. Research progress in relations between renin angiotensin system and diabetic cardiomyopathy. *Sheng Li Ke Xue Jin Zhan* **2011**, *42*, 269–275. [PubMed]
119. Fuentes-Antras, J.; Ioan, A.M.; Tunon, J.; Egido, J.; Lorenzo, O. Activation of toll-like receptors and inflammasome complexes in the diabetic cardiomyopathy-associated inflammation. *Int. J. Endocrinol.* **2014**, *2014*, 847827. [CrossRef] [PubMed]
120. Giacco, F.; Brownlee, M. Oxidative stress and diabetic complications. *Circ. Res.* **2010**, *107*, 1058–1070. [CrossRef]
121. Pal, P.B.; Sonowal, H.; Shukla, K.; Srivastava, S.K.; Ramana, K.V. Aldose Reductase Mediates NLRP3 Inflammasome-Initiated Innate Immune Response in Hyperglycemia-Induced Thp1 Monocytes and Male Mice. *Endocrinology* **2017**, *158*, 3661–3675. [CrossRef]
122. Grubic Rotkvic, P.; Cigrovski Berkovic, M.; Bulj, N.; Rotkvic, L.; Celap, I. Sodium-glucose cotransporter 2 inhibitors' mechanisms of action in heart failure. *World J. Diabetes* **2020**, *11*, 269–279. [CrossRef] [PubMed]
123. Verma, S.; McMurray, J.J.V. SGLT2 inhibitors and mechanisms of cardiovascular benefit: A state-of-the-art review. *Diabetologia* **2018**, *61*, 2108–2117. [CrossRef] [PubMed]
124. Garla, V.V.; Butler, J.; Lien, L.F. SGLT-2 Inhibitors in Heart Failure: Guide for Prescribing and Future Perspectives. *Curr. Cardiol. Rep.* **2021**, *23*, 59. [CrossRef] [PubMed]
125. Navale, A.M.; Paranjape, A.N. Glucose transporters: Physiological and pathological roles. *Biophys. Rev.* **2016**, *8*, 5–9. [CrossRef]
126. Ghezzi, C.; Hirayama, B.A.; Gorraitz, E.; Loo, D.D.; Liang, Y.; Wright, E.M. SGLT2 inhibitors act from the extracellular surface of the cell membrane. *Physiol. Rep.* **2014**, *2*, e12058. [CrossRef] [PubMed]
127. Al Jobori, H.; Daniele, G.; Adams, J.; Cersosimo, E.; Solis-Herrera, C.; Triplitt, C.; DeFronzo, R.A.; Abdul-Ghani, M. Empagliflozin Treatment Is Associated With Improved beta-Cell Function in Type 2 Diabetes Mellitus. *J. Clin. Endocrinol. Metab.* **2018**, *103*, 1402–1407. [CrossRef] [PubMed]

128. Merovci, A.; Mari, A.; Solis-Herrera, C.; Xiong, J.; Daniele, G.; Chavez-Velazquez, A.; Tripathy, D.; Urban McCarthy, S.; Abdul-Ghani, M.; DeFronzo, R.A. Dapagliflozin lowers plasma glucose concentration and improves beta-cell function. *J. Clin. Endocrinol. Metab.* **2015**, *100*, 1927–1932. [CrossRef] [PubMed]
129. Luna-Marco, C.; Iannantuoni, F.; Hermo-Argibay, A.; Devos, D.; Salazar, J.D.; Victor, V.M.; Rovira-Llopis, S. Cardiovascular benefits of SGLT2 inhibitors and GLP-1 receptor agonists through effects on mitochondrial function and oxidative stress. *Free Radic. Biol. Med.* **2024**, *213*, 19–35. [CrossRef]
130. Wang, C.; Qin, Y.; Zhang, X.; Yang, Y.; Wu, X.; Liu, J.; Qin, S.; Chen, K.; Xiao, W. Effect of Dapagliflozin on Indicators of Myocardial Fibrosis and Levels of Inflammatory Factors in Heart Failure Patients. *Dis. Markers* **2022**, *2022*, 5834218. [CrossRef]
131. Tian, J.; Zhang, M.; Suo, M.; Liu, D.; Wang, X.; Liu, M.; Pan, J.; Jin, T.; An, F. Dapagliflozin alleviates cardiac fibrosis through suppressing EndMT and fibroblast activation via AMPKalpha/TGF-beta/Smad signalling in type 2 diabetic rats. *J. Cell Mol. Med.* **2021**, *25*, 7642–7659. [CrossRef] [PubMed]
132. Katsurada, K.; Nandi, S.S.; Sharma, N.M.; Patel, K.P. Enhanced Expression and Function of Renal SGLT2 (Sodium-Glucose Cotransporter 2) in Heart Failure: Role of Renal Nerves. *Circ. Heart Fail.* **2021**, *14*, e008365. [CrossRef] [PubMed]
133. McMurray, J.J.V.; DeMets, D.L.; Inzucchi, S.E.; Kober, L.; Kosiborod, M.N.; Langkilde, A.M.; Martinez, F.A.; Bengtsson, O.; Ponikowski, P.; Sabatine, M.S.; et al. A trial to evaluate the effect of the sodium-glucose co-transporter 2 inhibitor dapagliflozin on morbidity and mortality in patients with heart failure and reduced left ventricular ejection fraction (DAPA-HF). *Eur. J. Heart Fail.* **2019**, *21*, 665–675. [CrossRef]
134. Gager, G.M.; von Lewinski, D.; Sourij, H.; Jilma, B.; Eyileten, C.; Filipiak, K.; Hulsmann, M.; Kubica, J.; Postula, M.; Siller-Matula, J.M. Effects of SGLT2 Inhibitors on Ion Homeostasis and Oxidative Stress associated Mechanisms in Heart Failure. *Biomed. Pharmacother.* **2021**, *143*, 112169. [CrossRef] [PubMed]
135. Faridvand, Y.; Kazemzadeh, H.; Vahedian, V.; Mirzajanzadeh, P.; Nejabati, H.R.; Safaie, N.; Maroufi, N.F.; Pezeshkian, M.; Nouri, M.; Jodati, A. Dapagliflozin attenuates high glucose-induced endothelial cell apoptosis and inflammation through AMPK/SIRT1 activation. *Clin. Exp. Pharmacol. Physiol.* **2022**, *49*, 643–651. [CrossRef] [PubMed]
136. Li, F.F.; Gao, G.; Li, Q.; Zhu, H.H.; Su, X.F.; Wu, J.D.; Ye, L.; Ma, J.H. Influence of Dapagliflozin on Glycemic Variations in Patients with Newly Diagnosed Type 2 Diabetes Mellitus. *J. Diabetes Res.* **2016**, *2016*, 5347262. [CrossRef] [PubMed]
137. Yu, Y.W.; Que, J.Q.; Liu, S.; Huang, K.Y.; Qian, L.; Weng, Y.B.; Rong, F.N.; Wang, L.; Zhou, Y.Y.; Xue, Y.J.; et al. Sodium-Glucose Co-transporter-2 Inhibitor of Dapagliflozin Attenuates Myocardial Ischemia/Reperfusion Injury by Limiting NLRP3 Inflammasome Activation and Modulating Autophagy. *Front. Cardiovasc. Med.* **2021**, *8*, 768214. [CrossRef] [PubMed]
138. Andreadou, I.; Efentakis, P.; Balafas, E.; Togliatto, G.; Davos, C.H.; Varela, A.; Dimitriou, C.A.; Nikolaou, P.E.; Maratou, E.; Lambadiari, V.; et al. Empagliflozin Limits Myocardial Infarction in Vivo and Cell Death in Vitro: Role of STAT3, Mitochondria, and Redox Aspects. *Front. Physiol.* **2017**, *8*, 1077. [CrossRef] [PubMed]
139. Lee, T.M.; Chang, N.C.; Lin, S.Z. Dapagliflozin, a selective SGLT2 Inhibitor, attenuated cardiac fibrosis by regulating the macrophage polarization via STAT3 signaling in infarcted rat hearts. *Free Radic. Biol. Med.* **2017**, *104*, 298–310. [CrossRef]
140. Yurista, S.R.; Sillje, H.H.W.; Oberdorf-Maass, S.U.; Schouten, E.M.; Pavez Giani, M.G.; Hillebrands, J.L.; van Goor, H.; van Veldhuisen, D.J.; de Boer, R.A.; Westenbrink, B.D. Sodium-glucose co-transporter 2 inhibition with empagliflozin improves cardiac function in non-diabetic rats with left ventricular dysfunction after myocardial infarction. *Eur. J. Heart Fail.* **2019**, *21*, 862–873. [CrossRef]
141. Daud, E.; Ertracht, O.; Bandel, N.; Moady, G.; Shehadeh, M.; Reuveni, T.; Atar, S. The impact of empagliflozin on cardiac physiology and fibrosis early after myocardial infarction in non-diabetic rats. *Cardiovasc. Diabetol.* **2021**, *20*, 132. [CrossRef] [PubMed]
142. Hsu, J.C.; Wang, C.Y.; Su, M.M.; Lin, L.Y.; Yang, W.S. Effect of Empagliflozin on Cardiac Function, Adiposity, and Diffuse Fibrosis in Patients with Type 2 Diabetes Mellitus. *Sci. Rep.* **2019**, *9*, 15348. [CrossRef] [PubMed]
143. Adel, S.M.H.; Jorfi, F.; Mombeini, H.; Rashidi, H.; Fazeli, S. Effect of a low dose of empagliflozin on short-term outcomes in type 2 diabetics with acute coronary syndrome after percutaneous coronary intervention. *Saudi Med. J.* **2022**, *43*, 458–464. [CrossRef] [PubMed]
144. Connelly, K.A.; Zhang, Y.; Desjardins, J.F.; Nghiem, L.; Visram, A.; Batchu, S.N.; Yerra, V.G.; Kabir, G.; Thai, K.; Advani, A.; et al. Load-independent effects of empagliflozin contribute to improved cardiac function in experimental heart failure with reduced ejection fraction. *Cardiovasc. Diabetol.* **2020**, *19*, 13. [CrossRef] [PubMed]
145. Wang, J.; Huang, X.; Liu, H.; Chen, Y.; Li, P.; Liu, L.; Li, J.; Ren, Y.; Huang, J.; Xiong, E.; et al. Empagliflozin Ameliorates Diabetic Cardiomyopathy via Attenuating Oxidative Stress and Improving Mitochondrial Function. *Oxidative Med. Cell Longev.* **2022**, *2022*, 1122494. [CrossRef]
146. Li, C.; Zhang, J.; Xue, M.; Li, X.; Han, F.; Liu, X.; Xu, L.; Lu, Y.; Cheng, Y.; Li, T.; et al. SGLT2 inhibition with empagliflozin attenuates myocardial oxidative stress and fibrosis in diabetic mice heart. *Cardiovasc. Diabetol.* **2019**, *18*, 15. [CrossRef]
147. Kim, S.R.; Lee, S.G.; Kim, S.H.; Kim, J.H.; Choi, E.; Cho, W.; Rim, J.H.; Hwang, I.; Lee, C.J.; Lee, M.; et al. SGLT2 inhibition modulates NLRP3 inflammasome activity via ketones and insulin in diabetes with cardiovascular disease. *Nat. Commun.* **2020**, *11*, 2127. [CrossRef]
148. Dekkers, C.C.J.; Petrykiv, S.; Laverman, G.D.; Cherney, D.Z.; Gansevoort, R.T.; Heerspink, H.J.L. Effects of the SGLT-2 inhibitor dapagliflozin on glomerular and tubular injury markers. *Diabetes Obes. Metab.* **2018**, *20*, 1988–1993. [CrossRef] [PubMed]

149. Hodrea, J.; Saeed, A.; Molnar, A.; Fintha, A.; Barczi, A.; Wagner, L.J.; Szabo, A.J.; Fekete, A.; Balogh, D.B. SGLT2 inhibitor dapagliflozin prevents atherosclerotic and cardiac complications in experimental type 1 diabetes. *PLoS ONE* **2022**, *17*, e0263285. [CrossRef]
150. Ye, Y.; Bajaj, M.; Yang, H.C.; Perez-Polo, J.R.; Birnbaum, Y. SGLT-2 Inhibition with Dapagliflozin Reduces the Activation of the Nlrp3/ASC Inflammasome and Attenuates the Development of Diabetic Cardiomyopathy in Mice with Type 2 Diabetes. Further Augmentation of the Effects with Saxagliptin, a DPP4 Inhibitor. *Cardiovasc. Drugs Ther.* **2017**, *31*, 119–132. [CrossRef]
151. Li, X.; Kerindongo, R.P.; Preckel, B.; Kalina, J.O.; Hollmann, M.W.; Zuurbier, C.J.; Weber, N.C. Canagliflozin inhibits inflammasome activation in diabetic endothelial cells—Revealing a novel calcium-dependent anti-inflammatory effect of canagliflozin on human diabetic endothelial cells. *Biomed. Pharmacother.* **2023**, *159*, 114228. [CrossRef] [PubMed]
152. Kang, S.; Verma, S.; Hassanabad, A.F.; Teng, G.; Belke, D.D.; Dundas, J.A.; Guzzardi, D.G.; Svystonyuk, D.A.; Pattar, S.S.; Park, D.S.J.; et al. Direct Effects of Empagliflozin on Extracellular Matrix Remodelling in Human Cardiac Myofibroblasts: Novel Translational Clues to Explain EMPA-REG OUTCOME Results. *Can. J. Cardiol.* **2020**, *36*, 543–553. [CrossRef] [PubMed]
153. Verma, S.; Mazer, C.D.; Yan, A.T.; Mason, T.; Garg, V.; Teoh, H.; Zuo, F.; Quan, A.; Farkouh, M.E.; Fitchett, D.H.; et al. Effect of Empagliflozin on Left Ventricular Mass in Patients With Type 2 Diabetes Mellitus and Coronary Artery Disease: The EMPA-HEART CardioLink-6 Randomized Clinical Trial. *Circulation* **2019**, *140*, 1693–1702. [CrossRef] [PubMed]
154. Brown, A.J.M.; Gandy, S.; McCrimmon, R.; Houston, J.G.; Struthers, A.D.; Lang, C.C. A randomized controlled trial of dapagliflozin on left ventricular hypertrophy in people with type two diabetes: The DAPA-LVH trial. *Eur. Heart J.* **2020**, *41*, 3421–3432. [CrossRef] [PubMed]
155. Hattori, S. Anti-inflammatory effects of empagliflozin in patients with type 2 diabetes and insulin resistance. *Diabetol. Metab. Syndr.* **2018**, *10*, 93. [CrossRef] [PubMed]
156. Sezai, A.; Sekino, H.; Unosawa, S.; Taoka, M.; Osaka, S.; Tanaka, M. Canagliflozin for Japanese patients with chronic heart failure and type II diabetes. *Cardiovasc. Diabetol.* **2019**, *18*, 76. [CrossRef] [PubMed]
157. Shigiyama, F.; Kumashiro, N.; Miyagi, M.; Ikehara, K.; Kanda, E.; Uchino, H.; Hirose, T. Effectiveness of dapagliflozin on vascular endothelial function and glycemic control in patients with early-stage type 2 diabetes mellitus: DEFENCE study. *Cardiovasc. Diabetol.* **2017**, *16*, 84. [CrossRef]
158. Tanaka, A.; Shimabukuro, M.; Machii, N.; Teragawa, H.; Okada, Y.; Shima, K.R.; Takamura, T.; Taguchi, I.; Hisauchi, I.; Toyoda, S.; et al. Effect of Empagliflozin on Endothelial Function in Patients With Type 2 Diabetes and Cardiovascular Disease: Results from the Multicenter, Randomized, Placebo-Controlled, Double-Blind EMBLEM Trial. *Diabetes Care* **2019**, *42*, e159–e161. [CrossRef]
159. Lee, Y.S.; Jun, H.S. Anti-diabetic actions of glucagon-like peptide-1 on pancreatic beta-cells. *Metabolism* **2014**, *63*, 9–19. [CrossRef]
160. Pyke, C.; Heller, R.S.; Kirk, R.K.; Orskov, C.; Reedtz-Runge, S.; Kaastrup, P.; Hvelplund, A.; Bardram, L.; Calatayud, D.; Knudsen, L.B. GLP-1 receptor localization in monkey and human tissue: Novel distribution revealed with extensively validated monoclonal antibody. *Endocrinology* **2014**, *155*, 1280–1290. [CrossRef]
161. Sharma, D.; Verma, S.; Vaidya, S.; Kalia, K.; Tiwari, V. Recent updates on GLP-1 agonists: Current advancements & challenges. *Biomed. Pharmacother.* **2018**, *108*, 952–962. [CrossRef]
162. Ussher, J.R.; Drucker, D.J. Glucagon-like peptide 1 receptor agonists: Cardiovascular benefits and mechanisms of action. *Nat. Rev. Cardiol.* **2023**, *20*, 463–474. [CrossRef]
163. Tan, Q.; Akindehin, S.E.; Orsso, C.E.; Waldner, R.C.; DiMarchi, R.D.; Muller, T.D.; Haqq, A.M. Recent Advances in Incretin-Based Pharmacotherapies for the Treatment of Obesity and Diabetes. *Front. Endocrinol.* **2022**, *13*, 838410. [CrossRef] [PubMed]
164. Gilbert, M.P.; Pratley, R.E. GLP-1 Analogs and DPP-4 Inhibitors in Type 2 Diabetes Therapy: Review of Head-to-Head Clinical Trials. *Front. Endocrinol.* **2020**, *11*, 178. [CrossRef]
165. Uccellatore, A.; Genovese, S.; Dicembrini, I.; Mannucci, E.; Ceriello, A. Comparison Review of Short-Acting and Long-Acting Glucagon-like Peptide-1 Receptor Agonists. *Diabetes Ther.* **2015**, *6*, 239–256. [CrossRef] [PubMed]
166. Peng, Y.; Lin, H.; Tian, S.; Liu, S.; Li, J.; Lv, X.; Chen, S.; Zhao, L.; Pu, F.; Chen, X.; et al. Glucagon-like peptide-1 receptor activation maintains extracellular matrix integrity by inhibiting the activity of mitogen-activated protein kinases and activator protein-1. *Free Radic. Biol. Med.* **2021**, *177*, 247–259. [CrossRef] [PubMed]
167. Li, Y.K.; Ma, D.X.; Wang, Z.M.; Hu, X.F.; Li, S.L.; Tian, H.Z.; Wang, M.J.; Shu, Y.W.; Yang, J. The glucagon-like peptide-1 (GLP-1) analog liraglutide attenuates renal fibrosis. *Pharmacol. Res.* **2018**, *131*, 102–111. [CrossRef] [PubMed]
168. Huang, L.; Lin, T.; Shi, M.; Chen, X.; Wu, P. Liraglutide suppresses production of extracellular matrix proteins and ameliorates renal injury of diabetic nephropathy by enhancing Wnt/beta-catenin signaling. *Am. J. Physiol. Renal Physiol.* **2020**, *319*, F458–F468. [CrossRef]
169. Wang, D.; Jiang, L.; Feng, B.; He, N.; Zhang, Y.; Ye, H. Protective effects of glucagon-like peptide-1 on cardiac remodeling by inhibiting oxidative stress through mammalian target of rapamycin complex 1/p70 ribosomal protein S6 kinase pathway in diabetes mellitus. *J. Diabetes Investig.* **2020**, *11*, 39–51. [CrossRef]
170. Picatoste, B.; Ramirez, E.; Caro-Vadillo, A.; Iborra, C.; Ares-Carrasco, S.; Egido, J.; Tunon, J.; Lorenzo, O. Sitagliptin reduces cardiac apoptosis, hypertrophy and fibrosis primarily by insulin-dependent mechanisms in experimental type-II diabetes. Potential roles of GLP-1 isoforms. *PLoS ONE* **2013**, *8*, e78330. [CrossRef]
171. Zhu, Q.; Luo, Y.; Wen, Y.; Wang, D.; Li, J.; Fan, Z. Semaglutide inhibits ischemia/reperfusion-induced cardiomyocyte apoptosis through activating PKG/PKCepsilon/ERK1/2 pathway. *Biochem. Biophys. Res. Commun.* **2023**, *647*, 1–8. [CrossRef] [PubMed]

172. Bin Dayel, A.F.; Alonazi, A.S.; Alrasheed, N.M.; Alamin, M.A.; Sarawi, W.S.; Alharbi, A.O.; Alabbad, N.A.; Albuaijan, D.A.; Alassiri, D.N.; Aljarbua, A.F.; et al. Role of the integrin-linked kinase/TGF-beta/SMAD pathway in sitagliptin-mediated cardioprotective effects in a rat model of diabetic cardiomyopathy. *J. Pharm. Pharmacol.* **2024**, *76*, 64–73. [CrossRef] [PubMed]
173. Zhao, T.; Chen, H.; Xu, F.; Wang, J.; Liu, Y.; Xing, X.; Guo, L.; Zhang, M.; Lu, Q. Liraglutide alleviates cardiac fibrosis through inhibiting P4halpha-1 expression in STZ-induced diabetic cardiomyopathy. *Acta Biochim. Biophys. Sin.* **2019**, *51*, 293–300. [CrossRef] [PubMed]
174. Zhang, Z.; Wang, X.; Yang, L.; Yang, L.; Ma, H. Liraglutide ameliorates myocardial damage in experimental diabetic rats by inhibiting pyroptosis via Sirt1/AMPK signaling. *Iran. J. Basic Med. Sci.* **2021**, *24*, 1358–1365. [CrossRef] [PubMed]
175. Noyan-Ashraf, M.H.; Momen, M.A.; Ban, K.; Sadi, A.M.; Zhou, Y.Q.; Riazi, A.M.; Baggio, L.L.; Henkelman, R.M.; Husain, M.; Drucker, D.J. GLP-1R agonist liraglutide activates cytoprotective pathways and improves outcomes after experimental myocardial infarction in mice. *Diabetes* **2009**, *58*, 975–983. [CrossRef]
176. Wu, L.; Wang, K.; Wang, W.; Wen, Z.; Wang, P.; Liu, L.; Wang, D.W. Glucagon-like peptide-1 ameliorates cardiac lipotoxicity in diabetic cardiomyopathy via the PPARalpha pathway. *Aging Cell* **2018**, *17*, e12763. [CrossRef] [PubMed]
177. Lyu, J.; Imachi, H.; Fukunaga, K.; Sato, S.; Kobayashi, T.; Saheki, T.; Japar, S.; Iwama, H.; Matsumura, Y.; Ozaki, M.; et al. Exendin-4 Increases Scavenger Receptor Class BI Expression via Activation of AMPK/FoxO1 in Human Vascular Endothelial Cells. *Curr. Issues Mol. Biol.* **2022**, *44*, 5474–5484. [CrossRef] [PubMed]
178. He, W.; Tong, G.; Fan, H.; Zhen, C.; Zeng, L.; Xue, L.; Chen, J.; Sun, Z.; He, P. Exendin-4 alleviates myocardial ischemia reperfusion injury by enhancing autophagy through promoting nuclear translocation of TFEB. *Exp. Cell Res.* **2023**, *423*, 113469. [CrossRef] [PubMed]
179. Nuamnaichati, N.; Mangmool, S.; Chattipakorn, N.; Parichatikanond, W. Stimulation of GLP-1 Receptor Inhibits Methylglyoxal-Induced Mitochondrial Dysfunctions in H9c2 Cardiomyoblasts: Potential Role of Epac/PI3K/Akt Pathway. *Front. Pharmacol.* **2020**, *11*, 805. [CrossRef]
180. Wei, H.; Bu, R.; Yang, Q.; Jia, J.; Li, T.; Wang, Q.; Chen, Y. Exendin-4 Protects against Hyperglycemia-Induced Cardiomyocyte Pyroptosis via the AMPK-TXNIP Pathway. *J. Diabetes Res.* **2019**, *2019*, 8905917. [CrossRef]
181. Wassef, M.A.E.; Tork, O.M.; Rashed, L.A.; Ibrahim, W.; Morsi, H.; Rabie, D.M.M. Mitochondrial Dysfunction in Diabetic Cardiomyopathy: Effect of Mesenchymal Stem Cell with PPAR-gamma Agonist or Exendin-4. *Exp. Clin. Endocrinol. Diabetes* **2018**, *126*, 27–38. [CrossRef] [PubMed]
182. Eid, R.A.; Khalil, M.A.; Alkhateeb, M.A.; Eleawa, S.M.; Zaki, M.S.A.; El-Kott, A.F.; Al-Shraim, M.; El-Sayed, F.; Eldeen, M.A.; Bin-Meferij, M.M.; et al. Exendin-4 Attenuates Remodeling in the Remote Myocardium of Rats After an Acute Myocardial Infarction by Activating beta-Arrestin-2, Protein Phosphatase 2A, and Glycogen Synthase Kinase-3 and Inhibiting beta-Catenin. *Cardiovasc. Drugs Ther.* **2021**, *35*, 1095–1110. [CrossRef] [PubMed]
183. Chen, J.; Xu, S.; Wang, L.; Zhou, W.; Li, P.; Deng, N.; Tang, Q.; Li, Y.; Wu, L.; Chen, J.; et al. Exendin-4 inhibits atrial arrhythmogenesis in a model of myocardial infarction-induced heart failure via the GLP-1 receptor signaling pathway. *Exp. Ther. Med.* **2020**, *20*, 3669–3678. [CrossRef] [PubMed]
184. Chen, J.; Wang, D.; Wang, F.; Shi, S.; Chen, Y.; Yang, B.; Tang, Y.; Huang, C. Exendin-4 inhibits structural remodeling and improves Ca(2+) homeostasis in rats with heart failure via the GLP-1 receptor through the eNOS/cGMP/PKG pathway. *Peptides* **2017**, *90*, 69–77. [CrossRef] [PubMed]
185. Wright, E.J.; Hodson, N.W.; Sherratt, M.J.; Kassem, M.; Lewis, A.L.; Wallrapp, C.; Malik, N.; Holt, C.M. Combined MSC and GLP-1 Therapy Modulates Collagen Remodeling and Apoptosis following Myocardial Infarction. *Stem Cells Int.* **2016**, *2016*, 7357096. [CrossRef] [PubMed]
186. Withaar, C.; Meems, L.M.G.; Markousis-Mavrogenis, G.; Boogerd, C.J.; Sillje, H.H.W.; Schouten, E.M.; Dokter, M.M.; Voors, A.A.; Westenbrink, B.D.; Lam, C.S.P.; et al. The effects of liraglutide and dapagliflozin on cardiac function and structure in a multi-hit mouse model of heart failure with preserved ejection fraction. *Cardiovasc. Res.* **2021**, *117*, 2108–2124. [CrossRef] [PubMed]
187. Huang, D.D.; Huang, H.F.; Yang, Q.; Chen, X.Q. Liraglutide improves myocardial fibrosis after myocardial infarction through inhibition of CTGF by activating cAMP in mice. *Eur. Rev. Med. Pharmacol. Sci.* **2018**, *22*, 4648–4656. [CrossRef] [PubMed]
188. Mitsuhashi, T.; Hibi, K.; Konishi, M.; Maejima, N.; Iwahashi, N.; Tsukahara, K.; Kosuge, M.; Ebina, T.; Umemura, S.; Kimura, K. Plasma Glucagon-Like Peptide-1 and Tissue Characteristics of Coronary Plaque in Non-Diabetic Acute Coronary Syndrome Patients. *Circ. J.* **2016**, *80*, 469–476. [CrossRef] [PubMed]
189. Trevisan, M.; Fu, E.L.; Szummer, K.; Norhammar, A.; Lundman, P.; Wanner, C.; Sjolander, A.; Jernberg, T.; Carrero, J.J. Glucagon-like peptide-1 receptor agonists and the risk of cardiovascular events in diabetes patients surviving an acute myocardial infarction. *Eur. Heart J. Cardiovasc. Pharmacother.* **2021**, *7*, 104–111. [CrossRef]
190. Trombara, F.; Cosentino, N.; Bonomi, A.; Ludergnani, M.; Poggio, P.; Gionti, L.; Baviera, M.; Colacioppo, P.; Roncaglioni, M.C.; Leoni, O.; et al. Impact of chronic GLP-1 RA and SGLT-2I therapy on in-hospital outcome of diabetic patients with acute myocardial infarction. *Cardiovasc. Diabetol.* **2023**, *22*, 26. [CrossRef]
191. Marfella, R.; Prattichizzo, F.; Sardu, C.; Rambaldi, P.F.; Fumagalli, C.; Marfella, L.V.; La Grotta, R.; Frige, C.; Pellegrini, V.; D'Andrea, D.; et al. GLP-1 receptor agonists-SGLT-2 inhibitors combination therapy and cardiovascular events after acute myocardial infarction: An observational study in patients with type 2 diabetes. *Cardiovasc. Diabetol.* **2024**, *23*, 10. [CrossRef] [PubMed]

192. Marso, S.P.; Daniels, G.H.; Brown-Frandsen, K.; Kristensen, P.; Mann, J.F.; Nauck, M.A.; Nissen, S.E.; Pocock, S.; Poulter, N.R.; Ravn, L.S.; et al. Liraglutide and Cardiovascular Outcomes in Type 2 Diabetes. *N. Engl. J. Med.* **2016**, *375*, 311–322. [CrossRef] [PubMed]
193. Paiman, E.H.M.; van Eyk, H.J.; van Aalst, M.M.A.; Bizino, M.B.; van der Geest, R.J.; Westenberg, J.J.M.; Geelhoed-Duijvestijn, P.H.; Kharagjitsingh, A.V.; Rensen, P.C.N.; Smit, J.W.A.; et al. Effect of Liraglutide on Cardiovascular Function and Myocardial Tissue Characteristics in Type 2 Diabetes Patients of South Asian Descent Living in the Netherlands: A Double-Blind, Randomized, Placebo-Controlled Trial. *J. Magn. Reson. Imaging* **2020**, *51*, 1679–1688. [CrossRef] [PubMed]
194. Zimmerman, R.S.; Hobbs, T.M.; Wells, B.J.; Kong, S.X.; Kattan, M.W.; Bouchard, J.; Chagin, K.M.; Yu, C.; Sakurada, B.; Milinovich, A.; et al. Association of glucagon-like peptide-1 receptor agonist use and rates of acute myocardial infarction, stroke and overall mortality in patients with type 2 diabetes mellitus in a large integrated health system. *Diabetes Obes. Metab.* **2017**, *19*, 1555–1561. [CrossRef] [PubMed]
195. Deacon, C.F. Dipeptidyl peptidase 4 inhibitors in the treatment of type 2 diabetes mellitus. *Nat. Rev. Endocrinol.* **2020**, *16*, 642–653. [CrossRef] [PubMed]
196. Fu, W.J.; Huo, J.L.; Mao, Z.H.; Pan, S.K.; Liu, D.W.; Liu, Z.S.; Wu, P.; Gao, Z.X. Emerging role of antidiabetic drugs in cardiorenal protection. *Front. Pharmacol.* **2024**, *15*, 1349069. [CrossRef] [PubMed]
197. Ishii, H.; Hayashino, Y.; Akai, Y.; Yabuta, M.; Tsujii, S. Dipeptidyl peptidase-4 inhibitors as preferable oral hypoglycemic agents in terms of treatment satisfaction: Results from a multicenter, 12-week, open label, randomized controlled study in Japan (PREFERENCE 4 study). *J. Diabetes Investig.* **2018**, *9*, 137–145. [CrossRef] [PubMed]
198. Nauck, M.A.; Meininger, G.; Sheng, D.; Terranella, L.; Stein, P.P.; Sitagliptin Study, G. Efficacy and safety of the dipeptidyl peptidase-4 inhibitor, sitagliptin, compared with the sulfonylurea, glipizide, in patients with type 2 diabetes inadequately controlled on metformin alone: A randomized, double-blind, non-inferiority trial. *Diabetes Obes. Metab.* **2007**, *9*, 194–205. [CrossRef] [PubMed]
199. Jermendy, G. Incretin-based antidiabetic treatment and diseases of the pancreas (pancreatitis, pancreas carcinoma). *Orv. Hetil.* **2016**, *157*, 523–528. [CrossRef]
200. Nicholson, G.; Hall, G.M. Diabetes mellitus: New drugs for a new epidemic. *Br. J. Anaesth.* **2011**, *107*, 65–73. [CrossRef]
201. Xie, D.; Wang, Q.; Huang, W.; Zhao, L. Dipeptidyl-peptidase-4 inhibitors have anti-inflammatory effects in patients with type 2 diabetes. *Eur. J. Clin. Pharmacol.* **2023**, *79*, 1291–1301. [CrossRef]
202. Pham, T.K.; Nguyen, T.H.T.; Yi, J.M.; Kim, G.S.; Yun, H.R.; Kim, H.K.; Won, J.C. Evogliptin, a DPP-4 inhibitor, prevents diabetic cardiomyopathy by alleviating cardiac lipotoxicity in db/db mice. *Exp. Mol. Med.* **2023**, *55*, 767–778. [CrossRef]
203. Moon, J.Y.; Woo, J.S.; Seo, J.W.; Lee, A.; Kim, D.J.; Kim, Y.G.; Kim, S.Y.; Lee, K.H.; Lim, S.J.; Cheng, X.W.; et al. The Dose-Dependent Organ-Specific Effects of a Dipeptidyl Peptidase-4 Inhibitor on Cardiovascular Complications in a Model of Type 2 Diabetes. *PLoS ONE* **2016**, *11*, e0150745. [CrossRef]
204. Arruda-Junior, D.F.; Salles, T.A.; Martins, F.L.; Antonio, E.L.; Tucci, P.J.F.; Gowdak, L.H.W.; Tavares, C.A.M.; Girardi, A.C. Unraveling the interplay between dipeptidyl peptidase 4 and the renin-angiotensin system in heart failure. *Life Sci.* **2022**, *305*, 120757. [CrossRef]
205. Wojcicka, G.; Pradiuch, A.; Fornal, E.; Stachniuk, A.; Korolczuk, A.; Marzec-Kotarska, B.; Nikolaichuk, H.; Czechowska, G.; Kozub, A.; Trzpil, A.; et al. The effect of exenatide (a GLP-1 analogue) and sitagliptin (a DPP-4 inhibitor) on asymmetric dimethylarginine (ADMA) metabolism and selected biomarkers of cardiac fibrosis in rats with fructose-induced metabolic syndrome. *Biochem. Pharmacol.* **2023**, *214*, 115637. [CrossRef]
206. Shao, S.; Xu, Q.; Yu, X.; Pan, R.; Chen, Y. Dipeptidyl peptidase 4 inhibitors and their potential immune modulatory functions. *Pharmacol. Ther.* **2020**, *209*, 107503. [CrossRef]
207. Adhikari, J.; Hirai, T.; Kawakita, E.; Iwai, K.; Koya, D.; Kanasaki, K. Linagliptin ameliorated cardiac fibrosis and restored cardiomyocyte structure in diabetic mice associated with the suppression of necroptosis. *J. Diabetes Investig.* **2023**, *14*, 844–855. [CrossRef]
208. Birnbaum, Y.; Tran, D.; Bajaj, M.; Ye, Y. DPP-4 inhibition by linagliptin prevents cardiac dysfunction and inflammation by targeting the Nlrp3/ASC inflammasome. *Basic Res. Cardiol.* **2019**, *114*, 35. [CrossRef]
209. Beraldo, J.I.; Benetti, A.; Borges-Junior, F.A.; Arruda-Junior, D.F.; Martins, F.L.; Jensen, L.; Dariolli, R.; Shimizu, M.H.; Seguro, A.C.; Luchi, W.M.; et al. Cardioprotection Conferred by Sitagliptin Is Associated with Reduced Cardiac Angiotensin II/Angiotensin-(1-7) Balance in Experimental Chronic Kidney Disease. *Int. J. Mol. Sci.* **2019**, *20*, 1940. [CrossRef]
210. Hong, S.K.; Choo, E.H.; Ihm, S.H.; Chang, K.; Seung, K.B. Dipeptidyl peptidase 4 inhibitor attenuates obesity-induced myocardial fibrosis by inhibiting transforming growth factor-betal and Smad2/3 pathways in high-fat diet-induced obesity rat model. *Metabolism* **2017**, *76*, 42–55. [CrossRef]
211. Chen, Y.F.; Zhang, L.J.; Liu, Q.H.; Li, X.W. Effects of Sitagliptin on myocardial remodeling and autophagy in diabetic mice and its mechanism. *Zhongguo Ying Yong Sheng Li Xue Za Zhi* **2021**, *37*, 534–537. [CrossRef]
212. Al-Rasheed, N.M.; Al-Rasheed, N.M.; Hasan, I.H.; Al-Amin, M.A.; Al-Ajmi, H.N.; Mahmoud, A.M. Sitagliptin attenuates cardiomyopathy by modulating the JAK/STAT signaling pathway in experimental diabetic rats. *Drug Des. Dev. Ther.* **2016**, *10*, 2095–2107. [CrossRef]
213. Zhang, X.; Zhang, Z.; Yang, Y.; Suo, Y.; Liu, R.; Qiu, J.; Zhao, Y.; Jiang, N.; Liu, C.; Tse, G.; et al. Alogliptin prevents diastolic dysfunction and preserves left ventricular mitochondrial function in diabetic rabbits. *Cardiovasc. Diabetol.* **2018**, *17*, 160. [CrossRef]

214. Zhang, X.; Zhang, Z.; Zhao, Y.; Jiang, N.; Qiu, J.; Yang, Y.; Li, J.; Liang, X.; Wang, X.; Tse, G.; et al. Alogliptin, a Dipeptidyl Peptidase-4 Inhibitor, Alleviates Atrial Remodeling and Improves Mitochondrial Function and Biogenesis in Diabetic Rabbits. *J. Am. Heart Assoc.* **2017**, *6*, e005945. [CrossRef]
215. Esser, N.; Zraika, S. Neprilysin inhibition: A new therapeutic option for type 2 diabetes? *Diabetologia* **2019**, *62*, 1113–1122. [CrossRef]
216. Potter, L.R. Natriuretic peptide metabolism, clearance and degradation. *FEBS J.* **2011**, *278*, 1808–1817. [CrossRef]
217. McMurray, J.J. Neprilysin inhibition to treat heart failure: A tale of science, serendipity, and second chances. *Eur. J. Heart Fail.* **2015**, *17*, 242–247. [CrossRef]
218. Jordan, J.; Stinkens, R.; Jax, T.; Engeli, S.; Blaak, E.E.; May, M.; Havekes, B.; Schindler, C.; Albrecht, D.; Pal, P.; et al. Improved Insulin Sensitivity With Angiotensin Receptor Neprilysin Inhibition in Individuals With Obesity and Hypertension. *Clin. Pharmacol. Ther.* **2017**, *101*, 254–263. [CrossRef]
219. Nougue, H.; Pezel, T.; Picard, F.; Sadoune, M.; Arrigo, M.; Beauvais, F.; Launay, J.M.; Cohen-Solal, A.; Vodovar, N.; Logeart, D. Effects of sacubitril/valsartan on neprilysin targets and the metabolism of natriuretic peptides in chronic heart failure: A mechanistic clinical study. *Eur. J. Heart Fail.* **2019**, *21*, 598–605. [CrossRef]
220. Suematsu, Y.; Miura, S.; Goto, M.; Matsuo, Y.; Arimura, T.; Kuwano, T.; Imaizumi, S.; Iwata, A.; Yahiro, E.; Saku, K. LCZ696, an angiotensin receptor-neprilysin inhibitor, improves cardiac function with the attenuation of fibrosis in heart failure with reduced ejection fraction in streptozotocin-induced diabetic mice. *Eur. J. Heart Fail.* **2016**, *18*, 386–393. [CrossRef]
221. Ge, Q.; Zhao, L.; Ren, X.M.; Ye, P.; Hu, Z.Y. LCZ696, an angiotensin receptor-neprilysin inhibitor, ameliorates diabetic cardiomyopathy by inhibiting inflammation, oxidative stress and apoptosis. *Exp. Biol. Med.* **2019**, *244*, 1028–1039. [CrossRef]
222. Gronholm, T.; Cheng, Z.J.; Palojoki, E.; Eriksson, A.; Backlund, T.; Vuolteenaho, O.; Finckenberg, P.; Laine, M.; Mervaala, E.; Tikkanen, I. Vasopeptidase inhibition has beneficial cardiac effects in spontaneously diabetic Goto-Kakizaki rats. *Eur. J. Pharmacol.* **2005**, *519*, 267–276. [CrossRef]
223. Malek, V.; Sharma, N.; Gaikwad, A.B. Simultaneous inhibition of neprilysin and activation of ACE2 prevented diabetic cardiomyopathy. *Pharmacol. Rep.* **2019**, *71*, 958–967. [CrossRef]
224. Torre, E.; Arici, M.; Lodrini, A.M.; Ferrandi, M.; Barassi, P.; Hsu, S.C.; Chang, G.J.; Boz, E.; Sala, E.; Vagni, S.; et al. SERCA2a stimulation by istaroxime improves intracellular Ca2+ handling and diastolic dysfunction in a model of diabetic cardiomyopathy. *Cardiovasc. Res.* **2022**, *118*, 1020–1032. [CrossRef]
225. Lou, S.; Zhu, W.; Yu, T.; Zhang, Q.; Wang, M.; Jin, L.; Xiong, Y.; Xu, J.; Wang, Q.; Chen, G.; et al. Compound SJ-12 attenuates streptozocin-induced diabetic cardiomyopathy by stabilizing SERCA2a. *Biochim. Biophys. Acta Mol. Basis Dis.* **2024**, *1870*, 167140. [CrossRef]
226. Xiong, X.; Zhang, X.; Zhang, Y.; Xie, J.; Bian, Y.; Yin, Q.; Tong, R.; Yu, D.; Pan, L. Sarco/endoplasmic reticulum Ca(2+) ATPase (SERCA)-mediated ER stress crosstalk with autophagy is involved in tris(2-chloroethyl) phosphate stress-induced cardiac fibrosis. *J. Inorg. Biochem.* **2022**, *236*, 111972. [CrossRef]
227. Katz, M.G.; Brandon-Warner, E.; Fargnoli, A.S.; Williams, R.D.; Kendle, A.P.; Hajjar, R.J.; Schrum, L.W.; Bridges, C.R. Mitigation of myocardial fibrosis by molecular cardiac surgery-mediated gene overexpression. *J. Thorac. Cardiovasc. Surg.* **2016**, *151*, 1191–1200.e3. [CrossRef]
228. Banks, T.E.; Rajapaksha, M.; Zhang, L.H.; Bai, F.; Wang, N.P.; Zhao, Z.Q. Suppression of angiotensin II-activated NOX4/NADPH oxidase and mitochondrial dysfunction by preserving glucagon-like peptide-1 attenuates myocardial fibrosis and hypertension. *Eur. J. Pharmacol.* **2022**, *927*, 175048. [CrossRef]

biomedicines

MDPI

Article

Glucose Variability in People with Type 1 Diabetes: Associations with Body Weight, Body Composition, and Insulin Sensitivity

Julia F. Semenova, Anton Yu. Yushin, Anton I. Korbut and Vadim V. Klimontov *

Laboratory of Endocrinology, Research Institute of Clinical and Experimental Lymphology—Branch of the Institute of Cytology and Genetics, Siberian Branch of Russian Academy of Sciences (RICEL—Branch of IC&G SB RAS), 630060 Novosibirsk, Russia; ekmxtyjr@yandex.ru (J.F.S.); antyush@yandex.ru (A.Y.Y.); korbutai@icgbio.ru (A.I.K.)

* Correspondence: klimontov@mail.ru

Abstract: The prevalence of overweight and obesity increases in people with type 1 diabetes (T1D). However, the impact of fat accumulation on glucose dynamics in T1D is poorly understood. We assessed continuous glucose monitoring (CGM) parameters in patients with T1D depending on their body weight, body composition, and insulin sensitivity. In 547 patients, including 238 overweight/obese individuals, CGM-derived time in range (TIR) and glucose variability (GV) were estimated. Body composition was assessed by DXA. Estimated glucose disposal rate (eGDR) was used as an indicator of insulin sensitivity. Overweight/obese patients, when compared to normal-weight ones, have a lower time below range (TBR) (<3 mmol/L), GV, and experienced fewer episodes of low glucose. In men, lower TIR, higher time above range (TAR), and GV reduction were associated with central adiposity assessed by total, trunk, and android fat mass. In women, gynoid fat mass only was associated with a lower TIR and higher TAR. The eGDR was a positive predictor of TIR and a negative predictor of TAR, TBR, and GV in men and women. In conclusion, adiposity in people with T1D is associated with a lower risk of CGM-confirmed hypoglycemia, higher TAR, and reduced GV. These features of daily glucose dynamics may be mediated by insulin resistance.

Keywords: type 1 diabetes; obesity; overweight; adiposity; insulin resistance; body composition; continuous glucose monitoring; time in range; glucose variability

1. Introduction

Type 1 diabetes (T1D) is a chronic disease with a high risk of complications and a negative impact on quality of life. In 2022, the total number of people living with T1D was estimated to be about 8.75 million worldwide [1]. Life expectancy of a 10-year-old individual diagnosed with T1D varies from a mean of 13 years in low-income countries to 65 years in high-income countries [2].

Current research demonstrates some trends in the natural history and phenotype of T1D. Nowadays, new cases of the disease are more often registered in adults [1,2]. Another current feature of T1D is the presence of overweight or obesity in a significant proportion of patients [3,4]. In youths with T1D, the prevalence of overweight and obesity varies from 15 to 36% [4]. In this cohort, a higher body mass index (BMI) and waist circumference (WC) correlate with lower insulin sensitivity [5]. Metabolic syndrome is increasingly detected in patients with T1D [6,7]. A recent meta-analysis of 27 studies revealed that 23.7% of T1D individuals are affected by metabolic syndrome [8].

It can be assumed that reduced insulin sensitivity in overweight and obese patients with T1D may affect their insulin requirement, the quality of glycemic control, and the risk of complications. Indeed, it was shown that an increased BMI in people with T1D is associated with a higher insulin dose and a worse cardiometabolic risk factor profile [9]. In the Diabetes Control and Complication Trial (DCCT), higher insulin resistance at baseline was associated with an increased subsequent risk of micro- and macrovascular diseases [10]. In the Diabetes Control and Complications Trial/Epidemiology of Diabetes Interventions and Complications (DCCT/EDIC) study, high body weight variability in people with T1D was related to an increased risk of major adverse events and all-cause mortality [11].

Accumulating evidence suggests that body weight and fat mass could be associated with both mean glucose and glucose variability (GV) levels across different stages of the metabolic continuum. In subjects with normal glucose tolerance, those who are overweight demonstrated slightly higher mean glucose estimated by continuous glucose monitoring (CGM) than individuals with normal weight; both fat mass and fat distribution were associated with mean glucose and amplitude-dependent GV parameters [12]. Results of a recent meta-analysis including 71 studies indicate that, in people with prediabetes, GV is increased, but is less clearly associated with adiposity and insulin sensitivity [13]. In patients with T1D, the presence of metabolic syndrome was reported to be associated with higher GV [14]. It was shown that GV is related to the adverse vascular profile in T1D patients, but only in those with concomitant insulin resistance [15].

Currently, there is very little data on the glucose dynamics in overweight and obese people with T1D, as well as on the relationships between GV and body composition in this cohort. Therefore, in this study, we examined CGM-derived time in the glucose ranges and a number of GV parameters in patients with T1D depending on body weight, body composition, and insulin sensitivity.

2. Materials and Methods

2.1. Design

Adult Caucasian men and women with insulin-treated T1D were included in this cross-sectional single-center comparative study. The list of exclusion criteria included: age under 18 years, type 2 diabetes (T2D) or other specific types of the disease, current hyperglycemic crises (diabetic ketoacidosis or hyperglycemic hyperosmolar states), pregnancy, end-stage renal disease, malignancies, and accompanied diseases, which may affect glucose metabolism. Since most patients also participated in the study of inflammatory markers [16], chronic inflammatory or autoimmune diseases, acute infections within three months prior to the study, treatment with glucocorticoids, non-steroidal anti-inflammatory drugs, or immunosuppressive agents also applied as exclusion criteria.

The search for potentially eligible patients was performed using an institutional database. After matching the inclusion and exclusion criteria, 570 individuals with T1D were included in the study. Patients with a BMI < 25 kg/m^2 and those with a BMI $\geq$ 25 kg/m^2 were considered as two separate groups.

Real-time CGM data for the last week were used for the calculation of mean glucose, time in the glucose ranges, and GV parameters. Insulin sensitivity was estimated indirectly by the estimated glucose disposal rate (eGDR). About a quarter of the study participants (n = 149) underwent dual-energy X-ray absorptiometry (DXA) to assess body composition parameters.

The study design is shown in Figure 1.

2.2. Methods

All patients underwent a detailed clinical examination with an assessment of metabolic status and screening/monitoring of complications.

Real-time CGM was performed with MMT-722 or MMT-754 monitoring systems, Enlite sensors, and CareLink® Pro software (2.5.524.0, v. 2.5A, Medtronic, Minneapolis, MN, USA). Patients were instructed to calibrate the systems at least 4 times a day. Median CGM duration was 6.7 days.

Time In the target Range (TIR: 3.9–10.0 mmol/L [70–180 mg/dL]); Time Above Range, Level 1 (TAR L-1: 10.0–13.9 mmol/L [180–250 mg/dL]); Time Above Range, Level 2 (TAR L-2: >13.9 mmol/L [>250 mg/dL]); Time Below Range, Level 1 (TBR L-1: 3.8–3.0 mmol/L,

[< 70–54 mg/dL]); and Time Below Range, Level 2 (TBR L-2: <3.0 mmol/L [<54 mg/dL]) were estimated according to the international guidelines [17,18].

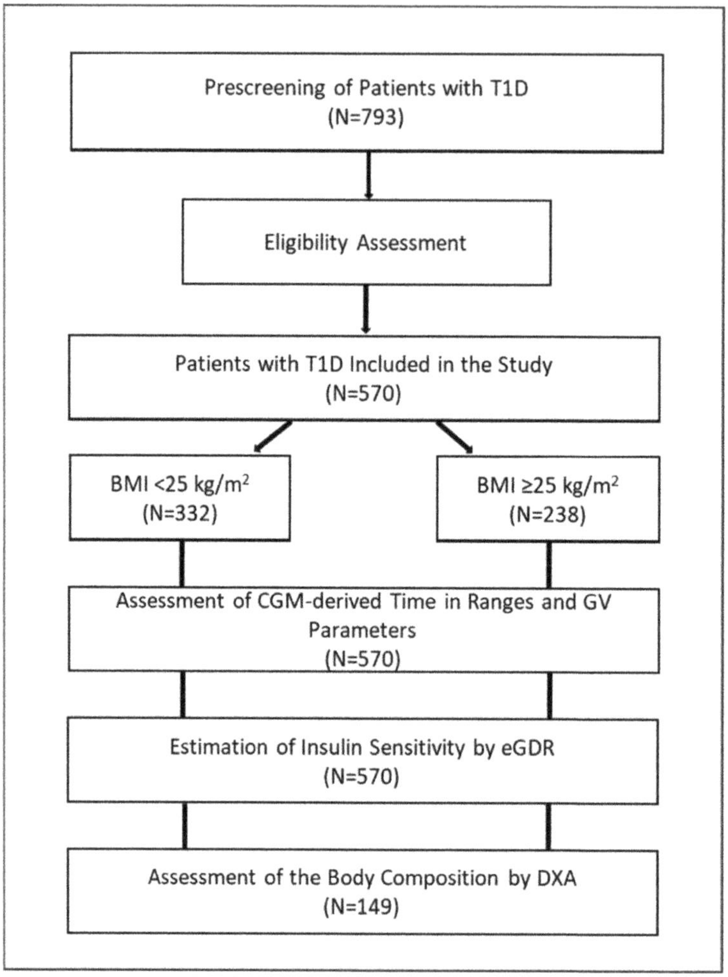

Figure 1. Study design. Abbreviations: BMI, body mass index; CGM, continuous glucose monitoring; DXA, dual-energy X-ray absorptiometry; eGDR, estimated glucose disposal rate; GV, glucose variability; T1D, type 1 diabetes.

The following GV indices were calculated: Coefficient of Variation (CV), Mean Amplitude of Glycemic Excursions (MAGE), Mean Absolute Glucose rate of change (MAG), and Lability Index (LI). Characteristics of these indices can be found in recent reviews [19,20]. In brief, CV is a measure of the dispersion of glucose values, MAGE is the mean differences from peaks to nadirs, and MAG and LI estimate the rate of change in glucose concentration. The GV parameters were estimated with the use of an EasyGV v. 9.0.R2 calculator [21].

Mean numbers of glucose episodes of <3.9 mmol/L (<70 mg/dL) and <3.0 mmol/L (<54 mg/dL) per 24 CGM hours were analyzed also.

eGDR was calculated with the use of the following formula: eGDR = 21.158 − (0.09 × WC) − (3.407 × hypertension) − (0.551 × HbA1c), where WC is the waist circumference (cm), hypertension (yes = 1/no = 0), and HbA1c = HbA1c (%) [22].

Body composition parameters were assessed by DXA with the use a Lunar Prodigy Advance densitometer and Body Composition software (GE healthcare, Madison, WI, USA). Specifically, we estimated total, trunk, android, gynoid fat masses, and lean mass, as described previously [23].

2.3. Statistical Analysis

Statistical analysis was performed using the STATISTICA 12 software package (Dell, Round Rock, TX, USA). We used the Kolmogorov–Smirnov criterion to test normality. The differences between the groups in quantitative parameters were assessed using the Mann–Whitney test. Spearman's rank correlation analysis and multiple stepwise regression analysis with a forward selection of variables were applied to test the associations between parameters. Medians, 25th and 75th percentiles, or minimum and maximum values are reported.

3. Results

3.1. Clinical Characteristics of Patients

The study included 570 patients, 211 men and 359 women, ranging from 18 to 73 years of age (median: 36 years). Diabetes duration varied from one to 55 years (median: 16 years). All patients received basal–bolus therapy with insulin analogs. Four-hundred subjects were managed with multiple daily injections (MDIs) and 170 individuals received a continuous subcutaneous insulin infusion (CSII) with the use of insulin pumps (mostly, MMT-722 or MMT-754, Medtronic, Minneapolis, MN, USA). Diabetic complications and/or associated diseases were verified in most patients: chronic kidney disease (n = 349), neuropathy (n = 349), diabetic retinopathy (n = 317), arterial hypertension (n = 216), impaired awareness of hypoglycemia (n = 200), non-alcoholic fatty liver disease (n = 187), peripheral artery disease (n = 84), diabetic foot (n = 44), and coronary artery disease (n = 29).

Three-hundred-and-thirty-two individuals had a BMI < 25 kg/m^2 and two-hundred-and-thirty-eight patients had a BMI ≥ 25 kg/m^2. In the second group, 156 subjects were overweight (BMI: 25–29.9 kg/m^2) and 82 subjects were obese (BMI ≥ 30 kg/m^2).

The clinical characteristics of the study groups are presented in Table 1. Patients with a BMI ≥ 25 kg/m^2, when compared to those with a BMI < 25 kg/m^2, were older, had a slightly longer diabetes duration, and were treated with higher insulin doses. Patients with a BMI ≥ 25 kg/m^2 demonstrated higher levels of total and LDL-cholesterol, triglycerides, uric acid, high-sensitivity C-reactive protein (hsCRP), and a lower estimated glomerular filtration rate (eGFR). No significant differences in glycated hemoglobin A1c (HbA1c) and albuminuria levels were found between the groups. The values of eGDR were markedly lower in overweight/obese patients.

Table 1. Clinical characteristics of study participants.

Characteristics	Groups of Patients with T1D		p
	BMI < 25 kg/m^2 N = 332	**BMI ≥ 25 kg/m^2 N = 238**	
Age, years	32 (25; 43)	41 (33; 54)	<0.0001
Sex, m/f, n (%)	96/236 (28.9/71.1)	115/123 (48.3/51.7)	<0.0001
BMI, kg/m^2	21.8 (20.0; 23.3)	28.5 (26.6; 31.0)	<0.0001
WC, cm	75 (70; 80)	96 (87; 103)	<0.001
Diabetes duration, years	15 (8.5; 22)	17 (10; 26)	0.017
Daily insulin dose, IU	42 (32; 52)	58 (45; 74)	<0.0001
Daily insulin dose, IU/kg	0.7 (0.5; 0.9)	0.7 (0.6; 0.9)	0.476
MDIs/CSII, n (%)	220/112 (66.3/33.7)	180/58 (75.6/24.4)	0.0001
HbA1c, %	8.1 (7.0; 9.3)	8.1 (7.3; 9.1)	0.827
HbA1c, mmol/L	64.6 (53.1; 78.6)	64.9 (55.9; 76.2)	0.827

Table 1. *Cont.*

Characteristics	Groups of Patients with T1D		p
	BMI < 25 kg/m² N = 332	BMI ≥ 25 kg/m² N = 238	
Total cholesterol, mmol/L	4.8 (4.1; 5.8)	5.2 (4.3; 5.9)	0.076
LDL-cholesterol, mmol/L	2.9 (2.4; 3.5)	3.2 (2.5; 3.9)	0.001
HDL-cholesterol, mmol/L	1.5 (1.3; 1.9)	1.4 (1.2; 1.6)	<0.0001
Triglycerides, mmol/L	0.93 (0.68; 1.27)	1.16 (0.86; 1.63)	<0.0001
Uric acid, μmol/L	233 (193; 287)	264 (222; 322)	<0.0001
hsCRP, mg/L	1.07 (0.52; 2.05)	2.12 (1.14; 4.22)	<0.0001
eGFR, mL/min/1.73 m²	91 (76; 105)	84 (71; 96)	0.0002
UACR, mg/mmol	2.2 (2.0; 5.89)	2.1 (2.0; 4.74)	0.307
eGDR, mg/kg/min	9.6 (7.2; 10.5)	5.3 (3.9; 7.9)	<0.0001

Continuous data are presented as medians (25% percentile; 75% percentile) and frequencies are presented as numbers of patients and percentages. Abbreviations: BMI, body mass index; eGDR, estimated glucose disposal rate; eGFR, estimated glomerular filtration rate; HbA1c, glycated hemoglobin A1c; HDL, high-density lipoprotein; hsCRP, high-sensitivity C-reactive protein; LDL, low-density lipoprotein; MDIs/CSII multiple daily injections/continuous subcutaneous insulin infusion; T1D, type 1 diabetes; UACR, urinary albumin-to-creatinine ratio; WC, waist circumference.

3.2. CGM Parameters in T1D Patients Depending on BMI and WC

Mean CGM glucose and TIR did not differ significantly between patients with a BMI ≥ 25 kg/m² and those with a BMI < 25 kg/m² (Table 2). Overweight/obese patients tended to have a higher TAR L-1 and lower TBR L-1; meanwhile, TBR-L2 was significantly lower in this group. There were no significant differences between the groups in CV and MAGE values. At the same time, lower MAG and LI values were revealed in overweight/obese individuals.

Table 2. CGM parameters in patients with T1D depending on BMI.

Parameter	Groups of Patients		p
	BMI < 25 kg/m² N = 332	BMI ≥ 25 kg/m² N = 238	
Mean glucose, mmol/L	7.9 (6.9; 9.2)	8.3 (7.2; 9.3)	0.143
TIR, %	74.5 (59.0; 85.3)	69.4 (58.6; 83.3)	0.423
TAR L-1, %	18.9 (9.3; 28.3)	21.1 (12.6; 30.4)	0.061
TAR L-2, %	2.6 (0.3; 9.3)	3.3 (0.5; 8.6)	0.389
TBR L-1, %	0.6 (0.0; 2.5)	0.6 (0.0; 1.7)	0.055
TBR L-2, %	0.0 (0.0; 0.2)	0.0 (0.0; 0.0)	0.017
CV, %	30.5 (27.0; 33.9)	29.6 (26.9; 33.8)	0.474
MAGE, mmol/L	3.9 (3.2; 4.8)	3.9 (3.3; 4.6)	0.299
MAG, mmol/L/h	2.1 (1.7; 2.5)	1.9 (1.7; 2.3)	0.001
LI, (mmol/L)²/h	3.2 (2.3; 4.7)	2.9 (2.2; 3.9)	0.013

Data are presented as medians [25% percentile; 75% percentile]. Abbreviations: BMI, body mass index; CGM, continuous glucose monitoring; CV, Coefficient of Variation; LI, Lability Index; MAG, Mean Absolute Glucose rate of change; MAGE, Mean Amplitude of Glycemic Excursions; TAR L-1, Time Above Range, Level 1; TAR L-2, Time Above Range, Level 2; TBR L-1, Time Below Range, Level 1; TBR L-2, Time Below Range, Level 2; TIR, Time In the target Range; T1D, type 1 diabetes.

Patients with a BMI ≥ 25 kg/m² experienced fewer episodes of low glucose levels per day than those with a BMI < 25 kg/m²: 0.33 (0.0; 0.86) and 0.21 (0.0; 0.56) episodes of glucose at <3.9 mmol/L, $p = 0.007$, and 0.0 (0.0; 0.13) and 0.0 (0.0; 0.0) episodes of glucose at <3.0 mmol/L, respectively, $p = 0.018$.

In the Spearman's rank correlation analysis, TBR L-2, MAG, and LI demonstrated weak negative correlations with BMI (Table 3). When men and women were considered separately, BMI correlated negatively with MAGE, MAG, and LI in men. In women, BMI demonstrated weak negative correlations with TBR L-2 and MAG, and a positive correlation with TAR L-1.

Table 3. Correlations of CGM parameters with BMI and WC in patients with T1D.

Parameter	BMI			WC		
	All	Men	Women	All	Men	Women
TIR	−0.01	0.1	−0.08	0.0	**0.2** *	−0.12
TAR L-1	0.06	−0.06	**0.13** *	0.02	**−0.17** *	**0.15** *
TAR L-2	0.02	−0.09	0.08	0.03	−0.15	**0.14** *
TBR L-1	−0.05	−0.03	−0.08	−0.08	−0.07	**−0.14** *
TBR L-2	**−0.11** **	−0.08	**−0.12** *	**−0.16** **	−0.11	**−0.21** **
CV	−0.04	−0.13	0.0	−0.04	**−0.17** *	−0.02
MAGE	−0.07	**−0.18** **	−0.02	−0.08	**−0.31** **	0.04
MAG	**−0.18** **	**−0.23** **	**−0.15** **	**−0.22** **	**−0.37** **	**−0.16** *
LI	**−0.15** **	**−0.24** **	−0.1	**−0.17** **	**−0.39** **	−0.06

Spearman's rank correlation coefficients (r) are presented. Significant coefficients are highlighted in bold: * $p < 0.05$; ** $p < 0.01$. Abbreviations: BMI, body mass index; CGM, continuous glucose monitoring; CV, Coefficient of Variation; LI, Lability Index; MAG, Mean Absolute Glucose rate of change; MAGE, Mean Amplitude of Glycemic Excursions; TAR L-1, Time Above Range, Level 1; TAR L-2, Time Above Range, Level 2; TBR L-1, Time Below Range, Level 1; TBR L-2, Time Below Range, Level 2; TIR, Time In the target Range; T1D, type 1 diabetes; WC, waist circumference.

Similarly to BMI, WC showed weak negative correlations with TBR L-2, MAG, and LI (Table 4). In men, WC correlated negatively with TAR L-1, CV, MAGE, MAG, and LI, and was associated positively with TIR. In women, WC showed weak negative correlations with TBR L-1, TBR L-2, and MAG, and demonstrated positive weak correlations with TAR L-1 and TAR L-2.

3.3. CGM Parameters in T1D Patients Depending on Body Composition

The assessment of body composition was performed on 149 subjects, 70 men and 79 women. Subjects with a BMI ≥ 25 kg/m^2 demonstrated higher total, trunk, android, and gynoid fat mass, as well as lean mass, when compared to those with a BMI < 25 kg/m^2 (Table 4).

Table 4. Parameters of body composition in patients with T1D depending on the BMI.

Parameter	Groups of Patients		p
	BMI < 25 kg/m^2 N = 85	BMI ≥ 25 kg/m^2 N = 64	
Total fat mass, kg	18.7 (14.3; 23.1)	30.6 (25.1; 34.4)	<0.0001
Total fat mass, %	30.6 (24.6; 36.9)	36.7 (31.6; 40.6)	<0.0001
Trunk fat mass, kg	8.2 (6.2; 11.5)	16.5 (13.4; 19.5)	<0.0001
Android fat mass, kg	1.2 (0.8; 1.7)	2.7 (2.2; 3.5)	<0.0001
Gynoid fat mass, kg	3.5 (2,7; 4.4)	4.6 (3.9; 5.7)	<0.0001
Lean mass, kg	43.1 (38.9; 51.7)	59.5 (46.7; 63.6)	<0.0001

Data are presented as medians [25% percentile; 75% percentile]. Abbreviations: BMI, body mass index; T1D, type 1 diabetes.

The values of TIR, TAR, and TBR did not correlate with the body composition parameters (Table 5). At the same time, MAG and LI demonstrated weak negative correlations with total, trunk, and android fat mass. MAGE correlated negatively with trunk fat mass only. No correlations were found between CGM-derived parameters and lean mass. In men, TIR correlated positively with total and trunk fat mass; TAR L-2 demonstrated negative correlations with total, trunk, android, and gynoid fat mass. In women, a positive correlation between CV and gynoid fat mass was found.

Table 5. Correlations between CGM metrics and body composition parameters in patients with T1D.

Parameter	TIR	TAR L-1	TAR L-2	TBR L-1	TBR L-2	CV	MAGE	MAG	LI
				All patients					
Total fat mass	0.05	−0.06	−0.07	−0.04	−0.07	−0.12	−0.11	**−0.22** **	**−0.19** *
Trunk fat mass	0.09	−0.11	−0.11	−0.04	−0.06	−0.14	**−0.17** *	**−0.26** **	**−0.24** **
Android fat mass	0.08	−0.09	−0.11	−0.06	−0.08	−0.15	−0.14	**−0.26** **	**−0.22** **
Gynoid fat mass	0.04	−0.05	−0.06	−0.06	−0.02	−0.11	−0.04	**−0.17** *	−0.12
Lean mass	−0.01	0.01	−0.01	0.07	0.01	0.01	0.01	−0.1	−0.05
				Men					
Total fat mass	**0.27** *	**−0.24** *	**−0.37** **	−0.02	0.01	**−0.27** *	**−0.43** **	**−0.36** **	**−0.49** **
Trunk fat mass	**0.25** *	−0.21	**−0.34** **	−0.04	−0.03	**−0.27** *	**−0.45** **	**−0.37** **	**−0.49** **
Android fat mass	0.22	−0.18	**−0.32** **	−0.04	−0.04	**−0.27** *	**−0.40** **	**−0.35** **	**−0.46** **
Gynoid fat mass	0.23	−0.21	**−0.34** **	0.02	0.04	−0.23	**−0.34** **	**−0.29** *	**−0.38** **
Lean mass	0.12	0.01	−0.19	−0.04	−0.08	−0.23	−0.22	−0.13	−0.25 *
				Women					
Total fat mass	−0.16	0.21	−0.03	−0.13	0.14	0.18	−0.12	0.07	0.07
Trunk fat mass	−0.03	0.09	−0.06	−0.11	0.03	0.08	−0.17	−0.01	−0.01
Android fat mass	−0.03	0.07	−0.11	−0.16	0.02	0.09	−0.18	−0.02	−0.02
Gynoid fat mass	−0.19	**0.24** *	−0.11	−0.07	0.19	**0.23** *	−0.12	0.08	0.08
Lean mass	0.01	−0.01	−0.03	−0.06	−0.06	0.08	−0.12	−0.0	−0.0

Spearman's rank correlation coefficients (r) are presented. Significant coefficients are highlighted in bold: * $p < 0.05$; ** $p < 0.01$. Abbreviations: CGM, continuous glucose monitoring; CV, Coefficient of Variation; LI, Lability Index; MAG, Mean Absolute Glucose rate of change; MAGE, Mean Amplitude of Glycemic Excursions; TAR L-1, Time Above Range, Level 1; TAR L-2, Time Above Range, Level 2; TBR L-1, Time Below Range, Level 1; TBR L-2, Time Below Range, Level 2; TIR, Time In the target Range; T1D, type 1 diabetes.

3.4. Relationships between CGM Parameters and eGDR

The values of eGDR correlated negatively with BMI (r = −0.62, $p < 0.0001$), WC (r = −0.73, $p < 0.0001$), total fat mass (r = −0.52, $p < 0.0001$), trunk fat mass and android fat mass (both r = −0.58, $p < 0.0001$), gynoid fat mass (r = −0.27, $p = 0.0009$), and lean mass (r = −0.41, $p < 0.0001$).

The correlations between eGDR and CGM parameters are presented in Table 6. In men, eGDR demonstrated positive correlations with TBR L-1, TBR L-2, MAG, and LI; weak negative correlations with TAR L-1 and TAR L-2 were found. In women, eGDR was related to TIR and MAG positively, and with TAR L-1, TAR L-2, TBR L-1, and TBR L-2 negatively. In addition, we found positive correlations between eGDR and a daily number of episodes of glucose <3.9 and <3 mmol/L (r = 0.22 and r = 0.28, respectively, both $p < 0.001$).

Table 6. Correlations of CGM parameters with eGDR in patients with T1D.

Parameter	All Patients	Men	Women
TIR	**0.19** **	0.10	**0.25** **
TAR L-1	**−0.23** **	**−0.14** *	**−0.30** **
TAR L-2	**−0.22** **	**−0.14** *	**−0.27** **
TBR L-1	**0.25** **	**0.25** **	**−0.27** **
TBR L-2	**0.24** **	**0.22** **	**−0.26** **
CV	−0.01	0.06	−0.03
MAGE	−0.03	0.03	0.08
MAG	**0.21** **	**0.29** **	**0.16** **
LI	**0.10** *	**0.17** *	0.06

Spearman's rank correlation coefficients (r) are presented. Significant coefficients are highlighted in bold: * $p < 0.05$; ** $p < 0.01$. Abbreviations: CGM, continuous glucose monitoring; CV, Coefficient of Variation; eGDR, estimated glucose disposal rate; LI, Lability Index; MAG, Mean Absolute Glucose rate of change; MAGE, Mean Amplitude of Glycemic Excursions; TAR L-1, Time Above Range, Level 1; TAR L-2, Time Above Range, Level 2; TBR L-1, Time Below Range, Level 1; TBR L-2, Time Below Range, Level 2; TIR, Time In the target Range; T1D, type 1 diabetes.

3.5. Multivariate Models

We assessed the associations of CGM metrics with clinical, anthropometric, body composition parameters, and eGDR in two sets of multivariate models.

In the first set, age, BMI, WC, diabetes duration, daily insulin dose, eGFR, and eGDR were included as independent variables. The results are presented in Table 7.

Table 7. Clinical and anthropometric predictors of CGM parameters in subjects with T1D in multivariate stepwise regression analysis (model set 1).

Parameter	Significant Predictors	R^2	F	p
	Men			
TIR	WC (β = 0.552), eGDR (β = 0.353)	0.15	7.73	0.0009
TAR L-1	WC (β = −0.542), eGDR (β = −0.334)	0.11	5.36	0.002
TAR L-2	WC (β = −0.37), eGDR (β = −0.325)	0.17	3.57	0.001
TBR L-2	eGDR (β = 0.321)	0.06	2.74	0.046
MAGE	WC (β = −0.539), eGDR (β = −0.275)	0.16	12.09	0.0002
MAG	Daily insulin dose (β = 0.244)	0.15	5.34	0.0005
LI	WC (β = −0.409)	0.16	8.28	0.0004
	Women			
TIR	Age (β = −0.16), BMI (β = 0.285), eGDR (β = 0.25)	0.08	9.92	<0.0001
TAR L-1	eGDR (β = −0.264)	0.08	2.76	0.009
TAR L-2	Age (β = −0.45), BMI (β = 0.285), eGDR (β = 0.25)	0.15	5.85	0.0002
TBR L-1	eGDR (β = 0.273), eGFR (β = 0.174)	0.11	4.19	0.0002
CV	BMI (β = 0.188), eGFR (β = −0.233)	0.06	3.05	0.01
MAGE	BMI (β = −0.261), eGDR (β = −0.214), eGFR (β = 0.26)	0.21	15.02	0.0003
MAG	WC (β = −0.32)	0.19	6.36	0.003
LI	BMI (β = −0.299), eGDR (β = −0.178), eGFR (β = 0.327)	0.11	7.11	<0.0001

Parameters of the models: β = beta coefficient, R^2 = R-Squared (or the coefficient of determination), F = F-statistic; p = p-value. Abbreviations: BMI, body mass index; CGM, continuous glucose monitoring; CV, Coefficient of Variation; eGDR, estimated glucose disposal rate; eGFR, estimated glomerular filtration rate; LI, Lability Index; MAG, Mean Absolute Glucose rate of change; MAGE, Mean Amplitude of Glycemic Excursions; TAR L-1, Time Above Range, Level 1; TAR L-2, Time Above Range, Level 2; TBR L-1, Time Below Range, Level 1; TBR L-2, Time Below Range, Level 2; TIR, Time In the target Range; T1D, type 1 diabetes; WC, waist circumference.

In men, WC turned out to be a predictor of TIR, TAR L-1, TAR L-2, MAGE, and LI. The values of eGDR were associated with TIR, TAR L-1, TAR L-2, TBR L-2, and MAGE. In these models, daily insulin dose predicted MAG. No reliable models were built for TBR L-1 and CV.

In women, BMI was associated with TIR, TAR L-2, CV, MAGE, and LI. An association between WC and MAG was found. eGDR predicted TIR, TAR L-1, TAR L-2, TBR L-1, MAGE, and LI. Age predicted TIR and TAR L-2, and eGFR was associated with TBR L-1, CV, MAGE, LI, and LBGI. No significant model for TBR L-2 was generated.

In the second set of multivariate models, BMI and WC were replaced by body composition parameters, namely total, trunk, android, gynoid fat mass, and lean mass. The results are summarized in Table 8.

In men, total fat mass was a negative predictor of TIR and LI, and a positive predictor of TAR L-2. Android fat mass was associated negatively with CV and MAGE. Trunk fat mass was a negative predictor of MAGE. eGDR demonstrated a positive association with MAG. Daily insulin dose was associated with TIR negatively, demonstrating positive relationships with TAR L-1 and TAR L-2. No reliable models were built for TBR L-1 and TBR L-2.

In women, gynoid fat mass was the negative predictor of TIR and positive predictor of TAR L-1 and TAR L-2. eGDF was associated negatively with TAR L-2 and demonstrated a positive association with TBR L-2. Daily insulin dose was associated positively with TBR L-1 and CV. We failed to generate models for MAGE and MAG. eGFR turned out to be the only predictor of LI.

Table 8. Clinical and body composition parameters as predictors of CGM metrics in subjects with T1D in multivariate stepwise regression analysis (model set 2).

Parameter	Significant Predictors	R^2	F	*p*
	Men			
TIR	Daily insulin dose (β = −0.31), total fat mass (β = 0.263)	0.17	5.95	0.004
TAR L-1	Daily insulin dose (β = 0.265)	0.15	3.32	0.03
TAR L-2	Daily insulin dose (β = 0.301), total fat mass (β = −0.36)	0.37	8.00	<0.0001
CV	Android fat mass (β = −0.34)	0.11	7.66	0.007
MAGE	Trunk fat mass (β = −2.1), android fat mass (β = −1.44)	0.32	8.76	<0.0001
MAG	eGDR (β = 0.444)	0.13	2.8	0.048
LI	Total fat mass (β = −1.7)	0.27	5.55	0.0007
	Women			
TIR	Gynoid fat mass (β = −0.46)	0.15	2.45	0.04
TAR L-1	Gynoid fat mass (β = 0.378)	0.15	2.50	0.04
TAR L-2	Gynoid fat mass (β = 0.573), eGDR (β = −0.36)	0.20	2.06	0.04
TBR L-1	Daily insulin dose (β = 0.310)	0.14	4.47	0.02
TBR L-2	eGDR (β = 0.413)	0.16	3.53	0.02
CV	Daily insulin dose (β = 0.346)	0.19	6.32	0.003
LI	eGFR (β = 0.652)	0.28	5.24	0.001

Parameters of the models: β = beta coefficient, R^2 = R-Squared (or the coefficient of determination), F = F-statistic; *p* = *p*-value. Abbreviations: CGM, continuous glucose monitoring; CV, Coefficient of Variation; eGDR, estimated glucose disposal rate; eGFR, estimated glomerular filtration rate; LI, Lability Index; MAG, Mean Absolute Glucose rate of change; MAGE, Mean Amplitude of Glycemic Excursions; TAR L-1, Time Above Range, Level 1; TAR L-2, Time Above Range, Level 2; TBR L-1, Time Below Range, Level 1; TBR L-2, Time Below Range, Level 2; TIR, Time In the target Range; T1D, type 1 diabetes.

4. Discussion

In this study, we assessed the associations of body weight, body composition, and insulin sensitivity to CGM-derived time in ranges and GV parameters in patients with T1D. To our knowledge, this is the first study demonstrating the relationships of adiposity and reduced insulin sensitivity with characteristics of glucose dynamics in these patients. For the in-depth analysis of CGM data, we calculated time in ranges (TIRs: TAR L-1, TAR L-2, TBR L-1, and TBR L-2), as well as GV indices, which characterize the dispersion of glucose values (CVs), the amplitude of glucose fluctuations (MAGEs), and the rate of change in glucose concentrations (MAGs, LI), as well as the number of low glucose episodes.

4.1. Main Findings

The principal finding of the study is an association of adiposity with a reduction in TIR, amplitude-dependent GV, and a risk of hypoglycemia. Specifically, we found that overweight/obese people with T1D when compared to those with BMI < 25 kg/m^2 have lower TBR L-2 (<3 mmol/L), MAG, and LI values, and experience fewer episodes of low glucose despite the higher daily insulin dose. Both BMI and WC showed weak negative correlations with TBR L-2, MAG, and LI.

Previously, an inverse correlation between BMI and CV in T1D patients was reported [24]. In youths with T1D, an association between BMI and hyperglycemic excursions, but not with CV and MAGE, was observed [25]. In disagreement with these data, a positive association was reported between hypoglycemia, CV, and BMI percentile in children and youths with T1D [26]. The discrepancy of the data may be explained by the different populations surveyed, as well as by the fact that BMI may not reflect the characteristics of body composition in obese individuals with different physical activities and sensitivity to insulin [27].

In this study, we tested the hypothesis that differences in body composition and insulin sensitivity may explain the patterns of glucose dynamics in T1D patients with overweight/obesity and normal body weight. Taking into account sex differences in weight and fat distribution, we analyzed men and women separately. When studying the relationships between CGM parameters and body composition, we identified correlations between total, trunk, android and gynoid fat mass with high glucose (TAR L-2), and amplitude-dependent GV parameters (CV, MAGE, MAG, and LI) in men. In the multivariate regression analysis, total fat mass was associated with high glucose (TAR L-2), while android fat mass turned out to be a predictor of CV and MAGE. In women, gynoid fat mass, but not other body composition parameters, correlated with TAR L-1 and CV, and predicted TIR and TAR in the multivariate model. Recently, Lipsky LM et al. reported an association between adiposity and TAR in youths with T1D. However, no relationships were found between body composition and GV estimated by MAGE and standard deviation [25].

A number of studies have shown that android fat or its ratio to gynoid fat is associated with decreased insulin sensitivity and related metabolic abnormalities. In subjects with normal glucose tolerance, android fat mass was positively associated with insulin resistance (HOMA-IR index) and demonstrated negative correlations with TBR and Low Blood Glucose Index [12]. Similarly, in obese children and adolescents, the android/gynoid ratio was related to HOMA-IR [28]. In young overweight males, preferential fat accumulation in the android area was associated with insulin resistance, impairment in lipid profile, and endothelial dysfunction [29]. A population-based study performed in Hangzhou, China, showed that android/gynoid ratio is positively associated with non-alcoholic fatty liver disease [30]. The latter, in turn, is closely related to insulin resistance [31].

In our study, we used eGDR as a validated score based on WC, hypertension, and HbA1c, which was introduced to measure insulin sensitivity in T1D [32,33]. A reduction in eGDR was found in overweight/obese patients indicating a decrease in insulin sensitivity. The eGDR values correlated negatively with BMI, WC, total, trunk, and android fat mass, and, to a lesser extent, gynoid fat mass. In agreement, Q. Zeng et al. reported negative associations of eGDR with visceral fat index and trunk fat mass in Chinese subjects with T1D [34]. In the multivariate models, we recognized eGDR to be a positive predictor of TIR and a negative predictor of TAR, TBR, and MAGE in men and women, and LI in women. Therefore, we can assume that the observed associations of body weight and fat mass accumulation with hyperglycemia and reduced GV are mediated through a decrease in insulin sensitivity.

Currently, the relationships between insulin sensitivity, CGM profiles, and, especially, GV are not well understood. Recently, I. Clinck et al. reported higher CGM-assessed TAR in patients with T1D with the lowest eGDR. In the regression analysis, a higher eGDR was associated with a higher TIR and TBR and a lower TAR. Our data confirm these results. Having studied a larger number of GV parameters, we also found a negative association between eGDR and GV. However, in the cited work, insulin sensitivity was assessed not only using the eGDR, but also by a hyperinsulinemic–euglycemic clamp. Interestingly, no significant relationships between CGM parameters and measured glucose disposal rate were found [35]. It was assumed that the enhancing effect of insulin on glucose fluctuations can be mitigated by insulin resistance [36]. In agreement, a reciprocal relationship between HOMA-IR and GV was revealed in subjects with prediabetes [37].

The results of our study show that total, trunk, and android fat mass values are related to CGM parameters in men, but not in women. This finding may be explained by sex differences in the association between abdominal fat accumulation and insulin sensitivity [38]. In Chinese adults, android fat percentage was more closely associated with metabolic syndrome components in men. In women, android fat percentage and gynoid fat percentage showed opposite effects on the levels of triglycerides, HDL-cholesterol, and WC [39]. In subjects with newly diagnosed T2D and individuals with prediabetes, android fat positively correlated with HOMA-IR in men, but not in women [40]. In transgender individuals receiving gender-affirming hormone therapy, android fat more strongly correlated with insulin resistance compared to gynoid fat [41].

Pathogenetic links between adiposity, insulin resistance, and T1D could be multi-directional. Patients with T1D have specific risk factors that contribute to weight gain. These include intensive insulin therapy, subcutaneous insulin administration leading to peripheral hyperinsulinemia, repetitive episodes of hypoglycemia, and the consequences of a fear of hypoglycemia in the form of frequent snacking and decreased physical activity. Diabetes-specific psychosocial burden (stress, depression, decreased quality of life, lack of support, etc.) can exacerbate obesity. Obesity triggers lipotoxicity, mitochondrial dysfunction, adipose tissue dysfunction, gut microbiome imbalance, low-grade inflammation, and, ultimately, reduces insulin sensitivity. In its turn, obesity-driven insulin resistance increases the requirement for exogenous insulin, forming a vicious circle. At the same time, the accelerator hypothesis postulates that obesity and insulin resistance can lead to glucotoxicity and accelerated apoptosis of pancreatic β-cells via immune and inflammatory mechanisms. Finally, some people with T1D may be genetically predisposed to obesity and insulin resistance, especially when they have a family history of T2D [4,42].

4.2. Clinical Implications

An increasing prevalence of overweight and obesity in people with T1D is a serious challenge. Although patients with insulin resistance may have a reduced risk of hypoglycemia, other factors associated with decreased sensitivity to insulin may have a detrimental effect on vascular health and disease outcomes. A 10.9-year follow-up of 26,125 T1D patients registered in the Swedish National Diabetes Registry showed an increase in the risk of major cardiovascular disease, heart failure, cardiovascular death, and mortality with increasing BMI. These associations were more apparent in men than in women [43]. In subjects with T1D, insulin resistance verified by the eGDR was associated with vascular complications independently from HbA1c [44,45]. The results of recent meta-analysis demonstrate that insulin resistance, as estimated by the eGDR, may be an additional risk factor for cardiovascular disease and all-cause mortality in T1D [46]. Data from our and other studies [9,47] indicate that overweight and obese T1D patients require higher insulin doses for glycemic control than their lean counterparts, which may pose an additional risk of complications and impede weight loss. Therefore, the prevention of overweight and obesity should become a part of the management strategy for T1D patients as well.

The features of metabolic changes in obese patients with T1D should be taken into account in clinical practice. Our results indicate that individuals with T1D who are overweight or obese are less likely to achieve glycemic control targets, especially in managing hyperglycemia, than patients with normal weight. Therefore, adiposity-driven insulin resistance should be considered as a barrier to the control of T1D. Currently, there are several options to manage or even eliminate this barrier. Lifestyle modification programs, including nutrition therapy, correction of dietary habits, and increased levels of physical activity, should be an essential part of comprehensive care for people with T1D and obesity [48]. Glucagon-like peptide-1 receptor agonists, dual glucagon-like peptide-1 and gastric inhibitory polypeptide agonists, sodium-glucose cotransporter-2 inhibitors, metformin, pramlintide, and some other drugs are discussed as promising therapeutic agents for the management of obesity and/or insulin resistance in patients with T1D [49,50]. Bariatric surgery may be a viable treatment for patients with T1D and severe obesity [51]. However, it should be noted that drug therapy and surgical treatment are not yet standard approaches to weight management in T1D.

4.3. Limitations of the Study and Future Remarks

Limitations of our study include cross-sectional design, patient recruitment in one clinical center, and short CGM duration. We did not differentiate between visceral and subcutaneous adipose tissue when assessing body composition. Insulin sensitivity was estimated indirectly by eGDR, but not by a clamp technique. We did not take into account the level of physical activity, dietary habits, stress, and other lifestyle and psychosocial factors of the study participants. It is likely that these factors could modify some of the associations between GV, body composition, and insulin sensitivity we observed. The lack of a control group does not allow us to compare associations between body composition and glucose dynamics in people with T1D with those in healthy individuals. The representativeness of the sample is limited to young and middle-aged adults with T1D without advanced complications and serious concomitant diseases. In addition, the study focuses on a Caucasian population, which may limit the generalizability of the findings to other ethnic groups.

The strengths of this study are the large sample size, comprehensive analysis of CGM data with a broad range of time-dependent and amplitude-dependent GV parameters, and the use of DXA to examine body composition. In an effort to provide insights into the whole story, we assessed glucose dynamics, anthropometric parameters, body composition, and insulin sensitivity in a sample of patients with T1D.

Future studies are needed for the identification of mechanisms underlying the associations of fat mass and fat distribution with glucose homeostasis in T1D patients. Prospective studies could answer the question of how changes in body weight and body composition affect insulin sensitivity and glucose dynamics in people living with T1D. In particular, the effect of weight loss and adiposity reduction on TIR and GV parameters in obese subjects with T1D is a great challenge.

5. Conclusions

The results of this study demonstrate that overweight and obese people with T1D have a lower risk of CGM-confirmed hypoglycemia and reduced GV than those with a BMI <25 kg/m^2. In men, central adiposity assessed by the total, trunk, and android fat mass is associated with higher glucose and lower GV. In women, gynoid fat mass, but no other body composition parameters, is related to hyperglycemia. The observed associations of body weight and body composition with the features of daily glucose dynamics may be mediated by insulin sensitivity.

Author Contributions: Conceptualization, V.V.K.; methodology, V.V.K.; investigation, J.F.S., A.Y.Y. and V.V.K.; data curation, A.Y.Y. and J.F.S.; formal analysis—A.I.K.; writing—original draft preparation, J.F.S. and A.Y.Y.; writing—review and editing, V.V.K.; supervision, project administration, and funding acquisition, V.V.K. All authors have read and agreed to the published version of the manuscript.

Funding: This research was funded by the Russian Science Foundation, grant number 20-15-00057-П.

Institutional Review Board Statement: This study was conducted in accordance with the Declaration of Helsinki and approved by the Ethics Committee of RICEL—a branch of IC&G SB RAS (protocol N. 158, date of approval 1 June 2020).

Informed Consent Statement: Written informed consent was obtained from each subject involved in the study.

Data Availability Statement: The source data are available from the corresponding authors upon reasonable request.

Conflicts of Interest: The authors declare no conflicts of interest. The funder had no role in the design of the study; in the collection, analysis, or interpretation of data; in the writing of the manuscript, or in the decision to publish the results.

References

1. Ogle, G.D.; Wang, F.; Gregory, G.A.; Maniam, J. Type 1 Diabetes Numbers in Children and Adults. IDF Atlas Report (2022). Available online: https://diabetesatlas.org/atlas/t1d-index-2022/ (accessed on 23 April 2024).
2. Gregory, G.A.; Robinson, T.I.G.; Linklater, S.E.; Wang, F.; Colagiuri, S.; De Beaufort, C.; Donaghue, K.C.; Magliano, D.J.; Maniam, J.; Orchard, T.J.; et al. Global Incidence, Prevalence, and Mortality of Type 1 Diabetes in 2021 with Projection to 2040: A Modelling Study. *Lancet Diabetes Endocrinol.* **2022**, *10*, 741–760. [CrossRef]
3. Van Der Schueren, B.; Ellis, D.; Faradji, R.N.; Al-Ozairi, E.; Rosen, J.; Mathieu, C. Obesity in People Living with Type 1 Diabetes. *Lancet Diabetes Endocrinol.* **2021**, *9*, 776–785. [CrossRef] [PubMed]
4. Kueh, M.T.W.; Chew, N.W.S.; Al-Ozairi, E.; Le Roux, C.W. The Emergence of Obesity in Type 1 Diabetes. *Int. J. Obes.* **2024**, *48*, 289–301. [CrossRef] [PubMed]

5. Chan, C.L.; Pyle, L.; Morehead, R.; Baumgartner, A.; Cree-Green, M.; Nadeau, K.J. The Role of Glycemia in Insulin Resistance in Youth with Type 1 and Type 2 Diabetes: Chan et Al. *Pediatr. Diabetes* **2017**, *18*, 470–477. [CrossRef] [PubMed]
6. Yayıcı Köken, Ö.; Kara, C.; Can Yılmaz, G.; Aydın, H.M. Prevalence of Obesity and Metabolic Syndrome in Children with Type 1 Diabetes: A Comparative Assessment Based on Criteria Established by the International Diabetes Federation, World Health Organisation and National Cholesterol Education Program. *J. Clin. Res. Pediatr. Endocrinol.* **2020**, *12*, 55–62. [CrossRef]
7. Mørk, F.B.; Madsen, J.O.B.; Pilgaard, K.A.; Jensen, A.K.; Klakk, H.; Tarp, J.; Bugge, A.; Heidemann, M.; Van Hall, G.; Pociot, F.; et al. The Metabolic Syndrome Is Frequent in Children and Adolescents with Type 1 Diabetes Compared to Healthy Controls. *Pediatr. Diabetes* **2022**, *23*, 1064–1072. [CrossRef] [PubMed]
8. Belete, R.; Ataro, Z.; Abdu, A.; Sheleme, M. Global Prevalence of Metabolic Syndrome among Patients with Type I Diabetes Mellitus: A Systematic Review and Meta-Analysis. *Diabetol. Metab. Syndr.* **2021**, *13*, 25. [CrossRef]
9. Braffett, B.H.; Dagogo-Jack, S.; Bebu, I.; Sivitz, W.I.; Larkin, M.; Kolterman, O.; Lachin, J.M. Association of Insulin Dose, Cardiometabolic Risk Factors, and Cardiovascular Disease in Type 1 Diabetes During 30 Years of Follow-up in the DCCT/EDIC Study. *Diabetes Care* **2019**, *42*, 657–664. [CrossRef]
10. Kilpatrick, E.S.; Rigby, A.S.; Atkin, S.L. Insulin Resistance, the Metabolic Syndrome, and Complication Risk in Type 1 Diabetes. *Diabetes Care* **2007**, *30*, 707–712. [CrossRef]
11. Petria, I.; Albuquerque, S.; Varoquaux, G.; Vie, J.-J.; Venteclef, N.; Mohammedi, K.; Roussel, R.; Camoin, M.; Perseghin, G.; Velho, G.; et al. Body-Weight Variability and Risk of Cardiovascular Outcomes in Patients with Type 1 Diabetes: A Retrospective Observational Analysis of Data from the DCCT/EDIC Population. *Cardiovasc. Diabetol.* **2022**, *21*, 247. [CrossRef]
12. Klimontov, V.V.; Semenova, J.F. Glucose Variability in Subjects with Normal Glucose Tolerance: Relations with Body Composition, Insulin Secretion and Sensitivity. *Diabetes Metab. Syndr.* **2022**, *16*, 102387. [CrossRef] [PubMed]
13. Hjort, A.; Iggman, D.; Rosqvist, F. Glycemic Variability Assessed Using Continuous Glucose Monitoring in Individuals without Diabetes and Associations with Cardiometabolic Risk Markers: A Systematic Review and Meta-Analysis. *Clin. Nutr.* **2024**, *43*, 915–925. [CrossRef] [PubMed]
14. Guo, K.; Zhang, L.; Ye, J.; Niu, X.; Jiang, H.; Gan, S.; Zhou, J.; Yang, L.; Zhou, Z. Metabolic Syndrome Associated with Higher Glycemic Variability in Type 1 Diabetes: A Multicenter Cross-Sectional Study in China. *Front. Endocrinol.* **2022**, *13*, 972785. [CrossRef] [PubMed]
15. Kietsiriroje, N.; Pearson, S.M.; O'Mahoney, L.L.; West, D.J.; Ariëns, R.A.; Ajjan, R.A.; Campbell, M.D. Glucose Variability Is Associated with an Adverse Vascular Profile but Only in the Presence of Insulin Resistance in Individuals with Type 1 Diabetes: An Observational Study. *Diabetes Vasc. Dis. Res.* **2022**, *19*, 147916412211032. [CrossRef]
16. Klimontov, V.V.; Mavlianova, K.R.; Orlov, N.B.; Semenova, J.F.; Korbut, A.I. Serum Cytokines and Growth Factors in Subjects with Type 1 Diabetes: Associations with Time in Ranges and Glucose Variability. *Biomedicines* **2023**, *11*, 2843. [CrossRef]
17. Danne, T.; Nimri, R.; Battelino, T.; Bergenstal, R.M.; Close, K.L.; DeVries, J.H.; Garg, S.; Heinemann, L.; Hirsch, I.; Amiel, S.A.; et al. International Consensus on Use of Continuous Glucose Monitoring. *Diabetes Care* **2017**, *40*, 1631–1640. [CrossRef]
18. Battelino, T.; Danne, T.; Bergenstal, R.M.; Amiel, S.A.; Beck, R.; Biester, T.; Bosi, E.; Buckingham, B.A.; Cefalu, W.T.; Close, K.L.; et al. Clinical Targets for Continuous Glucose Monitoring Data Interpretation: Recommendations from the International Consensus on Time in Range. *Diabetes Care* **2019**, *42*, 1593–1603. [CrossRef]
19. Kovatchev, B. Glycemic Variability: Risk Factors, Assessment, and Control. *J. Diabetes Sci. Technol.* **2019**, *13*, 627–635. [CrossRef]
20. Sun, B.; Luo, Z.; Zhou, J. Comprehensive Elaboration of Glycemic Variability in Diabetic Macrovascular and Microvascular Complications. *Cardiovasc. Diabetol.* **2021**, *20*, 9. [CrossRef]
21. Hill, N.R.; Oliver, N.S.; Choudhary, P.; Levy, J.C.; Hindmarsh, P.; Matthews, D.R. Normal Reference Range for Mean Tissue Glucose and Glycemic Variability Derived from Continuous Glucose Monitoring for Subjects without Diabetes in Different Ethnic Groups. *Diabetes Technol. Ther.* **2011**, *13*, 921–928. [CrossRef]
22. Lu, Z.; Xiong, Y.; Feng, X.; Yang, K.; Gu, H.; Zhao, X.; Meng, X.; Wang, Y. Insulin Resistance Estimated by Estimated Glucose Disposal Rate Predicts Outcomes in Acute Ischemic Stroke Patients. *Cardiovasc. Diabetol.* **2023**, *22*, 225. [CrossRef]
23. Klimontov, V.V.; Bulumbaeva, D.M.; Fazullina, O.N.; Lykov, A.P.; Bgatova, N.P.; Orlov, N.B.; Konenkov, V.I.; Pfeiffer, A.F.H.; Pivovarova-Ramich, O.; Rudovich, N. Circulating Wnt1-Inducible Signaling Pathway Protein-1 (WISP-1/CCN4) Is a Novel Biomarker of Adiposity in Subjects with Type 2 Diabetes. *J. Cell Commun. Signal.* **2020**, *14*, 101–109. [CrossRef] [PubMed]
24. Jin, S.-M.; Kim, T.-H.; Bae, J.C.; Hur, K.Y.; Lee, M.-S.; Lee, M.-K.; Kim, J.H. Clinical Factors Associated with Absolute and Relative Measures of Glycemic Variability Determined by Continuous Glucose Monitoring: An Analysis of 480 Subjects. *Diabetes Res. Clin. Pract.* **2014**, *104*, 266–272. [CrossRef] [PubMed]
25. Lipsky, L.M.; Gee, B.; Liu, A.; Nansel, T.R. Glycemic Control and Variability in Association with Body Mass Index and Body Composition over 18months in Youth with Type 1 Diabetes. *Diabetes Res. Clin. Pract.* **2016**, *120*, 97–103. [CrossRef] [PubMed]
26. Piona, C.; Marigliano, M.; Mancioppi, V.; Mozzillo, E.; Occhiati, L.; Zanfardino, A.; Iafusco, D.; Maltoni, G.; Zucchini, S.; Delvecchio, M.; et al. Glycemic Variability and Time in Range Are Associated with the Risk of Overweight and High LDL-Cholesterol in Children and Youths with Type 1 Diabetes. *Horm. Res. Paediatr.* **2023**, 1–7. [CrossRef]
27. Santi, A.; Bosch, T.A.; Bantle, A.E.; Alvear, A.; Wang, Q.; Hodges, J.S.; Dengel, D.R.; Chow, L.S. High Body Mass Index Masks Body Composition Differences in Physically Active Versus Sedentary Participants. *Metab. Syndr. Relat. Disord.* **2018**, *16*, 483–489. [CrossRef]

28. Aucouturier, J.; Meyer, M.; Thivel, D.; Taillardat, M.; Duché, P. Effect of Android to Gynoid Fat Ratio on Insulin Resistance in Obese Youth. *Arch. Pediatr. Adolesc. Med.* **2009**, *163*, 826–831. [CrossRef] [PubMed]
29. Sari, C.I.; Eikelis, N.; Head, G.A.; Schlaich, M.; Meikle, P.; Lambert, G.; Lambert, E. Android Fat Deposition and Its Association with Cardiovascular Risk Factors in Overweight Young Males. *Front. Physiol.* **2019**, *10*, 1162. [CrossRef] [PubMed]
30. Hsing, J.C.; Nguyen, M.H.; Yang, B.; Min, Y.; Han, S.S.; Pung, E.; Winter, S.J.; Zhao, X.; Gan, D.; Hsing, A.W.; et al. Associations Between Body Fat, Muscle Mass, and Nonalcoholic Fatty Liver Disease: A Population-Based Study. *Hepatol. Commun.* **2019**, *3*, 1061–1072. [CrossRef]
31. Zhong, H. Non-Alcoholic Fatty Liver Disease: Pathogenesis and Models. *Am. J. Transl. Res.* **2024**, *16*, 387–399. [CrossRef]
32. Epstein, E.J.; Osman, J.L.; Cohen, H.W.; Rajpathak, S.N.; Lewis, O.; Crandall, J.P. Use of the Estimated Glucose Disposal Rate as a Measure of Insulin Resistance in an Urban Multiethnic Population with Type 1 Diabetes. *Diabetes Care* **2013**, *36*, 2280–2285. [CrossRef] [PubMed]
33. Nyström, T.; Holzmann, M.J.; Eliasson, B.; Svensson, A.; Sartipy, U. Estimated Glucose Disposal Rate Predicts Mortality in Adults with Type 1 Diabetes. *Diabetes Obes. Metab.* **2018**, *20*, 556–563. [CrossRef]
34. Zeng, Q.; Chen, X.-J.; He, Y.-T.; Ma, Z.-M.; Wu, Y.-X.; Lin, K. Body Composition and Metabolic Syndrome in Patients with Type 1 Diabetes. *World J. Diabetes* **2024**, *15*, 81–91. [CrossRef]
35. Clinck, I.; Mertens, J.; Wouters, K.; Dirinck, E.; De Block, C. Insulin Resistance and CGM-Derived Parameters in People with Type 1 Diabetes: Are They Associated? *J. Clin. Endocrinol. Metab.* **2024**, dgae015. [CrossRef] [PubMed]
36. Huang, Y.; Heng, C.; Wei, J.; Jing, X.; Wang, X.; Zhao, G.; Hou, J.; Liu, Q.; Jiao, K. Influencing Factors of Glycemic Variability in Hospitalized Type 2 Diabetes Patients with Insulin Therapy: A Strobe-Compliant Article. *Medicine* **2017**, *96*, e8021. [CrossRef] [PubMed]
37. Dimova, R.; Chakarova, N.; Grozeva, G.; Kirilov, G.; Tankova, T. The Relationship between Glucose Variability and Insulin Sensitivity and Oxidative Stress in Subjects with Prediabetes. *Diabetes Res. Clin. Pract.* **2019**, *158*, 107911. [CrossRef]
38. Bantle, A.E.; Bosch, T.A.; Dengel, D.R.; Wang, Q.; Mashek, D.G.; Chow, L.S. DXA-Determined Regional Adiposity Relates to Insulin Resistance in a Young Adult Population with Overweight andObesity. *J. Clin. Densitom.* **2019**, *22*, 287–292. [CrossRef]
39. Bi, X.; Loo, Y.T.; Henry, C.J. Android Fat as a Determinant of Metabolic Syndrome: Sex Differences. *Nutrition* **2019**, *57*, 127–132. [CrossRef]
40. Ma, M.; Jiang, T.; Wen, Z.; Zhang, D.; Xiu, L. Gender Differences in Relation to Body Composition, Insulin Resistance, and Islet Beta Cell Function in Newly Diagnosed Diabetic or Pre-Diabetic Patients. *Diabetes Metab. Syndr. Obes.* **2023**, *16*, 723–732. [CrossRef]
41. Bretherton, I.; Spanos, C.; Leemaqz, S.Y.; Premaratne, G.; Grossmann, M.; Zajac, J.D.; Cheung, A.S. Insulin Resistance in Transgender Individuals Correlates with Android Fat Mass. *Ther. Adv. Endocrinol. Metab.* **2021**, *12*, 204201882098568. [CrossRef]
42. Bielka, W.; Przezak, A.; Molęda, P.; Pius-Sadowska, E.; Machaliński, B. Double diabetes-when type 1 diabetes meets type 2 diabetes: Definition, pathogenesis and recognition. *Cardiovasc. Diabetol.* **2024**, *23*, 62. [CrossRef] [PubMed]
43. Edqvist, J.; Rawshani, A.; Adiels, M.; Björck, L.; Lind, M.; Svensson, A.-M.; Gudbjörnsdottir, S.; Sattar, N.; Rosengren, A. BMI, Mortality, and Cardiovascular Outcomes in Type 1 Diabetes: Findings Against an Obesity Paradox. *Diabetes Care* **2019**, *42*, 1297–1304. [CrossRef] [PubMed]
44. Helliwell, R.; Warnes, H.; Kietsiriroje, N.; Campbell, M.; Birch, R.; Pearson, S.M.; Ajjan, R.A. Body Mass Index, Estimated Glucose Disposal Rate and Vascular Complications in Type 1 Diabetes: Beyond Glycated Haemoglobin. *Diabet. Med.* **2021**, *38*, e14529. [CrossRef]
45. Bhagadurshah, R.R.; Eagappan, S.; Kasthuri Santharam, R.; Subbiah, S. The Impact of Body Mass Index, Residual Beta Cell Function and Estimated Glucose Disposal Rate on the Development of Double Diabetes and Microvascular Complications in Patients with Type 1 Diabetes Mellitus. *Cureus* **2023**, *15*, e48979. [CrossRef]
46. Sun, R.; Wang, J.; Li, M.; Li, J.; Pan, Y.; Liu, B.; Lip, G.Y.H.; Zhang, L. Association of Insulin Resistance with Cardiovascular Disease and All-Cause Mortality in Type 1 Diabetes: Systematic Review and Meta-Analysis. *Diabetes Care* **2024**, dc240475. [CrossRef]
47. Cantley, N.W.; Lonnen, K.; Kyrou, I.; Tahrani, A.A.; Kahal, H. The Association between Overweight/Obesity and Double Diabetes in Adults with Type 1 Diabetes; a Cross-Sectional Study. *BMC Endocr. Disord.* **2021**, *21*, 187. [CrossRef]
48. Mottalib, A.; Kasetty, M.; Mar, J.Y.; Elseaidy, T.; Ashrafzadeh, S.; Hamdy, O. Weight Management in Patients with Type 1 Diabetes and Obesity. *Curr. Diab. Rep.* **2017**, *17*, 92. [CrossRef] [PubMed]
49. Kim, Y.J.; Hwang, S.D.; Lim, S. Effects of Sodium-Glucose Cotransporter Inhibitor/Glucagon-Like Peptide-1 Receptor Agonist Add-On to Insulin Therapy on Glucose Homeostasis and Body Weight in Patients with Type 1 Diabetes: A Network Meta-Analysis. *Front. Endocrinol.* **2020**, *11*, 553. [CrossRef] [PubMed]
50. Freeby, M.; Lane, K. Treating obesity in type 1 diabetes mellitus—Review of efficacy and safety. *Curr. Opin. Endocrinol. Diabetes Obes.* **2024**, *31*, 1–7. [CrossRef]
51. Dessify, B.; Wood, C.; Parker, D.; Carmichael, D.; Petrick, A.; Daouadi, M. Is there a role for bariatric surgery in patients with severe obesity and type 1 diabetes? *Surg. Obes. Relat. Dis.* **2022**, *18*, 177–181. [CrossRef]

biomedicines

Article

Exploring the Spectrum of Comorbidities Associated with Primary Aldosteronism: Insights from a Large Real-World Case-Control Study

Andreas Krieg [1,*], Sarah Krieg [2], Andreas Heuser [1], Ulrich Laverenz [1], Valentin-Alin Istrate [1], Matthias Schott [3] and Karel Kostev [4]

1 Department of General and Visceral Surgery, Thoracic Surgery and Proctology, University Hospital Herford, Medical Campus OWL, Ruhr University Bochum, 32049 Herford, Germany; andreas.heuser@rub.de (A.H.); ulrich.laverenz@klinikum-herford.de (U.L.); valentin-alin.istrate@klinikum-herford.de (V.-A.I.)

2 Department of Inclusive Medicine, University Hospital Ostwestfalen-Lippe, Bielefeld University, 33617 Bielefeld, Germany; sarah.krieg@mara.de

3 Division for Specific Endocrinology, Heinrich-Heine-University and University Hospital Duesseldorf, 40225 Duesseldorf, Germany; matthias.schott@med.uni-duesseldorf.de

4 Epidemiology, IQVIA, 60549 Frankfurt, Germany

* Correspondence: andreas.krieg@rub.de

Abstract: Background: Primary aldosteronism (PA) is a common cause of endocrine hypertension, characterized by excessive aldosterone secretion leading to hypertension, hypokalemia, and metabolic alkalosis. While historically diagnosed based on this classic triad of symptoms, current understanding reveals a more nuanced presentation. This study aimed to investigate the prevalence of PA-associated diseases in a large German population. **Methods**: Medical records from the IQVIA™ Disease Analyzer database were analyzed retrospectively. PA patients (n = 860) were matched with non-PA individuals (n = 4300) by age and sex. Associations between PA and predefined chronic diseases were examined using multivariable logistic regression. **Results**: PA was significantly associated with hypokalemia (7.8% vs. 1.6%, odds ratio (OR): 3.45; 95% confidence intervals (CIs): 2.41–4.96), hypertension (56.1% vs. 28.5%; OR: 2.37; 95% CIs: 2.00–2.81), hepatic steatosis (11.3% vs. 3.0%; OR: 1.85; 95% CIs: 1.34–2.57), gout (8.3% vs. 2.2%; OR: 1.64; 95% CIs: 1.15–2.35), chronic kidney disease (6.3% vs. 2.2%; OR: 1.59; 95% CIs: 1.10–2.31), diabetes mellitus not otherwise specified (7.9% vs. 2.9%; OR: 1.49; 95% CIs: 1.06–2.09), obesity (13.5% vs. 5.1%; OR: 1.38; 95% CIs: 1.05–1.82), and depression (14.8% vs. 6.2%; OR: 1.37; 95% CIs: 1.07–1.77). **Conclusions**: While the study design had limitations, including reliance on ICD codes for diagnosis, these findings underscore the critical need for early detection and personalized management strategies for PA to reduce associated risks and improve patient outcomes.

Keywords: Conn syndrome; primary aldosteronism; adrenal gland; hypertension; hypokalemia; hepatic steatosis; gout; chronic kidney disease; diabetes mellitus

1. Introduction

In 1956, Jerome Conn reported the case of a woman with a disorder he termed primary aldosteronism (PA), which included generalized weakness and transient paralysis, muscle spasms, hypertension, and hypokalemia. The term "primary" was used to distinguish this form of hyperaldosteronism from secondary forms that can occur in intravascular volume depletion, congestive heart failure, and cirrhosis [1].

PA is the most common cause of endocrine hypertension and occurs in approximately 4–13% of hypertensive patients in general practice [2–4]. PA is characterized by an autonomous and uncontrolled aldosterone secretion [5]. The resulting over-activation of the mineralocorticoid receptor leads to volume retention, hypertension, hypokalemia, and metabolic alkalosis. However, it is now known that hypokalemia occurs in only 46% of patients and the classic triad of arterial hypertension, hypokalemia, and metabolic alkalosis occurs in only a small proportion of patients, most of whom are severely affected [6,7]. The cause of uncontrolled aldosterone secretion is bilateral adrenal hyperplasia in two thirds of cases and unilateral adrenal adenoma in one third [5].

The subtyping between unilateral and bilateral disease is of particular importance in PA. Since a small adenoma of the adrenal cortex is typically responsible for the hypersecretion of aldosterone in unilateral disease, the treatment of choice for unilateral PA is minimally invasive (e.g., retroperitoneoscopic, laparoscopic) partial or total adrenalectomy [8–10]. In contrast, patients with proven bilateral hyperaldosteronism or those who are not candidates for surgery usually require lifelong therapy with mineralocorticoid receptor antagonists (MRAs) like spironolactone or eplerenone [8]. In many cases, additional antihypertensive therapy is required to adequately control blood pressure. The treatment with MRAs can be complemented or substituted with agents such as amiloride, which directly inhibit the epithelial sodium channel [11]. Furthermore, thiazide diuretics and calcium channel blockers can be combined with treatment with MRAs or amiloride. However, a low-salt diet and close monitoring of blood pressure and serum electrolytes are also key elements in the treatment plan [11].

Patients with PA have an approximately 3 to 12 times higher risk of cerebrovascular (e.g., stroke), cardiovascular (e.g., atrial fibrillation, coronary artery disease, left ventricular hypertrophy, heart failure) events, or chronic kidney disease compared to patients with essential hypertension [12–19]. Consequently, recommendations from various national and international medical societies, including the American College of Cardiology/American Heart Association [20] and the Endocrine Society [8], recommend that patients with refractory hypertension and hypertension with hypokalemia be evaluated for the presence of PA by measuring plasma aldosterone–renin activity or concentration. Additionally, metabolic disorders like type 2 diabetes and metabolic syndrome [19,21,22], psychiatric changes [23], and obstructive sleep apnea syndrome (OSAS) [24] are increasingly observed in patients with PA. Therefore, the Endocrine Society has already recommended that patients with OSAS should also be evaluated for the presence of PA [8].

Additional knowledge about the association of certain diseases with PA could help to modify screening strategies and provide a basis for earlier diagnosis, treatment, and prevention of PA sequelae in the general population. Thus, this study aimed to investigate the prevalence of potential PA-associated diseases compared with those observed in a control group of patients without PA and patients with hypertension but without PA in a large real-world German population.

2. Materials and Methods

2.1. Database

For this study, medical records (baseline demographics and diagnoses) from the IQVIA^{TM} Disease Analyzer database were used. Data from this repository were obtained directly and anonymously from electronically stored data systems used by primary-care physicians and specialists in private practice in Germany [25]. The database comprises approximately 3000 physicians selected by panel design according to predefined strata including specialty, federal state, community size category, and physician age. While previous research has shown the database to be representative for the country [25], it has been widely used in several studies of epidemiology including comorbidities [26,27].

2.2. Study Population

Our retrospective case-control study enrolled outpatients aged ≥18 years who had a first documented diagnosis of PA (ICD-10: E26.0) by a general practitioner (GP) between January 2015 and December 2023 (index date). Of note, this PA diagnosis did not necessarily have to be made by the GP, but could also be made by a specialist or in a hospital and then documented by the GP. Importantly, we must acknowledge that ICD codes were assigned by local protocols and may not have been standardized across the study. Only patients with data available from at least 12 months before the index date were included in the analysis. This inclusion criterion was necessary to ensure that PA was not documented prior to the index date and to allow analysis of diagnoses documented within 12 months of PA diagnosis. PA patients were matched 1:5 with non-PA individuals for age and sex. The index date for non-PA individuals was a random physician visit between January 2015 and December 2023 (Figure 1).

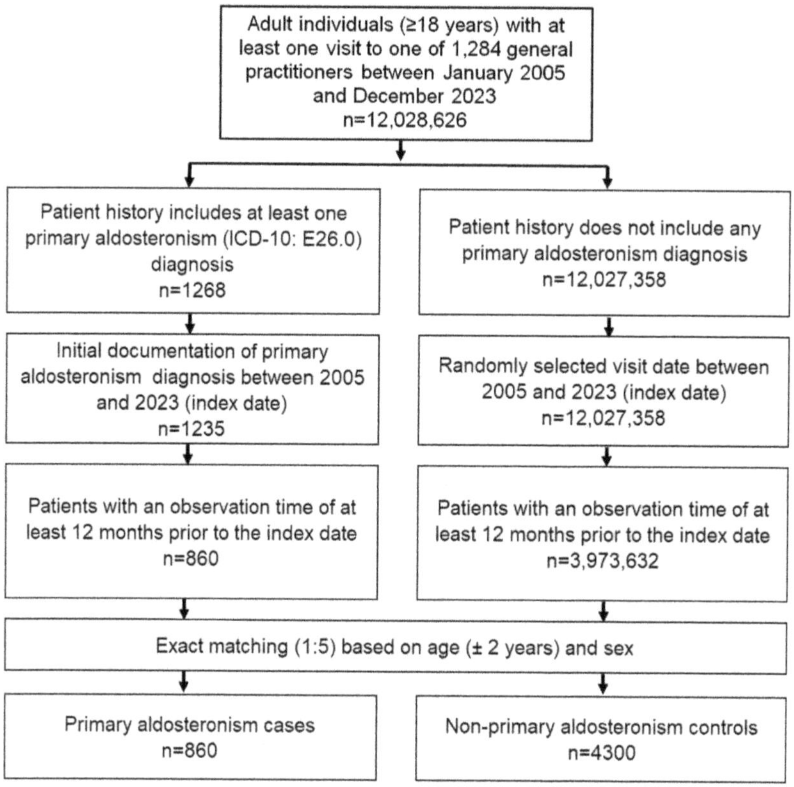

Figure 1. Stepwise selection of eligible study patients.

2.3. Study Outcomes and Covariates

The study outcomes were the prevalence of various disorders documented within the 365 days prior to the index date and the associations between these disorders and PA. All diagnoses or diagnosis classes occurring in at least 5% of the study patients were analyzed. These disorders included nontoxic goiter (ICD-10: E04), diabetes mellitus type 2 (ICD-10: E11), diabetes mellitus not otherwise specified (ICD-10: E14), obesity (ICD-10: E66), disorders of lipoprotein metabolism (ICD-10: E78), hypokalemia (ICD-10: E87.6), hypertension (ICD-10: I10), chronic ischemic heart disease (ICD-10: I25), depression (ICD-10: F32, F33), sleep disorders (ICD-10: G47), gastritis and duodenitis (ICD-10: K29), non-alcoholic fatty liver disease (NAFLD, ICD-10: K76.0), gout (ICD-10: M10), back pain (ICD-10: M54), and chronic kidney disease (ICD-10: N18). Additionally, the proportion of patients with prescriptions for spironolactone within the 365 days prior to the index date was evaluated.

2.4. Statistical Analyses

The prevalence of defined disorders was calculated for individuals with and without PA. Multivariable logistic regression models were used with all study disorders as dependent variables and PA as an outcome variable. Additionally, spironolactone was also investigated as a dependent variable. p values < 0.05 were considered statistically significant. Analyses were performed with SAS version 9.4 (SAS Institute, Cary, NC, USA).

2.5. Sensitivity Analyses

For sensitivity analysis, PA patients were matched 1:5 with non-PA individuals with hypertension diagnosis by age and sex. Both descriptive and regression analyses were repeated for new matched pairs.

3. Results

3.1. Baseline Characteristics of the Study Patients

Following a 1:5 matching, we enrolled 860 individuals with PA and 4300 without PA in our study. Baseline characteristics of the study patients are summarized in Table 1. In the entire study population, 51.1% of patients were female. The mean age in the PA group was 60.9 (SD: 14.5) years and 61.1 (SD: 14.7) years in the non-PA group.

Table 1. Age and sex characteristics of study patients with or without primary aldosteronism (PA) prior to and after 1:5 matching.

	Prior to Matching			After Matching		
Variable	Proportion Among Individuals with PA (n, %)	Proportion Among Individuals Without PA (n, %)	p-Value	Proportion Among Individuals with PA (n, %)	Proportion Among Individuals Without PA (n, %)	p-Value
N	860	3,973,632		860	4300	
Sex: female	439 (51.1)	2,102,813 (52.9)	0.271	439 (51.1)	2195 (51.1)	1.000
Sex: male	421 (48.9)	1,870,819 (47.1)		421 (48.9)	2105 (48.9)	
Age (mean, SD)	60.9 (14.5)	51.2 (20.0)	<0.001	60.9 (14.5)	61.1 (14.7)	0.685
Age ≤ 40	78 (9.1)	1,336,163 (33.6)	<0.001	78 (9.1)	406 (9.4)	0.945
Age 41–50	120 (14.0)	577,794 (14.5)		120 (14.0)	608 (14.1)	
Age 51–60	209 (24.3)	684,383 (17.2)		209 (24.3)	1030 (24.0)	
Age 61–70	208 (24.2)	569,630 (14.3)		208 (24.2)	1032 (24.0)	
Age > 70	245 (28.5)	805,662 (20.3)		245 (28.5)	1224 (28.5)	

3.2. Prevalence of Predefined Disorders

Among PA patients, hypertension was the disorder with the highest prevalence (56.1%), followed by lipoprotein metabolism disorders (26.1%), dorsalgia (21.9%), depression (14.8%), and obesity (13.5%). Hypertension (28.5%), lipoprotein metabolism disorders (15.1%), and dorsalgia (15.8%) were also the most common disorders in non-PA individuals, but the prevalence rates of these disorders were markedly lower in controls than in PA cases (Figure 2). In addition, 18.5% of the patients with PA and 2.6% of the controls were treated with spironolactone.

3.3. Association of PA with Predefined Disorders

Using multivariable logistic regression, we identified a significant positive association between PA and eight conditions: hypokalemia (7.8% vs. 1.6%, odds ratio (OR): 3.45; 95% confidence intervals (CIs): 2.41–4.96), hypertension (56.1% vs. 28.5%; OR: 2.37; 95% CIs: 2.00–2.81), hepatic steatosis (11.3% vs. 3.0%; OR: 1.85; 95% CIs: 1.34–2.57), gout (8.3% vs. 2.2%; OR: 1.64; 95% CIs: 1.15–2.35), chronic kidney disease (6.3% vs. 2.2%; OR: 1.59; 95%

CIs: 1.10–2.31), diabetes mellitus not otherwise specified (7.9% vs. 2.9%; OR: 1.49; 95% CIs: 1.06–2.09), obesity (13.5% vs. 5.1%; OR: 1.38; 95% CIs: 1.05–1.82), and depression (14.8% vs. 6.2%; OR: 1.37; 95% CIs: 1.07–1.77) (Table 2). Furthermore, spironolactone use was strongly positively associated with PA (OR: 7.46; 95% CIs: 5.54–10.05). To investigate whether the association between PA and gout was primarily due to PA and not to spironolactone therapy, only patients not receiving spironolactone therapy were examined for this association. However, this regression analysis did not reveal any direct association between PA and gout (OR: 1.23; 95% CIs: 0.74–2.03; $p = 0.429$).

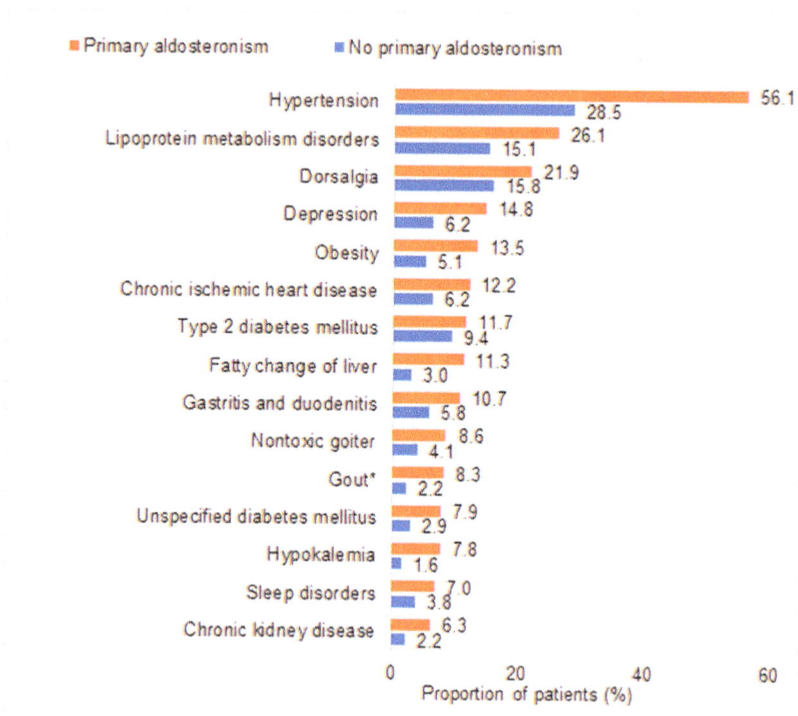

Figure 2. Prevalence of different disorders documented within 12 months prior to the index date. * A direct association between PA and gout could not be found in patients who were not treated with spironolactone.

Table 2. Association between primary aldosteronism (PA) and several disorders in individuals followed in general practices in Germany (reference group: all individuals without PA). * A direct association between PA and gout could not be found in patients who were not treated with spironolactone.

Diagnosis (ICD-10 Codes)	Odds Ratio for PA (95% CIs) #	*p*-Value
Hypokalemia (E87.6)	3.45 (2.41–4.96)	<0.001
Hypertension (I10)	2.37 (2.00–2.81)	<0.001
Fatty change of liver (K76.0)	1.85 (1.34–2.57)	<0.001
Gout (M10) *	1.64 (1.15–2.35)	0.007
Chronic kidney disease (N18)	1.59 (1.10–2.31)	0.014
Unspecified diabetes mellitus (E14)	1.49 (1.06–2.09)	0.021
Obesity (E66)	1.38 (1.05–1.82)	0.023

Table 2. *Cont.*

Diagnosis (ICD-10 Codes)	Odds Ratio for PA (95% CIs) #	p-Value
Depression (F32, F33)	1.37 (1.07–1.77)	0.014
Nontoxic goiter (E04)	1.30 (0.96–1.75)	0.088
Disorders of lipoprotein metabolism (E78)	1.20 (0.97–1.49)	0.091
Dorsalgia (M54)	1.18 (0.98–1.43)	0.088
Gastritis and duodenitis (K29)	1.13 (0.87–1.49)	0.362
Sleep disorders (G47)	1.11 (0.80–1.54)	0.516
Chronic ischemic heart disease (I25)	1.08 (0.83–1.41)	0.560
Type 2 diabetes mellitus (E11)	0.79 (0.61–1.01)	0.063

Multivariate logistic regression adjusted for all diagnoses listed in the table; $p < 0.05$ is considered statistically significant.

3.4. Sensitivity Analyses

Figure 3 shows the prevalence of chronic disorders among PA patients and age- and sex-matched non-PA patients with hypertension.

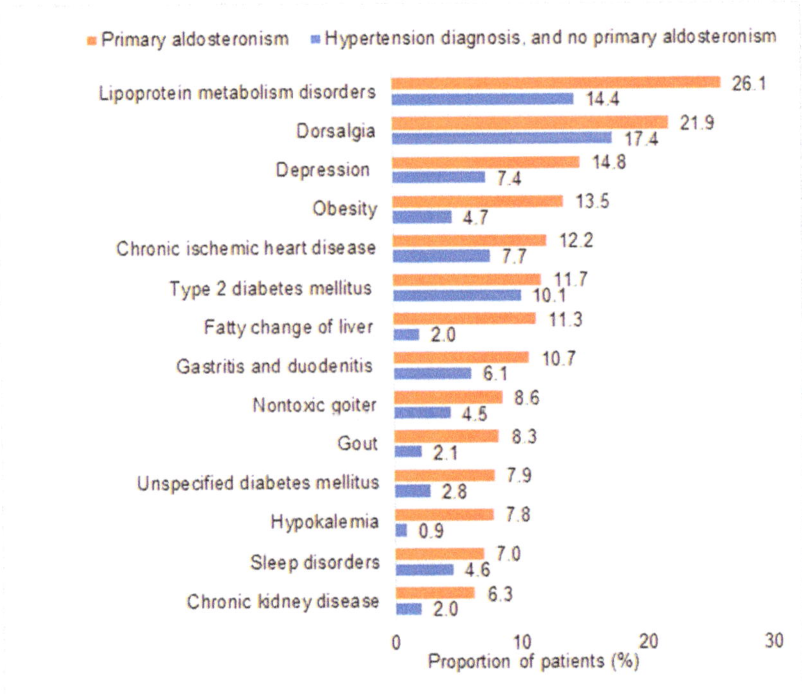

Figure 3. Prevalence of different disorders documented within 12 months prior to the index date (individuals with PA versus individuals with hypertension and without PA).

In regression analyses, a significant positive association was observed between PA and five disorders: hypokalemia (OR: 14.32; 95% CIs: 9.50–21.56), fatty change of liver (OR: 2.23; 95% CIs: 1.46–3.42), chronic kidney disease (OR: 2.73; 95% CIs: 1.77–4.23), obesity (OR: 5.07; 95% CIs: 3.94–6.54), and depression (OR: 1.99; 95% CIs: 1.52–2.59). Diabetes mellitus type 2 was negatively associated with PA (OR: 0.41; 95% CIs: 0.29–0.57) (Table 3). Note that only 3.0% of the controls were treated with spironolactone and spironolactone use was strongly positively associated with PA (OR: 9.49; 95% CIs: 7.14–12.62).

Table 3. Association between PA and several disorders in individuals followed in general practices in Germany (reference group: individuals with hypertension and without PA).

Diagnosis (ICD-10 Codes)	Odds Ratio for PA (95% CIs) *	p-Value
Hypokalemia (E87.6)	14.32 (9.50–21.56)	<0.001
Fatty change of liver (K76.0)	2.23 (1.46–3.42)	<0.001
Gout (M10)	1.56 (0.98–2.49)	0.056
Chronic kidney disease (N18)	2.73 (1.77–4.23)	<0.001
Unspecified diabetes mellitus (E14)	1.29 (0.85–1.95)	0.070
Obesity (E66)	5.07 (3.94–6.54)	<0.001
Depression (F32, F33)	1.99 (1.52–2.59)	<0.001
Nontoxic goiter (E04)	1.28 (0.91–1.79)	0.158
Disorders of lipoprotein metabolism (E78)	0.89 (0.70–1.12)	0.318
Dorsalgia (M54)	0.83 (0.67–1.03)	0.092
Gastritis and duodenitis (K29)	1.00 (0.72–1.37)	0.983
Sleep disorders (G47)	1.36 (0.97–1.92)	0.075
Chronic ischemic heart disease (I25)	0.97 (0.71–1.31)	0.829
Type 2 diabetes mellitus (E11)	0.41 (0.29–0.57)	<0.001

* Multivariate logistic regression adjusted for all diagnoses listed in the table; $p < 0.05$ is considered statistically significant.

4. Discussion

PA, caused by autonomous hypersecretion of aldosterone from the adrenal cortex, occurs in about 4–13% of hypertensive patients in general practice [2–4] and may be associated with hypokalemia, although this is seen in only about 46% of patients [7]. The aim of our study was to explore, in a real-world dataset, which chronic diseases were present prior to the diagnosis of PA and may therefore be strongly associated with PA. At this point, we must emphasize that there are other registries, such as the German Conn Registry [28] and the Spanish Primary Aldosteronism Registry of the Spanish Society of Endocrinology and Nutrition (SEEN) (SPAIN-ALDO Registry) [29]. Importantly, studies using data from these registries showed many of the associations we found in our dataset [30–34]. However, in contrast to our database, the German Conn Registry includes centers that specialize in patients with primary aldosteronism. Therefore, the purpose of our study was to provide an overview of patients treated by general practitioners rather than specialized centers.

In our study, hypertension and hypokalemia were observed in 56.1% and 7.8% of patients diagnosed with PA, respectively. These relatively low rates may be due to the fact that we could not specify whether the diagnosis was made as part of screening for hypertension or as part of the diagnosis of incidental adrenal tumor. It should be noted that hypertension and hypokalemia are not fundamental manifestations of PA, but, rather, depend on the severity and duration of exposure to renin–autonomous-aldosterone secretion and sodium retention [35]. Although hypertension is a common symptom of primary hyperaldosteronism and occurs in most patients, rare forms of normotensive PA have also been described in the literature [36]. In the context of normotensive PA, it has been postulated that these patients may be in an early stage of the disease, and presenting with mild or non-elevated blood pressure within the normal range [36].

However, this does not explain the relatively high prevalence of PA patients without a diagnosis of arterial hypertension that we observed in our cohort. Therefore, it cannot be excluded that some of the patients included in our study may have been receiving antihypertensive medication at the time of coding the diagnosis, which could have led to misclassification as normotensive. We also cannot exclude the possibility that different reference or cut-off values for hypokalemia and different definitions of blood pressure were used, and our database does not contain information on the method by which blood pressure was measured. Nevertheless, our multivariable analysis showed that both hypertension and hypokalemia were the most commonly associated conditions in patients with PA.

Using aldosterone–renin quotient (ARQ) screening, the prevalence of PA in primary-care patients treated for hypertension is approximately 4–13% [2–4]. Unfortunately, even today, many patients are not being screened. In this context, a retrospective cohort study of U.S. veterans with refractory hypertension between 2000 and 2017 found that only 1.6% of patients were screened for the presence of PA [37]. In addition, it is important to note that the rate of screening for the presence of PA was highly dependent on the specialty of the primary-care provider and that screening for the presence of PA was an important determinant of initiation of MRA therapy, and thus, blood-pressure control. In particular, in the study by Cohen et al., the screening rate was lowest in the group of general practitioners [37]. However, years of delay in diagnosis predispose the development of end-organ damage, and it is well known that patients diagnosed with PA have a higher incidence of cardiovascular morbidity and mortality as well as renal morbidity than patients of comparable age or blood pressure [19,38]. The cardiovascular effects of PA are both diverse and substantial, ranging from left ventricular hypertrophy, worsening of systolic and diastolic function, myocardial ischemia, vascular remodeling, arrhythmias, and sudden cardiac death [39]. The pathophysiological mechanisms leading to vascular damage are not limited to hypertension, which alone is a significant problem for the cardiovascular system. In addition, the induction of oxidative stress, endothelial inflammation, and vascular damage leading to fibrosis or podocyte damage plays a role in the pathogenesis of aldosterone-induced cardiac or chronic kidney disease [40–43]. Although PA patients in our study sample were almost twice as likely to have chronic ischemic heart disease, with a prevalence of 12.2%, this association was not significant in multivariable analysis. In contrast, chronic kidney disease had an almost 3-fold higher prevalence compared with the control group and patients with hypertension and no PA, which was also significant in the multivariable analysis.

To optimize and standardize the early detection, diagnosis, and treatment of PA, the Endocrine Society has developed a guideline [8]. According to these recommendations, patients should be evaluated for the presence of PA based on well-defined anamnestic and diagnostic criteria. These criteria are based on an increased prevalence of PA in defined risk groups, including OSAS. Unfortunately, our data search was unable to look specifically for the ICD-10 code G47.31, which is defined for OSAS. The lack of association with sleep disorders in our population could therefore be explained by the fact that our search for code G47 was only a general and therefore not a very detailed screen for sleep disorders.

The association between PA and depression observed in our study is also intensively discussed in the literature [23]. Numerous studies have already shown that elevated plasma aldosterone concentrations are associated with depression [44–46] and that adrenalectomy with normalization of aldosterone levels leads to a reduction in depressive symptoms [47].

In addition, PA is associated with decreased insulin sensitivity and secretion [48,49] and an increased incidence of metabolic syndrome and type 2 diabetes mellitus [19]. We also found a significant association between PA and obesity or unspecific diabetes mellitus (E14), but not with type 2 diabetes mellitus (E11) in our study population. Interestingly, there was a particularly strong association between the presence of NAFLD and PA. Our observations thus confirm studies conducted in much smaller populations [50,51].

Interestingly, patients with PA were 3.8 times and almost 4 times more likely to develop gout than the control group and the group of patients with hypertension but without PA, respectively. To our knowledge, an association between PA and gout has not been described in the literature to date. It is known that therapy with spironolactone, which is also used for PA, can lead to an increase in blood uric acid levels, which in turn can cause gout flares in predisposed patients. In our study population, 18.5% of the patients with PA, but only 2.6% of the controls, were treated with spironolactone. Therefore, it is tempting to speculate that the association we observed between PA and gout may have been affected by spironolactone therapy. To test the hypothesis that there might be a positive association between PA and gout, we excluded patients receiving spironolactone from a further regression analysis, limiting the analyses to patients not using this medication. However, no association was found, suggesting that the observed association between PA and gout may be at least partially explained by spironolactone therapy. Although we were able to confirm the association between PA and numerous chronic diseases in a relatively large patient population, we must point out some limitations, especially in the study design. As all diagnoses were based on ICD codes, we cannot exclude the possibility of misclassification. In addition, we cannot provide data on the validity of the diagnosis of PA, nor can we show which diagnostic tools were used to make the diagnosis of PA. ICD-10 classification does not allow us to differentiate between symptomatic and non-symptomatic diseases. Furthermore, patients identified with PA may represent only a small fraction of the patients in the German healthcare system who truly have PA. This may bias the differences between PA and non-PA individuals in the study with a consequence that PA cases identified are not fully representative of the clinical spectrum of PA. Finally, our database did not allow us to examine the effects of aldosterone antagonists or other medications, although spironolactone treatment was strongly positively associated with PA in our study.

Nevertheless, we believe that our study represents an important contribution to the literature because we were able to perform our investigations on a very large sample. In addition, the PA cases were age- and sex-matched to the control group.

5. Conclusions

In contrast to previous studies based on data from highly specialized centers, our study provides an overview of patients with PA and associated comorbidities who were treated by general practitioners. Through retrospective analysis of a large number of outpatients, the study confirmed a significant association between PA and various chronic diseases, including hypertension, hypokalemia, hepatic steatosis, gout, chronic kidney disease, obesity, and depression. Notably, PA patients exhibited a markedly higher likelihood of developing gout compared with the control group. While acknowledging limitations in the study design, such as reliance on ICD codes for diagnosis, the findings emphasize the critical need for early detection and individualized management strategies for PA to mitigate associated risks and improve patient outcomes.

Author Contributions: Conceptualization, A.K., S.K. and K.K.; methodology, A.K. and K.K.; software, A.K. and K.K.; validation, A.K., S.K., A.H. and U.L.; formal analysis, A.K., S.K., V.-A.I. and K.K.; investigation, K.K.; resources, A.K. and K.K.; data curation, K.K.; writing—original draft preparation, A.K., S.K. and K.K.; writing—review and editing, A.H., U.L., V.-A.I. and M.S.; visualization, A.K. and K.K.; supervision, A.K. and K.K.; project administration, A.K.; funding acquisition, A.K. All authors have read and agreed to the published version of the manuscript.

Funding: The article processing charge was funded by the Open Access Fund of the Ruhr University Bochum.

Institutional Review Board Statement: Ethical review and approval were waived for this study, due to the fact that the "Disease Analyzer" database, used for analysis, contains anonymized electronic patient records. Patient data were analyzed in aggregated form without individual data being available. The authors had no access to any identifying information at any time during the analysis of the data. The study was conducted according to Declaration of Helsinki guidelines.

Informed Consent Statement: German law allows the use of anonymous electronic medical records for research purposes under certain conditions. According to this legislation, it is not necessary to obtain informed consent from patients or approval from a medical ethics committee for this type of study that contains no directly identifiable data.

Data Availability Statement: The original contributions presented in the study are included in the article, further inquiries can be directed to the corresponding author.

Conflicts of Interest: Author Karel Kostev was employed by the company IQVIA. The remaining authors declare that the research was conducted in the absence of any commercial or financial relationships that could be construed as a potential conflict of interest.

References

1. Conn, J.W.; Louis, L.H. Primary aldosteronism, a new clinical entity. *Ann. Intern. Med.* **1956**, *44*, 1–15. [CrossRef] [PubMed]
2. Monticone, S.; Burrello, J.; Tizzani, D.; Bertello, C.; Viola, A.; Buffolo, F.; Gabetti, L.; Mengozzi, G.; Williams, T.A.; Rabbia, F.; et al. Prevalence and Clinical Manifestations of Primary Aldosteronism Encountered in Primary Care Practice. *J. Am. Coll. Cardiol.* **2017**, *69*, 1811–1820. [CrossRef] [PubMed]
3. Käyser, S.C.; Dekkers, T.; Groenewoud, H.J.; van der Wilt, G.J.; Carel Bakx, J.; van der Wel, M.C.; Hermus, A.R.; Lenders, J.W.; Deinum, J. Study Heterogeneity and Estimation of Prevalence of Primary Aldosteronism: A Systematic Review and Meta-Regression Analysis. *J. Clin. Endocrinol. Metab.* **2016**, *101*, 2826–2835. [CrossRef] [PubMed]
4. Buffolo, F.; Monticone, S.; Burrello, J.; Tetti, M.; Veglio, F.; Williams, T.A.; Mulatero, P. Is Primary Aldosteronism Still Largely Unrecognized? *Horm. Metab. Res.* **2017**, *49*, 908–914. [CrossRef]
5. Fuss, C.T.; Hahner, S.; Heinrich, D.A.; Adolf, C. Conn's syndrome-Frequent and still too rarely diagnosed to underdiagnosed. *Der Internist* **2022**, *63*, 25–33. [CrossRef]
6. Vonend, O.; Rump, L.C. Normokalemic primary hyperaldosteronism. *Dtsch. Med. Wochenschr. (1946)* **2006**, *131*, H24–H27. [CrossRef]
7. Douma, S.; Petidis, K.; Doumas, M.; Papaefthimiou, P.; Triantafyllou, A.; Kartali, N.; Papadopoulos, N.; Vogiatzis, K.; Zamboulis, C. Prevalence of primary hyperaldosteronism in resistant hypertension: A retrospective observational study. *Lancet* **2008**, *371*, 1921–1926. [CrossRef]
8. Funder, J.W.; Carey, R.M.; Mantero, F.; Murad, M.H.; Reincke, M.; Shibata, H.; Stowasser, M.; Young, W.F., Jr. The Management of Primary Aldosteronism: Case Detection, Diagnosis, and Treatment: An Endocrine Society Clinical Practice Guideline. *J. Clin. Endocrinol. Metab.* **2016**, *101*, 1889–1916. [CrossRef]
9. Walz, M.K.; Gwosdz, R.; Levin, S.L.; Alesina, P.F.; Suttorp, A.C.; Metz, K.A.; Wenger, F.A.; Petersenn, S.; Mann, K.; Schmid, K.W. Retroperitoneoscopic adrenalectomy in Conn's syndrome caused by adrenal adenomas or nodular hyperplasia. *World J. Surg.* **2008**, *32*, 847–853. [CrossRef]
10. Walz, M.K.; Peitgen, K.; Diesing, D.; Petersenn, S.; Janssen, O.E.; Philipp, T.; Metz, K.A.; Mann, K.; Schmid, K.W.; Neumann, H.P. Partial versus total adrenalectomy by the posterior retroperitoneoscopic approach: Early and long-term results of 325 consecutive procedures in primary adrenal neoplasias. *World J. Surg.* **2004**, *28*, 1323–1329. [CrossRef]
11. Reincke, M.; Bancos, I.; Mulatero, P.; Scholl, U.I.; Stowasser, M.; Williams, T.A. Diagnosis and treatment of primary aldosteronism. *Lancet Diabetes Endocrinol.* **2021**, *9*, 876–892. [CrossRef] [PubMed]
12. Carey, R.M.; Calhoun, D.A.; Bakris, G.L.; Brook, R.D.; Daugherty, S.L.; Dennison-Himmelfarb, C.R.; Egan, B.M.; Flack, J.M.; Gidding, S.S.; Judd, E.; et al. Resistant Hypertension: Detection, Evaluation, and Management: A Scientific Statement From the American Heart Association. *Hypertension* **2018**, *72*, e53–e90. [CrossRef] [PubMed]
13. Smith, S.M.; Huo, T.; Delia Johnson, B.; Bittner, V.; Kelsey, S.F.; Vido Thompson, D.; Noel Bairey Merz, C.; Pepine, C.J.; Cooper-Dehoff, R.M. Cardiovascular and mortality risk of apparent resistant hypertension in women with suspected myocardial ischemia: A report from the NHLBI-sponsored WISE Study. *J. Am. Heart Assoc.* **2014**, *3*, e000660. [CrossRef] [PubMed]
14. de la Sierra, A.; Segura, J.; Banegas, J.R.; Gorostidi, M.; de la Cruz, J.J.; Armario, P.; Oliveras, A.; Ruilope, L.M. Clinical features of 8295 patients with resistant hypertension classified on the basis of ambulatory blood pressure monitoring. *Hypertension* **2011**, *57*, 898–902. [CrossRef] [PubMed]
15. Daugherty, S.L.; Powers, J.D.; Magid, D.J.; Tavel, H.M.; Masoudi, F.A.; Margolis, K.L.; O'Connor, P.J.; Selby, J.V.; Ho, P.M. Incidence and prognosis of resistant hypertension in hypertensive patients. *Circulation* **2012**, *125*, 1635–1642. [CrossRef]
16. Egan, B.M.; Zhao, Y.; Axon, R.N.; Brzezinski, W.A.; Ferdinand, K.C. Uncontrolled and apparent treatment resistant hypertension in the United States, 1988 to 2008. *Circulation* **2011**, *124*, 1046–1058. [CrossRef]
17. Persell, S.D. Prevalence of resistant hypertension in the United States, 2003–2008. *Hypertension* **2011**, *57*, 1076–1080. [CrossRef]
18. Ohno, Y.; Sone, M.; Inagaki, N.; Yamasaki, T.; Ogawa, O.; Takeda, Y.; Kurihara, I.; Itoh, H.; Umakoshi, H.; Tsuiki, M.; et al. Prevalence of Cardiovascular Disease and Its Risk Factors in Primary Aldosteronism: A Multicenter Study in Japan. *Hypertension* **2018**, *71*, 530–537. [CrossRef]
19. Monticone, S.; D'Ascenzo, F.; Moretti, C.; Williams, T.A.; Veglio, F.; Gaita, F.; Mulatero, P. Cardiovascular events and target organ damage in primary aldosteronism compared with essential hypertension: A systematic review and meta-analysis. *Lancet Diabetes Endocrinol.* **2018**, *6*, 41–50. [CrossRef]
20. Whelton, P.K.; Carey, R.M.; Aronow, W.S.; Casey, D.E., Jr.; Collins, K.J.; Dennison Himmelfarb, C.; DePalma, S.M.; Gidding, S.; Jamerson, K.A.; Jones, D.W.; et al. 2017 ACC/AHA/AAPA/ABC/ACPM/AGS/APhA/ASH/ASPC/NMA/PCNA Guideline for the Prevention, Detection, Evaluation, and Management of High Blood Pressure in Adults: A Report of the American College of Cardiology/American Heart Association Task Force on Clinical Practice Guidelines. *Hypertension* **2018**, *71*, e13–e115. [CrossRef]

21. Fallo, F.; Pilon, C.; Urbanet, R. Primary aldosteronism and metabolic syndrome. *Horm. Metab. Res.* **2012**, *44*, 208–214. [CrossRef] [PubMed]
22. Fallo, F.; Veglio, F.; Bertello, C.; Sonino, N.; Della Mea, P.; Ermani, M.; Rabbia, F.; Federspil, G.; Mulatero, P. Prevalence and characteristics of the metabolic syndrome in primary aldosteronism. *J. Clin. Endocrinol. Metab.* **2006**, *91*, 454–459. [CrossRef] [PubMed]
23. Künzel, H.E. Psychopathological symptoms in patients with primary hyperaldosteronism—possible pathways. *Horm. Metab. Res.* **2012**, *44*, 202–207. [CrossRef] [PubMed]
24. Loh, H.H.; Sukor, N. Primary aldosteronism and obstructive sleep apnea: What do we know thus far? *Front. Endocrinol.* **2022**, *13*, 976979. [CrossRef]
25. Rathmann, W.; Bongaerts, B.; Carius, H.J.; Kruppert, S.; Kostev, K. Basic characteristics and representativeness of the German Disease Analyzer database. *Int. J. Clin. Pharmacol. Ther.* **2018**, *56*, 459–466. [CrossRef]
26. Loosen, S.H.; Roderburg, C.; Curth, O.; Gaensbacher, J.; Joerdens, M.; Luedde, T.; Konrad, M.; Kostev, K.; Luedde, M. The spectrum of comorbidities at the initial diagnosis of heart failure a case control study. *Sci. Rep.* **2022**, *12*, 2670. [CrossRef]
27. Jacob, L.; Gyasi, R.M.; Koyanagi, A.; Haro, J.M.; Smith, L.; Kostev, K. Prevalence of and Risk Factors for Adhesive Capsulitis of the Shoulder in Older Adults from Germany. *J. Clin. Med.* **2023**, *12*, 669. [CrossRef]
28. Schirpenbach, C.; Segmiller, F.; Diederich, S.; Hahner, S.; Lorenz, R.; Rump, L.C.; Seufert, J.; Quinkler, M.; Bidlingmaier, M.; Beuschlein, F.; et al. The diagnosis and treatment of primary hyperaldosteronism in Germany: Results on 555 patients from the German Conn Registry. *Dtsch. Arztebl. Int.* **2009**, *106*, 305–311. [CrossRef]
29. Araujo-Castro, M.; Paja Fano, M.; González Boillos, M.; Pla Peris, B.; Pascual-Corrales, E.; García Cano, A.M.; Parra Ramírez, P.; Rojas-Marcos, P.M.; Ruiz-Sanchez, J.G.; Vicente Delgado, A.; et al. Evolution of the cardiometabolic profile of primary hyperaldosteronism patients treated with adrenalectomy and with mineralocorticoid receptor antagonists: Results from the SPAIN-ALDO Registry. *Endocrine* **2022**, *76*, 687–696. [CrossRef]
30. Reincke, M.; Fischer, E.; Gerum, S.; Merkle, K.; Schulz, S.; Pallauf, A.; Quinkler, M.; Hanslik, G.; Lang, K.; Hahner, S.; et al. Observational study mortality in treated primary aldosteronism: The German Conn's registry. *Hypertension* **2012**, *60*, 618–624. [CrossRef]
31. Born-Frontsberg, E.; Reincke, M.; Rump, L.C.; Hahner, S.; Diederich, S.; Lorenz, R.; Allolio, B.; Seufert, J.; Schirpenbach, C.; Beuschlein, F.; et al. Cardiovascular and cerebrovascular comorbidities of hypokalemic and normokalemic primary aldosteronism: Results of the German Conn's Registry. *J. Clin. Endocrinol. Metab.* **2009**, *94*, 1125–1130. [CrossRef] [PubMed]
32. Reincke, M.; Meisinger, C.; Holle, R.; Quinkler, M.; Hahner, S.; Beuschlein, F.; Bidlingmaier, M.; Seissler, J.; Endres, S. Is primary aldosteronism associated with diabetes mellitus? Results of the German Conn's Registry. *Horm. Metab. Res.* **2010**, *42*, 435–439. [CrossRef] [PubMed]
33. Hanslik, G.; Wallaschofski, H.; Dietz, A.; Riester, A.; Reincke, M.; Allolio, B.; Lang, K.; Quack, I.; Rump, L.C.; Willenberg, H.S.; et al. Increased prevalence of diabetes mellitus and the metabolic syndrome in patients with primary aldosteronism of the German Conn's Registry. *Eur. J. Endocrinol.* **2015**, *173*, 665–675. [CrossRef] [PubMed]
34. Araujo-Castro, M.; Paja Fano, M.; Pla Peris, B.; González Boillos, M.; Pascual-Corrales, E.; García Cano, A.M.; Parra Ramírez, P.; Martín Rojas-Marcos, P.; Ruiz-Sanchez, J.G.; Vicente Delgado, A.; et al. Prevalence, risk factors and evolution of diabetes mellitus after treatment in primary aldosteronism. Results from the SPAIN-ALDO registry. *J. Endocrinol. Investig.* **2023**, *46*, 2343–2352. [CrossRef]
35. Vaidya, A.; Carey, R.M. Evolution of the Primary Aldosteronism Syndrome: Updating the Approach. *J. Clin. Endocrinol. Metab.* **2020**, *105*, 3771–3783. [CrossRef]
36. Jia, M.; Yu, H.; Liu, Z.; He, M.; Zhong, S.; Xu, X.; Song, X. Normotensive presentation in primary aldosteronism: A report of two cases. *J. Renin-Angiotensin-Aldosterone Syst. JRAAS* **2021**, *22*, 14703203211003780. [CrossRef]
37. Cohen, J.B.; Cohen, D.L.; Herman, D.S.; Leppert, J.T.; Byrd, J.B.; Bhalla, V. Testing for Primary Aldosteronism and Mineralocorticoid Receptor Antagonist Use Among U.S. Veterans: A Retrospective Cohort Study. *Ann. Intern. Med.* **2021**, *174*, 289–297. [CrossRef]
38. Hill, M.A.; Sowers, J.R. Mineralocorticoid antagonists and ENaC inhibitors in hyperaldosteronism. *J. Clin. Hypertens.* **2019**, *21*, 929–931. [CrossRef]
39. Byrd, J.B.; Turcu, A.F.; Auchus, R.J. Primary Aldosteronism: Practical Approach to Diagnosis and Management. *Circulation* **2018**, *138*, 823–835. [CrossRef]
40. Chen, Z.W.; Hung, C.S.; Wu, V.C.; Lin, Y.H. Primary Aldosteronism and Cerebrovascular Diseases. *Endocrinol. Metab.* **2018**, *33*, 429–434. [CrossRef]
41. Greene, E.L.; Kren, S.; Hostetter, T.H. Role of aldosterone in the remnant kidney model in the rat. *J. Clin. Investig.* **1996**, *98*, 1063–1068. [CrossRef] [PubMed]
42. Hollenberg, N.K. Aldosterone in the development and progression of renal injury. *Kidney Int.* **2004**, *66*, 1–9. [CrossRef] [PubMed]
43. Shibata, S.; Nagase, M.; Yoshida, S.; Kawachi, H.; Fujita, T. Podocyte as the target for aldosterone: Roles of oxidative stress and Sgk1. *Hypertension* **2007**, *49*, 355–364. [CrossRef] [PubMed]
44. Emanuele, E.; Geroldi, D.; Minoretti, P.; Coen, E.; Politi, P. Increased plasma aldosterone in patients with clinical depression. *Arch. Med. Res.* **2005**, *36*, 544–548. [CrossRef] [PubMed]

45. Murck, H.; Held, K.; Ziegenbein, M.; Künzel, H.; Koch, K.; Steiger, A. The renin-angiotensin-aldosterone system in patients with depression compared to controls--a sleep endocrine study. *BMC Psychiatry* **2003**, *3*, 15. [CrossRef]
46. Nowacki, J.; Wingenfeld, K.; Kaczmarczyk, M.; Chae, W.R.; Salchow, P.; Abu-Tir, I.; Piber, D.; Hellmann-Regen, J.; Otte, C. Steroid hormone secretion after stimulation of mineralocorticoid and NMDA receptors and cardiovascular risk in patients with depression. *Transl. Psychiatry* **2020**, *10*, 109. [CrossRef]
47. Murck, H.; Adolf, C.; Schneider, A.; Schlageter, L.; Heinrich, D.; Ritzel, K.; Sturm, L.; Quinkler, M.; Beuschlein, F.; Reincke, M.; et al. Differential effects of reduced mineralocorticoid receptor activation by unilateral adrenalectomy vs mineralocorticoid antagonist treatment in patients with primary aldosteronism—Implications for depression and anxiety. *J. Psychiatr. Res.* **2021**, *137*, 376–382. [CrossRef]
48. Gerards, J.; Heinrich, D.A.; Adolf, C.; Meisinger, C.; Rathmann, W.; Sturm, L.; Nirschl, N.; Bidlingmaier, M.; Beuschlein, F.; Thorand, B.; et al. Impaired Glucose Metabolism in Primary Aldosteronism Is Associated With Cortisol Cosecretion. *J. Clin. Endocrinol. Metab.* **2019**, *104*, 3192–3202. [CrossRef]
49. Adler, G.K.; Murray, G.R.; Turcu, A.F.; Nian, H.; Yu, C.; Solorzano, C.C.; Manning, R.; Peng, D.; Luther, J.M. Primary Aldosteronism Decreases Insulin Secretion and Increases Insulin Clearance in Humans. *Hypertension* **2020**, *75*, 1251–1259. [CrossRef]
50. Chen, Y.; Chen, X.; Chen, Q.; Yu, C. Non-Alcoholic Fatty Liver Disease and Hypokalemia in Primary Aldosteronism Among Chinese Population. *Front. Endocrinol.* **2021**, *12*, 565714. [CrossRef]
51. Fallo, F.; Dalla Pozza, A.; Tecchio, M.; Tona, F.; Sonino, N.; Ermani, M.; Catena, C.; Bertello, C.; Mulatero, P.; Sabato, N.; et al. Nonalcoholic fatty liver disease in primary aldosteronism: A pilot study. *Am. J. Hypertens.* **2010**, *23*, 2–5. [CrossRef] [PubMed]

biomedicines

MDPI

Article

Subclinical Hypothyroidism and Gestational Hypertensive Disorders in a Cohort of Romanian Pregnant Women with Gestational Diabetes Mellitus: A Pilot Study

Muntean Mihai [1], Săsăran Vladut [1,*], Pop Gheorghe Lucian [2], Muntean Elena Irina [3], Nyulas Victoria [4] and Mărginean Claudiu [1]

[1] Department of Obstetrics and Gynecology 2, University of Medicine Pharmacy Science and Technology George Emil Palade of Târgu Mureș, 540142 Târgu Mureș, Romania; munteanmihai@yahoo.com (M.M.); marginean.claudiu@gmail.com (M.C.)

[2] Department of Obstetrics and Gynecology, Polizu Hospital Clinic, University of Medicine Pharmacy Carl Davila, 050474 Bucharest, Romania; popluciangh@icloud.com

[3] Algcocalm SRL, 540360 Târgu Mureș, Romania; irinagauca@yahoo.com

[4] Department of Informatics and Medical Biostatistics, University of Medicine Pharmacy Science and Technology George Emil Palade of Târgu Mureș, 540142 Târgu Mureș, Romania; victoria.rus@umfst.ro

* Correspondence: vlad_sasaran0403@yahoo.com; Tel.: +40-741930348

Abstract: Objective: This study aimed to explore whether subclinical hypothyroidism (SCH) treated with levothyroxine in pregnancy complicated by gestational diabetes mellitus (GDM) is associated with an increased risk of gestational hypertensive disorders (GHDs) (gestational hypertension and preeclampsia). Methods: 96 pregnant women with GDM were enrolled in this study and grouped as per the European Thyroid Association criteria into the SCH (n = 21) and euthyroid groups (n = 75). All subjects were tested for anthropometric parameters, maternal glucose homeostasis parameters, lipid levels, thyroid function tests, and blood pressure. All GDM pregnant women received nutritional and insulin therapy where needed, and the SCH group received levothyroxine treatment. Then, the maternal and newborn outcomes were compared. Data were analyzed using Student's *t*-test, Mann–Whitney U, and Chi-square tests wherever applicable. *p* values of <0.05 were considered significant. Results: Patients with GDM and SCH had a pre-pregnancy BMI and BMI at inclusion in the study smaller than those of the euthyroid group ($p = 0.0004$, $p = 0.0009$). There were no significant differences between groups regarding the incidence of GHD, preterm prelabor rupture of membranes (PPROMs), macrosomia, low birth weight, and fetal distress ($p > 0.05$). Patients with GDM and SCH treated with levothyroxine had more premature delivery than the euthyroid group ($p = 0.03$). Conclusions: Subclinical hypothyroidism treated with levothyroxine in women with GDM does not increase the risk of gestational hypertensive disorders, but is associated with increased risk for prematurity.

Keywords: gestational diabetes mellitus; subclinical hypothyroidism; gestational hypertension; perinatal outcome

1. Introduction

Pregnancy is a challenging test for maternal thyroid function. Placental deiodinase type 3 degradation of thyroid hormones, renal iodide clearance, and serum thyroxine-binding globulin levels increase during pregnancy [1]. The consequences are an increased need for thyroid hormones T3 and T4 production throughout pregnancy, increased serum concentrations of total T4 and T3, increased free T4 (FT4) levels, decreased serum thyroid stimulating hormone (TSH) and thyroglobulin levels, and in iodine-deficient areas, thyroid hormone production decrease [2].

Thyroid hormones T4 and T3 are essential for fetal growth and neurodevelopment during pregnancy. The fetal thyroid gland begins to produce adequate quantities of thyroid hormones during the second trimester. Thus, the fetus depends on maternal thyroid hormones during pregnancy, especially during the first trimester [3].

Hypothyroidism's causes could be iodine deficiency, Hashimoto's thyroiditis, post thyroidectomy, secondary to medication (amiodarone), suppurative thyroiditis, lymphocytic hypophysitis, Sheehan's syndrome, and congenital hypothyroidism [4].

Subclinical hypothyroidism (SCH) represents an early stage of thyroid failure, typically diagnosed in the general population by a TSH level below 10 mU/l and a normal FT4 level [5,6]. The diagnosis is biochemical because the symptoms are mild and non-specific [7]. In recent years, significant progress has been made in the methods of diagnosing and treating thyroid disorders that occur during pregnancy [8].

A serum TSH level higher than the upper limit of the pregnancy-trimester-related reference range associated with an average serum FT4 concentration is defined as SCH in pregnancy [9]. The incidence of SCH in pregnancy in Europe is 10% [10]. The European Thyroid Association recommends using TSH levels higher than 2.5 mU/l for the first trimester, 3.0 mU/l for the second trimester, and 3.5 mU/l for the third trimester of pregnancy for diagnosing SCH when trimester-specific reference ranges are not available [9]. The Romanian Society of Endocrinology recommends using European Thyroid Association and American Thyroid Association recommendations for diagnosing and treating SCH in pregnancy [10]. In different countries, the incidence of this condition may vary depending on which cut-off values are used to define SCH.

Women with SCH with or without positive thyroid peroxidase antibodies (TPOAb) are at high risk of abortion [11], premature rupture of membranes, placental abruption, newborn death [12], gestational hypertension [13], preeclampsia [11,14,15], and gestational diabetes mellitus (GDM) [11,16], but some other studies have not found that SCH with or without positive TPOAb is associated with pregnancy complications [17–19].

Additionally, the impact of levothyroxine treatment in pregnant women with SCH is not clear. Some studies show that levothyroxine treatment may lower the risks of abortion and stillbirth [20], gestational hypertension, preterm delivery [21,22] GDM [23], low birth weight [24], and neonatal death [22]. Others have found that levothyroxine therapy does not influence obstetrical, neonatal outcomes, and childhood IQ score or neurodevelopmental outcomes [25,26], and others have found that treatment with levothyroxine is associated with a higher rate of preterm labor in women with SCH [20].

The incidence of GHD in Romania is 3.7% [27]. GHD is associated with a higher incidence of perinatal complications, like preterm birth, SGA neonates, stillbirths, and delivery by cesarean section [27].

Another complication of pregnancy is gestational diabetes mellitus (GDM) [28], which has a prevalence of 10.9% in Europe [29]. The American Diabetes Association (ADA) defined GDM as any glucose intolerance diagnosed during the second or third trimester of pregnancy [30]. GDM occurrence is associated with some risk factors, like heredo-colateral history of type 2 diabetes mellitus (T2DM), maternal age above 30–35 years, increased body mass index (BMI) greater than 25 kg/m^2, personal history of macrosomia (newborn with a birth weight > 4000 g), hypothyroidism, smoking, and other ethnicities than Caucasian [31,32]. Its pathophysiology involves insulin resistance, β-cell dysfunction, chronic inflammation, and low circulating adiponectin levels [32–34]. GDM induces a wide range of complications for mothers and newborns. Some of the short-term complications are polyhydramnios, gestational hypertension [35], pre-eclampsia, operative delivery, shoulder dystocia, birth canal trauma, macrosomia, neonatal hypoglycemia, and jaundice [28]. Long-term complications include the mother's increasing risk of T2DM, metabolic syndrome, and cardiovascular disease, and the offspring's long-term complications are increased risks of hyperglycemia, T2DM, obesity, and cardiovascular disease [28].

The prevalence of SCH and GDM described in the literature is 4.18% [19].

Although there are data from Romania on iodine deficiency and its treatment in pregnant women [36], there are no data on subclinical hypothyroidism or the evolution of these patients under treatment with levothyroxine.

This study aimed to explore the impact of SCH treated with levothyroxine on gestational hypertensive disorders (GHDs) (gestational hypertension and preeclampsia) in pregnant women diagnosed with GDM.

2. Material and Method

2.1. Study Design

The University of Medicine, Pharmacy, Science and Technology "G. E. Palade" of Târgu–Mures Ethics Committee authorized this study (decision number 1557/2022) in accordance with the principles of the Declaration of Helsinki (1964).

2.2. Description of Study Area and Duration of Study

This prospective case–control study was conducted at Obstetrics and Gynecology Clinic 2 in Târgu Mureș, Romania, between 1 January 2022 and 15 October 2024. Our cohort was consecutively selected and included pregnant women diagnosed with GDM.

2.3. Inclusion and Exclusion Criteria

The inclusion criteria were as follows: singleton pregnancy between 24 and 28 weeks of gestation (WG), Romanian ethnicity, diagnosis of GDM, age between 18 and 46 years, compliance with follow-up conditions, and delivery at the Obstetrics and Gynecology Clinic 2 Târgu Mureș. The exclusion criteria included the following: known patients with hypothyroidism with or without positive TPOAb, diagnosed before pregnancy or in the first trimester of pregnancy; patients with type 1 diabetes or T2DM diagnosed before pregnancy; pregnancies with chromosomal or fetal malformations; cases of intrauterine fetal death; and those who lacked informed consent.

Before enrollment in this study, written informed consent was obtained from all patients.

After applying the inclusion and exclusion criteria, we included 96 pregnant women with GDM in this study. Based on their TSH and FT4 results at the time of the oral glucose tolerance test (OGTT), they were divided into two groups: 75 euthyroid pregnant women with GDM and TSH levels < 3.0 mU/l and 21 pregnant women with GDM and TSH levels $\geq$ 3.0 mU/l, based on European Thyroid Association recommendations (Figure 1).

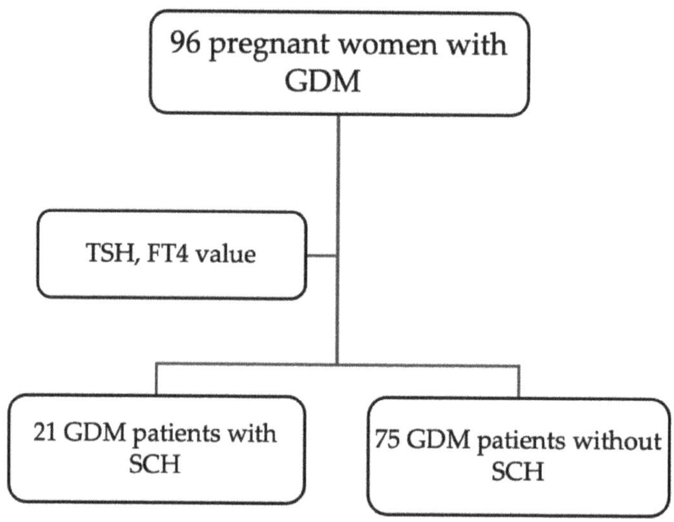

Figure 1. Flow chart of study participants at 24–28 WG. Note: GDM = gestational diabetes mellitus, FT4 = free T4, SCH = subclinical hypothyroidism, TSH = thyroid stimulating hormone.

2.4. Diagnosis of GDM

The International Association of Diabetes and Pregnancy Study Groups criteria were used to diagnose GDM. One or more abnormal glucose values above ≥92 mg/dl (≥5.2 mmol/l), 1 h ≥ 180 mg/dl (>10 mmol/l), or 2 h ≥ 153 mg/dl (>8.5 mmol/l) [37] were used for GDM diagnosis. Patients diagnosed with GDM were advised to engage in moderate physical activity, follow nutritional therapy, and monitor their glycemic status through three daily assessments of fasting and postprandial glucose levels for two weeks. A diabetologist prescribed insulin therapy at a dosage of 0.7–1.0 units/kg of body weight per day for women who did not achieve glycemic control through diet. The target glucose levels were fasting below 95 mg/dl and postprandial levels below 120 mg/dl at 2 h after eating [38]. The pregnant women continued to monitor their glucose levels until birth under the surveillance of the diabetologist.

2.5. Diagnosis of SCH

According to the European Thyroid Association, SCH is diagnosed if TSH levels in the second trimester (24–28 WG) are 3.0 mU/l [9]. Levothyroxine treatment was initiated after SCH was diagnosed at 24–28 WG at the OGTT time. An endocrinologist treated patients with SCH by administering 1.2 μg/kg/day of levothyroxine to achieve a TSH level below 2.5 mU/l. All patients undergoing levothyroxine treatment had their TSH levels checked at 4-week intervals. Their levothyroxine dosage was adjusted according to the endocrinologist's advice to achieve a TSH level of <3 mU/l in the second trimester and <3.5 mU/l in the third trimester of pregnancy. As our study did not assess thyroid peroxidase antibodies (TPOAb), we are considering including TPOAb testing in future studies.

After inclusion in the study, all pregnant women were scheduled for appointments for routine prenatal surveillance every two weeks or sooner if clinically indicated until delivery as part of routine prenatal care.

Upon inclusion in this study, at 24–28 WG, we collected demographic characteristics like maternal age, gestation, parity, smoking, chronic hypertension, and heredo-collateral history of T2DM; we performed anthropometric measurements and obtained a fasting blood sample. At delivery, we reviewed the medical records of each patient. We recorded information on pregnancy complications (gestational hypertension, preeclampsia, placental abruption, premature delivery < 37 weeks, preterm prelabor rupture of membranes (PPROM) < 37 weeks, macrosomia, low birth weight, and fetal distress), mode of delivery, and anthropometric measurements of the mothers and newborns.

2.6. Maternal and Neonatal Complications

We defined maternal and neonatal complications as follows:

Gestational hypertension (GH) = a systolic blood pressure reading of 140 mm Hg or higher, or a diastolic blood pressure reading of 90 mm Hg or higher, or both, on two separate occasions at least 4 h apart after 20 weeks of pregnancy in a woman who previously had normal blood pressure [39].

Preeclampsia = gestational hypertension and proteinuria ≥ 300 mg/24 h urine collection [39].

Placental abruption = the premature separation of the placenta from the uterine wall after 20 WG and before birth [40].

Premature delivery = birth at less than 37 completed WG, according to ICD 10 definitions (O60).

Preterm prelabor rupture of membranes (PPROM) = membrane rupture before labor that occurs before 37 WG [41].

Macrosomia = birth weight ≥ 4000 g [42].

Low birth weight = birth weight below 2500 g [43].

Fetal distress = Cardiotocographic signs of fetal compromise in labor [44].

2.7. Anthropometric Measurements

In this study, we included maternal pre-pregnancy BMI, BMI at 24–28 WG, and at birth. Maternal pre-pregnancy BMI (kg/m^2) was calculated from pre-pregnancy medical records or where it was impossible to patient-reported pre-pregnancy weight and height measured during the first prenatal visit during the first trimester of pregnancy. BMI at 24–28 WG was measured during OGTT, and weight at birth was measured at admission to the hospital before birth. The patient's height (cm) was measured using a wall tape measure without shoes and estimated to the nearest 1 mm. The patient's weight was measured using a Beurer PS digital scale (Beurer Gmbh, Ulm, Germany) and subtracting 0.5 kg as the weight of the patient's clothing. Newborn anthropometric measurements (weight, length, and ponderal index at birth) were performed in the first 30 min after birth. Ponderal index was calculated as 100 × [birthweight (g)/length (cm^3)].

Systolic blood pressure (SBP) and diastolic blood pressure (DBP) were measured according to the American College of Obstetricians and Gynecologists Practice Bulletin no 202 recommendations at the inclusion in this study [39].

2.8. Biochemical Analyses

We obtained maternal blood samples during OGTT in a fasting state between 8 and 10 a.m. using the classic peripheral blood collection technique before any treatment for GDM was administered.

We measured the fasting glucose level, 1 h glucose level, and 2 h glucose level after administering 75 g of glucose orally from maternal blood at 24–28 WG. Additionally, we also assessed TSH, FT4, C-reactive protein (CRP) level, HbA1c, HOMA-IR, total cholesterol (TC), high-density lipoprotein cholesterol (HDL-C), low-density lipoprotein cholesterol (LDL-C), and triglycerides (TG).

The Atellica Solution CH 930 device (Siemens Healthcare GmbH, Forchheim, Germany) was used to determine glucose levels in blood using spectrophotometry, CRP and glycosylated hemoglobin using turbidimetry, TC, HDL-C, LDL-C, and TG values using photometry, and TSH and FT4 using chemiluminescent microparticle immunoassay. The formula used to estimate IR HOMA was: [(fasting insulin (mU/l) × fasting glucose (mmol/l)]/22.5 [45].

2.9. Statistical Analysis

GraphPad Prism version 9.0 software (GraphPad Software, Boston, MA, USA) was used for statistical analyses. The median (IQR) and mean ± standard deviation were used to express continuous data. Percentages were used to express categorical data. When dealing with regularly distributed continuous variables, Student's *t*-test was utilized, and when dealing with non-normally distributed data, the Mann–Whitney test was chosen. Clinical characteristics of SCH and control participants were compared using the chi-square test or Fisher's exact testing for categorical data. A two-tailed *p*-value of less than 0.05 was accepted as statistically significant.

The power sample was calculated with G*Power sample size calculation software (version 3.1.9.7.), which indicated that for a power of 80% and a high effect size of 0.7, a sample ratio of 1/3 requires 72 patients for the control group and 21 patients for the testing group.

3. Results

3.1. Demographic, Anthropometric Characteristics, and Laboratory Results at 24–28 Weeks of Pregnancy

Our study found that patients with SCH were older than patients from the euthyroid group, but without significant differences ($p = 0.25$). There were no significant differences between groups regarding gestation ($p = 0.61$), parity ($p = 0.55$), smoking ($p = 0.14$), heredo-colateral history of T2DM ($p = 0.79$), chronic hypertension ($p > 0.99$), and gestational age at inclusion in this study ($p = 0.73$). Patient characteristics are shown in Table 1.

We found that patients from the euthyroid group had higher pre-pregnancy BMI (28.54 kg/m^2, 95% CI 27.25–29.84 kg/m^2 (p = 0.0004)), BMI (31.14 kg/m^2, 95% CI 29.9–32.39 kg/m^2 (p = 0.0009)), and CRP values (0.8 mg/dl, 95% CI 0.65–0.94 (p = 0.01)) at inclusion in this study compared with patients from the SCH group. There were no differences between groups regarding SBP, DBP values, glucose homeostasis parameters, and lipid values. The serum values of TSH in the SCH group were significantly greater than those in the euthyroid group (3.82 mU/l, 95%CI 3.5–4.13 (p < 0.0001)). There were no differences in FT4 values between the groups (p = 0.27).

Table 1. Demographic and anthropometric characteristics, and laboratory results at 24–28 weeks of pregnancy.

Parameters	Euthyroid Group n = 75	SCH Group n = 21	p-Value
Age, years, Mean, (SD)	31.49 ± 5.33	32.71 ± 3.88	0.25
Gestation, Mean, (SD)	2.47 ± 1.15	2.46 ± 1.59	0.61
Parity, Mean, (SD)	1.87 ± 0.82	1.66 ± 0.48	0.55
Smoking, %	19 (25.33%)	2 (9.52%)	0.14
Heredo-colateral history of T2DM, %	23 (30.66%)	7 (33.33%)	0.79
Chronic hypertension, %	3 (4%)	0	>0.99
Gestational age, weeks, Mean, (SD)	25.95 ± 1.33	25.86 ± 1.31	0.73
Pre-pregnancy BMI, kg/m^2, Mean, (SD)	28.54 ± 5.63	25.04 ± 3.03	0.0004
BMI, kg/m^2, Mean, (SD)	31.14 ± 5.41	27.84 ± 3.22	0.0009
SBP, mmHg, Mean, (SD)	109.5 ± 11.89	113.8 ± 13.14	0.18
DBP, mmHg, Mean, (SD)	70.28 ± 8.39	73.86 ± 7.15	0.059
CRP, mg/dl, Mean, (min-max)	0.8 ± 0.63	0.43 ± 0.19	0.01
Fasting glucose level, mg/dl, Mean, (SD)	97.15 ± 13.5	98.33 ± 12.17	0.48
1 h glucose level, mg/dl, Mean, (SD)	176.7 ± 34.01	181.0 ± 36.93	0.76
2 h glucose level, mg/dl, Mean, (SD)	136.9 ± 34.03	149.3 ± 38.08	0.40
HbA1c, %, Mean, (SD)	5.4 ± 0.56	5.33 ± 0.35	0.89
IR HOMA, Mean, (min-max)	5.83 ± 12.23	3.85 ± 3.15	0.28
T-cholesterol, mg/dl, mean, SD	235.8 ± 45.64	246.1 ± 29.25	0.21
HDL cholesterol, mg/dl, mean, SD	65.89 ± 13.99	69.33 ± 20.71	0.89
LDL cholesterol, mg/dl, mean, SD	141.2 ± 41.98	140.7 ± 27.46	0.95
Triglycerides, mg/dl, mean, SD	226 ± 74.75	245.4 ± 75.74	0.19
TSH mU/l, mean, SD	1.72 ± 0.61	3.82 ± 0.69	<0.0001
FT4, ng/dl, SD	0.91 ± 0.2	0.96 ± 0.11	0.27

Note: SCH = subclinical hypothyroidism; T2DM = type 2 diabetes mellitus; GDM = gestational diabetes mellitus, BMI = body mass index; SBP = systolic blood pressure, DBP = diastolic blood pressure, CRP = C reactive protein; HbA1c = glycosylated hemoglobin; IR HOMA = homeostasis model of assessment for insulin resistance; T-cholesterol = total cholesterol; HDL cholesterol = high-density lipoprotein cholesterol; LDL cholesterol = low-density lipoprotein cholesterol; TSH = thyroid stimulating hormone; FT4 = free T4; SD = standard deviation.

3.2. Maternal and Newborn Demographic, Anthropometric Characteristics, Results at Birth

There was no difference between groups concerning gestational age at birth ($p = 0.42$), cesarean section rate ($p = 0.45$), newborn weight at birth ($p = 0.58$), and newborn ponderal index ($p = 0.43$). However, patients from the euthyroid group had a higher BMI at birth than patients from the SCH group (33.08 kg/m^2, 95% CI 31.8–34.36 kg/m^2 ($p = 0.005$)). The patient's characteristics are shown in Table 2.

Table 2. Maternal and newborn demographic and anthropometric characteristics, and results at birth.

Parameters	Euthyroid Group n = 75	SCH Group n = 21	*p*-Value
Gestational age, weeks, Mean, (SD)	38.35 ± 1.38	38.62 ± 1.35	0.42
BMI, kg/m^2, Mean, (SD)	33.08 ± 5.54	30.04 ± 3.73	0.005
Cesarean section, n, %	41(54.66%)	14(66.66%)	0.45
Newborn weight, grams, Mean, (SD)	3482 ± 517.8	3408 ± 557	0.58
Ponderal index	2.27 ± 0.21	2.23 ± 0.21	0.43

Note: SCH = subclinical hypothyroidism; BMI = body mass index; SD = standard deviation.

3.3. Maternal and Perinatal Outcomes

The incidence of GH in the euthyroid group was 17.33%, and in the SCH group, it was 28.57%.

We found no differences between the groups regarding the incidence of GHD, PPROM, macrosomia, low birth weight, and fetal distress. In both groups, there were no cases of placental abruption. However, patients from the SCH group had more premature deliveries ($p = 0.03$) than those in the euthyroid group. The patients' characteristics are shown in Table 3.

Table 3. Maternal and perinatal outcomes.

Parameters	Euthyroid Group n = 75	SCH Group n = 21	*p*-Value
GH, n, %	13(17.33%)	6(28.57%)	0.35
Preeclampsia, n, %	0	1(4.76%)	0.21
Placental abruption, n, %	0	0	N/A
Premature delivery < 37 weeks, n, %	1(1.33%)	3(14.28%)	0.03
PPROM, n, %	2(2.66%)	0	>0.99
Macrosomia, n, %	15(20%)	2(9.52%)	0.34
Low birth weight, n, %	4(5.33%)	2(9.52%)	0.60
Fetal distress, n, %	5(6.66%)	1(4.76%)	>0.99

Note: SCH = subclinical hypothyroidism; GH = gestational hypertension; PPROM = preterm prelabor rupture of membranes.

Regarding the relationship between TSH levels at inclusion in the study and premature birth, we found that TSH levels above 4.2 mU/l had an excellent predictive ability to predict premature delivery with an AUROC of 0.94 (95% CI 0.75 to 0.99) (Figure 2).

Table 4 shows the results of multivariate regression analyses assessing premature delivery. We found that a higher TSH level at study inclusion had an OR of 7.46 for premature delivery. Increased maternal age and GH were associated with OR of 1.46 and 7.0 for premature delivery, but without statistical significance ($p = 0.06$ and respectively 0.14). Figure 3 shows the forest plot for premature delivery.

Table 4. Multivariate regression results for premature delivery.

Parameter	OR (95%CI)	p-Value
Mother's age	1.46 (0.97–2.20)	0.06
TSH	7.46 (1.04–53.36)	0.04
Pre-pregnancy BMI	1.01 (0.67–1.52)	0.93
CRP value	0.01 (0.0–131.40)	0.37
C-section delivery	0.19 (0.01–2.62)	0.21
GH	7.0 (0.49–98.6)	0.14

Note: BMI = body mass index, CRP = C reactive protein, C = cesarean, GH = gestational. Hypertension, TSH = thyroid stimulating hormone.

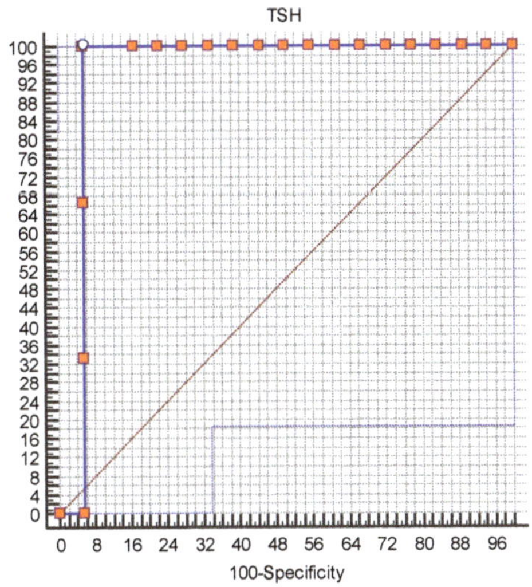

Figure 2. ROC curve for premature birth. Note: ROC curve for TSH levels at 24–28 WG for prediction of premature birth.

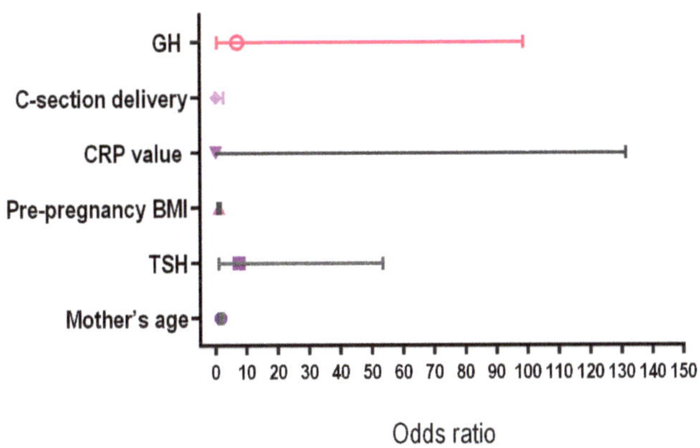

Figure 3. Forest plot for premature delivery. Note: BMI = body mass index, CRP = C reactive protein, C = cesarean, TSH = thyroid stimulating hormone.

4. Discussions

Pregnancy can affect thyroid function, and there are changes in TSH, FT4, and FT3 serum levels during pregnancy as pregnancy advances [2]. Thyroid hormones are essential for fetal growth and neurodevelopment [3]. There are variations in thyroid hormone levels according to ethnicity, country, and detection methods [9]. Iodine deficiency is the most important cause of hypothyroidism in Eastern Europe [46]. There is no trimester-specific reference range for thyroid hormones for Romanian pregnant women, so we used a trimester-specific reference range from the European Thyroid Association Guidelines to diagnose SCH in the second trimester of pregnancy [9].

Pregnant women with SCH can develop GDM [11,16] and hypertensive disorders [11,14,15], and also GDM pregnant women are at increased risk of hypertensive disorders [28], increasing the risk for adverse outcomes for the pregnant women, fetus, and newborn. Additionally, there is conflicting evidence regarding the usefulness of levothyroxine treatment of SCH in pregnancy [20–26].

This is the first study to evaluate the impact of SCH and levothyroxine treatment on maternal and neonatal outcomes of a cohort of Romanian GDM-diagnosed pregnant women.

In our cohort, there were no differences between groups regarding age at inclusion in this study (32.71 ± 3.88 vs. 31.49 ± 5.33 years, $p = 0.25$). Pregnant women with GDM and SCH from the Durcame et al. [47] study were 28.8 ± 4.6 years. This difference can be explained by postponing getting pregnant in our study group and increasing thyroid dysfunction caused by aging [48]. We did not find any differences between the groups regarding gestation, parity, smoking, heredo-colateral history of T2DM, and gestational age at the inclusion in this study. The same results were found by Durcame et al. [47] and Chen et al. [49].

Pregnant women with GDM and SCH from our cohort were overweight before pregnancy and at inclusion in this study. The pregnant women from the euthyroid group had significantly greater pre-pregnancy BMI ($p = 0.0004$) and BMI at inclusion in this study ($p = 0.0009$). Additionally, pregnant women from the SCH group had substantially lower CRP values than pregnant women from the euthyroid group ($p = 0.01$). The greater CRP serum values in the euthyroid group than those in the SCH group are in the context of low-grade chronic inflammation of greater BMI values of these patients [50]. On the contrary, Durcame et al. [47] found in their study that pregnant women with SCH were obese grade 1 at admission to the study, and the pregnant women from the euthyroid group were overweight ($p = 0.20$). Additionally, Croce et al. [51] found that TSH was significantly higher in obese women with negative TPOAb compared with overweight and normal-weight pregnant women in the first trimester of pregnancy. However, Knight et al. [52] did not find a positive correlation between SCH and BMI in the first trimester of pregnancy.

We did not find any differences between groups regarding SBP, DBP, glucose metabolism parameters, or lipid values in the second trimester of pregnancy. Only triglyceride values in both groups exceeded the reference values for healthy pregnant women in the second trimester [53] Ryckman et al. [54] showed in their meta-analysis that triglyceride levels were elevated from the first trimester until the third trimester of pregnancy of women who will develop GDM during pregnancy, suggesting the role of metabolic dysfunction early in pregnancy or even before pregnancy in GDM appearance. Wang et al. [55] found in their study that pregnant women with SCH and dyslipidemia in the first trimester of pregnancy were older (>35 years) or overweight/obese and had a greater incidence of GH, preeclampsia/eclampsia, GDM, and low birth weight. Lower thyroid hormone and higher TSH values encountered in hypothyroidism increase T-cholesterol, LDL-cholesterol, and triglyceride values by decreasing lipoprotein lipase function, reducing the activity of cholesterol 7α-hydroxylase and ATP-binding cassette transporter G5/8, and increasing Niemann–Pick C1-like 1 protein concentration; however, these changes are seen in patients with overt hypothyroidism [56].

Regarding TSH levels in the second trimester of pregnancy, they were significantly higher in the SCH group ($p < 0.0001$), with no differences for FT4 levels ($p = 0.27$). Regarding the TSH levels used to diagnose SCH, we used the European Thyroid Association's reference range (TSH > 3.0 mU/l in the second trimester of pregnancy). In the literature, there is no general agreement regarding the TSH levels used to diagnose SCH; more thresholds are used; therefore, there are contradictory conclusions. Cakmak et al. [11] used values of >2.5 mU/l and Durcame et al. [47] used the reference levels of the European Thyroid Association, but Fatima et al. [57] used the range of 4.4–10 mU/l to diagnose SCH.

Our patient groups had no differences concerning gestational age, newborn weight, or ponderal index at birth. Regarding mode of delivery, 66.66% of patients from the SCH group gave birth by cesarean section, but without statistical difference from the euthyroid group ($p = 0.45$). Also, Durcame et al. [47] found no differences between GDM pregnant women with and without SCH regarding gestational age at birth, mode of delivery, and newborn weight.

Regarding maternal complications during pregnancy, we did not find significant differences between groups regarding GH, preeclampsia, PPROM, and placental abruption.

The rate of GH in our cohort of GDM pregnant women with and without SCH (28.57% and 17.33%) was more significant than the incidence of GH found by Walker et al. [58] in a cohort of pregnant women without GDM or SCH (6.3%). This difference is because our cohort patients were older and had a greater BMI than those in the Walker et al. [58] group. In our cohort, we did not have cases of placental abruption.

Regarding GDM, GH, and preeclampsia, Kvetny et al. [59] and Bryson et al. [60] found that GH and preeclampsia appeared more frequently in women with GDM, and BMI was higher in women with GH or preeclampsia and GDM compared with controls [60]. Bryson et al. [60] found that GDM increased the risk of developing hypertensive disease during pregnancy by 1.5-fold, and this was greater in different ethnic groups with less prenatal care. From pathophysiologic points, GDM and hypertensive disorders of pregnancy share similar abnormalities, like insulin resistance, central obesity, dyslipidemia, oxidative stress, endothelial dysfunction, chronic inflammation (neutrophil activation, abnormal cytokines), and abnormal levels of adipokines (low levels of adiponectin, high levels of leptin) [61].

Regarding the role of SCH in hypertensive disorders of pregnancy (HDP), some researchers, like Cakmak et al. [11], found a significantly higher incidence ($p = 0.004$) of GH in a cohort of 930 pregnant women with untreated SCH compared with 7986 control patients, matched for age and BMI; Han et al. [14], in their meta-analysis, found that a TSH level > of 3 mU/l, regardless of trimester of pregnancy, was associated with increased risk by 1.67 times of HDP. Lai et al. [13] suggested that SCH in early pregnancy is a risk factor for GH later in pregnancy. Tolosa et al. [15], in their meta-analysis, found that SCH, defined as TSH levels above the 97.5th percentile of the reference range and FT4 levels within the reference range (2.5th–97.5th percentile), was associated with a higher risk of preeclampsia. Some previous studies concluded that alteration in thyroid hormones seen in SCH could increase the risk of hypertensive disorders of pregnancy by endothelial dysfunction resulting from a reduction in nitric oxide availability [62], impaired cardiac contractility, impaired diastolic function, and increased serum cholesterol [63]. On the contrary, other studies did not show that SCH was associated with an increased risk of gestational hypertension. Furukawa et al. [17] did not find an increased risk of GH in 167 pregnant women with SCH (median TSH 3.4 mU/l) and a mean BMI of 22 ± 3.7 Kg/m^2. The fact that they did not have obese patients in the SCH group is the reason why they did not find an increased risk of GH associated with SCH in pregnancy.

Regarding premature delivery, we observed significantly more premature delivery in the SCH group ($p = 0.03$). Stagnaro-Green et al. [64] found an increased risk of very preterm birth (<32 weeks) associated with high TSH levels. Still, they did not observe the same association in the case of moderately preterm deliveries. Lee et al. [65] found that a TSH level > 4 mU/l was associated with a 2.17-fold increased risk of prematurity. Also, we found that a level of TSH > 4.2 mU/l in the second trimester of pregnancy was associated with an OR of 7.46 (95% CI 1.04–53.36) for premature birth. One explanation for higher rates of premature births in our SCH group could be related to vascular disease etiology: endothelial dysfunction in the context of lower nitric oxide levels in SCH patients [62] and the failure of the physiologic transformation of the myometrial segment of spiral arteries, along with placental vascular lesions induced by maternal vascular poor perfusion [66,67]. Another explanation for a higher premature birth rate could be the association of GDM and SCH with gestational hypertensive disease, along with an increased rate of medically induced premature delivery [68].

Regarding newborn outcomes, we found no differences between groups in the incidences of macrosomia, low birth weight, and fetal distress. Durcame et al. [47] also found no differences between mothers with and without SCH in macrosomia and low birth weight incidence.

All GDM pregnant women in our study received nutritional and insulin therapy where needed. Pregnant women diagnosed with SCH were treated by an endocrinologist with 1.2 μg/kg/day of levothyroxine until birth to achieve a serum TSH level below 2.5 mU/l. We did not find an increased risk of GHD in our SCH group treated with levothyroxine, but our results must be interpreted with caution due to our small sample of GDM patients with SCH. We found an increased risk of premature birth in the SCH group treated with levothyroxine. Sankoda et al. [69] found in their meta-analysis that levothyroxine treatment during pregnancy with SCH was associated with a reduced risk of preterm birth when TSH levels were >4.0 mU/l, but no significant effect when TSH levels were between 2.5 and 4.0 mU/l. According to our findings, Sitoris et al. [23] found that pregnant women with untreated SCH (TSH > 3.74 mIU/l) and without TPOAb had a higher rate of GDM and pre-eclampsia compared with women without SCH. Additionally, they found that if the levothyroxine treatment was initiated even after the first trimester, the pregnant women did not develop these complications. In their meta-analysis, Ding et al. [21] found that pregnant women with SCH diagnosed after American Thyroid Association criteria (TSH > 4.0mIU/l) and treated with levothyroxine had lower risks of pregnancy loss, preterm birth, and gestational hypertension. In contrast, Yamamoto et al. [25] in their meta-analysis, which included only three randomized trials, found no benefit of levothyroxine treatment on gestational hypertension, pre-eclampsia, preterm delivery, mode of delivery, neonatal intensive care unit admission, birth weight, and gestational age at delivery.

We did not assess iodine levels and TPOAb status during the second trimester of pregnancy, which can impact thyroid function and pregnancy outcome as a confounding factor. Shenhav et al. [70] found that iodine deficiency in the third trimester of pregnancy can alter thyroid function, and He et al. [71] found that TPOAb positivity in pregnant women with and without thyroid dysfunction was associated with an increased risk of preterm delivery.

The principal strength of our study is that the same multidisciplinary team managed all women with GDM and SCH in our center throughout the study. This avoided significant variation regarding diagnosing GDM and SCH, the need for treatment (insulin and levothyroxine therapy), and perinatal management. We utilized standardized protocols to minimize outcome variations due to differences in clinical practice. We measured weight and height during the second trimester and at birth for BMI calculation instead of relying on the weight and height reported by the patient. This study is one of the first conducted in Romania to explore the GHD in pregnant women diagnosed with GDM and SCH treated with levothyroxine and underline that GDM patients with SCH treated with levothyroxine have no increased risk of GHD, PPROM, macrosomia, and LBW, but have a higher risk of premature delivery compared with GDM patients without SCH.

Our study has some limitations. All our patients were from the same area, and the small sample may have reduced the statistical power of our research. We did not assess the iodine and TPOAb status of our patients as iodine deficiency in pregnancy can influence thyroid function, and positive TPOAb during pregnancy can increase the risk of adverse pregnancy outcomes, including premature birth. We did not have long-term information about the neurodevelopment of the offspring. This study reflects our experience with the interdisciplinary approach of women with GDM and SCH. Our findings can only be applied to other perinatal centers that employ similar practices. The rate of GH in our GDM with SCH group (28.57%) is higher than that in the literature (10.9%) [72] and should be explained by the small sample of women with SCH (n = 21) in our study.

Future research could explore the TPOAb status and thyroid function of GDM patients since autoimmune disorders increase the risk of GDM. Another potential direction is to conduct long-term follow-up studies on the neurodevelopment of children born to mothers with GDM and SCH.

5. Conclusions

In conclusion, our results suggest that subclinical hypothyroidism treated with levothyroxine in women with GDM does not increase the risk of gestational hypertensive disorders but is associated with an increased risk of prematurity. Given the small sample size of this study's patients, our findings need to be confirmed in large prospective studies.

Author Contributions: Conceptualization, M.M., S.V. and M.C.; Methodology, M.M., P.G.L., M.E.I. and M.C.; Software, N.V.; Validation, M.M.; Formal analysis, M.M., P.G.L., N.V. and M.C.; Investigation, M.M., S.V. and M.E.I.; Resources, M.M., P.G.L., M.E.I. and M.C.; Data curation, N.V.; Writing—original draft, M.M., S.V., P.G.L. and M.E.I.; Writing—review & editing, M.M., S.V., P.G.L., N.V. and M.C.; Visualization, M.M. and M.C.; Supervision, M.C.; Project administration, M.M. and M.C.; Funding acquisition, M.M. All authors have read and agreed to the published version of the manuscript.

Funding: This research received no external funding.

Institutional Review Board Statement: The University of Medicine, Pharmacy, Science and Technology "G. E. Palade" of Târgu–Mures Ethics Committee authorized this study (decision number 1557/2022) in accordance with the principles of the Declaration of Helsinki (1964).

Informed Consent Statement: Informed consent was obtained from all subjects involved in the study.

Data Availability Statement: The data that support the findings of this study are available from the corresponding author V.S. upon reasonable request.

Conflicts of Interest: The authors declare no conflict of interest.

References

1. Toloza, F.J.; Abedzadeh-Anaraki, S.; Maraka, S. Subclinical Hypothyroidism in Pregnancy. *Curr. Opin. Endocrinol. Diabetes Obes.* **2019**, *26*, 225–231. [CrossRef] [PubMed]
2. Lazarus, J.H. Thyroid Function in Pregnancy. *Br. Med. Bull.* **2011**, *97*, 137–148. [CrossRef]
3. Eng, L.; Lam, L. Thyroid Function during the Fetal and Neonatal Periods. *Neoreviews* **2020**, *21*, e30–e36. [CrossRef] [PubMed]
4. Sullivan, S.A. Hypothyroidism in Pregnancy. *Clin. Obstet. Gynecol.* **2019**, *62*, 308–319. [CrossRef] [PubMed]
5. Cooper, D.S.; Biondi, B. Subclinical Thyroid Disease. *Lancet* **2012**, *379*, 1142–1154. [CrossRef]
6. Gietka-Czernel, M.; Glinicki, P. Subclinical Hypothyroidism in Pregnancy: Controversies on Diagnosis and Treatment. *Pol. Arch. Intern. Med.* **2021**, *131*, 266–275. [CrossRef]
7. Negro, R.; Stagnaro-Green, A. Diagnosis and Management of Subclinical Hypothyroidism in Pregnancy. *Bmj* **2014**, *349*, g4929. [CrossRef]
8. Chen, A.; Luo, Z.; Zhang, J.; Cao, X. Emerging Research Themes in Maternal Hypothyroidism: A Bibliometric Exploration. *Front. Immunol.* **2024**, *15*, 1370707. [CrossRef]
9. Lazarus, J.; Brown, R.S.; Daumerie, C.; Hubalewska-Dydejczyk, A.; Negro, R.; Vaidya, B. 2014 European Thyroid Association Guidelines for the Management of Subclinical Hypothyroidism in Pregnancy and in Children. *Eur. Thyroid J.* **2014**, *3*, 76–94. [CrossRef]
10. Negro, R.; Attanasio, R.; Papini, E.; Guglielmi, R.; Grimaldi, F.; Toscano, V.; Niculescu, D.A.; Paun, D.L.; Poiana, C. A 2018 Italian and Romanian Survey on Subclinical Hypothyroidism in Pregnancy. *Eur. Thyroid J.* **2018**, *7*, 294–301. [CrossRef]
11. Cakmak, B.D.; Turker, U.A.; Temur, M.; Ustunyurt, E. Pregnancy Outcomes of Antibody Negative and Untreated Subclinical Hypothyroidism. *J. Obstet. Gynaecol. Res.* **2019**, *45*, 810–816. [CrossRef] [PubMed]
12. Maraka, S.; Ospina, N.M.S.; O'Keeffe, D.T.; Espinosa De Ycaza, A.E.; Gionfriddo, M.R.; Erwin, P.J.; Coddington, C.C., III; Stan, M.N.; Murad, M.H.; Montori, V.M. Subclinical Hypothyroidism in Pregnancy: A Systematic Review and Meta-Analysis. *Thyroid* **2016**, *26*, 580–590. [CrossRef] [PubMed]

13. Lai, H.; Zhan, Z.-Y.; Liu, H. Association between Thyroid Hormone Parameters during Early Pregnancy and Gestational Hypertension: A Prospective Cohort Study. *J. Int. Med. Res.* **2020**, *48*, 0300060520904814. [CrossRef] [PubMed]
14. Han, Y.; Wang, J.; Wang, X.; Ouyang, L.; Li, Y. Relationship between Subclinical Hypothyroidism in Pregnancy and Hypertensive Disorder of Pregnancy: A Systematic Review and Meta-Analysis. *Front. Endocrinol.* **2022**, *13*, 823710. [CrossRef]
15. Toloza, F.J.; Derakhshan, A.; Männistö, T.; Bliddal, S.; Popova, P.V.; Carty, D.M.; Chen, L.; Taylor, P.; Mosso, L.; Oken, E. Association between Maternal Thyroid Function and Risk of Gestational Hypertension and Pre-Eclampsia: A Systematic Review and Individual-Participant Data Meta-Analysis. *Lancet Diabetes Endocrinol.* **2022**, *10*, 243–252. [CrossRef]
16. Li, P.; Lin, S.; Cui, J.; Chen, X.; Meng, Z.; Fan, J. Impact of Early Pregnancy Subclinical Hypothyroidism on Gestational Diabetes Mellitus: A Retrospective Study of 7,536 Cases. *J. Womens Health* **2022**, *31*, 293–298. [CrossRef]
17. Furukawa, S.; Miyakawa, K.; Shibata, J.; Iwashita, M. Women with Subclinical Hypothyroidism Are at Low Risk of Poor Pregnancy Outcome in Japan. *Tohoku J. Exp. Med.* **2017**, *242*, 167–172. [CrossRef]
18. Mir, F.; Chiti, H.; Mazloomzadeh, S. Short-Term Adverse Pregnancy Outcomes in Women with Subclinical Hypothyroidism: A Comparative Approach of Iranian and American Guidelines. *J. Thyroid Res.* **2022**, *2022*, 9315250. [CrossRef]
19. Dash, P.; Tiwari, R.; Nayak, S.; Jena, S.K.; Mangaraj, M. Prevalence of Subclinical Hypothyroidism in Pregnancy and Its Association with Anti-Thyroperoxidase Antibody and the Occurrence of Gestational Diabetes Mellitus. *Cureus* **2022**, *14*, e21087. [CrossRef]
20. Nazarpour, S.; Ramezani Tehrani, F.; Amiri, M.; Bidhendi Yarandi, R.; Azizi, F. Levothyroxine Treatment and Pregnancy Outcomes in Women with Subclinical Hypothyroidism: A Systematic Review and Meta-Analysis. *Arch. Gynecol. Obstet.* **2019**, *300*, 805–819. [CrossRef]
21. Ding, Z.; Liu, Y.; Maraka, S.; Abdelouahab, N.; Huang, H.-F.; Fraser, W.D.; Fan, J. Pregnancy and Neonatal Outcomes with Levothyroxine Treatment in Women with Subclinical Hypothyroidism Based on New Diagnostic Criteria: A Systematic Review and Meta-Analysis. *Front. Endocrinol.* **2021**, *12*, 797423. [CrossRef] [PubMed]
22. Bein, M.; Yu, O.H.Y.; Grandi, S.M.; Frati, F.Y.; Kandil, I.; Filion, K.B. Levothyroxine and the Risk of Adverse Pregnancy Outcomes in Women with Subclinical Hypothyroidism: A Systematic Review and Meta-Analysis. *BMC Endocr. Disord.* **2021**, *21*, 34. [CrossRef]
23. Sitoris, G.; Veltri, F.; Jelloul, E.; Kleynen, P.; Rozenberg, S.; Poppe, K.G. Impact of Thyroid Hormone Treatment on Maternal Pregnancy Outcomes in Women with Subclinical Hypothyroidism without TPOAb: A Retrospective Cross-Sectional Study. *Thyroid Res.* **2023**, *16*, 29. [CrossRef]
24. Maraka, S.; Singh Ospina, N.M.; O'Keeffe, D.T.; Rodriguez-Gutierrez, R.; Espinosa De Ycaza, A.E.; Wi, C.-I.; Juhn, Y.J.; Coddington, C.C., III; Montori, V.M.; Stan, M.N. Effects of Levothyroxine Therapy on Pregnancy Outcomes in Women with Subclinical Hypothyroidism. *Thyroid* **2016**, *26*, 980–986. [CrossRef]
25. Yamamoto, J.M.; Benham, J.L.; Nerenberg, K.A.; Donovan, L.E. Impact of Levothyroxine Therapy on Obstetric, Neonatal and Childhood Outcomes in Women with Subclinical Hypothyroidism Diagnosed in Pregnancy: A Systematic Review and Meta-Analysis of Randomised Controlled Trials. *BMJ Open* **2018**, *8*, e022837. [CrossRef] [PubMed]
26. Jiao, X.-F.; Zhang, M.; Chen, J.; Wei, Q.; Zeng, L.; Liu, D.; Zhang, C.; Li, H.; Zou, K.; Zhang, L. The Impact of Levothyroxine Therapy on the Pregnancy, Neonatal and Childhood Outcomes of Subclinical Hypothyroidism during Pregnancy: An Updated Systematic Review, Meta-Analysis and Trial Sequential Analysis. *Front. Endocrinol.* **2022**, *13*, 964084. [CrossRef] [PubMed]
27. Panaitescu, A.M.; Ciobanu, A.M.; Popescu, M.R.; Huluta, I.; Botezatu, R.; Peltecu, G.; Gica, N. Incidence of Hypertensive Disorders of Pregnancy in Romania. *Hypertens. Pregnancy* **2020**, *39*, 423–428. [CrossRef]
28. McIntyre, H.D.; Catalano, P.; Zhang, C.; Desoye, G.; Mathiesen, E.R.; Damm, P. Gestational Diabetes Mellitus. *Nat. Rev. Dis. Primer* **2019**, *5*, 47. [CrossRef] [PubMed]
29. Dłuski, D.F.; Ruszała, M.; Rudziński, G.; Pożarowska, K.; Brzuszkiewicz, K.; Leszczyńska-Gorzelak, B. Evolution of Gestational Diabetes Mellitus across Continents in 21st Century. *Int. J. Environ. Res. Public Health* **2022**, *19*, 15804. [CrossRef]
30. American Diabetes Association. Diabetes and Employment. *Diabetes Care* **2009**, *32* (Suppl. 1), S80–S84. [CrossRef]
31. Giannakou, K.; Evangelou, E.; Yiallouros, P.; Christophi, C.A.; Middleton, N.; Papatheodorou, E.; Papatheodorou, S.I. Risk Factors for Gestational Diabetes: An Umbrella Review of Meta-Analyses of Observational Studies. *PLoS ONE* **2019**, *14*, e0215372. [CrossRef] [PubMed]
32. Gajera, D.; Trivedi, V.; Thaker, P.; Rathod, M.; Dharamsi, A. Detailed Review on Gestational Diabetes Mellitus with Emphasis on Pathophysiology, Epidemiology, Related Risk Factors, and Its Subsequent Conversion to Type 2 Diabetes Mellitus. *Horm. Metab. Res.* **2023**, *55*, 295–303. [CrossRef] [PubMed]
33. SkórzyŦ, E.; Kimber-Trojnar, Ż.; Olszewska, A.; Zaborowski, T. An Interplay between Obesity and Inflammation in Gestational Diabetes Mellitus. *Curr. Pharm. Biotechnol.* **2016**, *17*, 603–613.
34. Moyce Gruber, B.L.; Dolinsky, V.W. The Role of Adiponectin during Pregnancy and Gestational Diabetes. *Life* **2023**, *13*, 301. [CrossRef] [PubMed]
35. Mihai, M.; Vladut, S.; Sonia-Teodora, L.; Mihaela, S.L.; Victoria, N.; Elena, M.I.; Claudiu, M. Correlation between Overweight, Obesity, Gestational Diabetes Mellitus, Adipokines (Adipolin and Adiponectin), and Adverse Pregnancy Outcomes: A Pilot Study. *Medicina* **2024**, *60*, 1544. [CrossRef]
36. Ittermann, T.; Albrecht, D.; Arohonka, P.; Bilek, R.; De Castro, J.J.; Dahl, L.; Filipsson Nystrom, H.; Gaberscek, S.; Garcia-Fuentes, E.; Gheorghiu, M.L. Standardized Map of Iodine Status in Europe. *Thyroid* **2020**, *30*, 1346–1354. [CrossRef]

37. Metzger, B.E.; Gabbe, S.G.; Persson, B.; Lowe, L.P.; Dyer, A.R.; Oats, J.J.; Buchanan, T.A. International Association of Diabetes and Pregnancy Study Groups Recommendations on the Diagnosis and Classification of Hyperglycemia in Pregnancy: Response to Weinert. *Diabetes Care* **2010**, *33*, e98. [CrossRef]
38. Mazaki-Tovi, S.; Romero, R.; Vaisbuch, E.; Erez, O.; Mittal, P.; Chaiworapongsa, T.; Kim, S.K.; Pacora, P.; Yeo, L.; Gotsch, F. Dysregulation of Maternal Serum Adiponectin in Preterm Labor. *J. Matern. Fetal Neonatal Med.* **2009**, *22*, 887–904. [CrossRef]
39. Espinoza, J.; Vidaeff, A.; Pettker, C.M.; Simhan, H. Gestational Hypertension and Preeclampsia. *Obstet. Gynecol.* **2019**, *133*, E1–E25.
40. Tikkanen, M. Placental Abruption: Epidemiology, Risk Factors and Consequences. *Acta Obstet. Gynecol. Scand.* **2011**, *90*, 140–149. [CrossRef]
41. American College of Obstetricians and Gynecologists. Prelabor Rupture of Membranes: ACOG Practice Bulletin, Number 217. *Obstet. Gynecol.* **2020**, *135*, e80–e97. [CrossRef] [PubMed]
42. American College of Obstetricians and Gynecologists. Practice Bulletin No. 173: Fetal Macrosomia. *Obstet. Gynecol.* **2016**, *128*, e195–e209.
43. World Health Organization. *WHO Recommendations for Care of the Preterm or Low Birth Weight Infant*; World Health Organization: Geneva, Switzerland, 2022.
44. Tharmaratnam, S. Fetal Distress. *Best Pract. Res. Clin. Obstet. Gynaecol.* **2000**, *14*, 155–172. [CrossRef] [PubMed]
45. Wallace, T.M.; Levy, J.C.; Matthews, D.R. Use and Abuse of HOMA Modeling. *Diabetes Care* **2004**, *27*, 1487–1495. [CrossRef]
46. Delange, F. Iodine Deficiency in Europe and Its Consequences: An Update. *Eur. J. Nucl. Med. Mol. Imaging* **2002**, *29*, S404–S416. [CrossRef]
47. Ducarme, G.; Desroys du Roure, V.; Le Thuaut, A.; Crespin-Delcourt, I. Subclinical Hypothyroidism Is Not Associated with Neonatal Morbidity in Women with Gestational Diabetes Mellitus: A Case–Control Study. *Arch. Gynecol. Obstet.* **2021**, *303*, 1153–1159. [CrossRef]
48. Bremner, A.P.; Feddema, P.; Leedman, P.J.; Brown, S.J.; Beilby, J.P.; Lim, E.M.; Wilson, S.G.; O'Leary, P.C.; Walsh, J.P. Age-Related Changes in Thyroid Function: A Longitudinal Study of a Community-Based Cohort. *J. Clin. Endocrinol.* **2012**, *97*, 1554–1562. [CrossRef]
49. Chen, L.-M.; Du, W.-J.; Dai, J.; Zhang, Q.; Si, G.-X.; Yang, H.; Ye, E.-L.; Chen, Q.-S.; Yu, L.-C.; Zhang, C. Effects of Subclinical Hypothyroidism on Maternal and Perinatal Outcomes during Pregnancy: A Single-Center Cohort Study of a Chinese Population. *PLoS ONE* **2014**, *9*, e109364. [CrossRef]
50. Christian, L.M.; Porter, K. Longitudinal Changes in Serum Proinflammatory Markers across Pregnancy and Postpartum: Effects of Maternal Body Mass Index. *Cytokine* **2014**, *70*, 134–140. [CrossRef]
51. Croce, L.; Beneventi, F.; Ripepi, F.; De Maggio, I.; Malovini, A.; Bellingeri, C.; Coperchini, F.; Teliti, M.; Rotondi, M.; Spinillo, A. Relationship between Maternal Obesity and First-Trimester TSH in Women with Negative Anti-TPO Antibodies. *Eur. Thyroid J.* **2024**, *13*, e230213. [CrossRef]
52. Knight, B.A.; Shields, B.M.; Hattersley, A.T.; Vaidya, B. Maternal Hypothyroxinaemia in Pregnancy Is Associated with Obesity and Adverse Maternal Metabolic Parameters. *Eur. J. Endocrinol.* **2016**, *174*, 51–57. [CrossRef] [PubMed]
53. Dathan-Stumpf, A.; Vogel, M.; Jank, A.; Thiery, J.; Kiess, W.; Stepan, H. Reference Intervals of Serum Lipids in the Second and Third Trimesters of Pregnancy in a Caucasian Cohort: The LIFE Child Study. *Arch. Gynecol. Obstet.* **2019**, *300*, 1531–1539. [CrossRef] [PubMed]
54. Ryckman, K.; Spracklen, C.; Smith, C.; Robinson, J.; Saftlas, A. Maternal Lipid Levels during Pregnancy and Gestational Diabetes: A Systematic Review and Meta-analysis. *Bjog Int. J. Obstet. Gynaecol.* **2015**, *122*, 643–651. [CrossRef]
55. Wang, X.; Zhang, E.; Tian, Z.; Zhao, R.; Huang, K.; Gao, S.; Su, S.; Xie, S.; Liu, J.; Luan, Y. The Association between Dyslipidaemia in the First Trimester and Adverse Pregnancy Outcomes in Pregnant Women with Subclinical Hypothyroidism: A Cohort Study. *Lipids Health Dis.* **2024**, *23*, 13. [CrossRef]
56. Liu, H.; Peng, D. Update on Dyslipidemia in Hypothyroidism: The Mechanism of Dyslipidemia in Hypothyroidism. *Endocr. Connect.* **2022**, *11*, e210002. [CrossRef] [PubMed]
57. Fatima, S.S.; Rehman, R.; Butt, Z.; Asif Tauni, M.; Fatima Munim, T.; Chaudhry, B.; Khan, T.A. Screening of Subclinical Hypothyroidism during Gestational Diabetes in Pakistani Population. *J. Matern. Fetal Neonatal Med.* **2016**, *29*, 2166–2170. [CrossRef]
58. Walker, R.L.; Hemmelgarn, B.; Quan, H. Incidence of Gestational Hypertension in the Calgary Health Region from 1995 to 2004. *Can. J. Cardiol.* **2009**, *25*, e284–e287. [CrossRef]
59. Kvetny, J.; Poulsen, H.F. Incidence of Gestational Hypertension in Gestational Diabetes Mellitus. *Arch. Gynecol. Obstet.* **2003**, *267*, 153–157. [CrossRef]
60. Bryson, C.L.; Ioannou, G.N.; Rulyak, S.J.; Critchlow, C. Association between Gestational Diabetes and Pregnancy-Induced Hypertension. *Am. J. Epidemiol.* **2003**, *158*, 1148–1153. [CrossRef]
61. Sibai, B.M.; Ross, M.G. Hypertension in Gestational Diabetes Mellitus: Pathophysiology and Long-Term Consequences. *J. Matern. Fetal Neonatal Med.* **2010**, *23*, 229–233. [CrossRef]
62. Taddei, S.; Caraccio, N.; Virdis, A.; Dardano, A.; Versari, D.; Ghiadoni, L.; Salvetti, A.; Ferrannini, E.; Monzani, F. Impaired Endothelium-Dependent Vasodilatation in Subclinical Hypothyroidism: Beneficial Effect of Levothyroxine Therapy. *J. Clin. Endocrinol. Metab.* **2003**, *88*, 3731–3737. [CrossRef]

63. Floriani, C.; Gencer, B.; Collet, T.-H.; Rodondi, N. Subclinical Thyroid Dysfunction and Cardiovascular Diseases: 2016 Update. *Eur. Heart J.* **2018**, *39*, 503–507. [CrossRef]
64. Stagnaro-Green, A.; Chen, X.; Bogden, J.D.; Davies, T.F.; Scholl, T.O. The Thyroid and Pregnancy: A Novel Risk Factor for Very Preterm Delivery. *Thyroid* **2005**, *15*, 351–357. [CrossRef] [PubMed]
65. Lee, S.Y.; Cabral, H.J.; Aschengrau, A.; Pearce, E.N. Associations between Maternal Thyroid Function in Pregnancy and Obstetric and Perinatal Outcomes. *J. Clin. Endocrinol. Metab.* **2020**, *105*, e2015–e2023. [CrossRef] [PubMed]
66. Romero, R.; Dey, S.K.; Fisher, S.J. Preterm Labor: One Syndrome, Many Causes. *Science* **2014**, *345*, 760–765. [CrossRef] [PubMed]
67. Rao, M.; Zeng, Z.; Zhou, F.; Wang, H.; Liu, J.; Wang, R.; Wen, Y.; Yang, Z.; Su, C.; Su, Z. Effect of Levothyroxine Supplementation on Pregnancy Loss and Preterm Birth in Women with Subclinical Hypothyroidism and Thyroid Autoimmunity: A Systematic Review and Meta-Analysis. *Hum. Reprod. Update* **2019**, *25*, 344–361. [CrossRef]
68. Guida, J.P.d.S.; Dias, T.Z.; Lajos, G.J.; Nomura, M.L.; Pacagnella, R.d.C.; Tedesco, R.P.; Rehder, P.M.; Haddad, S.; Sousa, M.H.; Passini, R. Hypertensive Disorders during Pregnancy as a Major Cause of Preterm Birth and Adverse Perinatal Outcomes: Findings from a Brazilian National Survey. *Einstein São Paulo* **2024**, *22*, eAO0514. [CrossRef]
69. Sankoda, A.; Suzuki, H.; Imaizumi, M.; Yoshihara, A.; Kobayashi, S.; Katai, M.; Hamada, K.; Hidaka, Y.; Yoshihara, A.; Nakamura, H. Effects of Levothyroxine Treatment on Fertility and Pregnancy Outcomes in Subclinical Hypothyroidism: A Systematic Review and Meta-Analysis of Randomized Controlled Trials. *Thyroid* **2024**, *34*, 519–530. [CrossRef]
70. Shenhav, S.; Benbassat, C.; Gefel, D.; Zangen, S.; Rosen, S.R.; Avrahami-Benyounes, Y.; Almashanu, S.; Groisman, L.; Rorman, E.; Fytlovich, S. Can Mild-to-Moderate Iodine Deficiency during Pregnancy Alter Thyroid Function? Lessons from a Mother–Newborn Cohort. *Nutrients* **2022**, *14*, 5336. [CrossRef]
71. He, X.; Wang, P.; Wang, Z.; He, X.; Xu, D.; Wang, B. Endocrinology in Pregnancy: Thyroid Antibodies and Risk of Preterm Delivery: A Meta-Analysis of Prospective Cohort Studies. *Eur. J. Endocrinol.* **2012**, *167*, 455–464. [CrossRef]
72. Wilson, K.L.; Casey, B.M.; McIntire, D.D.; Halvorson, L.M.; Cunningham, F.G. Subclinical Thyroid Disease and the Incidence of Hypertension in Pregnancy. *Obstet. Gynecol.* **2012**, *119*, 315–320. [CrossRef] [PubMed]

biomedicines

MDPI

Article

Effect of Vitamin D Deficiency on Arterial Stiffness in Pregnant Women with Preeclampsia and Pregnancy-Induced Hypertension and Implications for Fetal Development

Mircea Iurciuc [1], Florina Buleu [1,2,*], Stela Iurciuc [1], Izabella Petre [2,3], Daian Popa [4,5], Radu Dumitru Moleriu [6], Anca Bordianu [7], Oana Suciu [8], Rabia Tasdemir [2], Ramona-Elena Dragomir [9], Madalina Otilia Timircan [2,3] and Ion Petre [4,6]

1 Department of Cardiology, "Victor Babes" University of Medicine and Pharmacy, E. Murgu Square No. 2, 300041 Timisoara, Romania; iurciuc.mircea@umft.ro (M.I.); iurciuc.stela@umft.ro (S.I.)
2 County Emergency Clinical Hospital "Pius Brinzeu", 300732 Timisoara, Romania; petre.izabella@umft.ro (I.P.); rabia.tasdemir@gmail.com (R.T.); madalina-otilia.timircan@umft.ro (M.O.T.)
3 Department XII of Obstetrics and Gynaecology, "Victor Babes" University of Medicine and Pharmacy, 300041 Timisoara, Romania
4 Doctoral School, "Victor Babes" University of Medicine and Pharmacy, 300041 Timisoara, Romania; daian-ionel.popa@umft.ro (D.P.); petre.ion@umft.ro (I.P.)
5 Department of Surgery, Emergency Discipline, "Victor Babes" University of Medicine and Pharmacy, 300041 Timisoara, Romania
6 Department of Functional Sciences, Medical Informatics and Biostatistics Discipline, "Victor Babes" University of Medicine and Pharmacy, 300041 Timisoara, Romania; radu.moleriu@umft.ro
7 Department of Plastic Surgery and Reconstructive Microsurgery Bagdasar-Arseni, Emergency Hospital Bucharest, University of Medicine and Pharmacy "Carol Davila", 010825 Bucharest, Romania; anca.bordianu@gmail.com
8 Department of Microbiology, "Victor Babeș" University of Medicine and Pharmacy, Eftimie Murgu Sq. No. 2, 300041 Timisoara, Romania; suciu.oana@umft.ro
9 Doctoral School, "Carol Davila" University of Medicine and Pharmacy, 020021 Bucharest, Romania; ramona.dragomir@drd.umfcd.ro
* Correspondence: florina.buleu@umft.ro; Tel.: +40-724-351-393

Abstract: Background and objectives: Over the past few years, researchers have focused on the importance of vitamin D in the health of pregnant women and in reducing the chances of developmental disorders occurring in fetuses. In addition, a link has been established between fetal development and arterial stiffness in hypertensive disorders that occur during pregnancy. Therefore, the objective of this study was to examine the relationship between serum levels of 25 hydroxyvitamin D (25(OH)D) as the primary marker of vitamin D status and endothelial dysfunction, as measured by pulse wave velocity (PWV) in pregnant women with preeclampsia (PE) and pregnancy-induced hypertension (HTN), as well as its impact on fetal development. Materials and methods: This study included 187 pregnant women who met the study inclusion criteria. Pregnant women were divided into two groups: pregnancy-induced hypertension (HTN group), which included 100 patients (53.48%), and preeclampsia (PE group), which included 87 patients (46.52%). Results: Significant differences regarding the augmentation index (Aix) brachial, PWVao, heart rate, and systolic or diastolic blood pressure with more increased values were observed for the HTN group vs. the preeclampsia group in the current research ($p < 0.001$). Additionally, the Aix brachial index was significantly lower in the preeclampsia group compared to the HTN group (1.76 ± 0.71 for the HTN group vs. 0.62 ± 0.5 for the preeclampsia group, $p < 0.001$). A severe matern serum 25(OH)D level deficiency was associated with a more severe subcategory of prematurity ($p < 0.001$) and with increased chances of newborn preterm birth ($p < 0.05$). Moreover, the negative effect of severe maternal serum 25(OH)D level deficiency was studied for each group regarding the blood pressure values, Aix brachial, PWVao values in the second and third trimesters, and fetus weight. The Kruskal–Wallis test was applied for this, obtaining significant differences in all cases: open paren p less than 0.05 and closed. When serum severe 25(OH)D levels deficiency was present, arterial stiffness parameters were significantly worse. Conclusions: The findings of this research revealed notable connections between vitamin

D deficiency and increased arterial rigidity in pregnant women with preeclampsia and pregnancy-induced hypertension. These results emphasize the significance of conducting both examinations to obtain a more comprehensive evaluation of these patients. Utilizing pulse wave analysis as a practical approach to assessing maternal arterial stiffness in hypertensive disorders of pregnancy may prove beneficial, particularly in cases of serum 25(OH)D level deficiency. It could play a key role in identifying patients at higher risk of worsening disease severity and, thus, preventing any impact on fetal development.

Keywords: vitamin D deficit; arterial stiffness; preeclampsia; pregnancy-induced hypertension; developmental disorders in the fetus

1. Introduction

One prevalent public health problem, vitamin D deficiency, often goes unnoticed and remains untreated [1]. This deficiency has been associated with an increased risk of various health disorders, including hypertension, diabetes, metabolic syndrome, cancers, congestive heart failure, autoimmune diseases, and chronic vascular inflammation [1–3].

A unique category, however, is pregnant women, who experience subtle changes in their metabolism and endocrine functions. The nutritional intake, which must meet the needs of both the pregnant woman and the developing fetus [4], also impacts circulating 25(OH)D concentrations, with lower plasma concentrations in vegetarians and vegans compared to meat and fish consumers [5]. Unfortunately, because of rapid changes in modern lifestyles, the prevalence of lower serum 25(OH)D concentrations during pregnancy has increased and become a global concern [6]; therefore, evidence that supports the effective use of vitamin D supplementation is important [7]. Extensive clinical research has proved the crucial role of vitamin D in the well-being of pregnant women and newborns. Deficient levels of this vitamin during pregnancy can have detrimental effects on the health of both the mother and the pregnancy itself, including hypertensive disorders of pregnancy, premature rupture of membranes, premature delivery [6], and gestational diabetes mellitus [8,9].

Furthermore, vitamin D deficiency during pregnancy can significantly impact the growth and development of the fetus, particularly in terms of bone development, potentially leading to adverse effects on weight [10,11]. The Rostami et al. study also found that preterm birth was not only associated with vitamin D deficiency but was also indirectly related to low blood levels of 25(OH)D and increased risks [12]. Therefore, circulating 25(OH)D serum levels are considered the primary marker of prenatal vitamin D status.

Vitamin D deficiency has been linked to arterial stiffness, a well-known indicator of cardiovascular disease and a marker of subclinical atherosclerosis [1]. In pregnant women, arterial stiffness is a crucial measure of vascular health that has shown promising results in predicting the occurrence of hypertensive disorders during pregnancy, such as preeclampsia and pregnancy-induced hypertension [13]. A recent comprehensive analysis and meta-analyses in this field have revealed an elevation in arterial stiffness indices among women who develop hypertensive disorders during pregnancy, emphasizing the potential of measuring arterial stiffness as an early predictive marker [14]. Evidence is accumulating that arterial stiffness measurements can identify women who will later develop hypertensive disorders during pregnancy [15].

The significance of vitamin D in developing endothelial dysfunction is widely recognized. However, its role as a contributing factor to arterial stiffness in pregnancy-induced hypertension and preeclampsia, particularly in Romania, where information on vitamin D deficiency during pregnancy is limited, has not been thoroughly examined. This study aimed to assess if vitamin D deficiency is related to arterial stiffness (measured by pulse wave velocity) in pregnant women with preeclampsia and pregnancy-induced hypertension and if there is a correlation between lower serum 25(OH)D levels and fetal development.

2. Material and Methods

2.1. Study Design and the Selection of Participants

The study was carried out in the Obstetrics and Gynaecology Departments of the Emergency Clinical Hospital "Pius Brînzeu" in Timișoara and included 187 pregnant women who met the study inclusion criteria. Before participating, all patients gave informed consent per the principles outlined in the Declaration of Helsinki. The Emergency Clinical Hospital Ethics Committee "Pius Brînzeu" Timișoara approved this study (decision no. 54/20 April 2017).

Our study focused exclusively on pregnant women between 18 and 45 who were in their first or second pregnancy and had stable clinical and hemodynamic conditions. Only those in the second trimester of pregnancy and non-smokers were eligible for inclusion. To ensure the integrity of our study's design, we excluded women with a history of arterial hypertension, intrauterine fetal growth restriction, placental abruption, or those taking medication that could potentially impact blood pressure. Additionally, we excluded individuals with multiple pregnancies, coronary artery disease, valvular heart disease, congenital heart disease, heart failure, cardiomyopathy, arrhythmias or conduction disorders on electrocardiography, chronic kidney or liver diseases, cancer, a history of alcohol or drug abuse, hematological disease, ongoing infection, systemic inflammatory conditions, or any autoimmune disease such as systemic lupus erythematosus or antiphospholipid antibody syndrome. Furthermore, we excluded individuals with hyperlipidemia, pre-existing diabetes mellitus, hypercholesterolemia, peripheral arterial disease, thyroid function abnormalities, significant anemia (defined as a hemoglobin level of 9 g/dL or less), or known psychiatric comorbidities. Lastly, pregnancies with aneuploidy or significant fetal abnormalities were also excluded from our study.

Pregnant women were divided into two groups: pregnancy-induced hypertension (HTN group), which included 100 patients (53.48%), and preeclampsia (PE group), which included 87 patients (46.52%). The patients from both groups were selected with similar characteristics: age, body mass index (BMI), environment, and habits.

No pregnant women in the study had taken vitamin D supplements independently of calcium and other multivitamin/micronutrient supplements. Therefore, that season, to not influence the serum 25(OH)D level, only pregnant women from whom the blood sampling was taken between March 1 and November 1 were included in the study. Moreover, anamnestically, none of the pregnant women were exposed to excessive sunlight due to the cardiologist's recommendations.

2.2. Newborns Assessment

The classification of preterm birth, according to the World Health Organization (WHO), is based on the duration of gestation. Specifically, any birth that occurs before completing 37 weeks of gestation or fewer than 259 days since the woman's last menstrual period (LMP) is considered preterm. They are subdivided based on gestational age (GA) to categorize preterm births further. The widely accepted definition of preterm birth categorizes it into three groups: extremely preterm (less than 28 weeks), very preterm (28 to less than 32 weeks), and moderate to late preterm (32 to 37 weeks). This classification is recognized and commonly used in the field [16].

The Apgar score is a standardized assessment of a newborn's condition immediately after birth. It consists of five parts. Each category is weighted equally and assigned a 0, 1, or 2 value. The components are then added to produce a score recorded 1 and 5 min after birth. A score from 7 to 10 is considered safe, 4 to 6 is moderately abnormal, and 0 to 3 is considered low in term and late preterm infants [17].

2.3. Preeclampsia and Pregnancy-Induced Hypertension Definitions

The criteria for diagnosing preeclampsia were established based on the guidelines provided by the International Society for the Study of Hypertension in Pregnancy (ISSHP) [18]. To meet this definition, women who were previously normotensive must have a systolic blood pressure of 140 mmHg or higher and a diastolic blood pressure of 90 mmHg or higher on two separate occasions, at least four hours apart after reaching the 20-week mark of gestation. Additionally, proteinuria of 300 mg or more in a 24-h urine collection or two readings of at least ++ on dipstick analysis of midstream or catheter urine specimens (if a 24-h collection is unavailable) is required alongside hypertension.

Pregnancy-induced hypertension, also known as gestational hypertension, is a condition characterized by high blood pressure, specifically a systolic BP of 140 or higher and a diastolic BP of 90 or higher, that develops after 20 weeks of pregnancy. This condition occurs without proteinuria or abnormalities in blood tests or hematological markers. It is important to note that gestational hypertension typically does not coincide with restrictions in fetal growth [18]

2.4. 25-Hydroxyvitamin D Analysis

The DIAsource 25-OH Vitamin D Total Elisa 90kit by DIAsource Immunoassays SA in Louvain-la-Neuve, Belgium, was explicitly used to determine the serum levels of 25(OH)D. Reproducibility and accuracy were evaluated with two low and high concentrations samples. Their concentrations were measured in 10 different runs in duplicate for reproducibility and a single run for repeatability precision. According to the company's application notes, we used the Free 25OH Vitamin D serum control to calibrate and validate the measurements. The limit of blank (LOB) was calculated to be 2.012 ng/mL. The limit of detection (LOD) was calculated as the LOB—1.645 standard deviation of a low-concentration sample tested in 10 different runs. The LOD was calculated to be 3.035 ng/mL. The interpretation of the values is as follows: levels equal to or greater than 30 ng/mL are considered sufficient, levels between 21 ng/mL and 29 ng/mL are deemed insufficient, mild deficiency is defined by levels between 10 ng/mL and 20 ng/mL, moderate deficiency is indicated by levels greater than five ng/mL but less than ten ng/mL, and severe deficiency is defined by levels less than five ng/mL [19].

2.5. Measurement of Arterial Stiffness

According to the European Society of Cardiology, arterial stiffness can be accurately assessed using pulse wave velocity, the gold standard [20]. This study conducted carotid-femoral PWV measurements using the MedexpertArteriograph device version 3.0.0.3, manufactured by TensioMedKft., Budapest, Hungary. This device determined the central pressure and augmentation index and measured pulse wave propagation velocity in the aorta (PWVao). To ensure the utmost precision, pregnant participants were instructed to lie supine for 10 min in a quiet room before the measurements. The readings obtained from this accredited medical device included central pressure pulse (PP), augmentation index, and pulse wave propagation velocity in the aorta. Following the guidelines outlined in the expert consensus document on arterial stiffness, a single examiner conducted multiple measurements using the prescribed determination method. To ensure accurate results, participants were required to abstain from smoking, caffeine-containing foods, or drinks for at least 3 h before the measurements. Additionally, alcohol consumption was prohibited for at least 10 h before the investigation. Similar to blood pressure, arterial diameter and stiffness exhibit a circadian rhythm, with an increase observed during sleep. As a result, participants were instructed to stay awake during the assessment to avoid interfering with these parameters. Throughout the measurements, participants maintained silence. According to multiple sources, the accepted measurement for pulse wave velocity in adult females is typically 7.4 m/s. However, it is essential to acknowledge that younger, physically active women generally have lower baseline values, averaging around 6.1 m/s (with a range from 4.6 to 7.5 m/s). As women grow older, these values gradually rise due to various factors such as changes in the vascular endothelium, elevated blood pressure, related health conditions, and even pregnancy [21,22].

2.6. Statistical Analysis

The data were gathered using the Microsoft Excel 2021 program; the JASPv18.3 program was used for the statistical analysis. After the inclusion and exclusion criteria were applied, 187 patients underwent the study, split into two groups: patients with hypertension or preeclampsia. The Shapiro–Wilk test was used to obtain a non-normal distribution for testing the data distribution; for this, only non-parametrical tests were used in the following analysis. The Mann–Whitney test was applied to determine whether the two groups' differences were significant. When more than two different groups are analyzed, the Kruskal–Wallis test is used. The Pearson coefficient (r) and the Spearman coefficient (R) were calculated to test the association between variables, and a linear correlation/regression model was applied to determine the significance of the data. The significance was set at $\alpha = 0.05$ for the whole study.

3. Results

The mean values of the numerical variables were tested by applying a Mann–Whitney test, obtaining significant differences in the quantity of serum 25(OH)D levels for mother and newborn, Aix brachial: [%], PWVao [m/s], in the second and third trimester, heart rate (beat/minute) (HR), systolic (mmHg) (Sys) and diastolic (mmHg)(Dia) blood pressure, gestational period (weeks), APGAR score, fetus weight (grams); and insignificant differences ($p > 0.05$) or mother age and mother body mass index. The entire analysis is presented in Table 1. The analyzed parameters have significantly above-average values in the HTN group.

Table 1. Descriptive statistics were run between the studied groups. The p-value was obtained after applying a Mann—Whitney test, obtaining significant differences in open paren p less than 0.05 and close paren in most cases. The essential results are highlighted in grey.

Variables	Group	N	Mean	SD	SE	Coefficient of Variation	p Value
Mother's age, years	HTN	100	37.56	2.65	0.26	0.07	$p = 0.989$
	Preeclampsia	87	37.58	2.65	0.28	0.07	
Mother serum 25(OH)D level, ng/mL	HTN	100	18.77	7.29	0.73	0.39	$p < 0.001$
	Preeclampsia	87	13.85	6.46	0.69	0.47	
Newborn serum 25(OH)D level, ng/mL	HTN	100	22.77	10.89	1.09	0.47	$p < 0.001$
	Preeclampsia	87	16.48	5.96	0.64	0.36	
BMI (kg/m^2)	HTN	100	30.33	2.71	0.27	0.09	$p = 0.861$
	Preeclampsia	87	30.41	2.70	0.29	0.09	
Aix brachial: [%] Trim II	HTN	100	1.76	0.71	0.07	0.41	$p < 0.001$
	Preeclampsia	87	0.62	0.50	0.05	0.80	
Aix brachial: [%] Trim III	HTN	100	4.09	1.37	0.14	0.34	$p < 0.001$
	Preeclampsia	87	3.08	0.94	0.10	0.31	
PWVao [m/s] Trim II	HTN	100	11.79	1.01	0.10	0.07	$p < 0.001$
	Preeclampsia	87	9.85	0.86	0.09	0.09	
PWVao [m/s] Trim III	HTN	100	13.43	1.15	0.12	0.09	$p < 0.001$
	Preeclampsia	87	11.07	1.23	0.13	0.11	
HR [beats/min]	HTN	100	95.79	8.31	0.83	0.09	$p < 0.001$
	Preeclampsia	87	84.08	6.17	0.66	0.07	

Table 1. *Cont.*

Variables	Group	N	Mean	SD	SE	Coefficient of Variation	*p* Value
Sys [mmHg]	HTN	100	208.40	16.49	1.65	0.08	$p < 0.001$
	Preeclampsia	87	180.92	11.29	1.21	0.06	
Dia [mmHg]	HTN	100	129.69	9.18	0.92	0.07	$p < 0.001$
	Preeclampsia	87	110.70	5.85	0.63	0.05	
Gestational period [weeks]	HTN	100	34.24	3.19	0.32	0.09	$p < 0.001$
	Preeclampsia	87	32.72	2.99	0.32	0.09	
APGAR score [at 1 min]	HTN	100	7.61	2.14	0.21	0.28	$p = 0.007$
	Preeclampsia	87	7.03	1.94	0.21	0.28	
Fetus weight [gram]	HTN	100	2953.70	528.86	52.87	0.18	$p < 0.001$
	Preeclampsia	87	1989.89	714.63	76.62	0.36	

The newborn serum 25(OH)D levels in each group were compared based on the prematurity stage using a Kruskal–Wallis test. We observed severe deficient serum levels associated with a more severe prematurity subcategory. Further, vitamin D deficiency in pregnant women was associated with premature birth. Moreover, when the linear correlation model was applied, after calculating the Spearman coefficient, a significant, strong, positive, and direct association was obtained (for the HTN group, a $p < 0.001$, r = 0.78 and $p < 0.001$, r = 0.83 for the preeclampsia group). In addition, newborns with severe lower serum 25(OH)D levels were highly premature, with even lower levels when they were birthed by pregnant women with preeclampsia (Figure 1).

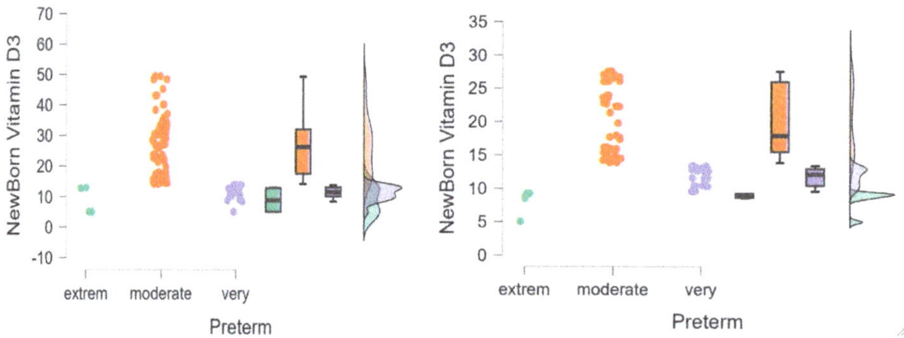

(a) (b)

Figure 1. The data from the Kruskal–Wallis test regarding the relation between serum 25(OH)D level and the prematurity subcategory in both groups are represented using raincloud plots: (**a**) The relation between the serum 25(OH)D level and the prematurity subcategory in the HTN group. (**b**) The relation between the serum 25(OH)D level and the prematurity subcategory in the preeclampsia group.

A linear regression model was applied in both groups to test the possible association between the lower serum 25(OH)D levels in mothers and their newborns, between mothers and their blood pressure values, between lower serum 25(OH)D levels in newborns and their weight on birth, and between lower serum 25(OH)D levels in mothers and their age or BMI.

A significant, robust, and positive association was found in the case of serum 25(OH)D level dependence between mother and newborn ($|r| > 0.75$, $p < 0.05$); a weak positive association was obtained between serum 25(OH)D level and the mother's systolic blood pressure ($|r| < 0.25$, $p < 0.05$); a week true median negative indirect significant correlation was obtained between serum 25(OH)D level in newborns and their weight at birth. All the results are presented in Table 2.

Table 2. The regression analysis uses the numerical variables from the study. The Pearson coefficient was calculated using the sample to determine the direction of the association. The significant results are highlighted in grey.

Association between	Results	
	HTN Group	**Preeclampsia Group**
serum 25(OH)D level in mothers and newborn	$r = 0.75$, $p < 0.001$	$r = 0.91$, $p < 0.001$
serum 25(OH)D level in mothers and systolic blood pressure	$r = 0.23$, $p = 0.047$	$r = 0.27$, $p = 0.013$
serum 25(OH)D level in mothers and diastolic blood pressure	$r = 0.12$, $p > 0.05$	$r = 0.17$, $p > 0.05$
serum 25(OH)D level in newborns and their weight at birth	$r = -0.26$, $p = 0.02$	$r = -0.38$, $p < 0.001$
serum 25(OH)D level in mothers and their age	$r = -0.09$, $p > 0.05$	$r = -0.11$, $p > 0.05$
serum 25(OH)D level in mothers and their BMI	$r = -0.16$, $p > 0.05$	$r = -0.13$, $p > 0.05$

Moreover, for each group, the negative effect of lower serum 25(OH)D level on the mother's body was studied regarding the blood pressure values, Aix brachial [%], PWVao [m/s] values in the second and third trimesters, and fetus weight. The Kruskal–Wallis test was applied for this, obtaining significant differences in all cases ($p < 0.05$). When a severe serum 25(OH)D level was present, the analyzed parameters worsened significantly.

4. Discussion

The occurrence of hypertensive disorders during pregnancy, such as preeclampsia and pregnancy-induced hypertension, continues to be a significant complication with an impact on both mother and fetus all over the world [18]. Ensuring optimal healthcare for the prevention and treatment of these disorders in pregnant women remains a top priority in overall health policy [23,24], as they are known to be one of the leading causes of maternal deaths globally [25–29]. Early prediction of these disorders is crucial to effectively monitor at-risk pregnant women and prevent the development of serious complications. Current clinical guidelines, both nationally and internationally, recommend assessing a combination of maternal risk factors, placental biomarkers, and arterial stiffness to predict the risk of preeclampsia and pregnancy-induced hypertension [20,30,31]. However, the accuracy of these markers is limited due to high variability in detection rates and false positives, especially during early pregnancy [32]. There is a growing interest in utilizing arterial stiffness measurements as a predictive tool during pregnancy, as they have shown the ability to detect changes in vessel hemodynamics that differentiate normotensive and non-normotensive pregnancies [14,21].

Significant differences in hemodynamic and arterial stiffness parameters were observed between pregnant women groups (HTN group vs. preeclampsia group) in the current research ($p < 0.001$). These parameters include Aix brachial, PWVao, heart rate, and systolic or diastolic blood pressure. Pregnant women from the HTN group exhibited higher values for these parameters than the preeclampsia group. Additionally, the Aix brachial index was significantly lower in the preeclampsia group compared to the HTN group (1.77 ± 0.71 for the HTN group vs. 0.62 ± 0.5 for the preeclampsia group, $p < 0.001$). This index reflects the aorta's ability to receive blood. In a healthy pregnancy, there is an increase in compliance in the arterial system. However, our study found that women with pregnancy-induced hypertension did not demonstrate this physiological adaptation when compared to pregnant women with preeclampsia.

Previous studies have also shown peripheral and aortic arterial stiffness in individuals with preeclampsia [33,34]. It has been observed that pregnant women who experienced hypertensive disorders during pregnancy exhibit increased arterial stiffness postpartum [35]. However, when Kim et al. conducted their study, they discovered no variation in the longitudinal alteration of arterial stiffness between women with preeclampsia and those with normal blood pressure within a year after delivery [36]. To the best of our knowledge, this is the initial evidence indicating that pregnancy-induced hypertension leads to greater arterial stiffness compared to preeclampsia, as demonstrated by our results. No other research from the literature compared these two hypertensive disorders. One study assesses arterial stiffness in pregnancies complicated by hypertensive disorders: preeclampsia and chronic hypertension. Women with chronic hypertension exhibited elevated systemic vascular resistance, similar to those with preeclampsia. However, the impact on arterial stiffness was comparatively lesser in cases with chronic hypertension [37].

Evidence suggests that increased arterial stiffness plays a role in the development of early gestational age in normotensive pregnant women. This indicates a connection between fetal growth and maternal endothelial function [38]. When comparing pregnancies affected by hypertensive disorders with and without a small gestational age neonate, it was found that both groups had significantly higher Aix measured by PWV compared to uncomplicated normotensive pregnancies. The highest Aix values were observed in pregnancies complicated by hypertensive disorders and a small for gestational age neonate, indicating a worsening of arterial stiffness with a more severe clinical presentation [39]. These findings likely indicate reduced vascular compliance and increased systemic vascular resistance in pregnancies affected by preeclampsia or pregnancy-induced hypertension.

The severity of hypertensive disorders of pregnancy can be indicated not only by the gestational age at which preeclampsia or pregnancy-induced hypertension occurs but also by the presence of fetal growth restriction [40]. Our findings reveal a significant correlation ($p < 0.05$) between serum 25(OH)D level deficiency in the mother and newborn, accompanied by a low APGAR score and fetal growth restriction. These results provide compelling evidence for the link between serum 25(OH)D level deficit and the severity of preeclampsia and pregnancy-induced hypertension.

A noteworthy finding from our study is a statistically significant correlation between serum 25(OH)D level deficiency in newborns and their birth weight, indicating a negative indirect relationship ($p < 0.001$). This observation aligns with previous research in the field. For instance, Mahfod et al. [41] reported a significant decrease in fetal weight among pregnant women with fetal growth restriction, consistent with the findings of Khalessi et al. [42], who suggested that maternal vitamin D deficiency could elevate the risk of low birth weight in neonates.

This study found that maternal serum vitamin D levels in highly preterm infants decreased significantly. This coincides with research by Zhao et al., who demonstrated an inverse relationship between maternal 25-hydroxyvitamin D concentrations and the likelihood of low birth weight, preterm birth, and early gestational age. However, their meta-analysis found no significant association between maternal vitamin D levels and macrosomia or intrauterine growth restriction [43].

Since the results have been inconsistent, there should be prudence when interpreting observational studies examining the relationship between vitamin D and preeclampsia. Many of these studies considered factors such as maternal age, body mass index, season, and gestational trimester at the time of sample collection. Some studies, including our own, also exclude smoking pregnant women as a variable [44], and others bring evidence suggesting that pregnant women who smoke have lower levels of 25(OH)D regardless of sun exposure season [45]. Benachi et al. conducted a study that found no significant association between vitamin D insufficiency in the first trimester and preeclampsia. However, they discovered that women with sufficient vitamin D levels during the third trimester and those who maintained sufficient levels in both the first and third trimesters had a significantly reduced risk of developing preeclampsia [46].

The results of our study emphasized the potential of measuring arterial stiffness as an early predictive tool in pregnancy together with serum 25(OH)D level. It is becoming increasingly evident that these measurements can effectively identify women who will develop hypertensive disorders later on.

We also believe that further research is crucial to understanding the impact of vitamin levels throughout pregnancy. New research should focus on detecting deficiencies in the early stages of pregnancy, specifically in the first weeks, and determining if these deficiencies can be swiftly restored to normal levels. By doing so, we can potentially improve pregnancy outcomes and address arterial stiffness, which is linked to restricted fetal growth in patients with hypertensive disorders during pregnancy.

5. Study Limitations

However, it is essential to note that this type of research had a few limitations. It requires a large sample size and an adequate number of participants. Additionally, it would be beneficial to exclusively study populations with a multi-generational history of preeclampsia or pregnancy-induced hypertension in each pregnancy. This targeted approach would provide valuable insights into how vitamin D influences arterial stiffness in this specific group of pregnant women. It is worth mentioning that previous studies, including the reviewed literature, have primarily focused on apparently healthy groups without documented comorbidities [8]. However, it is crucial to acknowledge that these comorbidities have been identified as significant disease burdens over the years [47]. Furthermore, due to the fact that the period of data collection in this study did not comprise all seasons (only from 1 March to 1 November), we could not account for seasonal variability. However, it appears that the influence of seasonality on UV radiation is more pronounced in regions with high latitudes and limited exposure to sunlight in winter, as opposed to lower latitudes [48], which is the region where this study was carried out. Figueiredo et al. performed adjusted multiple analyses to determine if seasons have an impact on serum 25(OH)D concentrations: they observed that pregnant women who started the study in spring ($p < 0.001$), winter ($p < 0.001$), or fall ($p = 0.028$) showed a longitudinal increase, whereas women who started the study in summer did not [49].

6. Conclusions

We demonstrated that in pregnant women with preeclampsia and pregnancy-induced hypertension, increased arterial stiffness may be involved, in part, in the pathogenesis of preterm birth, suggesting an association between fetal development and maternal endothelial dysfunction. Pulse wave analysis may be a clinically applicable method for assessing maternal arterial stiffness. It may be more relevant to intrauterine fetal growth when associated with lower serum 25(OH)D levels.

Author Contributions: Conceptualization, F.B., M.I., S.I., I.P. (Izabella Petre) and I.P. (Ion Petre). Data curation, D.P., R.D.M. and I.P. (Izabella Petre); Investigation, F.B., M.I., S.I., R.T. and M.O.T.; Methodology, F.B., I.P. (Izabella Petre), S.I. and M.I.; Software, I.P. (Ion Petre), R.D.M., D.P. and R.-E.D.; Supervision, M.I., S.I., A.B., O.S. and I.P. (Izabella Petre); Validation, I.P. (Ion Petre) and M.I.; Visualization, S.I., A.B. and I.P. (Izabella Petre); Writing—original draft, F.B., M.I., S.I., D.P. and I.P. (Izabella Petre); Writing—review and editing, F.B., M.I., S.I. and I.P. (Ion Petre). All authors have read and agreed to the published version of the manuscript.

Funding: We would like to acknowledge "Victor Babes" University of Medicine and Pharmacy Timisoara for their support in covering the costs of publication for this research paper.

Institutional Review Board Statement: The study conformed to the Declaration of Helsinki and was approved by the Ethics Committee of the Emergency Clinical Hospital "Pius Brinzeu" Timisoara Timișoara, Romania (decision no. 54/20 April 2017).

Informed Consent Statement: Informed consent was obtained from all patients involved in the study.

Data Availability Statement: The datasets are not publicly available, but de-identified data may be provided upon request by the corresponding author.

Conflicts of Interest: The authors declare no conflicts of interest.

References

1. Mozos, I.; Marginean, O. Links between Vitamin D Deficiency and Cardiovascular Diseases. *BioMed Res. Int.* **2015**, *2015*, 109275. [CrossRef]
2. Sirbu, E.; Buleu, F.; Tudor, A.; Dragan, S. Vitamin D and disease activity in rheumatoid arthritis patients: A retrospective study in a Romanian cohort. *Acta Biochim. Pol.* **2020**, *67*, 267–272. [CrossRef] [PubMed]
3. Amrein, K.; Scherkl, M.; Hoffmann, M.; Neuwersch-Sommeregger, S.; Köstenberger, M.; Tmava Berisha, A.; Martucci, G.; Pilz, S.; Malle, O. Vitamin D deficiency 2.0: An update on the current status worldwide. *Eur. J. Clin. Nutr.* **2020**, *74*, 1498–1513. [CrossRef]
4. Marshall, N.E.; Abrams, B.; Barbour, L.A.; Catalano, P.; Christian, P.; Friedman, J.E.; Hay, W.W., Jr.; Hernandez, T.L.; Krebs, N.F.; Oken, E.; et al. The importance of nutrition in pregnancy and lactation: Lifelong consequences. *Am. J. Obs. Gynecol.* **2022**, *226*, 607–632. [CrossRef] [PubMed]
5. Crowe, F.L.; Steur, M.; Allen, N.E.; Appleby, P.N.; Travis, R.C.; Key, T.J. Plasma concentrations of 25-hydroxyvitamin D in meat eaters, fish eaters, vegetarians and vegans: Results from the EPIC-Oxford study. *Public Health Nutr.* **2011**, *14*, 340–346. [CrossRef]
6. Zhang, H.; Wang, S.; Tuo, L.; Zhai, Q.; Cui, J.; Chen, D.; Xu, D. Relationship between Maternal Vitamin D Levels and Adverse Outcomes. *Nutrients* **2022**, *14*, 4230. [CrossRef]
7. Holick, M.F. A Call to Action: Pregnant Women In-Deed Require Vitamin D Supplementation for Better Health Outcomes. *J. Clin. Endocrinol. Metab.* **2018**, *104*, 13–15. [CrossRef]
8. Giourga, C.; Papadopoulou, S.K.; Voulgaridou, G.; Karastogiannidou, C.; Giaginis, C.; Pritsa, A. Vitamin D Deficiency as a Risk Factor of Preeclampsia during Pregnancy. *Diseases* **2023**, *11*, 158. [CrossRef] [PubMed]
9. Wei, S.Q.; Qi, H.P.; Luo, Z.C.; Fraser, W.D. Maternal vitamin D status and adverse pregnancy outcomes: A systematic review and meta-analysis. *J. Matern.-Fetal Neonatal Med.* **2013**, *26*, 889–899. [CrossRef]
10. Avram, C.; Bucur, O.M.; Zazgyva, A.; Avram, L.; Ruta, F. Vitamin Supplementation in Pre-Pregnancy and Pregnancy among Women-Effects and Influencing Factors in Romania. *Int. J. Environ. Res. Public Health* **2022**, *19*, 8503. [CrossRef]
11. Dragomir, R.E.; Toader, D.O.; Gheoca Mutu, D.E.; Dogaru, I.A.; Răducu, L.; Tomescu, L.C.; Moleriu, L.C.; Bordianu, A.; Petre, I.; Stănculescu, R. Consequences of Maternal Vitamin D Deficiency on Newborn Health. *Life* **2024**, *14*, 714. [CrossRef] [PubMed]
12. Rostami, M.; Tehrani, F.R.; Simbar, M.; Bidhendi Yarandi, R.; Minooee, S.; Hollis, B.W.; Hosseinpanah, F. Effectiveness of Prenatal Vitamin D Deficiency Screening and Treatment Program: A Stratified Randomized Field Trial. *J. Clin. Endocrinol. Metab.* **2018**, *103*, 2936–2948. [CrossRef] [PubMed]
13. Mihaela Viviana Ivan, I.P. Brigitha Vlaicu, Adrian Apostol, Dan Tesloianu, Mircea Munteanu, Radmila Costachescu, Lavinia Cristina Moleriu, Lazar Fulger, The Use of Pulse Wave Velocity in Predicting Pre-Eclampsia in High-Risk Women. *Rev. Chim.* **2018**, *69*, 3.
14. Forrest, M.; Bourgeois, S.; Pichette, É.; Caughlin, S.; Kuate Defo, A.; Hales, L.; Labos, C.; Daskalopoulou, S.S. Arterial stiffness measurements in pregnancy as a predictive tool for hypertensive disorders of pregnancy and preeclampsia: Protocol for a systematic review and meta-analysis. *Eur. J. Obs. Gynecol. Reprod. Biol. X* **2022**, *13*, 100141. [CrossRef] [PubMed]
15. Cooper, K.M.; Barrett, T.; McBride, C.A.; Badger, G.J.; Steiner, J.; LeWinter, M.M.; Bernstein, I.M. Subclinical cardiac stiffness is associated with arterial stiffness in healthy young nulligravid women: Potential links to preeclampsia. *Pregnancy Hypertens* **2019**, *18*, 49–54. [CrossRef] [PubMed]
16. Quinn, J.A.; Munoz, F.M.; Gonik, B.; Frau, L.; Cutland, C.; Mallett-Moore, T.; Kissou, A.; Wittke, F.; Das, M.; Nunes, T.; et al. Preterm birth: Case definition & guidelines for data collection, analysis, and presentation of immunisation safety data. *Vaccine* **2016**, *34*, 6047–6056. [PubMed]
17. Simon, L.V.; Shah, M.; Bragg, B.N. *APGAR Score*; [Internet]; StatPearls Publishing: Treasure Island, FL, USA, 2024. Available online: https://www.ncbi.nlm.nih.gov/books/NBK470569/ (accessed on 11 May 2024).
18. Brown, M.A.; Magee, L.A.; Kenny, L.C.; Karumanchi, S.A.; McCarthy, F.P.; Saito, S.; Hall, D.R.; Warren, C.E.; Adoyi, G.; Ishaku, S. Hypertensive Disorders of Pregnancy. *Hypertension* **2018**, *72*, 24–43. [CrossRef] [PubMed]
19. Holick, M.F. Vitamin D status: Measurement, interpretation, and clinical application. *Ann. Epidemiol.* **2009**, *19*, 73–78. [CrossRef] [PubMed]
20. Williams, B.; Mancia, G.; Spiering, W.; Agabiti Rosei, E.; Azizi, M.; Burnier, M.; Clement, D.L.; Coca, A.; de Simone, G.; Dominiczak, A.; et al. 2018 ESC/ESH Guidelines for the management of arterial hypertension. *Eur. Heart J.* **2018**, *39*, 3021–3104. [CrossRef]
21. Turi, V.; Dragan, S.; Iurciuc, M.; Moleriu, L.; Bungau, S.; Tit, D.M.; Toader, D.-O.; Diaconu, C.C.; Behl, T.; Petre, I. Arterial Function in Healthy Pregnant Women vs. Non-Pregnant Women—A 10-Year Study. *Diagnostics* **2020**, *10*, 374. [CrossRef]
22. Petre, I.; Iurciuc, S.; Buleu, F.; Petre, I.; Moleriu, R.D.; Popa, D.; Turi, V.; Bordianu, A.; Tasdemir, R.; Craciun, L.M.; et al. The Impact of Medical Physical Training and a Structured Personalized Exercise Training Program on Hemodynamic Parameters and Arterial Stiffness in Pregnant Women. *Biomedicines* **2024**, *12*, 986. [CrossRef] [PubMed]

23. Ward, Z.J.; Atun, R.; King, G.; Sequeira Dmello, B.; Goldie, S.J. A simulation-based comparative effectiveness analysis of policies to improve global maternal health outcomes. *Nat. Med.* **2023**, *29*, 1262–1272. [CrossRef] [PubMed]
24. Ward, Z.J.; Atun, R.; King, G.; Dmello, B.S.; Goldie, S.J. Global maternal mortality projections by urban/rural location and education level: A simulation-based analysis. *eClinicalMedicine* **2024**, *72*, 102653. [CrossRef]
25. Musarandega, R.; Nyakura, M.; Machekano, R.; Pattinson, R.; Munjanja, S.P. Causes of maternal mortality in Sub-Saharan Africa: A systematic review of studies published from 2015 to 2020. *J. Glob. Health* **2021**, *11*, 04048. [CrossRef] [PubMed]
26. Alipour, J.; Payandeh, A.; Karimi, A. Prevalence of maternal mortality causes based on ICD-MM: A systematic review and meta-analysis. *BMC Pregnancy Childbirth* **2023**, *23*, 821. [CrossRef] [PubMed]
27. Aukes, A.M.; Arion, K.; Bone, J.N.; Li, J.; Vidler, M.; Bellad, M.B.; Charantimath, U.; Goudar, S.S.; Hoodbhoy, Z.; Katageri, G.; et al. Causes and circumstances of maternal death: A secondary analysis of the Community-Level Interventions for Pre-eclampsia (CLIP) trials cohort. *Lancet Glob. Health* **2021**, *9*, e1242–e1251. [CrossRef] [PubMed]
28. Aftab, F.; Ahmed, I.; Ahmed, S.; Ali, S.M.; Amenga-Etego, S.; Ariff, S.; Bahl, R.; Baqui, A.H.; Begum, N.; Bhutta, Z.A.; et al. Direct maternal morbidity and the risk of pregnancy-related deaths, stillbirths, and neonatal deaths in South Asia and sub-Saharan Africa: A population-based prospective cohort study in 8 countries. *PLoS Med.* **2021**, *18*, e1003644. [CrossRef] [PubMed]
29. Leal, L.F.; Malta, D.C.; Souza, M.F.M.; Vasconcelos, A.M.N.; Teixeira, R.A.; Veloso, G.A.; Lansky, S.; Ribeiro, A.L.P.; França, G.V.A.; Naghavi, M. Maternal Mortality in Brazil, 1990 to 2019: A systematic analysis of the Global Burden of Disease Study 2019. *Rev. Soc. Bras. Med. Trop.* **2022**, *55* (Suppl. S1), e0279. [CrossRef] [PubMed]
30. National Institute for Health and Care Excellence: Guidelines. In *Hypertension in Pregnancy: Diagnosis and Management*; National Institute for Health and Care Excellence (NICE): London, UK, 2019. Available online: https://www.ncbi.nlm.nih.gov/books/NBK546004/ (accessed on 11 May 2024).
31. Narcisa Carmen Mladin Micoara, D.L. Stelian Ioan Morariu, Camelia Anisoara Ciacli, Lavinia Cristina Moleriu, George Toth, Lavinia Stelea, Izabella Petre, Dana Chiriac, Ioana Ionita, Maria Puschita, Biomarkers in Diagnosing Preeclampsia and Their Correlation with Blood Pressure. *Rev. Chim.* **2017**, *68*, 4.
32. Poon, L.C.; Shennan, A.; Hyett, J.A.; Kapur, A.; Hadar, E.; Divakar, H.; McAuliffe, F.; da Silva Costa, F.; von Dadelszen, P.; McIntyre, H.D.; et al. The International Federation of Gynecology and Obstetrics (FIGO) initiative on pre-eclampsia: A pragmatic guide for first-trimester screening and prevention. *Int. J. Gynaecol. Obs.* **2019**, *145* (Suppl. S1), 1–33. [CrossRef]
33. Orabona, R.; Sciatti, E.; Vizzardi, E.; Bonadei, I.; Valcamonico, A.; Metra, M.; Frusca, T. Elastic properties of ascending aorta in women with previous pregnancy complicated by early-or late-onset pre-eclampsia. *Ultrasound Obstet. Gynecol.* **2016**, *47*, 316–323. [CrossRef] [PubMed]
34. Hernández-Mora, F.J.; Cerda-Guerrero, C.K.; García-Benavides, L.; Cervantes-Pérez, E.; Ramírez-Ochoa, S.; Vázquez-Beltrán, J.C.; Cervantes-Guevara, G.; Ledezma-Hurtado, E.; Nápoles-Echauri, A.; González-Ojeda, A.; et al. Comparison of Central Aortic Pressure between Women with Preeclampsia and Normotensive Postpartum Women from an Urban Region of Western Mexico. *Medicina* **2023**, *59*, 1343. [CrossRef] [PubMed]
35. Yinon, Y.; Kingdom, J.C.; Odutayo, A.; Moineddin, R.; Drewlo, S.; Lai, V.; Cherney, D.Z.; Hladunewich, M.A. Vascular dysfunction in women with a history of preeclampsia and intrauterine growth restriction: Insights into future vascular risk. *Circulation* **2010**, *122*, 1846–1853. [CrossRef] [PubMed]
36. Kim, S.; Lim, H.J.; Kim, J.R.; Oh, K.J.; Hong, J.S.; Suh, J.W. Longitudinal change in arterial stiffness after delivery in women with preeclampsia and normotension: A prospective cohort study. *BMC Pregnancy Childbirth* **2020**, *20*, 685. [CrossRef] [PubMed]
37. Tihtonen, K.M.H.; Kööbi, T.; Uotila, J.T. Arterial stiffness in preeclamptic and chronic hypertensive pregnancies. *Eur. J. Obstet. Gynecol. Reprod. Biol.* **2006**, *128*, 180–186. [CrossRef] [PubMed]
38. Tomimatsu, T.; Fujime, M.; Kanayama, T.; Mimura, K.; Koyama, S.; Kanagawa, T.; Kimura, T. Maternal arterial stiffness in normotensive pregnant women who subsequently deliver babies that are small for gestational age. *Eur. J. Obstet. Gynecol. Reprod. Biol.* **2013**, *169*, 24–27. [CrossRef] [PubMed]
39. Perry, H.; Gutierrez, J.; Binder, J.; Thilaganathan, B.; Khalil, A. Maternal arterial stiffness in hypertensive pregnancies with and without small-for-gestational-age neonate. *Ultrasound Obstet. Gynecol.* **2020**, *56*, 44–50. [CrossRef] [PubMed]
40. Bonamy, A.-K.E.; Parikh, N.I.; Cnattingius, S.; Ludvigsson, J.F.; Ingelsson, E. Birth characteristics and subsequent risks of maternal cardiovascular disease: Effects of gestational age and fetal growth. *Circulation* **2011**, *124*, 2839–2846. [CrossRef]
41. Hanadi Salah Mahfod, M.M.E.B. Mai Mostafa Zaitoun, Hala Sherif El-sayed, The Relation between Vitamin D Deficiency and Fetal Growth Restriction in Pregnant Women. *Egypt. J. Hosp. Med.* **2022**, *89*, 7.
42. Khalessi, N.; Kalani, M.; Araghi, M.; Farahani, Z. The Relationship between Maternal Vitamin D Deficiency and Low Birth Weight Neonates. *J. Fam. Reprod Health* **2015**, *9*, 113–117.
43. Zhao, R.; Zhou, L.; Wang, S.; Yin, H.; Yang, X.; Hao, L. Effect of maternal vitamin D status on risk of adverse birth outcomes: A systematic review and dose-response meta-analysis of observational studies. *Eur. J. Nutr.* **2022**, *61*, 2881–2907. [CrossRef] [PubMed]
44. Shand, A.; Nassar, N.; Von Dadelszen, P.; Innis, S.; Green, T. Maternal vitamin D status in pregnancy and adverse pregnancy outcomes in a group at high risk for pre-eclampsia. *BJOG Int. J. Obstet. Gynaecol.* **2010**, *117*, 1593–1598. [CrossRef]
45. Lokki, A.I.; Heikkinen-Eloranta, J.; Öhman, H.; Heinonen, S.; Surcel, H.-M.; Nielsen, H.S. Smoking during pregnancy reduces vitamin D levels in a Finnish birth register cohort. *Public Health Nutr.* **2020**, *23*, 1273–1277. [CrossRef] [PubMed]

46. Benachi, A.; Baptiste, A.; Taieb, J.; Tsatsaris, V.; Guibourdenche, J.; Senat, M.-V.; Haidar, H.; Jani, J.; Guizani, M.; Jouannic, J.-M.; et al. Relationship between vitamin D status in pregnancy and the risk for preeclampsia: A nested case-control study. *Clin. Nutr.* **2020**, *39*, 440–446. [CrossRef] [PubMed]
47. Chien, M.C.; Huang, C.Y.; Wang, J.H.; Shih, C.L.; Wu, P. Effects of vitamin D in pregnancy on maternal and offspring health-related outcomes: An umbrella review of systematic review and meta-analyses. *Nutr. Diabetes* **2024**, *14*, 35. [CrossRef] [PubMed]
48. Brustad, M.; Edvardsen, K.; Wilsgaard, T.; Engelsen, O.; Aksnes, L.; Lund, E. Seasonality of UV-radiation and vitamin D status at 69 degrees north. *Photochem. Photobiol. Sci.* **2007**, *6*, 903–908. [CrossRef]
49. Figueiredo, A.C.C.; Cocate, P.G.; Adegboye, A.R.A.; Franco-Sena, A.B.; Farias, D.R.; de Castro, M.B.T.; Brito, A.; Allen, L.H.; Mokhtar, R.R.; Holick, M.F.; et al. Changes in plasma concentrations of 25-hydroxyvitamin D and 1,25-dihydroxyvitamin D during pregnancy: A Brazilian cohort. *Eur. J. Nutr.* **2018**, *57*, 1059–1072. [CrossRef]

biomedicines

MDPI

Article

The Impact of Medical Physical Training and a Structured Personalized Exercise Training Program on Hemodynamic Parameters and Arterial Stiffness in Pregnant Women

Izabella Petre [1,2], Stela Iurciuc [3,*], Florina Buleu [2,3], Ion Petre [4,5], Radu Dumitru Moleriu [5], Daian Popa [4,6], Vladiana Turi [7], Anca Bordianu [8], Rabia Tasdemir [2], Laura Maria Craciun [3], Luciana Marc [9,10], Flavia Mirela Barna [11] and Mircea Iurciuc [3]

1 Department XII of Obstetrics and Gynaecology, "Victor Babes" University of Medicine and Pharmacy, 300041 Timisoara, Romania; petre.izabella@umft.ro
2 County Emergency Clinical Hospital "Pius Brinzeu", 300732 Timisoara, Romania; florina.buleu@umft.ro (F.B.); rabia.tasdemir@gmail.com (R.T.)
3 Department of Cardiology, "Victor Babes" University of Medicine and Pharmacy, 300041 Timisoara, Romania; maria-laura.craciun@umft.ro (L.M.C.); iurciuc.mircea@umft.ro (M.I.)
4 Doctoral School, "Victor Babes" University of Medicine and Pharmacy, 300041 Timisoara, Romania; petre.ion@umft.ro (I.P.); daian-ionel.popa@umft.ro (D.P.)
5 Department of Functional Sciences, Medical Informatics and Biostatistics Discipline, "Victor Babes" University of Medicine and Pharmacy, 300041 Timisoara, Romania; radu.moleriu@umft.ro
6 Department of Surgery, Emergency Discipline, "Victor Babes" University of Medicine and Pharmacy, 300041 Timisoara, Romania
7 Department of Internal Medicine, "Victor Babes" University of Medicine and Pharmacy, 300041 Timisoara, Romania; turi.vladiana@umft.ro
8 Department of Plastic Surgery and Reconstructive Microsurgery Bagdasar-Arseni, Emergency Hospital Bucharest, University of Medicine and Pharmacy "Carol Davila", 010825 Bucharest, Romania; anca.bordianu@gmail.com
9 Centre for Molecular Research in Nephrology and Vascular Disease, Faculty of Medicine, "Victor Babes" University of Medicine and Pharmacy, 300041 Timisoara, Romania; marc.luciana@umft.ro
10 Department of Internal Medicine II, "Victor Babes" University of Medicine and Pharmacy, 300041 Timisoara, Romania
11 Department of Finance, Faculty of Economics and Business Administration, West University of Timisoara, 300115 Timisoara, Romania; flavia.barna@e-uvt.ro
* Correspondence: iurciuc.stela@umft.ro; Tel.: +40-726-307-293

Abstract: Introduction: In developed countries, heart disease is the primary cause of maternal mortality during pregnancy. Arterial stiffness, an independent risk factor for atherosclerosis and a predictor of cardiovascular complications, can be assessed using the augmentation index (AIx) and pulse wave velocity (PWV). In this prospective study, we aimed to evaluate diverse hemodynamic parameters and arterial stiffness in pregnant women before and after participating in a structured, personalized exercise training program. Materials and methods: Forty healthy pregnant women, non-smokers, who agreed to participate daily for 12 weeks in a physical exercise training program under the supervision of a team made up of an obstetrician, a cardiologist, and a physiotherapist were included. Anthropometric characteristics, arterial function, and physical activity data were collected from the participants at two different time points: at the beginning of the exercise training program (T0) and at the end, after 12 weeks (T1). Results: Upon conducting a statistical analysis, it was discovered that there were noteworthy disparities ($p = 0.05$) in body mass index, brachial AIx, systolic blood pressure, and pulse pressure values between the two time points. The regression analysis for the AIx brachial values and the PWVao values from Trim II (T0) and Trim III (T1) showed major differences between these two time points; the association between the AIx brachial values in the second and third trimesters of pregnancy revealed a strong direct significant correlation ($p < 0.001$), and the correlation between the PWVao values in the second (T0) and third trimester (T1) of pregnancy was weak and insignificant ($p = 0.12$). Conclusions: The findings of our study indicate that a personalized exercise training program positively impacts the physical and psychological well-being of pregnant women, leading to a reduction in PWV.

Keywords: personalized exercise training program; arterial stiffness; pulse wave velocity; augmentation index; pregnancy; cardiovascular risk

1. Introduction

In addition to traditional risk factors for cardiovascular disease, women face an extra burden of gender-specific risk factors. Milestones in a woman's reproductive life history can influence or reveal short- and long-term cardiometabolic and cardiovascular pathways [1].

During pregnancy, the maternal cardiovascular system undergoes necessary adjustments to accommodate physiological changes. Normal pregnancy is characterized by significant increases in plasma volume and cardiac output, primarily due to arterial vasodilation. These adaptations play a crucial role in ensuring a successful pregnancy. The expansion of the aorta is linked to the arterial vasodilation that occurs during pregnancy [2]. It was also demonstrated that the physiological increase in cardiac output and circulating blood volume could secondarily increase the value of measures of arterial stiffness [3]. Research has shown that elevated arterial stiffness during pregnancy contributes to the development of conditions like pregnancy-induced hypertension and fetal growth restriction [4]. But, also in a study where 541 healthy normotensive pregnant women were analyzed, no significant changes in arterial stiffness were observed as pregnancy progressed [5].

Throughout normal pregnancy, the body experiences a marked increase in vascular volume and cardiac output to meet its metabolic demands. However, in this situation, low aortic stiffness prevents substantial increases in pulse pressure (PP) and systolic blood pressure (SBP). In individuals who are not pregnant, arterial stiffness typically intensifies as one moves from the aorta to the peripheral arteries, which is essential for minimizing the energy carried by the forward wave to the microcirculation [6]. Over the years, many studies have associated the severity and occurrence of arterial stiffness with various pathologies with cardiovascular impact [7] or even with health outcomes on longer-term follow-up [8]. Studies have shown that aortic stiffness is consistently elevated in pregnancy-associated hypertension compared to healthy pregnant women [9].

There is growing evidence that exercise improves systemic endothelial function and arterial stiffness in a variety of patients, from children to older adults, and in a variety of diseases or as a preventive therapy for gestational hypertensive disorders [10,11]. Surprisingly, the effects of exercise on the vasculature of healthy pregnant women have been poorly studied, and there are almost no data on individualized exercise programs [12]. To our knowledge, only one study has examined the effects of exercise training on endothelial function during healthy pregnancy more than a decade ago. The study used a different method of measuring arterial stiffness (flow-mediated dilation (FMD)) not the gold standard carotid–femoral pulse wave velocity (PWV), which was improved by 30% when moderate-intensity training was initiated between weeks 16 and 20 of pregnancy [13]. Regarding arterial stiffness, significant improvements in PWV were observed with prenatal exercise early after birth, but this has not been studied during pregnancy [14].

However, the impact of physical activity on arterial stiffness in healthy pregnant women, which could potentially decrease distal pulsatility and protect the microcirculatory system, remains uncertain.

Despite the European guidelines on the management of cardiovascular disease in pregnancy [15], the implementation of strategies to improve adherence to methods to decrease pregnancy-related cardiovascular disease mortality remains sub-optimal, especially in developing countries [16].

Moreover, there is no global consensus on the reduction in cardiovascular risk via physical activity in pregnant women [17], or what kind of exercise can be performed by pregnant women, as there was evaluated in different cardiovascular pathologies or even in healthy subjects [18–25], especially analyzing the impact on endothelial dysfunction.

So, this study aimed to assess the impact of a personalized exercise training program on hemodynamic parameters and arterial stiffness in pregnant women and to determine if this training regimen improves hemodynamic parameters.

2. Material and Methods

2.1. Study Design and the Selection of Participants

This research was conducted at the Obstetrics and Gynaecology Departments of the Emergency Clinical Hospital "Pius Brînzeu" in Timisoara, involving 40 pregnant women who met the inclusion criteria for the study. These women had healthy pregnancies with only one fetus each. Before participating, all patients gave informed consent, adhering to the principles outlined in the Declaration of Helsinki [26]. This study was approved by the Ethics Committee of the Emergency Clinical Hospital "Pius Brînzeu" Timișoara (decision no. 54/20 April 2017).

Only pregnant women aged ≥18 years and ≤45 years, with gestational age in the second trimester of pregnancy, in their first pregnancy or second pregnancy, in stable clinical and hemodynamic conditions, and who expressed a desire to perform physiotherapy exercises and non-smoker were included. Pregnant women with a family history of cardiovascular disease or diagnosed before pregnancy with cardiovascular disease, aged below 18 years and more than 45 years, multiparous (more than 3 pregnancies), with hypertension or other pregnancy-induced diseases, gestational diabetes or pregnant women classified as at risk of pregnancy or who developed other pregnancy complications were excluded.

2.2. Clinical and Biochemical Evaluation

Demographic information, anthropometric parameters (including age, height, weight, and body mass index (BMI)), personal and family medical history, cardiovascular risk factors, medications, and laboratory values (total cholesterol, triglycerides, complete blood count, blood glucose) were gathered at inclusion in the exercise training program by using a photometric method (Siemens Dimension RXL-MAX, Dade Behring, Erlangen, Germany). Additionally, arterial function evaluations were conducted at the beginning and end of the 12-week program.

Blood pressure (BP) and heart rate (HR) were determined according to the European Guidelines on Cardiovascular Disease Prevention in clinical practice [27] using a manual sphygmomanometer (Riester, Jungingen, Germany), and the values obtained were compared with the values measured automatically by the Medexpert Arteriograph.

2.3. Measurement of Arterial Stiffness

Using the Medexpert Arteriograph device version 3.0.0.3, created by TensioMed Kft. in Budapest, Hungary, we could non-invasively measure the pulse wave velocity (PWV). This accredited medical device provided precise readings of the central pressure pulse (PP), augmentation index (AIx), and pulse wave propagation velocity in the aorta (PWVao). To ensure the greatest accuracy, pregnant women were instructed to remain in a supine position for 10 min in a quiet room before measurements.

The same examiner followed the determination method outlined in the expert consensus document on arterial stiffness, conducting repeated measurements. To maintain consistency, participants were required to abstain from smoking, caffeine-containing foods, or drinks for at least 3 h before the measurements. Additionally, alcohol consumption was halted at least 10 h before the investigation. As arterial diameter and stiffness exhibit circadian variation, which increases during sleep, participants were instructed not to fall asleep during the assessment. Throughout the measurements, participants refrained from speaking.

Based on information from various sources, the standard measurement of pulse wave velocity in adult women is 7.4 m/s. However, it is essential to note that baseline values tend to be lower in young, fit women, with an average of 6.1 (ranging from 4.6 to 7.5) m/s.

As women age, these values gradually increase either due to physiological changes in the vascular endothelium, increased blood pressure, or other associated pathologies, or even during pregnancy [28].

2.4. Personalized Exercise Training Program

The exercise training program was developed by a team that included an obstetrician in collaboration with a cardiologist and a physiotherapist. The included pregnant women participated daily for 12 weeks in this individualized physical training program under the supervision of a physiotherapist.

Exercise training program exercises performed by the pregnant women created and used in this study are described in Table 1. The existence of an average age of 25 years and, consequently, an adequate physical condition allowed the use of medium-intensity exercise sets on the Borg scale in this study [29].

Table 1. Description of the physical exercises performed during the intervention program.

Position	Exercise	Sets	Repetitions
Standing up	Circular movements of the head to the left and to the right	1	10
Standing up	Hands on the shoulders, raise arms and inhale, exhale on bringing hands back to the shoulders	1	10
Standing up	Legs pulled apart, with a straight back, both hands on hips, turn the trunk to the left, and then turn the trunk to the right and exhale	1	10
Standing up	Back straight, arms extended forward, heels on the floor, bend knees, extend knees, and exhale.	2	10 (1 min break between the series)
Standing up	With 2-kg weights in hands, do alternative back and forth lunges.	2	10 (1 min break between the series)
Standing up	With 2-kg weights in hands, bring the arm up to 90 degrees and exhale slowly when bringing the arm back down.	2	10 (1 min break between the series)
Standing up	With 2-kg weights in hands, flex forearms on the arms; let the air out slowly as you bring forearm back down.	2	10 (1 min break between the series)
Standing up	With arms raised at 90 degrees and elbows bent, bring arms together in front of you, and then take arms back and exhale	1	10
Standing up	Extend arms forward as you lift up each leg out laterally and exhale	1	10
Sitting on a fitness ball	With 2-kg weights attached to the ankles, lift each leg and inhale, bring leg back down slowly, and exhale.	1	10 for each leg
Sitting on a fitness ball	Using a strip, bring leg to the back, eyes following the arm, bring leg in the initial position, and exhale	1	10 for each leg
Sitting on a fitness ball	With both hands-on hips, rotate the trunk laterally	1	10 for each leg
Warning signs to stop physical activity during pregnancy	Vaginal bleeding, shortness of breath, dizziness, headache, precordial chest pain, easy fatigability, target heart rate > 145 bpm, decreased fetal movement, uterine contractions, pain in the lower back, abdomen, or pelvic area (potentially indicating pre-term labor)		

2.5. Statistical Analysis

The SPSS software (SPSS 22.0 Inc., Chicago, IL, USA) and JASP v18.3 were used for statistical analysis. Results for variables were presented as means ± standard deviation or percentages. Group comparisons were conducted using the two-tailed Student *t*-test, respectively, the Mann–Whitney test, or the ANOVA test/Kruskal–Wallis test, depending on the situation. A p-value of less than 0.05 was considered statistically significant. At the end of our analysis, a regression model was included to test the possible association between the studied variables; and the results were plotted using a scatter representation. The database has only numerical variables, so, we can calculate the central tendency and dispersion parameters for the entire database. For representing the data in the descriptive analysis, a boxplot or histogram chart was used. The data distribution was tested using the Shapiro–Wilk test (for a p value below 0.05, non-parametrical tests were applied).

3. Results

3.1. Description of the Patient's Lot

Forty pregnant patients in the second trimester of pregnancy were included in this study, whose mean values at inclusion in the exercise program for the variables age, height, weight, and BMI are represented in Table 2. We can say that our sample comprised young subjects, with a mean value for the age of 25 years, and women who practiced sports regularly (Table 2).

Table 2. Descriptive data on pregnant women at baseline (T0, n = 40).

UPN	AGE (Years)	Pregnancy	Cardiovascular Risk Factors	Medical History	At Baseline (T0)			
					Gestational Week	Height (cm)	Weight (cm)	BMI (kg/m^2)
#1	18	G1P0	No	No	15 weeks 5 days	155	40	16.6
#2	19	G1P0	No	No	23 weeks 4 days	169	67	23.5
#3	19	G1P0	No	No	16 weeks 5 days	169	75	26.3
#4	19	G1P0	No	No	19 weeks 4 days	170	59	20.4
#5	19	G1P0	No	No	20 weeks 2 days	164	58	21.6
#6	20	G1P0	Obesity	No	15 weeks 3 days	160	88	34.4
#7	20	G1P0	No	No	16 weeks 6 days	175	65	21.2
#8	20	G1P0	No	No	21 weeks 5 days	167	65	23.3
#9	20	G1P0	No	No	18 weeks 5 days	152	54	23.4
#10	20	G2P1	No	No	16 weeks 5 days	155	69	28.7
#11	21	G1P0	No	No	23 weeks 3 days	169	76	26.6
#12	21	G1P0	No	No	22 weeks 6 days	157	73	29.6
#13	21	G1P0	No	No	18 weeks 6 days	161	75	28.9
#14	21	G1P1	No	No	16 weeks 5 days	170	81	28
#15	21	G1P0	No	No	19 weeks 4 days	168	75	26.6
#16	21	G1P0	No	No	21 weeks 1 days	164	69	25.7
#17	21	G1P0	No	No	20 weeks 4 days	162	98	37.3
#18	21	G1P0	No	No	16 weeks 2 days	167	52	18.6
#19	21	G1P0	No	No	14 weeks 6 days	168	68	24.1
#20	22	G1P0	No	No	20 weeks 7 days	185	87.5	25.5
#21	22	G1P0	Obesity	No	22 weeks 6 days	178	101	31.9
#22	22	G1P0	No	No	23 weeks 5 days	168	81	28.7
#23	22	G1P0	No	No	17 weeks 5 days	160	69	27
#24	23	G1P0	Obesity	No	20 weeks 4 days	165	96	35.3
#25	24	G1P0	No	No	16 weeks 3 days	168	78	27.6
#26	24	G1P0	No	No	16 weeks 5 days	164	68	25.3
#27	24	G1P0	Obesity	No	20 weeks 3 days	160	98	38.3
#28	25	G1P0	No	No	19 weeks 6 days	168	78	27.6
#29	26	G1P0	Obesity	Cholecystectomy	17 weeks 4 days	168	97	34.4
#30	27	G1P0	No	No	22 weeks 1 day	164	68	25.3

Table 2. *Cont.*

UPN	AGE (Years)	Pregnancy	Cardiovascular Risk Factors	Medical History	At Baseline (T0)			
					Gestational Week	Height (cm)	Weight (cm)	BMI (kg/m^2)
#31	27	G1P0	No	No	16 weeks 6 days	167	73	26.2
#32	28	G1P0	Obesity	No	20 weeks 4 days	151	74	32.5
#33	28	G1P0	No	No	18 weeks 3 days	158	51	20.4
#34	28	G1P0	No	No	17 weeks 5 days	172	65	22
#35	30	G1P0	No	Appendectomy	21 weeks 2 days	165	61	22.4
#36	35	G1P0	No	No	19 weeks 5 days	168	68	24.1
#37	35	G1P0	No	No	16 weeks 5 days	185	87.4	25.5
#38	43	G1P0	No	Chronic Gastritis	17 weeks 6 days	164	61	22.7
#39	44	G2P1	No	No	18 weeks 5 days	152	55	23.5
#40	45	G1P0	No	No	20 weeks 2 days	169	64	22.2

UPN, unic patient number.

3.2. Analysis of Arterial Function Parameters before and after Performing the Exercise Training Program

The analyzed pregnant women ($n = 40$) had an active life and practiced sports regularly. We gathered information about the subject's age, height, weight, body mass index (BMI), AIx brachial values, PWVao values, systolic (Sys) and diastolic (Dia) blood pressure, and heartbeats minute in the second (at baseline, T0) and third trimester of pregnancy (after finished exercise training program, T1) (Trim II and Trim III).

All the characteristics of arterial function variables measured with arteriography at inclusion and after performing the exercise training program are presented in the next table (Table 3).

Table 3. Arterial function parameters measure with arteriograph at T0 and T1 ($n = 40$); in the case where the data are normally distributed, a parametrical test was applied—the *t*-paired test (*), respectively, where the data are not normally distributed, a non-parametrical test was applied—the Wilcoxon Signed-Rank test (**). The level of significance is $\alpha = 0.05$. The significant results are highlighted in grey.

Statistics	AIx Brachial [%]		PWVao [m/s]		SBP [mmHg]		DBP [mmHg]		HR [bpm]	
	T0	T1	T0	T1	T0	T1	T0	T1	T0	T1
p Value	$p = 0.02$ (**)		$p < 0.001$ (*)		$p = 0.001$ (**)		$p = 0.006$ (**)		$p = 0.095$ (**)	
Mean	−53.94	−52.66	8.54	7.62	120.55	117.80	72.18	70.33	72.63	71.55
Standard Error	2.33	2.37	0.12	0.11	2.16	1.79	1.66	1.61	1.42	1.27
Median	−56	−55.75	8.55	7.5	123	120	69.5	68.5	72.5	71
Mode	−61.3	−30	7.9	6.8	124	120	66	60	75	62
Standard Deviation	14.77	14.98	0.77	0.69	13.65	11.30	10.52	10.20	9.01	8.03
Sample Variance	218.01	224.48	0.59	0.48	186.41	127.75	110.76	104.02	81.11	64.41
Range	49.3	58.7	2.9	2.6	52	45	45	35	36	33
Minimum	−78.7	−78.7	6.9	6.5	96	100	53	55	57	57
Maximum	−29.4	−20	9.8	9.1	148	145	98	90	93	90
Count	40	40	40	40	40	40	40	40	40	40

All the characteristics of arterial function variables measured with arteriography at inclusion and after performing the exercise training program, as well as the significance obtained after applying the t-paired/Wilcoxon Signed-Rank test, are presented in Table 3. A significant improvement ($p < 0.05$) was obtained in four out of five parameters.

Regarding the evolution of the AIx brachial and PWVao values, we observed a decreased in these arterial stiffness parameters in all healthy pregnant women ($n = 40$), as can be seen in Figures 1 and 2.

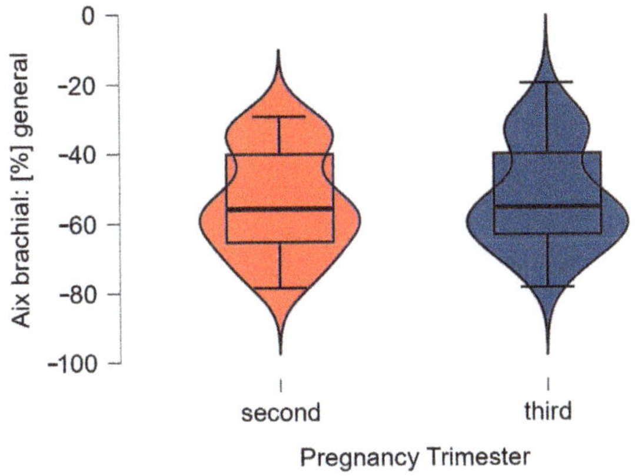

Figure 1. The data distribution of AIx brachial values in the second (T0) and third trimester of pregnancy (T1) ($n = 40$), using a boxplot representation with violin effect.

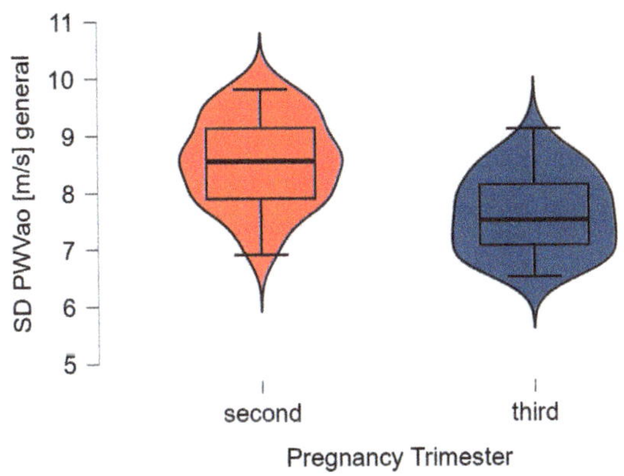

Figure 2. The data distribution of the PWVao values in the second (T0) and third trimester of pregnancy (T1) ($n = 40$), using a boxplot representation with violin effect.

The regression analysis for the AIx brachial values and the PWVao values from Trim II (T0) and Trim III (T1) showed major differences between these two time points, but we also wanted to test if these variables have a relation between them. For this purpose, we have run a regression analysis in which we considered the values from Trim II as predictors and the values from Trim III as responses. The association of the sample was calculated with the Pearson coefficient. The results obtained are the following: pregnancy revealed a strong direct significant correlation between the AIx brachial values in the second and third trimesters of pregnancy $\left(r = 0.97,\ R^2 = 0.95,\ p < 0.001\right)$ and that the correlation between the PWVao values in the second and third trimester of pregnancy is weak and insignificant $\left(r = -0.25,\ R^2 = 0.06,\ p = 0.12 > 0.05\right)$.

In conclusion, the AIx brachial values are constantly decreasing for the whole sample, while for PWVao values, the decreasing process does not have the same dynamic in the whole sample. This relation between the two variables is presented in Figures 3 and 4.

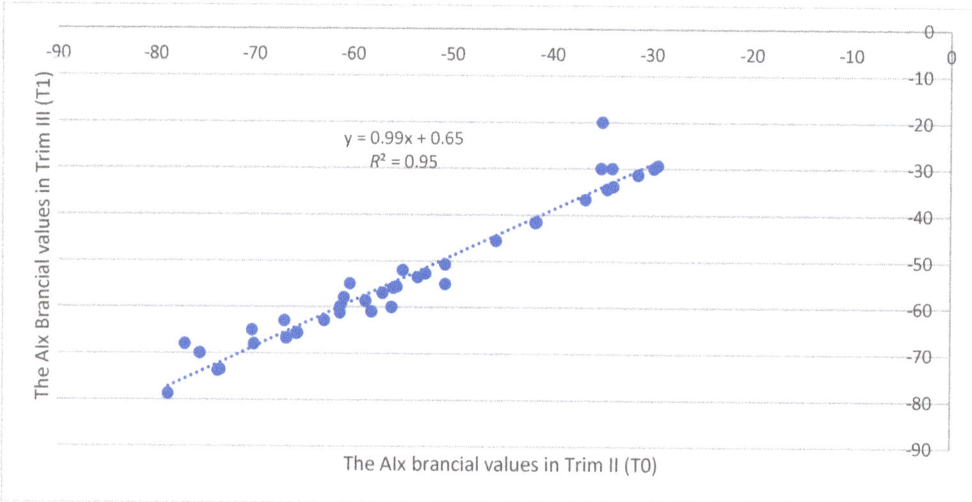

Figure 3. The association between the AIx brachial values in Trim II (T0) and Trim III (T1) (n = 40).

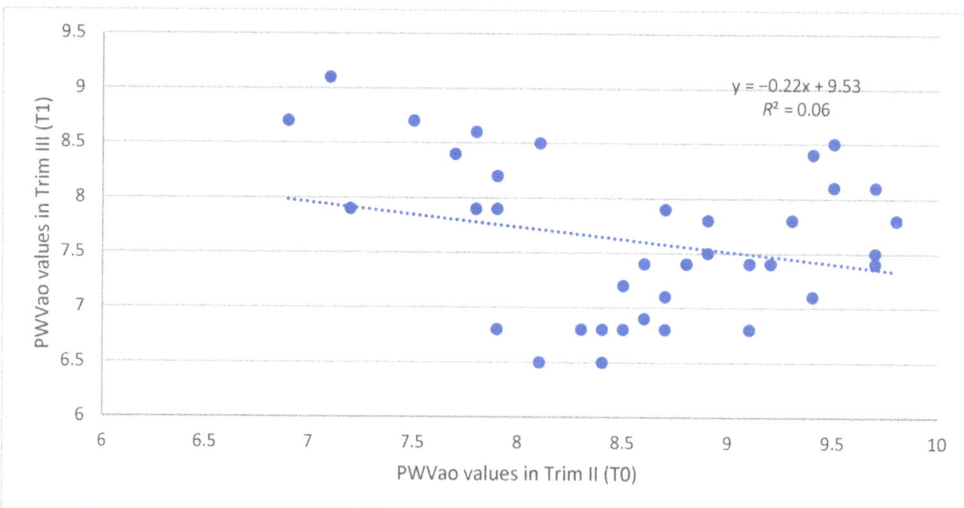

Figure 4. The association between the PWVao values in Trim II (T0) and Trim III (T1) (n = 40).

4. Discussion

The present study concerns a special group of subjects, pregnant women, who, according to the guideline for the management of cardiovascular disease during pregnancy from the European Society of Cardiology, are at very high cardiovascular risk [15]. Additionally, it is essential to note that pregnancy alone is linked to a significant three to four-fold increase in the occurrence of acute myocardial infarction compared to women of the same age who are not pregnant [30–32].

The etiology of cardiovascular disease in pregnancy differs from that of the general population; most pregnant women develop coronary artery disease that has non-atherosclerotic mechanisms, followed closely by pregnancy-related spontaneous coronary artery dissection (43% pregnancy-related cardiovascular disease), and coronary arteries in pregnant women are angiographically normal [33,34]. The mechanisms of acute myocardial infarction in pregnant women with angiographically normal coronary arteries remain unclear and include transient coronary spasm [35] due to either increased vascular reactivity and/or arterial stiffness that occurs physiologically in pregnancy [28,36,37].

So, in this study, we examined endothelial dysfunction as a marker of subclinical arterial stiffness among healthy pregnant women and the impact of a personalized exercise training program on it. This study has three major findings. Our main finding was the reduction in PWV values with significant differences between the two times studied (T0 at inclusion in the exercise training program and T1 at the finished of the exercise training program). Secondly, the benefit of this program is reducing and normalizing cardiovascular risk factors (blood pressure, women's weight, pulse pressure, etc.). Thirdly, the performance in the diagnosis and monitoring of endothelial dysfunction with the help of PWV measurement in pregnant women. dysfunction. Another added value of the current study is that this program was developed, initiated, and continued in a local hospital and led by a team that included an obstetrician, a cardiologist, and a physiotherapist.

Specialty studies show how physical activity has been a subject of considerable research and attention during pregnancy and they highlight the importance of physical activity in order to promote a healthy status. An appropriate level of physical activity or an exercise program during pregnancy is very useful. Choosing to continue and maintain this health status is a recent research area in maternal and child health, and pregnant women can choose different levels of physical activity [38]. Clapp et al. found that women who continued to exercise during pregnancy maintained their training regimens and their fitness levels well above the cardiovascular risk index, and their level of risk is well below those present in both the general population and the number of women who temporarily interrupted their exercise during pregnancy. Further, they also observed that pregnant women who engage in weight-bearing exercise throughout their pregnancy preserve their overall fitness and maintain a low cardiovascular risk profile during the perimenopausal phase [39].

The American College of Obstetricians and Gynecologists (ACOG) released its initial findings and suggestions regarding physical activity during pregnancy in 2002. According to the ACOG, pregnant women without any medical or obstetric complications should engage in at least 30 min of moderate-intensity exercise. Conducting a thorough clinical examination before providing exercise recommendations to pregnant women is essential. Unless there are any reasons to avoid exercise, it is recommended to engage in moderate-intensity exercises regularly. Additionally, pregnant women should be educated on the signs indicating the need to stop physical training [40]. When developing a physical exercise program, it is crucial to consider the type and intensity of the exercise [41].

The American College of Obstetricians and Gynecologists [42], the Society of Obstetricians and Gynecologists of Canada (SOGC) [43], and the Royal College of Obstetricians and Gynecologists of Australia and New Zealand (RANZCOG) [44] guidelines were analyzed in a review [17] regarding recommending exercise during pregnancy. All these guidelines universally agreed that women who do not have any contraindications should be encouraged to engage in regular aerobic and strength-conditioning exercises during pregnancy. The ACOG recommends that pregnant women aim for 150 min of exercise per week, which can be broken down into 20–30 min per day. The RAZCOG suggests that pregnant women can aim for 150–300 or 70–150 min of vigorous exercise per week (with each session not exceeding 60 min). The SOGC does not officially recommend exercise duration during pregnancy. It is important to note that exercising during pregnancy can positively affect both the mother's and the fetus's health.

At the same time, physical inactivity is considered a significant risk factor for maternal mortality. Furthermore, regular exercise during pregnancy has not been linked to adverse perinatal outcomes [45,46]. Pregnant women who adhered to the recommended physical activity guidelines of engaging in 150 min of moderate-to-vigorous physical activity per week experienced lower central and peripheral PWV levels [47].

Our research yielded a significant and noteworthy distinction in the values of systolic blood pressure, diastolic blood pressure, and heart rate when comparing two distinct periods: before and after a 12-week exercise program during pregnancy. A similar study, which involved 56 women with healthy, singleton, low-risk pregnancies (30 in the control group and 26 in the exercise group), utilized magnetocardiogram recordings to demonstrate that exercising during pregnancy can enhance cardiac autonomic control [48]. A recent systematic review and meta-analysis that investigated the effects of aerobic and resistance exercise on blood pressure during pregnancy while experiencing clinical conditions such as gestational diabetes mellitus and obesity during pregnancy observed that exercise has the potential to decrease the typical rise in blood pressure associated with these conditions. These discoveries carry significant importance for pregnant women who are at risk of developing gestational hypertension and pre-eclampsia [49].

The findings from our study, which demonstrate a decrease in arterial stiffness and improvements in hemodynamic parameters, align with the existing data reported in the literature. At the onset of the second trimester of pregnancy, the exercise and control groups exhibited no significant disparity in PWV values when assessing arterial stiffness. However, upon analyzing the same group of pregnant women one month after delivery, those who engaged in regular exercise throughout their pregnancy displayed a significantly lower PWV compared to their second-trimester measurements (1145.9 $\pm$ 88.1 cm/s vs. 1122.7 $\pm$ 100.2 cm/s, respectively; insignificant). Conversely, the control group, which did not partake in exercise, maintained a PWV of 1116.7 $\pm$ 87.9 cm/s, indicating an increase in arterial stiffness [14]. In a separate study, 191 women with high-risk singleton pregnancies were examined to assess the predictive capabilities of arterial stiffness parameters in early pre-eclampsia compared to peripheral blood pressure, angiogenic biomarkers, and uterine artery Doppler. Within this group of expectant mothers, a total of 7.3% experienced the development of pre-eclampsia. The likelihood of pre-eclampsia increased by 64% ($p <$ 0.05) for every one m/s rise in first trimester PWV, while a 1-millisecond increase in time to wave reflection resulted in an 11% decrease in the odds of pre-eclampsia ($p < 0.01$). The researchers assert that arterial stiffness is a superior predictor of pre-eclampsia compared to other analyzed methods, demonstrating its early detection and heightened efficacy [50].

The regression analysis for the AIx brachial values and the PWVao values from Trim II (T0) and Trim III (T1) showed major differences between these two time points as follows: pregnancy revealed a strong direct significant correlation between the AIx brachial values in the second and third trimester of pregnancy $\left(r = 0.97,\ R^2 = 0.95,\ p < 0.001\right)$ and that the correlation between the PWVao values in the second and third trimester of pregnancy is weak and insignificant $\left(r = -0.25,\ R^2 = 0.06,\ p = 0.12\right)$.

While our study highlights the advantages of personalized exercise training programs for healthy pregnant women in their second trimester, there is still room for improvement. It is crucial to address the identified gaps and take action to enhance general exercise programs for pregnant women, regardless of their cardiovascular risk factors. Various barriers hinder the implementation of these exercise programs, and we will focus on a few encountered in our study. These include patients' willingness to participate, inequalities in access and availability of exercise facilities, and the need for more collaboration between obstetricians, cardiologists, and physiotherapists, possibly due to limited experience [51,52].

Initiating prevention measures for cardiovascular disease is crucial at the earliest stages for individuals of all genders. We believe that women in particular should take advantage of cardiac consultations during pregnancy, perimenopause, and menopause to evaluate their cardiovascular risk. It is widely known that early onset of menopause is associated with an increased likelihood of developing cardiovascular disease, making it a significant red flag during medical check-ups [1]. One method to identify potential major adverse cardiac events (MACEs) is via screening mammography, which can assess breast density in overweight women and serve as a predictive tool [53]. Indeed, tissue over-expressed inflammatory cytokines and oxidative stress molecules leading to cardiac dysfunction and worse prognosis were observed [54]. Overweight and metabolic distress could cause MACEs in women via over-inflammation [55].

Limitations of the Study

One limitation of this study is its reliance on data collected from a single regional hospital in Romania, which restricts the generalizability of the findings to other contexts due to variations in healthcare policies [51]. However, it is important to note that the study's focus on healthy pregnant women, who are the majority of the pregnant population, ensures the relevance of the findings to a significant portion of the healthcare community. Another constraint is the lack of homogeneity in the age distribution of the analyzed group, as only pregnant women under the age of 40 were included, with a significantly higher proportion being under the age of 30 also the sample size, which is quite small, underlining the need for future studies with a larger sample to support the results of this research.

By excluding pregnant women who possess any of the numerous high-risk factors that have the potential to impact arterial stiffness, selection bias is effectively minimized. Consequently, the chances of encountering selection bias are meager, enabling the normal ranges we have delineated to apply to low-risk women across different populations.

The exclusion of pregnant women with any of a long list of high-risk factors (which could affect arterial stiffness) should effectively reduce selection bias. As a result, the likelihood of encountering selection bias is minimal, allowing the normal ranges we outline to be relevant for low-risk women in various populations. It is also recognized that the accuracy of all self-reported information could not be fully verified in terms of perceived correct exercise intensity (intensity perception may differ from one pregnant woman to another), but we believe that we have eliminated these reasons by objectively tracking the warning signs for discontinuation of physical activity (see Table 1).

5. Conclusions

Our study results showed that physical training, coordinated by a medical team that consisted of an obstetrician, a physiotherapist, and a cardiologist, improves the hemodynamic parameters (SBP, PP, and HR) of the healthy pregnant woman during pregnancy, and that the PWV is a reliable method to measured arterial stiffness in this type of patients. Strictly supervised physical training may reduce pregnancy-induced hypertension.

Additionally, regular exercise in healthy pregnant women decreased arterial stiffness, suggesting that regular exercise may help prevent hypertensive disorders during pregnancy and that our personalized exercise training program may be used to reduce blood pressure and prevent the development of arterial rigidity during pregnancy. We believe that this personalized exercise training program and, moreover, assessment by a multidisciplinary medical team represents an opportunity for the early detection of risk factors, refinement of CVD risk assessment, and implementation of primary prevention in women.

However, further studies are required to determine whether this adaptation to exercise can effectively reduce the risk of adverse outcomes associated with gestational conditions characterized by impaired autonomic control, such as diabetes, hypertension, pre-eclampsia, and excessive weight gain.

Author Contributions: Conceptualization, I.P. (Izabella Petre), S.I., M.I. and F.B. (Florina Buleu); Data curation, I.P. (Ion Petre), R.D.M., F.M.B. and D.P.; Investigation, I.P. (Izabella Petre), V.T., R.T. and L.M.; Methodology, I.P. (Izabella Petre), S.I. and M.I.; Software, I.P. (Ion Petre), R.D.M., D.P. and F.M.B. (Flavia Mirela Barna); Supervision, A.B., S.I., and M.I.; Validation, I.P. (Izabella Petre) and M.I.; Visualization, V.T., A.B. and L.M.; Writing—original draft, I.P. (Izabella Petre), S.I. and V.T.; Writing—review and editing, I.P. (Izabella Petre), S.I., F.B. (Florina Buleu), A.B., L.M.C., L.M. and M.I. All the authors have equal contributions to this paper. All authors have read and agreed to the published version of the manuscript.

Funding: We would like to acknowledge "Victor Babes" University of Medicine and Pharmacy Timisoara for their support in covering the costs of publication for this research paper.

Institutional Review Board Statement: The study conformed to the Declaration of Helsinki and was approved by the Ethics Committee of the Emergency Clinical Hospital "Pius Brinzeu" Timisoara Timișoara, Romania (decision no. 54/20 April 2017).

Informed Consent Statement: Informed consent was obtained from all patients involved in the study.

Data Availability Statement: The data and materials can be provided upon reasonable request to the corresponding author.

Conflicts of Interest: The authors declare no conflicts of interest.

References

1. O'Kelly, A.C.; Michos, E.D.; Shufelt, C.L.; Vermunt, J.V.; Minissian, M.B.; Quesada, O.; Smith, G.N.; Rich-Edwards, J.W.; Garovic, V.D.; El Khoudary, S.R.; et al. Pregnancy and Reproductive Risk Factors for Cardiovascular Disease in Women. *Circ. Res.* **2022**, *130*, 652–672. [CrossRef] [PubMed]
2. Soma-Pillay, P.; Nelson-Piercy, C.; Tolppanen, H.; Mebazaa, A. Physiological changes in pregnancy. *Cardiovasc. J. Afr.* **2016**, *27*, 89–94. [CrossRef] [PubMed]
3. Wykrętowicz, M.; Krauze, T.; Guzik, P.; Piskorski, J.; Markwitz, W.; Wykrętowicz, A.; Wysocki, H. Arterial stiffness, central hemodynamics and wave reflection in normal pregnancy and control nonpregnant women. *Eur. J. Obs. Gynecol. Reprod. Biol.* **2011**, *159*, 49–52. [CrossRef] [PubMed]
4. Khalil, A.; Garcia-Mandujano, R.; Maiz, N.; Elkhouli, M.; Nicolaides, K.H. Longitudinal changes in maternal hemodynamics in a population at risk for pre-eclampsia. *Ultrasound Obstet. Gynecol.* **2014**, *44*, 197–204. [CrossRef] [PubMed]
5. Khalil, A.; Jauniaux, E.; Cooper, D.; Harrington, K. Pulse wave analysis in normal pregnancy: A prospective longitudinal study. *PLoS ONE* **2009**, *4*, e6134. [CrossRef] [PubMed]
6. Tucker, T. Physics Linkages Between Arterial Morphology, Pulse Wave Reflection and Peripheral Flow. *Artery Res.* **2023**, *29*, 46–71. [CrossRef]
7. Iurciuc, M.; Gaita, D.; Iurciuc, S.; Avram, C.; Fira-Mladinescu, O.; Oravitan, M.; Mancas, S. The evolution of arterial stiffness and hemodynamic parameters following an rehabilitation program. *J. Hypertens* **2008**, *26*, S492.
8. Vasan, R.S.; Pan, S.; Xanthakis, V.; Beiser, A.; Larson, M.G.; Seshadri, S.; Mitchell, G.F. Arterial Stiffness and Long-Term Risk of Health Outcomes: The Framingham Heart Study. *Hypertension* **2022**, *79*, 1045–1056. [CrossRef]
9. Turi, V.; Iurciuc, S.; Crețu, O.M.; Tit, D.M.; Bungau, S.; Apostol, A.; Moleriu, R.D.; Bustea, C.; Behl, T.; Diaconu, C.C.; et al. Arterial function in hypertensive pregnant women. Is arterial stiffness a marker for the outcomes in pregnancy? *Life Sci.* **2021**, *264*, 118723. [CrossRef]
10. Witvrouwen, I.; Mannaerts, D.; Van Berendoncks, A.M.; Jacquemyn, Y.; Van Craenenbroeck, E.M. The Effect of Exercise Training During Pregnancy to Improve Maternal Vascular Health: Focus on Gestational Hypertensive Disorders. *Front. Physiol.* **2020**, *11*, 450. [CrossRef]
11. Do, N.C.; Vestgaard, M.; Nørgaard, S.K.; Damm, P.; Mathiesen, E.R.; Ringholm, L. Prediction and prevention of preeclampsia in women with preexisting diabetes: The role of home blood pressure, physical activity, and aspirin. *Front. Endocrinol.* **2023**, *14*, 1166884. [CrossRef] [PubMed]
12. Lan, Y.S.; Khong, T.K.; Yusof, A. Effect of Exercise on Arterial Stiffness in Healthy Young, Middle-Aged and Older Women: A Systematic Review. *Nutrients* **2023**, *15*, 308. [CrossRef] [PubMed]
13. Ramírez-Vélez, R.; Aguilar de Plata, A.C.; Escudero, M.M.; Echeverry, I.; Ortega, J.G.; Salazar, B.; Rey, J.J.; Hormiga, C.; López-Jaramillo, P. Influence of regular aerobic exercise on endothelium-dependent vasodilation and cardiorespiratory fitness in pregnant women. *J. Obstet. Gynaecol. Res.* **2011**, *37*, 1601–1608. [CrossRef]
14. Kawabata, I.; Nakai, A.; Sekiguchi, A.; Inoue, Y.; Takeshita, T. The effect of regular exercise training during pregnancy on postpartum brachial-ankle pulse wave velocity, a measure of arterial stiffness. *J. Sports Sci. Med.* **2012**, *11*, 489–494. [PubMed]
15. Regitz-Zagrosek, V.; Roos-Hesselink, J.W.; Bauersachs, J.; Blomström-Lundqvist, C.; Cífková, R.; De Bonis, M.; Iung, B.; Johnson, M.R.; Kintscher, U.; Kranke, P.; et al. 2018 ESC Guidelines for the management of cardiovascular diseases during pregnancy: The Task Force for the Management of Cardiovascular Diseases during Pregnancy of the European Society of Cardiology (ESC). *Eur. Heart J.* **2018**, *39*, 3165–3241. [CrossRef]
16. Iurciuc, M.; Gaita, D.; Iurciuc, S.; Avram, C.; Craciun, L.; Avram, A. From guideline to clinical practice-reinforced primary care at high-risk patients. *Circulation* **2012**, *125*, E732.
17. Tsakiridis, I.; Bakaloudi, D.R.; Oikonomidou, A.C.; Dagklis, T.; Chourdakis, M. Exercise during pregnancy: A comparative review of guidelines. *J. Perinat. Med.* **2020**, *48*, 519–525. [CrossRef]
18. Craciun, L.M.; Buleu, F.; Pah, A.M.; Badalica-Petrescu, M.; Bodea, O.; Man, D.E.; Cosor, O.C.; Iurciuc, S.; Dragan, S.; Rada, M. The Benefits of a Comprehensive Cardiac Rehabilitation Program for Patients with Acute Coronary Syndrome: A Follow-Up Study. *J. Pers. Med.* **2023**, *13*, 1516. [CrossRef] [PubMed]
19. Saz-Lara, A.; Cavero-Redondo, I.; Álvarez-Bueno, C.; Notario-Pacheco, B.; Ruiz-Grao, M.C.; Martínez-Vizcaíno, V. The Acute Effect of Exercise on Arterial Stiffness in Healthy Subjects: A Meta-Analysis. *J. Clin. Med.* **2021**, *10*, 291. [CrossRef]
20. Sacre, J.W.; Jennings, G.L.R.; Kingwell, B.A. Exercise and Dietary Influences on Arterial Stiffness in Cardiometabolic Disease. *Hypertension* **2014**, *63*, 888–893. [CrossRef]
21. Zang, Y.; Ding, X.; Zhao, M.X.; Zhang, X.; Zhang, L.; Wu, S.; Sun, L. Arterial stiffness acute changes following aerobic exercise in males with and without hypertension. *J. Clin. Hypertens.* **2022**, *24*, 430–437. [CrossRef] [PubMed]

22. Avram, C.; Iurciuc, M.; Craciun, L.; Avram, A.; Iurciuc, S.; Oancea, C.; Gaita, D. Dietary and physical activity counseling in high-risk asymptomatic patients with metabolic syndrome-A primary care intervention. *J. Food Agric. Environ.* **2011**, *9*, 16–19.
23. Iurciuc, M.; Gaita, D.; Iurciuc, S.; Avram, C.; Duda-Seiman, D.; Ciorica, G.; Cobzariu, I.; Oravitan, M.; Ursoniu, S. The importance of arterial stiffness in a rehabilitation program at hypertensive person. *J. Hypertens.* **2009**, *27*, S287–S288.
24. Iurciuc, M.; Avram, C.; Iurciuc, S.; Franculescu, C.; Vlad, A.; Mancas, S. Comprehensive rehabilitation programs may improve some of the ambulatory blood pressure parameter. In Proceedings of the 17th European Congress of Physical and Rehabilitation Medicine, Venice, Italy, 23–27 May 2010; pp. 253–255.
25. Iurciuc, M.; Gaita, D.; Iurciuc, S.; Dragan, S.; Duda-Seiman, D.; Dumitrasciuc, M.; Avram, A.; Mancas, S. The benefit of exercise training on arterial stiffness at hypertensive patients. *Eur. Heart J.* **2007**, *28*, 523.
26. Helsinki, D.O. Recommendations guiding physicians in biomedical research involving human subjects. *JAMA* **1997**, *277*, 925–926.
27. Visseren, F.L.; Mach, F.; Smulders, Y.M.; Carballo, D.; Koskinas, K.C.; Bäck, M.; Benetos, A.; Biffi, A.; Boavida, J.-M.; Capodanno, D. 2021 ESC Guidelines on cardiovascular disease prevention in clinical practice: Developed by the Task Force for cardiovascular disease prevention in clinical practice with representatives of the European Society of Cardiology and 12 medical societies With the special contribution of the European Association of Preventive Cardiology (EAPC). *Eur. J. Prev. Cardiol.* **2022**, *29*, 5–115. [PubMed]
28. Turi, V.; Dragan, S.; Iurciuc, M.; Moleriu, L.; Bungau, S.; Tit, D.M.; Toader, D.-O.; Diaconu, C.C.; Behl, T.; Petre, I. Arterial Function in Healthy Pregnant Women vs. Non-Pregnant Women—A 10-Year Study. *Diagnostics* **2020**, *10*, 374. [CrossRef]
29. Scherr, J.; Wolfarth, B.; Christle, J.W.; Pressler, A.; Wagenpfeil, S.; Halle, M. Associations between Borg's rating of perceived exertion and physiological measures of exercise intensity. *Eur. J. Appl. Physiol.* **2013**, *113*, 147–155. [CrossRef] [PubMed]
30. James, A.H.; Jamison, M.G.; Biswas, M.S.; Brancazio, L.R.; Swamy, G.K.; Myers, E.R. Acute myocardial infarction in pregnancy: A United States population-based study. *Circulation* **2006**, *113*, 1564–1571. [CrossRef]
31. Merlo, A.C.; Rosa, G.M.; Porto, I. Pregnancy-related acute myocardial infarction: A review of the recent literature. *Clin. Res. Cardiol.* **2022**, *111*, 723–731. [CrossRef]
32. Tweet, M.S.; Lewey, J.; Smilowitz, N.R.; Rose, C.H.; Best, P.J.M. Pregnancy-Associated Myocardial Infarction. *Circ. Cardiovasc. Interv.* **2020**, *13*, e008687. [CrossRef] [PubMed]
33. Elkayam, U.; Jalnapurkar, S.; Barakkat, M.N.; Khatri, N.; Kealey, A.J.; Mehra, A.; Roth, A. Pregnancy-associated acute myocardial infarction: A review of contemporary experience in 150 cases between 2006 and 2011. *Circulation* **2014**, *129*, 1695–1702. [CrossRef] [PubMed]
34. Tweet, M.S.; Hayes, S.N.; Codsi, E.; Gulati, R.; Rose, C.H.; Best, P.J.M. Spontaneous Coronary Artery Dissection Associated With Pregnancy. *J. Am. Coll. Cardiol.* **2017**, *70*, 426–435. [CrossRef] [PubMed]
35. Roth, A.; Elkayam, U. Acute myocardial infarction associated with pregnancy. *J. Am. Coll. Cardiol.* **2008**, *52*, 171–180. [CrossRef] [PubMed]
36. Pereira, M.M.; Torrado, J.; Sosa, C.; Diaz, A.; Bia, D.; Zócalo, Y. Center-To-Periphery Arterial Stiffness Gradient Is Attenuated and/or Reversed in Pregnancy-Associated Hypertension. *Front. Cardiovasc. Med.* **2021**, *8*, 766723. [CrossRef] [PubMed]
37. Pandey, A.K.; Siwach, S.; Sangwan, V.; Sharma, S.; Das, A. Assessment of maternal vascular stiffness indices in three trimesters of normal pregnancy. *Indian. J. Physiol. Pharmacol.* **2014**, *58*, 197–205. [PubMed]
38. Chan, C.W.H.; Au Yeung, E.; Law, B.M.H. Effectiveness of Physical Activity Interventions on Pregnancy-Related Outcomes among Pregnant Women: A Systematic Review. *Int. J. Env. Res. Public. Health* **2019**, *16*, 1840. [CrossRef] [PubMed]
39. Clapp, J.F., 3rd. Long-term outcome after exercising throughout pregnancy: Fitness and cardiovascular risk. *Am. J. Obs. Gynecol.* **2008**, *199*, 489.e1–489.e6. [CrossRef] [PubMed]
40. ACOG Committee on Obstetric Practice. Committee opinion #267: Exercise during pregnancy and the postpartum period. *Obs. Gynecol* **2002**, *99*, 171–173.
41. Artal, R.; O'Toole, M. Guidelines of the American College of Obstetricians and Gynecologists for exercise during pregnancy and the postpartum period. *Br. J. Sports Med.* **2003**, *37*, 6–12; discussion 12. [CrossRef]
42. ACOG. Physical Activity and Exercise During Pregnancy and the Postpartum Period: ACOG Committee Opinion, Number 804. *Obstet. Gynecol.* **2020**, *135*, e178–e188. [CrossRef] [PubMed]
43. Mottola, M.F.; Davenport, M.H.; Ruchat, S.-M.; Davies, G.A.; Poitras, V.J.; Gray, C.E.; Garcia, A.J.; Barrowman, N.; Adamo, K.B.; Duggan, M.; et al. 2019 Canadian guideline for physical activity throughout pregnancy. *Br. J. Sports Med.* **2018**, *52*, 1339–1346. [CrossRef] [PubMed]
44. The Royal College of Obstetricians and Gynecologists of Australia and New Zealand. Exercise during Pregnancy. Available online: https://ranzcog.edu.au/wp-content/uploads/2022/05/Exercise-during-pregnancy.pdf (accessed on 25 September 2023).
45. Clapp, J.F., 3rd; Lopez, B.; Harcar-Sevcik, R. Neonatal behavioral profile of the offspring of women who continued to exercise regularly throughout pregnancy. *Am. J. Obs. Gynecol.* **1999**, *180 Pt 1*, 91–94. [CrossRef] [PubMed]
46. Davenport, M.H.; Meah, V.L.; Ruchat, S.M.; Davies, G.A.; Skow, R.J.; Barrowman, N.; Adamo, K.B.; Poitras, V.J.; Gray, C.E.; Jaramillo Garcia, A.; et al. Impact of prenatal exercise on neonatal and childhood outcomes: A systematic review and meta-analysis. *Br. J. Sports Med.* **2018**, *52*, 1386–1396. [CrossRef] [PubMed]
47. Matenchuk, B.A.; Fujii, K.; Skow, R.J.; Sobierajski, F.; MacKay, C.; Steinback, C.D.; Davenport, M.H. The effects of physical activity on arterial stiffness during pregnancy: An observational study. *Appl. Physiol. Nutr. Metab.* **2022**, *47*, 234–242. [CrossRef] [PubMed]

48. May, L.E.; Knowlton, J.; Hanson, J.; Suminski, R.; Paynter, C.; Fang, X.; Gustafson, K.M. Effects of Exercise During Pregnancy on Maternal Heart Rate and Heart Rate Variability. *PMR* **2016**, *8*, 611–617. [CrossRef] [PubMed]
49. Giles, C.; Johnston, R.; Kubler, J.; Spathis, J.; Beetham, K. The effects of aerobic and resistance exercise on blood pressure in uncomplicated and at risk pregnancies: A systematic review and meta-analysis. *Women's Health* **2023**, *19*, 17455057231183573. [CrossRef] [PubMed]
50. Phan, K.; Gomez, Y.H.; Gorgui, J.; El-Messidi, A.; Gagnon, R.; Abenhaim, H.A.; Rahme, E.; Daskalopoulou, S.S. Arterial stiffness for the early prediction of pre-eclampsia compared with blood pressure, uterine artery Doppler and angiogenic biomarkers: A prospective cohort study. *BJOG Int. J. Obstet. Gynaecol.* **2023**, *130*, 932–940. [CrossRef] [PubMed]
51. Petre, I.; Barna, F.; Gurgus, D.; Tomescu, L.C.; Apostol, A.; Petre, I.; Furau, C.; Năchescu, M.L.; Bordianu, A. Analysis of the Healthcare System in Romania: A Brief Review. *Healthcare* **2023**, *11*, 2069. [CrossRef]
52. Ilea, C.D.N.; Daina, L.G.; Bungau, S.; Tit, D.M.; Uivarosan, D.; Moleriu, L.; Petre, I.; Bungau, C.; Petre, I. Sustainable Management, Instable Legislation Regarding Wages, and Employee Satisfaction/Motivation in Two Romanian Hospitals. *Sustainability* **2020**, *12*, 909. [CrossRef]
53. Sardu, C.; Gatta, G.; Pieretti, G.; Viola, L.; Sacra, C.; Di Grezia, G.; Musto, L.; Minelli, S.; La Forgia, D.; Capodieci, M.; et al. Pre-Menopausal Breast Fat Density Might Predict MACE During 10 Years of Follow-Up: The BRECARD Study. *JACC Cardiovasc. Imaging* **2021**, *14*, 426–438. [CrossRef] [PubMed]
54. Sardu, C.; Gatta, G.; Pieretti, G.; Onofrio, N.; Balestrieri, M.L.; Scisciola, L.; Cappabianca, S.; Ferraro, G.; Nicoletti, G.F.; Signoriello, G.; et al. SGLT2 breast expression could affect the cardiovascular performance in pre-menopausal women with fatty vs. non fatty breast via over-inflammation and sirtuins' down regulation. *Eur. J. Intern. Med.* **2023**, *113*, 57–68. [CrossRef] [PubMed]
55. Sardu, C.; Paolisso, G.; Marfella, R. Impact of Sex Differences in Incident and Recurrent Coronary Events and All-Cause Mortality. *J. Am. Coll. Cardiol.* **2021**, *77*, 829–830. [CrossRef] [PubMed]

biomedicines

MDPI

Review

Iron Deficiency as a Factor of Worse Prognosis in Patients with Acute Myocardial Infarction

Aleksander Misiewicz *, Krzysztof Badura, Oliwia Matuszewska-Brycht, Jan Krekora and Jarosław Drożdż

2nd Department of Cardiology, Medical University of Lodz, 92-213 Lodz, Poland
* Correspondence: aleksander.misiewicz@umed.lodz.pl; Tel.: +48-607-272-539

Abstract: Acute coronary syndromes (ACS) are a leading cause of death and impairment in the adult population. Precise identification and modification of risk factors is crucial for a favorable clinical outcome. In this review, we aim to provide a comprehensive overview of the significance of iron deficiency (ID) in patients with ACS, particularly myocardial infarction (MI). The paper evaluates the impact of ID on the prognosis of ACS patients, highlighting its potential influence on myocardial healing, regeneration and cardiovascular events during the follow-up period. The findings suggest that iron deficiency may have a negative impact on the prognosis of patients with MI, resulting in worse quality of life, physical capacity and higher rehospitalization rates in comparison to patients with normal iron status. Iron supplementation in patients with MI could be beneficial and may have an effect on myocardial healing and left ventricular remodeling.

Keywords: iron deficiency; myocardial infarction; acute coronary syndrome; transferrin saturation; ferritin; cardiovascular disease; reactive oxygen species; oxidative stress

1. Introduction

Cardiovascular diseases are consistently the leading cause of death around the globe. In 2019, they were responsible for almost 18 million of deaths, accounting for 32% of deaths worldwide. The most common diagnoses among this group are myocardial infarction (MI) and stroke [1]. Despite the far-reaching expenditures on treatment and prevention programs, acute coronary syndromes (ACS) still constitute a great burden on healthcare systems and patients themselves. The most common risk factors for coronary artery disease are obesity, hypertension, diabetes, dyslipidemia and nicotinism [2]. In contrast to acute heart failure, the assessment of iron parameters in patients with ACS is not a part of a regular practice, yet iron plays a key role in the transport and storage of oxygen, as well as intracellular respiration. Therefore, its proper concentration and availability seem to be crucial in ischemic processes such as MI. Iron deficiency is the most common deficiency in the human population [3] and its non-invasive diagnosis is based on laboratory markers—ferritin (Fer) and transferrin saturation (TSAT). Values of Fer < 100 µg/L correspond to resource depletion and absolute iron deficiency (ID), and the range of Fer 100–300 µg/L along with TSAT < 20% correspond to functional ID [4,5]. The criteria presented above are widely used in patients with heart failure (HF), with their effectiveness proven in clinical trials [6–8]. The aim of this paper is to highlight the importance of ID, its incidence and prognostic value in patients with ACS, as well as to indicate potential areas of development on the basis of the available literature.

https://doi.org/10.3390/biomedicines13040769

2. Materials and Methods

Most scientific papers published to date seem to confirm the negative impact of iron deficiency on the prognosis of patients with myocardial infarction. We evaluated publications on iron deficiency in myocardial infarction written in English. We analyzed MEDLINE and Google Scholar databases between November 2023 and June 2024 using key words and terms, such as: "Iron deficiency" AND ("myocardial infarction" OR "acute coronary syndrome") AND "iron deficiency" AND "prognostic value" OR "iron supplementation" AND ("myocardial infarction" OR "acute coronary syndrome"). We included studies with human patients with ACS stratified by iron status, in most cases with regard to TSAT and Fer concentration values, with and without anemia, regardless of iron supplementation. We excluded papers which did not answer the question of the review, for example, those which examined only patients with anemia or focused on patients with heart failure. Nine studies, one of which was a systematic review, fulfilled the above-mentioned criteria. The search process is summarized in Figure 1. At the time of this research there were no clinical trials available which assessed the effect of iron supplementation in patients after MI with confirmed ID.

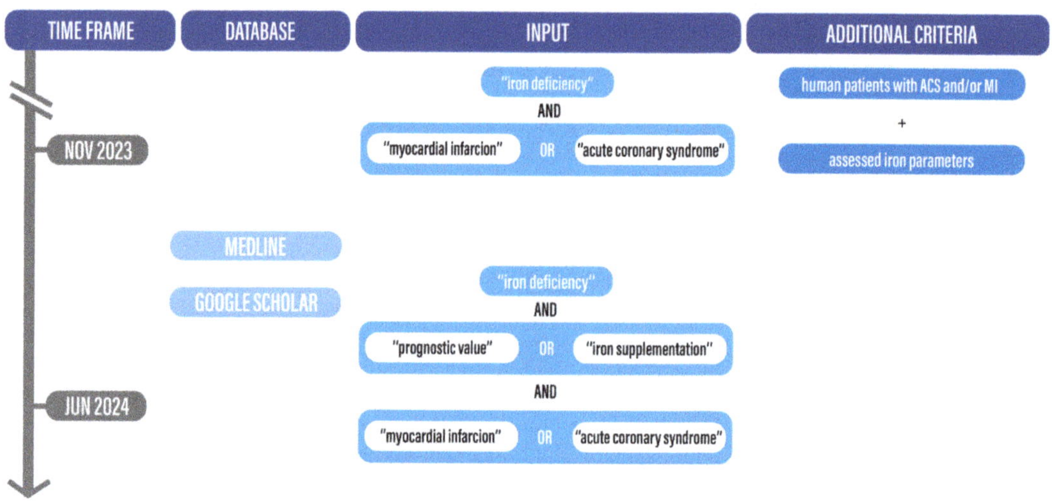

Figure 1. Data collection strategy.

3. Pathophysiology of Iron Deficiency in Patients with Coronary Artery Disease

3.1. Physiology of Iron Metabolism

In the human body, iron is mostly absorbed within the small intestine through enterocytes. Without parenteral iron supplementation, absorbed iron originates from ingestion of iron-rich foods and oral iron supplementation. Ingested iron is present in the following biological forms: (1) heme-bound Fe^{2+}; (2) non-heme Fe^{3+}; and (3) Fe^{2+} from oral iron supplementation [9]. Iron solubility increases in the acid mucus within the stomach, where insoluble Fe^{3+}, a form normally present in neutral pH, is reduced to soluble Fe^{2+} [10]. Additionally, Fe^{3+} is reduced to Fe^{2+} by ferroreductases localized within the luminal membrane of enterocytes [9]. According to iron solubility, only the reduced form (Fe^{2+}) can be transported through biological membranes.

Iron absorption occurs via several pathways. Heme-bound Fe^{2+} is transported to enterocyte cytosol via a heme transporter, whereas Fe^{2+} is transported through the divalent metal transporter 1 (DMT1). Within the enterocyte, oxidation occurs, which is catalyzed by heme-oxidase and leads to porphobilinogen formation and Fe^{2+} release. In cytosol, Fe^{2+} may undergo oxidation to Fe^{3+} again with subsequent binding with Fer, which constitutes a main iron storage molecule and its localized mostly in cytosol; however, mitochondrial and nuclear forms have also been reported [9,10].

To fulfill metabolic needs, Fe^{2+} can be transported into blood via ferroportin 1 (FPN1). Within the bloodstream, iron is transported by transferrin, which constitutes a specialized protein with an ability to bind the Fe^{3+} form. Thus, Fe^{2+} is converted to Fe^{3+} by hephaestin [9,10], before binding with transferrin. Iron release from enterocytes is regulated by hepcidin, an acute-phase protein secreted by the liver in response to inflammation. Hepcidin leads to FPN1 endocytosis with subsequent ubiquitination and FPN1 lysis.

Apart from the absorption and iron release from enterocytes, iron homeostasis is maintained by peripheral iron intake. Fe^{3+}-saturated transferrin (Tf) binds with transferrin receptor 1 (TfR1), which is followed by endocytosis. Fe^{3+} is released and reduced within endosomes to Fe^{2+} which can be used in biological processes, e.g., enzyme synthesis or oxygenated again and stored by Fer.

3.2. Etiology and Pathogenesis of Iron Deficiency in Cardiovascular Disease

ID occurs in approximately 50% of patients with established cardiovascular disease. Moreover, up to 60% of patients with coronary artery disease have been shown to suffer from ID [11]. Recent data indicate that systemic iron deficiency, even without anemia, worsens mortality and prognosis in acute and chronic heart diseases [12]. Several factors contribute to ID in CVD, comprising enhanced inflammation, malnutrition and comorbidities such as heart failure leading to kidney dysfunction and reduced iron absorption within the intestine [11,13]. The consequences of iron deficiency at the cellular level include mitochondrial dysfunction, the impairment of non-mitochondrial energy production pathways, a reduction in myoglobin and oxygen stores, an increase in reactive oxygen species (ROS), an increase in abnormalities during replication and repair of the cell DNA, and an increase in abnormal immune responses [14], which further contribute to tissue damage caused by ischemia [15–17].

3.3. Iron Deficiency and Ischemia-Related Cardiomyocyte Damage

Iron content within cardiomyocytes is highly dependent on influx and outflow balance, which is mainly maintained by TfR1, DMT1 and the hepcidin–ferroportin axis [18]. Iron importation is enhanced due to the activation of TfR1 and DMT1 in iron-deficient cardiomyocytes, whereas the transcription of ferroportin (FPN) is decreased. Moreover, hepcidin, whose expression is increased in ID, is responsible for FPN inhibition and degradation. Finally, intracellular iron storage is decreased with the aim to increase the cytosolic iron pool via the decreased expression and increased degradation of ferritin [12].

The potentially poor outcomes of patients with ACS and concomitant ID (see Section 3.1) may be related to metabolic changes that occur in myocardial ID. ID may be associated with enhanced oxidative stress, as it constitutes an essential component of ROS-neutralizing enzymes. Endothelial nitric oxide synthase (eNOS) and soluble guanylate cyclase (sGC) belong to the eNOS/sGC/protein kinase-G (PKG) pathway and contain protoporphyrin IX, which includes iron within its structure [12]. The decreased synthesis of eNOS and sGC and subsequent eNOS/sGC/PKG pathway inhibition may be associated with enhanced oxidative stress after reperfusion, due to ischemia–reperfusion injury [19,20]. This phenomenon may explain the larger infarct size and decreased contractility of iron-deficient cardiomyocytes.

ROS constitute well-known factors leading to cellular damage. This phenomenon also involves cardiomyocytes, where cardiac troponin release is associated with redox state dysregulation due to enhanced ROS formation and decreased degradation. Oxidative stress leads to cardiomyocyte maladaptation due to electrophysiological and mechanical impairment.

Electrophysiological impairment is associated with ROS-mediated function reverse of the Na^+/Ca^{2+} exchanger (NCX), and increased influx of Ca^{2+} through Ca^{2+} L-type channels. Moreover, oxidative stress affects the sarcoplasmic reticulum (SER), which is involved in calcium balance maintenance. Oxidative stress decreases sarcoplasmic reticulum Ca^{2+}-adenosine triphosphatase 2 (SERCA2) function, leading to decreased Ca^{2+} influx to SER, whereas the function of ryanodine receptor 2 (RyR2) is enhanced [21]. These processes lead to calcium overload. It should be noted that an increased Ca^{2+} level within cardiomyocytes, often associated with impaired function of NCX and RyR2, may lead to malignant arrythmias via a mechanism of triggered activity: early depolarizations and delayed afterdepolarizations [22].

Mechanical function impairment of cardiomyocytes, manifesting as impaired systolic and diastolic function, is mainly caused by an enhanced formation of the tissue inhibitor of metalloproteinases and a decrease in metalloproteinase synthesis, which lead to myocardial fibrosis. Moreover, calcium overload is associated with decreased sensitivity of myofilaments which leads to impaired contractility [21].

Figure 2 summarizes the pathophysiological mechanisms leading to cardiac dysfunction in enhanced oxidative stress.

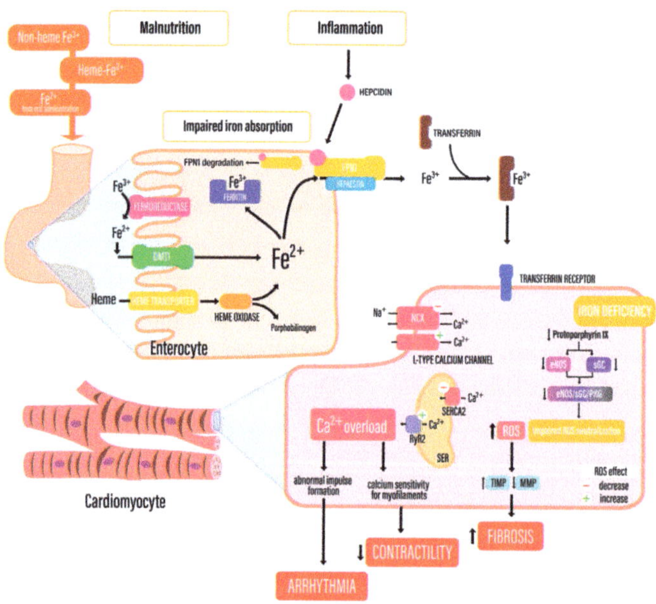

Figure 2. Iron metabolism and mechanisms of cardiac damage in iron deficiency. DMT1—divalent metal transporter 1; FPN1—ferroportin 1; Na^+/Ca^{2+} exchanger; MMP—metalloproteinase; ROS—reactive oxygen species; RyR2—ryanodine receptor 2; SER—sarcoplasmic reticulum; SERCA2—sarcoplasmic reticulum Ca^{2+}-adenosine triphosphatase 2; TIMP—tissue inhibitor of metalloproteinase.

4. Diagnosis

It has been shown that preexisting anemia occurs in 27.7% of patients presenting with ACS and constitutes a risk factor of all-cause mortality [RR 2.08 (95% CI 1.70–2.55)] [23]. Recent World Health Organization guidelines define cutoffs to diagnose anemia in individuals between 15 and 65 years old as <12 g/dL for non-pregnant women and <13 g/dL for men. The simplified definition commonly used in clinical practice defines anemia as <12 g/dL in women and <13 g/dL in men.

It should be noted that iron deficiency may be present with or without concomitant anemia. In isolated ID, Hb levels persist within the normal range.

ID can be diagnosed following two diagnostic pathways: invasive and non-invasive. As the invasive pathway is based on bone marrow biopsy, it is rarely used in clinical practice due to a higher risk of complications when compared to standardized laboratory tests using blood serum. Thus, the non-invasive pathway is preferred in clinical practice, whereas a bone marrow biopsy should be performed only after unclear laboratory test results for a definitive diagnosis [24]. To date, two laboratory parameters are supported by clinical studies to reflect iron status in cardiovascular diseases—Fer and TSAT. Serum Fer, secreted by macrophages, Kupfer cells and hepatocytes have an ability to carry labile extracellular iron. Levels of serum Fer are decreased in absolute iron deficiency. TSAT represents the calculated total serum iron/total iron binding capacity (TIBC) × 100. TIBC can be calculated as transferrin × 1389.

In order to assess the iron status of patients with CVD, both Fer and TSAT from blood serum should be assessed. Fer < 100 mcg/L allows clinicians to diagnose absolute iron deficiency, whereas Fer levels between 100 and 300 mcg/L associated with decreased TSAT < 20% suggest functional iron deficiency. It should be noted that Fer concentrations and TSAT may be influenced by several factors. Moreover, different cutoffs of each parameter may be applicable according to comorbidities such as chronic kidney disease or liver cirrhosis [25]. The iron status assessment pathways have been presented in Figure 3.

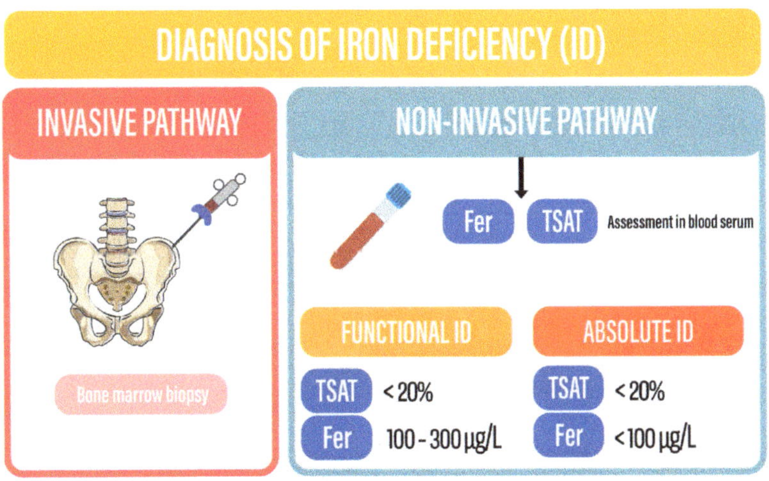

Figure 3. Diagnosis of iron deficiency. Fer—ferritin; ID—iron deficiency; TSAT—transferrin saturation.

5. Iron Deficiency and Prognosis in Acute Coronary Syndromes

The data included in the present review resulted from observational, mainly prospective studies. The main characteristics of and differences between cited original studies can be found in Table 1.

The study by Cosentino et al. [26] assessed the iron status of consecutive patients with ST-elevated myocardial infarction (STEMI) undergoing percutaneous coronary angioplasty. The iron-deficient group of patients accounted for 56% of the population and was characterized by a higher prevalence of type 2 diabetes, anemia, higher concentrations of high-sensitivity cardiac troponins and circulating mitochondrial DNA on admission.

Cardiac magnetic resonance imaging (CMR) did not reveal significant differences between patients with and without ID pertaining to left and right ventricular volumes and ejection fractions. Patients with ID had a larger area at risk, a similar infarct size, and, as a result, a higher myocardial salvage index in comparison to patients with a normal iron status. Paradoxically, patients with ID had a better in-hospital course and a lower incidence of the primary composite endpoint consisting of in-hospital mortality and Killip–Kimball class ≥ 3, even after adjustment for major confounders [odds ratio (OR) 0.50, 95% confidence interval CI 0.27–0.93; $p = 0.02$] [26]. Analogical results had been drawn in a post hoc substudy based on the CULPRIT-SHOCK trial—a randomized multicenter study, which included patients with AMI treated with percutaneous intervention (PCI), complicated by cardiogenic shock. In this case, ID without anemia was associated with a lower probability of death from any cause or renal replacement therapy [OR 0.63 (CI 0.31–1.08); $p = 0.06$] during a 30-day follow-up period in comparison to nonanemic patients with a regular iron status [27].

Contrary to the above-mentioned findings are the results from the research conducted by Fujinaga et al. [28], in which 352 nonanemic patients with STEMI who underwent successful PCI were stratified by serum iron concentration on admission. Patients with low iron concentration (<70 mg/dL) constituted 48% of the population and were older, more frequently women (36% vs. 17%, $p < 0.001$), had elevated C-reactive protein (CRP) (31 vs. 12%, $p < 0.001$), higher Killip–Kimball class (>II; 30 vs. 20%, $p = 0.04$), higher plasma BNP (286 ± 315 vs. 184 ± 227 pg/mL, $p = 0.001$) and higher incidence of in-hospital death (6.5 vs. 1.6%, $p = 0.03$) in comparison to those without ID. LVEF was similar in both groups [28].

Another study with a short-term observation period was conducted by Merono et al. [29] and aimed to test patient-assessed quality of life (QOL) and exercise capacity among patients with ACS. Iron deficiency was found in 57% of patients included in the study at baseline and persisted in 46% of the population on the 30th day of follow-up. The patients with ID were older, had lower hemoglobin concentrations and higher inflammatory parameters. Exercise tolerance in the group with ID was lower in both the Bruce protocol treadmill test and the 6 min walk test compared to the patients without ID (7.9 ± 2.9 vs. 9.3 ± 2.6 METS; $p = 0.003$; 277 vs. 423 m; $p = 0.009$, respectively). Similarly, patients' perceived QOL in the ID group was much lower (OR: 1.9; 95% CI: 1.1–3.3; $p < 0.001$). Prior aspirin intake was independently associated with ID [OR 3.254 (CI 1.373–7.716); $p = 0.007$]. The results of the experiment showed no correlation between iron deficiency and increased cardiovascular morbidity or mortality during short-term follow-up [29].

Table 1. A review of original publications examining iron deficiency in a population with ACS—short-term follow-up.

Author	Cosentino N [26]	Obradovic D [27]	Fujinaga H. (Abstract Only) [28]	Merono O [29]	Silva C [30]	González-D'Gregorio J [31]	Zeller T [5]	Jenča D [32]
Year	2019	2024	2013	2016	2021	2018	2018	2024
Study type	prospective observational	randomized trial	prospective observational	prospective observational	retrospective	prospective observational cohort	prospective observational cohort	prospective observational cohort
Population	420	427	352	244–>226	817	252	836	1156
ID (%)	237 (56%)	72 (~17%) [patients with ID without anemia]	169 (48%)	139–>102 (57%–>46%)	298 (36%)	n/s	243 (29.1%)	357 (31%)
Observation time	ACS-related hospitalization	30 days	ACS-related hospitalization	30 days	2 years	IQR: 2–5.4 years	4 years	1224 days
Conclusions	ID in ACS is associated with better in-hospital prognosis [OR 0.50 (CI 0.27–0.93)].	ID in AMI complicated by cardiogenic shock is associated with lower probability of death from any cause or renal replacement therapy [OR 0.63 (CI 0.31–1.08)].	ID on admission is associated with elevated CRP and higher Killip–Kimball class, and predicts poor outcomes after primary PCI in nonanemic STEMI patients.	ID is associated with worse exercise tolerance [OR 2.9 (CI 1.4–5.5)] and lower quality of life [OR: 1.9 (CI: 1.1–3.3)] but has no effect on mortality during short-term follow-up.	ID is an independent predictor of death / development of heart failure in ACS patients [HR 1.66 (CI 1.11–2.50)].	Lower TSAT levels are independently associated with an increased risk of long-term mortality [HR 1.54 (CI 1.03–2.30)].	Iron deficiency is associated with unfavorable medium-term outcomes (independent of systolic heart function), the extent of myocardial necrosis and anemia [HR 1.52 (CI 1.03–2.26)].	Iron deficiency is a common burden in patients with first ACS without past CAD history and, depending on measured parameters, is associated with all-cause mortality.

ACS—acute coronary syndrome; AMI—acute myocardial infarction; CAD—coronary artery disease; CI—confidence interval; HR—hazard ratio; ID—iron deficiency; IQR—interquartile range; n/s—not specified; OR—odds ratio; PCI—percutaneous intervention; STEMI—ST-elevated myocardial infarction; TSAT—transferrin saturation.

However, these outcomes do not indicate that ID does not affect the long-term prognosis of ACS patients. In the study by Silva et al. [30], consecutive patients with ACS were included. The ID group accounted for 36% of the study population and consisted of older patients with a higher prevalence of comorbidities, and in whom coronary artery bypass grafting was more common, in comparison to patients without ID. Patients with ID had worse baseline clinical conditions, characterized by an increased prevalence of higher Killip–Kimball class (class II-IV 21.8% vs. 12.1%, respectively, $p < 0.001$), anemia (20.1% vs. 8.5%, respectively, $p < 0.001$), glomerular filtration rate below 60 mL/min (30.2% vs. 17.9%, respectively, $p < 0.001$), triple-vessel disease (26.6% vs. 16.5%, respectively, $p < 0.001$), and left ventricular ejection fraction below 40% (34.2% vs. 22.3%, respectively, $p < 0.001$). Follow-up time averaged 738.77 days, during which patients were evaluated for all-cause mortality, death from cardiovascular causes, occurrence of stroke, reinfarction, heart failure exacerbation (New York Heart Association [NYHA] class III and IV), angina (Canadian Cardiovascular Society class > I) and rehospitalization. The group with ID had a higher incidence of the aforementioned adverse events, notably higher any-cause mortality (12.6% vs. 6.3%, $p = 0.004$), more frequent heart failure exacerbation (10.5% to 5.3%, $p = 0.011$) and rehospitalization (13.7% vs. 9.8%, $p = 0.048$) compared to controls. Moreover, the patients burdened with ID had a higher all-cause mortality rate regardless of the presence of anemia [30].

Another publication examining the prognosis of patients with ID was the study by Gonzales-D'Gregorio et al. [31], which focused on the follow-up of patients aged > 65 years with ACS (STEMI, NSTEMI or UA). TSAT and ferritin were stratified into quartiles yielding the following ranges for TSAT: Q1TSAT: 2.8–11.8% (n = 63), Q2TSAT: 11.8–17.2% (n = 63), Q3TSAT: 17.2–24.6% (n = 63), Q4TSAT: 25–95% (n = 63); for ferritin: Q1fer: 9–81 ng/mL (n = 63), Q2fer: 82–147 ng/mL (n = 63), Q3fer: 148–258 ng/mL (n = 63), Q4fer: 259–1609 ng/mL (n = 63). The median follow-up was 4.7 years, during which 121 (48%) patients died. Patients in the lower quartiles of TSAT were more likely to suffer from STEMI and had higher NT-proBNP serum concentrations on admission. There were no significant differences in frailty index (Fried score), GRACE score, Charlson Comorbidity Index, left ventricular systolic function or management strategy between the patients across the ferritin and TSAT quartiles. After multivariate adjustment, TSAT as a continuous variable was inversely and nonlinearly associated with the risk of long-term mortality ($p = 0.002$), with an exponential increase in risk from values of 20% and below. Lower TSAT values (Q1TSAT vs. Q2–Q4TSAT) were found to be strongly associated with the risk of death in anemic patients (HR: 2.13; 95% CI: 1.31–3.48; $p = 0.002$), but had a neutral effect in nonanemic subjects (HR: 0.80; 95% CI: 0.36–1.70; $p = 0.539$). Ferritin serum concentrations and the current definition of ID were not independently associated with mortality in this paper [31].

In the study conducted by Zeller et al. [5], iron deficiency was present in 29% of 836 participants with ACS, more common in women (42.8%, $p < 0.001$) and co-present with anemia (42.5%, $p < 0.001$). Both studied iron parameters positively correlated with male gender, dyslipidemia and troponin I serum concentration. During a mean follow-up time of 4 years, 111 patients died of cardiovascular reasons or had non-fatal myocardial infarction. ID was an independent predictor for both endpoints after adjustment for age, sex and cardiovascular death risk factors (HR 1.52; 95% CI: 1.03–2.26; $p = 0.037$) [5].

Similar conclusions were drawn by Jenča et al. [32] in a prospective observational cohort study. A total of 1156 consecutive patients with no previous history of coronary artery disease and diagnosed type I MI were included. Blood samples were collected in the morning on the first day after hospital admission and serum iron concentration, ferritin, transferrin, soluble transferrin receptor (sTFR), TIBC and TSAT were determined. The median follow-up time amounted to 1224 days (IQR 626–1782), during which 194 (16.8%) patients died. Each evaluated ID criterion, except for ferritin, was independently associated with all-cause mortality.

Due to conflicting results from formerly published papers on the issue of ID in ACS, researchers have suggested new criteria, named "Prague ID", based on serum iron concentration and sTfR. The combination of iron $\leq$ 12.8 µmol/L and sTfR $\geq$ 3.0 mg/L showed the best association with total mortality risk, also after adjustment for the GRACE score and other confounders [32].

There is only one systematic review on the prognostic value of ID in patients with ACS available to date. Reinhold et al. [33] summarized seven papers, three of which were conference abstracts. According to their findings, ID was present in 43% (n = 1226) of all patients with ACS and was associated with worse patient prognosis during mid- to long-term follow-up. Due to the differences in outcome measures and follow-up periods of each analyzed study, a meta-analysis could not be performed. Conclusions drawn from this research are similar to ones already mentioned in this paper, due to being based on similar source data [33].

Figure 4 summarizes factors leading to iron deficiency in ACS patients and potential mechanisms that may influence prognosis.

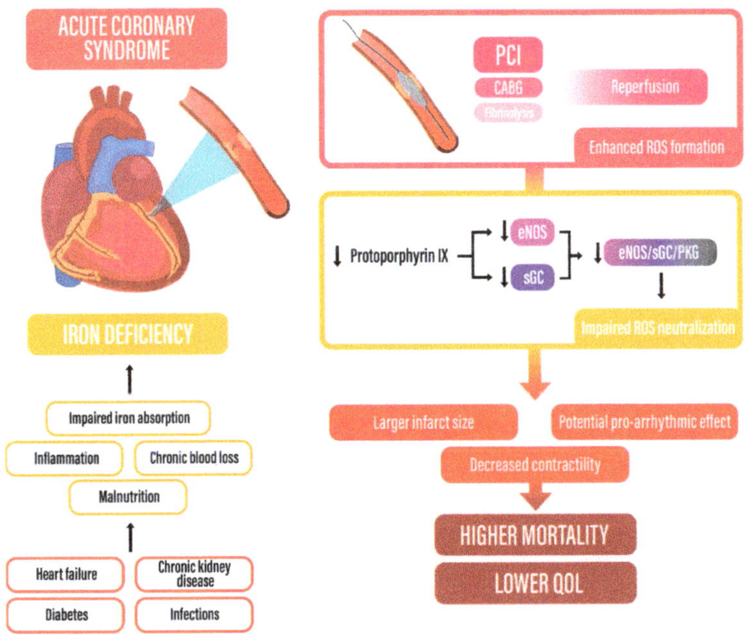

Figure 4. Iron deficiency in acute coronary syndromes—summarizing figure. CABG—coronary artery bypass grafting; eNOS—endothelial nitric oxide synthase; PCI—percutaneous coronary intervention; PKG—protein kinase G; ROS—reactive oxygen species; sGC—soluble guanylate cyclase.

6. Iron Supplementation and ACS

In light of the available scientific literature, no clinical trials have been established to date which investigate the effect of iron supplementation in ACS patients with known ID. There was an experiment conducted by Florian et al. [16] to test the effect of iron supplementation in post-MI patients, known as the NIMINI-3 trial. The prospective non-randomized unblinded study involved 39 patients with established STEMI undergoing primary percutaneous coronary intervention with successful reperfusion, of which 17 were assigned to the group receiving parenteral iron in the form of ultrasmall superparamagnetic iron-oxide (USPIO) and 22 to the group receiving placebo. Patients underwent myocardial MRI up to 1 week and 3 months after ACS. Iron administration occurred within 24 h after the imaging was performed. During follow-up, none of the patients had relevant cardiovascular events. A significant increase in left ventricular ejection fraction was observed in both groups, with a greater effect in the iron-treated group (USPIO: 53 ± 10%–59 ± 9%; $p = 0.002$; control: 54 ± 6%–57 ± 10%; $p = 0.005$). In both groups the infarct size was significantly reduced in the follow-up MRI with a predominance of the study group (USPIO: 27 ± 8% to 17 ± 9%; $p < 0.001$ vs. control: 27 ± 12% to 20 ± 11%; $p < 0.001$). It seems that USPIO-based intravenous iron administration in patients with STEMI is associated with more favorable healing and left ventricular remodeling. The limitations of the study were the small patients groups and the lack of iron parameter analysis and ID diagnosis [16]. The results of this experiment seem to be supported by the findings of Mohanty et al. [34] and Huang et al. [17] which have shown a positive, statistically significant correlation between serum iron concentration and LVEF improvement 6 months after STEMI/NSTEMI [17,34]. Deeper relationships between cardiac remodeling and ischemia are the subject of research in the work of Inserte et al. [35] The paper reports on a prospective observational study on humans and an interventional experiment on mice. In total, 141 patients, who were tested for their iron status with their first anterior STEMI, were treated with PCI and underwent CMR at the beginning and at the end of the 6-month observation period. ID was defined according to the current consensus. Patients with ID had significantly larger mean infarct size and more extensive microvascular obstruction than those with normal iron status ($p < 0.05$). They also showed a greater increase in LV volume at the end of the follow-up, with similar changes in LVEF. Adverse LV remodeling occurred in 37.8% of patients with ID and 14.1% of those without ID ($p = 0.004$). The pathophysiological background was tested in the second part of the study, where mice were parted into two groups, based on a 4-week diet period. Some mice in the study group were given intravenous iron supplementation. Mice were subjected to MI by left descending coronary artery ligation. The myocardium of mice fed with an ID diet was subdued to increased oxidative and nitrosative stress, significantly reducing the antioxidant capacity in comparison to controls ($p = 0.008$). The infarct size was significantly larger in the study group (58.1% ± 3.0% vs. 40.4% ± 3.7% of area at risk; $p = 0.004$). Iron supplementation prevented the above-mentioned issues [35].

7. Discussion

ID is a common condition in patients with acute coronary syndrome. The results of the papers summarized in our study seem to be contradictory. The influence of ID on short-term prognosis according to the current data is ambiguous. Research conducted by Cosentino et al. [26] and Obradowic et al. [27] included highly specific groups of patients—with STEMI and with ACS and multivessel disease complicated by cardiogenic shock, respectively. Iron parameters were assessed either by admission or during coronarography. Important to note is the fact that TSAT and Fer are both reactants whose concentrations vary during acute conditions. Transferrin saturation decreases, but ferritin, as an intracellular protein, increases its presence in circulation after cellular damage [36]. In this case, low ferritin concentration may relate to less myocardial damage, and consequently, better short-term prognosis, which would also be supported by Jenca et al. [32] Taking into consideration the limited group of patients and early iron parameter assessment in these two papers, conclusions drawn pertaining to better prognoses during short-term follow-up should be regarded with caution. The findings of Fujinaga et al. [28] are available only in abstract form, in which data contributing to the study population, recruitment and methods are strictly limited, and the sole examination of iron serum concentration decreases the impact of the presented results. Only in the study by Merono et al. [29] were iron parameters assessed 5 days after ACS, during initial stabilization. Consecutive patients were recruited, but only those who had undergone the above-mentioned iron examination were further evaluated. ID had no effect on mortality in short-term follow-up, but was associated with worse QOL and exercise tolerance, which may relate to the increased prevalence of chronic diseases and, due to this, possible recurrent inflammation in this group, which impedes iron absorption and affects regular serum iron concentrations [37,38]. In consequence, it may lead to increased ROS concentration and impede heart muscle contractility, due to calcium influx and its overload in cardiomyocytes.

However, current evidence supports the importance of ID as a factor of worse prognosis in patients with ACS. Papers assessing mid- to long-term follow-up seem to agree on ID in relation to the increased occurrence of major adverse cardiovascular events regardless of age, gender and other comorbidities. In research conducted by Silva et al. [30] and D'Gregorio et al. [31], lower TSAT was associated with age and an increased incidence of comorbidities. ID was more common in patients suffering from STEMI and who had higher concentrations of hsCRP, which also supports the thesis of iron being an anti-inflammatory agent reducing atherosclerosis [39]. Iron acts as a protective agent in cardiomyocytes—increasing overall antioxidative capacity, reducing adverse effects of hypoxia and diminishing cellular damage [40]. Increased calcium concentration in cardiomyocytes during ID conditions is related to increased fibrosis, which in the long term could lead to adverse LV remodeling. In the work by Jenca et al. [32], newly developed PragueID criteria based on soluble transferrin receptor and iron serum concentrations showed the best association with total mortality risk in comparison to TSAT and Fer. Their presence in blood serum appeared to be more stable during acute conditions, which could facilitate more reliable ID diagnosis. This new criteria may also be used in the healthy population, as ID in this group has been proven to be a major risk factor associated with increased all-cause mortality [41].

At this moment in time, there are not enough data to support regular iron supplementation in patients with ACS with confirmed ID, even though we already have some evidence that it may be related to better tissue healing and LV remodeling prevention [16]. In the FAIR-HF trial, more than 60% of the patients included suffered from heart failure caused by ischemic heart disease. The administration of intravenous ferric carboxymaltose was beneficial in all cases regardless of the hemoglobin concentration [7]. The potentially positive effect of iron supplementation could also be supported by necessary pharmacotherapy after ACS, namely dual antiplatelet therapy, which is a major risk factor for potential bleeding and cause of—naturally—iron deficiency [42].

8. Conclusions

ID is a common condition in patients with ACS. Although its influence on short-term follow-up appears to be uncertain, ID seems to be independently associated with worse patient prognosis during mid- to long-term follow-up. Transferrin saturation, contrary to ferritin, is not upregulated during acute conditions, which may be crucial in the non-invasive diagnosis of ID. TSAT appears to have a greater predictive value of death and other adverse events compared to ferritin or serum iron concentration, but there are new, promising, precise markers used for non-invasive ID diagnosis in the works. Iron supplementation in ACS patients may have a beneficial effect on myocardial healing and left ventricular remodeling after myocardial infarction, but further research, especially on human models, is needed to support this relationship.

Author Contributions: Conceptualization, methodology, investigation, project administration, resources, writing—original draft preparation, writing—review and editing—A.M.; investigation, visualization, writing—review and editing—K.B.; validation, writing—review and editing—O.M.-B.; writing—review and editing, formal analysis—J.K.; writing—review and editing, supervision—J.D. All authors have read and agreed to the published version of the manuscript.

Funding: There was no external funding of this research.

Institutional Review Board Statement: Not applicable.

Informed Consent Statement: Not applicable.

Conflicts of Interest: The authors declare no conflict of interest.

Abbreviations

The following abbreviations are used in this manuscript:

ACS	acute coronary syndrome
AMI	acute myocardial infarction
CABG	coronary artery bypass grafting
CAD	coronary artery disease
CI	confidence interval
CMR	cardiac magnetic resonance imaging
CRP	C-reactive protein
CVD	cardiovascular diseases
DMT1	divalent metal transporter 1
eNOS	endothelial nitric oxide synthase
EF	ejection fraction
Fer	ferritin
FPN	transcription ferroportin
FPN1	transcription ferroportin 1
HF	heart failure
HR	hazard ratio
ID	iron deficiency
IQR	interquartile range
LV	left ventricle
LVEF	left ventricular ejection fraction
MI	myocardial infarction
MMP	metalloproteinase
NCX	Na^+/Ca^{2+} exchanger
n/s	not specified
NSTEMI	non-ST-elevated myocardial infraction
NT-proBNP	N-terminal pro B-type natriuretic peptide
NYHA	New York Heart Association
OR	odds ratio
PCI	percutaneous intervention
PKG	protein kinase-G
QOL	quality of life
ROS	reactive oxygen species
RR	risk ratio
RyR2	ryanodine receptor 2
SER	sarcoplasmic reticulum
SERCA 2	sarcoplasmic reticulum Ca^{2+}-adenosine triphosphatase
sGC	soluble guanylate cyclase
STEMI	ST-elevated myocardial infarction
sTFR	soluble transferrin receptor
Tf	transferrin

TfR1	transferrin receptor 1
TIBC	total iron binding capacity
TIMP	tissue inhibitor of metalloproteinase
TSAT	transferrin saturation
UA	unstable angina

References

1. WHO Factsheet on Cardiovascular Diseases. Available online: https://www.who.int/news-room/fact-sheets/detail/cardiovascular-diseases-(cvds) (accessed on 1 July 2024).
2. Visseren, F.L.J.; Mach, F.; Smulders, Y.M.; Carballo, D.; Koskinas, K.C.; Bäck, M.; Benetos, A.; Biffi, A.; Boavida, J.-M.; Capodanno, D.; et al. 2021 ESC Guidelines on Cardiovascular Disease Prevention in Clinical Practice. *Eur. Heart J.* **2021**, *42*, 3227–3337. [CrossRef] [PubMed]
3. Pasricha, S.R.; Tye-Din, J.; Muckenthaler, M.U.; Swinkels, D.W. Iron Deficiency. *Lancet* **2021**, *397*, 233–248. [PubMed]
4. Pasricha, S.S.; Flecknoe-Brown, S.C.; Allen, K.J.; Gibson, P.R.; McMahon, L.P.; Olynyk, J.K.; Roger, S.D.; Savoia, H.F.; Tampi, R.; Thomson, A.R.; et al. Diagnosis and Management of Iron Deficiency Anaemia: A Clinical Update. *Med. J. Aust.* **2010**, *193*, 525–532. [CrossRef]
5. Zeller, T.; Waldeyer, C.; Ojeda, F.; Schnabel, R.B.; Schäfer, S.; Altay, A.; Lackner, K.J.; Anker, S.D.; Westermann, D.; Blankenberg, S.; et al. Adverse Outcome Prediction of Iron Deficiency in Patients with Acute Coronary Syndrome. *Biomolecules* **2018**, *8*, 60. [CrossRef]
6. Ponikowski, P.; Kirwan, B.-A.; Anker, S.D.; McDonagh, T.; Dorobantu, M.; Drozdz, J.; Fabien, V.; Filippatos, G.; Göhring, U.M.; Keren, A.; et al. Ferric Carboxymaltose for Iron Deficiency at Discharge after Acute Heart Failure: A Multicentre, Double-Blind, Randomised, Controlled Trial. *Lancet* **2020**, *396*, 1895–1904. [CrossRef]
7. Anker, S.D.; Comin Colet, J.; Filippatos, G.; Willenheimer, R.; Dickstein, K.; Drexler, H.; Lüscher, T.F.; Bart, B.; Banasiak, W.; Niegowska, J.; et al. Ferric Carboxymaltose in Patients with Heart Failure and Iron Deficiency. *N. Engl. J. Med.* **2009**, *361*, 2436–2448. [CrossRef]
8. Kalra, P.R.; Cleland, J.G.F.; Petrie, M.C.; Thomson, E.A.; Kalra, P.A.; Squire, I.B.; Ahmed, F.Z.; Al-Mohammad, A.; Cowburn, P.J.; Foley, P.W.X.; et al. Intravenous Ferric Derisomaltose in Patients with Heart Failure and Iron Deficiency in the UK (IRONMAN): An Investigator-Initiated, Prospective, Randomised, Open-Label, Blinded-Endpoint Trial. *Lancet* **2022**, *400*, 2199–2209. [CrossRef]
9. von Haehling, S.; Jankowska, E.A.; van Veldhuisen, D.J.; Ponikowski, P.; Anker, S.D. Iron Deficiency and Cardiovascular Disease. *Nat. Rev. Cardiol.* **2015**, *12*, 659–669. [CrossRef]
10. Toyokuni, S.; Yanatori, I.; Kong, Y.; Zheng, H.; Motooka, Y.; Jiang, L. Ferroptosis at the Crossroads of Infection, Aging and Cancer. *Cancer Sci.* **2020**, *111*, 2665–2671. [CrossRef]
11. Savarese, G.; von Haehling, S.; Butler, J.; Cleland, J.G.F.; Ponikowski, P.; Anker, S.D. Iron Deficiency and Cardiovascular Disease. *Eur. Heart J.* **2023**, *44*, 14–27. [CrossRef]
12. Corradi, F.; Masini, G.; Bucciarelli, T.; De Caterina, R. Iron Deficiency in Myocardial Ischaemia: Molecular Mechanisms and Therapeutic Perspectives. *Cardiovasc. Res.* **2023**, *119*, 2405–2420. [CrossRef] [PubMed]
13. Rymer, J.A.; Rao, S.V. Anemia and Coronary Artery Disease. *Coron. Artery Dis.* **2018**, *29*, 161–167. [CrossRef] [PubMed]
14. Jankowska, E.A.; Von Haehling, S.; Anker, S.D.; MacDougall, I.C.; Ponikowski, P. Iron Deficiency and Heart Failure: Diagnostic Dilemmas and Therapeutic Perspectives. *Eur. Heart J.* **2013**, *34*, 816–829. [PubMed]
15. Andrews, N.C. Disorders of Iron Metabolism. *N. Engl. J. Med.* **1999**, *341*, 1986–1995. [CrossRef]
16. Florian, A.; Ludwig, A.; Rösch, S.; Yildiz, H.; Klumpp, S.; Sechtem, U.; Yilmaz, A. Positive Effect of Intravenous Iron-Oxide Administration on Left Ventricular Remodelling in Patients with Acute ST-Elevation Myocardial Infarction—A Cardiovascular Magnetic Resonance (CMR) Study. *Int. J. Cardiol.* **2014**, *173*, 184–189. [CrossRef]
17. Huang, C.H.; Chang, C.C.; Kuo, C.L.; Huang, C.S.; Chiu, T.W.; Lin, C.S.; Liu, C.S. Serum Iron Concentration, but Not Hemoglobin, Correlates with TIMI Risk Score and 6-Month Left Ventricular Performance after Primary Angioplasty for Acute Myocardial Infarction. *PLoS ONE* **2014**, *9*, e104495. [CrossRef]
18. Lakhal-Littleton, S. Mechanisms of Cardiac Iron Homeostasis and Their Importance to Heart Function. *Free Radic. Biol. Med.* **2019**, *133*, 234–237. [CrossRef]
19. Bice, J.S.; Burley, D.S.; Baxter, G.F. Novel Approaches and Opportunities for Cardioprotective Signaling Through 3′,5′-Cyclic Guanosine Monophosphate Manipulation. *J. Cardiovasc. Pharmacol. Ther.* **2014**, *19*, 269–282. [CrossRef]
20. Inserte, J.; Garcia-Dorado, D. The cGMP/PKG Pathway as a Common Mediator of Cardioprotection: Translatability and Mechanism. *Br. J. Pharmacol.* **2015**, *172*, 1996–2009. [CrossRef]
21. van der Pol, A.; van Gilst, W.H.; Voors, A.A.; van der Meer, P. Treating Oxidative Stress in Heart Failure: Past, Present and Future. *Eur. J. Heart Fail.* **2019**, *21*, 425–435. [CrossRef]
22. Badura, K.; Buławska, D.; Dąbek, B.; Witkowska, A.; Lisińska, W.; Radzioch, E.; Skwira, S.; Młynarska, E.; Rysz, J.; Franczyk, B. Primary Electrical Heart Disease—Principles of Pathophysiology and Genetics. *Int. J. Mol. Sci.* **2024**, *25*, 1826. [CrossRef] [PubMed]

23. Jung, C.; Rezar, R.; Wischmann, P.; Masyuk, M.; Datz, C.; Bruno, R.R.; Kelm, M.; Wernly, B. The Role of Anemia on Admission in Acute Coronary Syndrome—An Umbrella Review of Systematic Reviews and Meta-Analyses. *Int. J. Cardiol.* **2022**, *367*, 1–10. [CrossRef] [PubMed]
24. Killip, S.; Bennett, J.M.; Chambers, M.D. Iron Deficiency Anemia. *Am. Fam. Physician* **2007**, *75*, 671–678. [PubMed]
25. Badura, K.; Janc, J.; Wąsik, J.; Gnitecki, S.; Skwira, S.; Młynarska, E.; Rysz, J.; Franczyk, B. Anemia of Chronic Kidney Disease—A Narrative Review of Its Pathophysiology, Diagnosis, and Management. *Biomedicines* **2024**, *12*, 1191. [CrossRef]
26. Cosentino, N.; Campodonico, J.; Pontone, G.; Guglielmo, M.; Trinei, M.; Sandri, M.T.; Riggio, D.; Baggiano, A.; Milazzo, V.; Moltrasio, M.; et al. Iron Deficiency in Patients with ST-Segment Elevation Myocardial Infarction Undergoing Primary Percutaneous Coronary Intervention. *Int. J. Cardiol.* **2020**, *300*, 14–19. [CrossRef]
27. Obradovic, D.; Loncar, G.; Zeymer, U.; Pöss, J.; Feistritzer, H.J.; Freund, A.; Jobs, A.; Fuernau, G.; Desch, S.; Ceglarek, U.; et al. Impact of Anaemia and Iron Deficiency on Outcomes in Cardiogenic Shock Complicating Acute Myocardial Infarction. *Eur. J. Heart Fail.* **2024**, *26*, 448–457. [CrossRef]
28. Fujinaga, H.; Okumura, T.; Harada, K. Iron Deficiency Predicts Poor Outcomes after Primary Intervention in Nonanemic Patients with Stemi. *J. Am. Coll. Cardiol.* **2013**, *61*, E206. [CrossRef]
29. Meroño, O.; Cladellas, M.; Ribas-Barquet, N.; Poveda, P.; Recasens, L.; Bazán, V.; García-García, C.; Ivern, C.; Enjuanes, C.; Orient, S.; et al. Iron Deficiency Is a Determinant of Functional Capacity and Health-Related Quality of Life 30 Days After an Acute Coronary Syndrome. *Rev. Española De Cardiol. Engl. Ed.* **2017**, *70*, 363–370. [CrossRef]
30. Silva, C.; Martins, J.; Campos, I.; Arantes, C.; Braga, C.G.; Salomé, N.; Gaspar, A.; Azevedo, P.; Álvares Pereira, M.; Marques, J.; et al. Prognostic Impact of Iron Deficiency in Acute Coronary Syndromes. *Rev. Port. De Cardiol. Engl. Ed.* **2021**, *40*, 525–536. [CrossRef]
31. González-D'Gregorio, J.; Miñana, G.; Núñez, J.; Núñez, E.; Ruiz, V.; García-Blas, S.; Bonanad, C.; Mollar, A.; Valero, E.; Amiguet, M.; et al. Iron Deficiency and Long-Term Mortality in Elderly Patients with Acute Coronary Syndrome. *Biomark. Med.* **2018**, *12*, 987–999. [CrossRef]
32. Jenča, D.; Melenovský, V.; Mrázková, J.; Šramko, M.; Kotrč, M.; Želízko, M.; Adámková, V.; Piťha, J.; Kautzner, J.; Wohlfahrt, P. Iron Deficiency and All-Cause Mortality after Myocardial Infarction. *Eur. J. Intern. Med.* **2024**, *126*, 102–108. [CrossRef] [PubMed]
33. Reinhold, J.; Papadopoulou, C.; Baral, R.; Vassiliou, V.S. Iron Deficiency for Prognosis in Acute Coronary Syndrome—A Systematic Review and Meta-Analysis. *Int. J. Cardiol.* **2021**, *328*, 46–54. [CrossRef] [PubMed]
34. Mohanty, N.K.; Dash, B.K.; Satpathy, C.; Banerjee, M.; Routray, S. Prognostic Impact of Iron Metabolism Changes in Patients with Acute Coronary Syndrome and Its Correlation with TIMI Risk Score and 6-Month Left Ventricular Performance. *Indian J. Cardiovasc. Dis. Women* **2024**, *9*, 195–200. [CrossRef]
35. Inserte, J.; Barrabés, J.A.; Aluja, D.; Otaegui, I.; Bañeras, J.; Castellote, L.; Sánchez, A.; Rodríguez-Palomares, J.F.; Pineda, V.; Miró-Casas, E.; et al. Implications of Iron Deficiency in STEMI Patients and in a Murine Model of Myocardial Infarction. *JACC Basic. Transl. Sci.* **2021**, *6*, 567–580. [CrossRef] [PubMed]
36. Van Der Schouw, Y.T.; Van Der Veeken, P.M.W.C.; Kok, F.J.; Koster, J.F.; Schouten, E.G.; Hofman, A. Original Contribution Iron Status in the Acute Phase and Six weeks after Myocardial Infarction. *Free. Radic. Biol. Med.* **1990**, *8*, 47–53. [CrossRef]
37. Makrecka-Kuka, M.; Krumschnabel, G.; Gnaiger, E. High-Resolution Respirometry for Simultaneous Measurement of Oxygen and Hydrogen Peroxide Fluxes in Permeabilized Cells, Tissue Homogenate and Isolated Mitochondria. *Biomolecules* **2015**, *5*, 1319–1338. [CrossRef]
38. Alayash, A. Hemoglobin-Based Blood Substitutes and the Treatment of Sickle Cell Disease: More Harm than Help? *Biomolecules* **2017**, *7*, 2. [CrossRef]
39. Madaudo, C.; Coppola, G.; Parlati, A.L.M.; Corrado, E. Discovering Inflammation in Atherosclerosis: Insights from Pathogenic Pathways to Clinical Practice. *Int. J. Mol. Sci.* **2024**, *25*, 6016. [CrossRef]
40. Dziegala, M.; Kasztura, M.; Kobak, K.; Bania, J.; Banasiak, W.; Ponikowski, P.; Jankowska, E.A. Influence of the Availability of Iron during Hypoxia on the Genes Associated with Apoptotic Activity and Local Iron Metabolism in Rat H9C2 Cardiomyocytes and L6G8C5 Skeletal Myocytes. *Mol. Med. Rep.* **2016**, *14*, 3969–3977. [CrossRef]
41. Schrage, B.; Rübsamen, N.; Schulz, A.; Münzel, T.; Pfeiffer, N.; Wild, P.S.; Beutel, M.; Schmidtmann, I.; Lott, R.; Blankenberg, S.; et al. Iron Deficiency Is a Common Disorder in General Population and Independently Predicts All-Cause Mortality: Results from the Gutenberg Health Study. *Clin. Res. Cardiol.* **2020**, *109*, 1352–1357. [CrossRef]
42. Erriquez, A.; Campo, G.; Guiducci, V.; Escaned, J.; Moreno, R.; Casella, G.; Menozzi, M.; Cerrato, E.; Sacchetta, G.; Menozzi, A.; et al. Complete vs Culprit-Only Revascularization in Older Patients with Myocardial Infarction and High Bleeding Risk. *JAMA Cardiol.* **2024**, *9*, 565. [CrossRef] [PubMed]

biomedicines

MDPI

Article

Cardiovascular Risk Factors in Socioeconomically Disadvantaged Populations in a Suburb of the Largest City in Western Romania

Andreea Dumitrescu [1,2], Gabriela Mut Vitcu [1], Svetlana Stoica [1,3,4,*], Septimiu Radu Susa [5] and Emil Robert Stoicescu [6,7,8]

1 Neoclinic Concept SRL, Calea Dorobantilor 3, 300134 Timisoara, Romania; andreea.dumitrescu@e-uvt.ro (A.D.); gabriela.mut@cardioprevent.org (G.M.V.)
2 Department of Kinetotherapy, Faculty of Physical Education and Sport, West Univestity of Timisoara, 300223 Timisoara, Romania
3 Cardiology University Clinic, Department VI, "Victor Babes" University of Medicine and Pharmacy Timisoara, Eftimie Murgu Square No. 2, 300041 Timisoara, Romania
4 Research Centre of Timisoara Institute of Cardiovascular Diseases, "Victor Babes" University of Medicine and Pharmacy Timisoara, Eftimie Murgu Square No. 2, 300041 Timisoara, Romania
5 Doctoral School, "Victor Babes" University of Medicine and Pharmacy Timisoara, Eftimie Murgu Square 2, 300041 Timisoara, Romania; septimiu.susa@umft.ro
6 Radiology and Medical Imaging University Clinic, 'Victor Babes' University of Medicine and Pharmacy Timisoara, Eftimie Murgu Square No. 2, 300041 Timisoara, Romania; stoicescu.emil@umft.ro
7 Research Center for Pharmaco-Toxicological Evaluations, 'Victor Babes' University of Medicine and Pharmacy Timisoara, Eftimie Murgu Square No. 2, 300041 Timisoara, Romania
8 Field of Applied Engineering Sciences, Specialization Statistical Methods and Techniques in Health and Clinical Research, Faculty of Mechanics, 'Politehnica' University Timisoara, Mihai Viteazul Boulevard No. 1, 300222 Timisoara, Romania
* Correspondence: svetlana.mosteoru@umft.ro; Tel.: +40-72-4174030

Abstract: *Background and Objectives*: Cardiovascular disease (CVD) remains a major public health issue worldwide, disproportionately affecting socioeconomically disadvantaged populations due to the social determinants of health (SDOHs). In Western Romania, these populations are particularly vulnerable to CVD. This study aims to investigate the prevalence and impact of cardiovascular risk factors (CVRFs) among socioeconomically disadvantaged individuals in Western Romania and identify the primary CVRFs contributing to the high incidence of CVD within this population. *Materials and Methods*: A retrospective observational design was employed, utilizing data from the medical records of 1433 eligible individuals. The inclusion criteria were based on Eurostat's EU-SILC benchmarks, focusing on severe material deprivation, at-risk-of-poverty rates, and low work intensity. Data on demographics, familial and personal medical history, smoking status, blood pressure, glucose, cholesterol, triglycerides, and HbA1c levels were collected. *Results*: Of the 1433 subjects, 34.75% were male, with a median age of 52 years. Significant conditions included diabetes (7.39%), coronary disease (3.83%), arterial hypertension (35.58%), and dyslipidemia (21.28%). Median ages were higher for those with diabetes (65 vs. 51 years, $p < 0.0001$), coronary disease (64 vs. 51 years, $p < 0.0001$), arterial hypertension (65 vs. 43 years, $p < 0.0001$), and dyslipidemia (66 vs. 47 years, $p < 0.0001$). BMI (Body Mass Index) classifications showed 33.77% were overweight, 21.21% obese, and 15.07% morbidly obese. Smokers were younger than non-smokers (48 vs. 54 years, $p < 0.0001$). *Conclusions*: The findings highlight the significant prevalence of CVRFs among socioeconomically disadvantaged populations in Western Romania. Socioeconomically disadvantaged populations exhibit a significantly higher prevalence of cardiovascular risk factors such as diabetes, impaired glucose regulation, hypertension, and dyslipidemia compared to their before known status.

Keywords: cardiovascular disease; socioeconomic disparities; socioeconomically disadvantaged populations; cardiovascular risk factors; Western Romania; hypertension; diabetes; dyslipidemia; obesity; public health interventions

1. Introduction

Cardiovascular disease (CVD) remains a significant public health challenge worldwide, with disproportionate risks observed in certain populations due to various social determinants of health (SDOHs) [1,2]. These determinants, including socioeconomic status (SES), have a profound influence on health outcomes, particularly in the context of CVD. Globally, SES is a well-documented predictor of cardiovascular health, where lower SES is consistently associated with higher CVD risk and poorer outcomes [3,4].

Romania has the highest percentage of people at risk of poverty or social exclusion among EU (European Union) member states, with 34.5% of its population affected, according to Eurostat data. In 2021, 95.4 million people across the EU, representing 21.7% of the population, were at risk of poverty or social exclusion. This includes those facing severe material and social deprivation or living in households with very low work intensity. Romania's figures are notably higher than the EU average, with other countries like Bulgaria (32%), Greece, and Spain (both 28%) also having significant portions of their populations at risk. In contrast, the lowest rates were observed in Czechia (11%), Slovenia (13%), and Finland (14%) [5].

Focusing on the local context, West Romania is one of the regions with lower rates of people at risk of poverty or social exclusion among Romania's regions (29.5%) [6]. In the West Development Region of Romania, with a population of 2,014,732, approximately 29.5% are at risk of poverty or social deprivation. This translates to roughly 594,346 people facing such challenges in this region [7]. But this region still presents a particularly vulnerable population, where the intersection of low income, limited education, housing instability, and restricted access to healthcare creates a complex web of risks for CVD [8–10]. Social determinants of health (SDOHs) play a crucial role in shaping cardiovascular health and contributing to disparities in risk factors, outcomes, and clinical care for CVD. These determinants span six domains: economic stability, education, food, neighborhood and physical environment, healthcare system, and community and social context [11,12].

In West Romania, as well as in all of the country, factors such as income, education, housing stability, and access to healthcare intersect to create a complex web of risk [13–16]. Addressing these social determinants is crucial for improving cardiovascular health. Furthermore, disadvantaged populations often grapple with unhealthy behaviors that contribute to CVD. These include smoking, poor dietary choices, physical inactivity, and substance abuse [1,8,17].

Access to healthcare services is another pivotal factor that influences cardiovascular health outcomes in this region [2,4]. Financial constraints, lack of health insurance, and inadequate primary care facilities are significant barriers that hinder effective prevention and management of CVD. Community-based programs offer potential solutions to bridge these gaps, emphasizing the need for targeted interventions [17].

By focusing on this region, this study aims to investigate the prevalence and impact of cardiovascular risk factors (CVRFs) among socioeconomically disadvantaged populations in Western Romania. Specifically, it seeks to identify the association between SES and the presence of various CVRFs, such as diabetes, hypertension, dyslipidemia, and smoking, within this population. This study also aims to highlight the extent of undiagnosed conditions and the disparity in health outcomes due to limited access to healthcare and unhealthy lifestyle choices. Ultimately, this research study seeks to inform targeted public health interventions to reduce these disparities and improve cardiovascular health outcomes in socioeconomically disadvantaged communities.

2. Materials and Methods

2.1. General Information

This article presents the results from the project conducted by European Social Fund through the Operational Programme Human Capital (POCU) and by the Timisoara Local Action Group, with the main aim of improving the health and quality of life of vulnerable people. Project title: "Detection of cardiovascular problems and awareness of the population regarding medical problems"; SMIS code: 149707. The duration of this study was two years (November 2021–November 2023).

This study was conducted in partnership with "Neoclinic Concept" Clinique, where all eligible patients included in this study were evaluated by two cardiologists with over 10 years of experience. Our target group for this investigation consisted of the residents of Freidorf (~10,000 habitants), a suburban region located in Timisoara, the major city in Western Romania.

2.2. Sample Size

This study's sample size was carefully determined to ensure the representativeness of the socioeconomically disadvantaged population of the West Development Region of Romania, where 29.5% of the 2,014,732 regional population is at risk of poverty or social exclusion. All eligible subjects have been included from a population of around 10,000 inhabitants. The sample was chosen to capture the variability and prevalence of cardiovascular risk factors (CVRFs) and to achieve adequate statistical power for detecting significant differences in these factors, with a 95% confidence level and 80% power. Additionally, the sample size balanced the need for robust statistical analysis with practical and ethical considerations, including resource limitations and patient confidentiality.

2.3. Selection Criteria

The inclusion criteria were based on Eurostat's EU-SILC (European Union Statistics on Income and Living Conditions) benchmarks [18]. The inclusion criteria were as follows:

(a) Severe material deprivation rate (SMD): population unable to afford at least four out of nine predefined material items essential for an adequate quality of life. These items include housing, heating, durable goods, and access to healthcare.

(b) At-risk-of-poverty rate: people who are at risk of falling below the poverty threshold (typically set at 60% of the national median equivalized disposable income). Eurostat provides information on at-risk-of-poverty rates for various demographic groups, including age, gender, and household composition.

(c) Low work intensity indicator: we analyzed data related to low work intensity, focusing on people aged 18–59 years living in households where adults (aged 18–59, excluding students aged 18–24) worked a working time equal to or less than 20% of their total combined work-time potential during the previous year [18].

2.4. Study Design and Analysis

This analysis employed a retrospective observational design, where data were gathered from the medical records of eligible individuals. The research gained ethical approval from the Ethics Committee of "Neoclinic Concept" Clinique (approval number 1/2024).

The analysis of subject records was conducted to gather demographic information, including age, gender, place of origin, weight, and height. Additionally, we collected information on familial history of diabetes mellitus and cardiovascular disease, as well as personal pathologies such as diabetes mellitus, cardiovascular disease, blood pressure, and dyslipidemia. All of this information was recorded based on their medical history documentation. Smoking status analysis, systolic and diastolic blood pressure measurement, glucose level, cholesterol level, triglycerides, and HbA1c level were obtained in the course of the cardiological examination. All investigations and measurements of medical test values were carried out in the same laboratory at "Neoclinic Concept" Clinique, using the same equipment settings. The anamnesis, data collection, and cardiology consultations were consistently performed by one of the two cardiologists with over 10 years of experience (A.D., S.S).

The cut-offs for all values were selected according to international guidelines. For systolic and diastolic blood pressure, we used the "2023 ESH Guidelines for the management of arterial hypertension" [19]. The cut-off for fasting glucose level was defined according to the American Diabetes Association [20]. The specific cut-off values for HDL, LDLc, and fasting triglyceride measurements were chosen according to the Adult Treatment Panel III (ATP III) Update [21,22].

2.5. Statistical Analysis

The statistical analysis was performed using MedCalc® Statistical Software version 22.030, created by MedCalc® Software Ltd. in Ostend, Belgium. The software can be viewed at the URL https://www.medcalc.org and was accessed on 15 June 2024.

The data related to identification, clinical, and paraclinical aspects were carefully documented in a secured computerized database using Microsoft® Excel® for Microsoft 365 MSO (Version 2406 Build 16.0.17726.20078) 64-bit, which was released on 11 June 2024.

This study included a summary of patient demographics, clinical characteristics, and laboratory data. The results were presented by first summarizing the patient demographics, clinical characteristics, and laboratory data. The distribution of data was assessed using the Shapiro–Wilk test to determine whether the data followed a normal distribution. Based on the results of this test, non-parametric statistical methods were primarily employed due to significant departures from normal distribution. Specifically, the Mann–Whitney test was used to compare non-parametric parameters, while the independent t-test was applied for parametric parameters. Differences between groups were considered statistically significant if the *p*-value was less than or equal to 0.05. The results were presented as median values with interquartile ranges (IQR) for non-parametric data and as means with standard deviations for parametric data. This approach allowed for a clear and accurate presentation of the data, highlighting significant differences where applicable.

3. Results

3.1. Demographic Features

Out of a total of 1433 subjects included, 498 were male (34.75%). The median age for entire lot was 52 with IQR between 38 and 64.50. The median age for male and female gender are 51 and 52, respectively. The Mann–Whitney test suggested that there was no significant difference in medians between the two samples ($p = 0.17$). All included subjects were from the same urban area, the Freidorf suburb. The conditions that were investigated include hereditary–collateral antecedents (HCAs), such as diabetes and cardiovascular diseases, as well as personal pathologic antecedents (PPAs) such as diabetes, coronary disease, blood pressure, and dyslipidemia. The prevalence of these conditions is presented in Table 1.

Table 1. The prevalence of the investigated conditions.

Condition	Number of Subjects	Percentage
HCA (diabetes)	115	8.02%
HCA (cardiovascular)	126	8.79%
PPA (diabetes)	106	7.39%
PPA (coronary disease)	55	3.83%
PPA (blood pressure)	510	35.58%
PPA (dyslipidemia)	305	21.28%

HCA—hereditary–collateral antecedent; PPA—personal pathologic antecedent.

Table 2 presents the classification of parameter categories according to the subjects' analyzed values. The patient data reveal a diverse range of BMI classifications. The median value of BMI is 28, with an interquartile range between 24.04 and 32. The highest value is 56 kg/m^2, while the lowest one is 15.05 kg/m^2. A small percentage of patients, 2.30%, fall into the underweight category with a BMI of less than 18.5. A significant proportion of the patients, 27.63%, have a normal weight, with BMIs ranging from 18.5 to 24.9. The largest group, comprising 33.77% of the patients, is classified as overweight, with BMIs between 25 and 29.9. Additionally, 21.21% of patients are categorized as obese, having BMIs from 30 to 34.9. Lastly, 15.07% of patients are considered morbidly obese, with BMIs exceeding 35.

Table 2. Classification of parameter categories according to subjects' analyzed values.

Category	Parameter	No of Subjects (Percentage)
	BMI	
Underweight	<18.5 kg/m^2	33 (2.30%)
Normal weight	18.5–24.9 kg/m^2	396 (27.63%)
Overweight	25–29.9 kg/m^2	484 (33.77%)
Obese	30–34.9 kg/m^2	304 (21.21%)
Morbidly obese	≥35 kg/m^2	216 (15.07%)
	Smoker status	
Non-smoker		830 (58.49%)
Active smoker		450 (31.71%)
Ex-smoker	Smoke-free for at least 28 days	139 (9.79%)
	Systolic blood pressure	
Optimal	<120 mmHg	394 (27.84%)
Normal	120–129 mmHg	282 (19.92%)
High normal	130–139 mmHg	251 (17.73%)
Grade 1 hypertension	140–159 mmHg	319 (22.54%)
Grade 2 hypertension	160–179 mmHg	117 (8.26%)
Grade 3 hypertension	≥180 mmHg	52 (3.67%)
	Diastolic blood pressure	
Optimal	<80 mmHg	400 (28.24%)
Normal	80–84 mmHg	263 (18.57%)
High normal	85–89 mmHg	220 (15.53%)
Grade 1 hypertension	90–99 mmHg	315 (22.24%)
Grade 2 hypertension	100–109 mmHg	155 (10.94%)
Grade 3 hypertension	≥110 mmHg	63 (4.68%)
	Fasting blood glucose level	
Normal	<100 mg/dL	381 (31.90%)
Alteration in fasting glucose	100–125 mg/dL	617 (51.67%)
Alteration in fasting glucose (diabetes category)	≥126 mg/dL	196 (16.41%)
	HDL level	
Low	<40 mg/dL	218 (18.07%)
Intermediate	40–59 mg/dL	637 (52.81%)
High	≥60 mg/dL	351 (29.10%)
	LDLc level	
Optimal	< 100 mg/ dL	451 (37.83%)
Near optimal/above optimal	100–129 mg/dL	331 (27.76%)
Borderline high	130–159 mg/dL	238 (19.96%)
High	160–189 mg/dL	127 (10.65%)
Very high	≥190 mg/dL	45 (3.77%)
	Fasting triglyceride level	
Normal	<150 mg/dL	840 (69.65%)
Mild hypertriglyceridemia	150–499 mg/dL	352 (29.18%)
Moderate hypertriglyceridemia	500–886 mg/dL	11 (0.91%)
Very high or severe hypertriglyceridemia	>886 mg/dL	3 (0.24%)

BMI—body mass index.

The median systolic blood pressure is 130, with an IQR between 117 and 145 mmHg. The median diastolic blood pressure is 85, with an IQR between 77 and 94 mmHg.

The blood glucose levels range from 62 to 377 mg/dL, suggesting significant variability among patients. The median value is 105.50 mg/dL, with an IQR between 97 and 118 mg/dL.

The total cholesterol level ranges from 86 to 404 mg/dL. The median value is 195 mg/dL, with an IQR between 164 and 225 mg/dL. HDL levels range from 18 to 127 mg/dL, with a median of 52 mg/dL (42, 61). LDLc levels range from 15 to 258 mg/dL, with a median of 113 mg/dL (IQR 88, 140).

Fasting triglyceride levels vary from 24 to 2333 mg/dL. The median value is 111 mg/dL, with an IQR of 77–163 mg/dL.

HbA1c levels vary from 4.80 to 14.50%. The median percentage is 6.2%, with an IQR between 5.70 and 7.

3.2. Age Distribution and Its Association with Hereditary and Personal Pathologic Antecedents

The ages of subjects with and without diabetes as an HCA have different median values (49 vs. 52), with a 95% confidence interval for the median difference between 1 and 7. The interquartile range also differs (36 to 55.75 vs. 38 to 65), indicating variability in the data. The Mann–Whitney test suggests a statistically significant difference between the groups ($p = 0.014$), with the second group having higher average ranks. The graphical representation is presented in Figure 1.

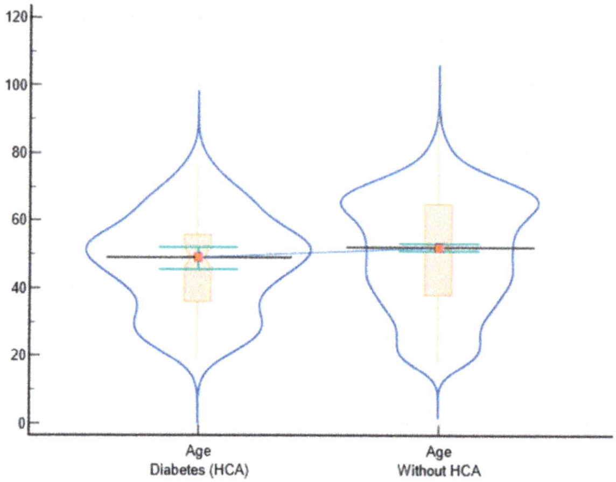

Figure 1. Graphical representation of age between subjects with and without HCA diabetes including notched box-and-whisker and violin plot representations (notched box-and-whisker, as well as horizontal lines, markers, connecting lines, and error bars, to indicate 95% confidence intervals for medians).

The ages of subjects with and without cardiovascular diseases as an HCA have different median values (48 vs. 52), with a 95% confidence interval for the median difference between 1 and 7. The interquartile range also differs (36 to 59 vs. 38.75 to 65), indicating variability in the data. The Mann–Whitney test suggests a statistically significant difference between the groups ($p = 0.006$), with the second group having higher average ranks.

The median age of individuals diagnosed with diabetes was 65 years (57, 70), whereas the median age of individuals without diabetes was 51 years (37, 64). The disparity is extremely significant, as indicated by a p-value of less than 0.0001.

The median age of individuals diagnosed with coronary disease was 64 years (57.50, 69.75), whereas those without the condition had a median age of 51 years (38, 64). The observed difference was extremely significant, as indicated by a p-value of less than 0.0001.

The median age of individuals diagnosed with blood pressure was 65 years (57, 70), whereas the median age of individuals without hypertension was 43 years (32, 55). The difference was extremely significant, as indicated by a p-value of less than 0.0001.

The median age of individuals diagnosed with dyslipidemia was 66 years (58, 70), while those without dyslipidemia had a median age of 47 years (34, 60). The observed difference was extremely significant, with a p-value of less than 0.0001.

The median age of smokers was 48 years (36, 62), while the median age of non-smokers was 54 years (40, 65). The difference was highly significant, with a p-value of less than 0.0001. Table 3 presents the differences between the ages of the subjects according to the investigated conditions.

Table 3. Age of subjects according to investigated conditions.

Condition	Age of Subjects with Condition	Age of Subjects without Condition	*p*-Value
HCA (diabetes)	49; (36, 55.75)	52; (38, 65)	0.014
HCA (cardiovascular)	48; (36, 59)	52; (38.75, 65)	0.006
PPA (diabetes)	65; (57, 70)	51; (37, 64)	<0.001
PPA (coronary disease)	64; (57.50, 69.75)	51; (38, 64)	<0.001
PPA (blood pressure)	65; (57, 70)	43; (32, 55)	<0.001
PPA (dyslipidemia)	66; (58, 70)	47; (34, 60)	<0.001
Smoker status	48; (36, 62)	54; (40, 65)	<0.001

HCA—hereditary–collateral antecedent; PPA—personal pathologic antecedent. Data are presented as medians (IQRs).

3.3. Body Mass Index (BMI) Comparison across Hereditary and Personal Pathologic Conditions

Subjects with diabetes (both HCA and PPA) have a higher average BMI compared to those without diabetes, with significant differences. For cardiovascular conditions (HCA), there is no significant difference in BMI between subjects with and without the condition. Subjects with coronary disease (PPA) and blood pressure (PPA) also have higher average BMIs compared to those without these conditions, with significant differences. Similarly, subjects with dyslipidemia (PPA) have a higher average BMI compared to those without, with significant differences. Lastly, smokers have a slightly lower average BMI compared to non-smokers, with a significant difference. Table 4 presents the difference between BMI of subjects according to their condition status.

Table 4. BMI of subjects according to condition status.

Condition	BMI of Subjects with Condition	BMI of Subjects without Condition	*p*-Value
HCA (diabetes)	29.62; (25.77, 34.56)	27.74; (24, 32)	0.011
HCA (cardiovascular)	28.30; (23.70, 32.87)	28; (24.15, 32)	0.847
PPA (diabetes)	31.63; (28.53, 36.07)	27.64; (24, 31.80)	<0.001
PPA (coronary disease)	29.36; (25.95, 34.58)	27.93; (24.02, 32)	0.033
PPA (blood pressure)	30; (27, 34.44)	26.53; (23, 31.04)	<0.001
PPA (dyslipidemia)	29.40; (26.37, 34)	27.10; (23.70, 31.96)	<0.001
Smoker status	27.66; (23.90; 31.71)	28; (24.52, 32.36)	0.031

HCA—hereditary–collateral antecedent; PPA—personal pathologic antecedent.

3.4. Gender-Based Variations in Cardiovascular and Metabolic Risk Factors

The data showed that males generally have higher BMI (Figure 2), systolic (Figure 3) and diastolic blood pressure, blood glucose levels (Figure 4), and fasting triglyceride levels compared to females. However, females tended to have higher HDL levels. There were no significant differences in total cholesterol and LDLc levels between males and females. HbA1c levels were slightly higher in males, but the difference was not statistically significant. The comparison between male and female participants according to parameter variabilities is presented in Table 5.

Table 5. Comparison between male and female participants according to parameter variabilities.

Parameter	Male Gender	Female Gender	*p*-Value
BMI	28.70; (25, 32.11)	27.43; (23.87, 32)	0.021
Systolic blood pressure	134; (121, 150)	128; (115,144)	<0.001
Diastolic blood pressure	86; (80, 96)	85; (76, 92)	0.001
Blood glucose level	108; (100, 120)	103; (95, 116)	<0.001
Total cholesterol level	191; (160.75, 221)	196; (166, 228)	0.062
HDL level	45; (38, 55)	54; (45, 64)	<0.001
LDLc level	111; (87, 143)	114; (88, 140)	0.562
Fasting triglyceride level	125; (86, 191.25)	107; (74, 153.25)	<0.001
HbA_{1c}	6.2; (5.80, 7.45)	6.1; (5.70, 6.87)	0.487

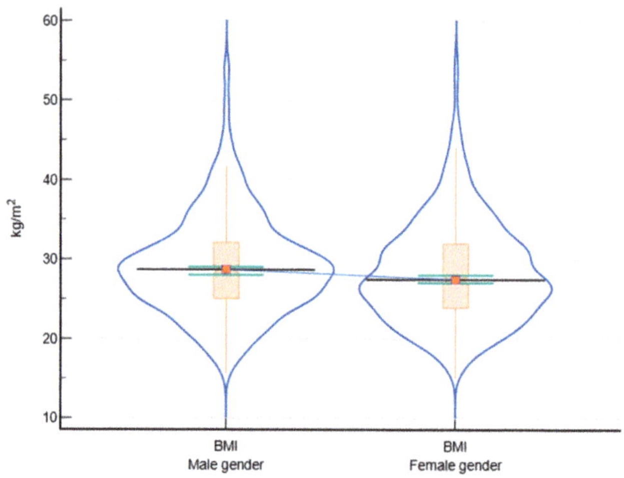

Figure 2. Graphical depiction of BMI between male and female participants, including notched box-and-whisker and violin plot representations (notched box-and-whisker, as well as horizontal lines, markers, connecting lines, and error bars, indicate 95% confidence intervals for medians).

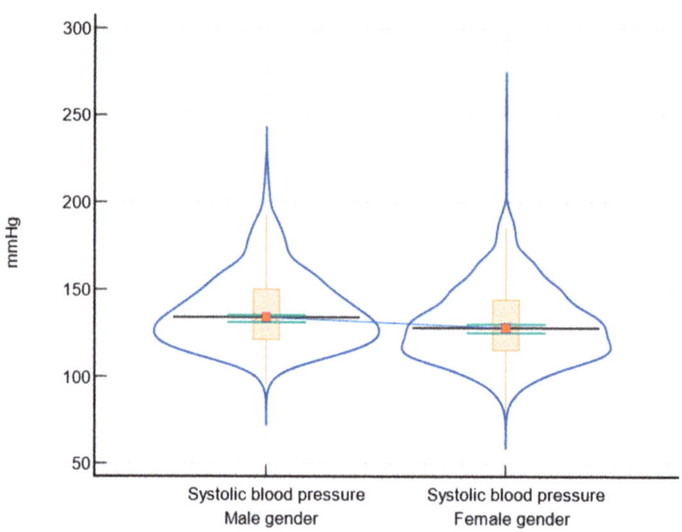

Figure 3. Graphical representation of systolic blood pressure between male and female participants, including notched box-and-whisker and violin plot representations (notched box-and-whisker, as well as horizontal lines, markers, connecting lines, and error bars, indicate 95% confidence intervals for medians).

3.5. Prevalence and Distribution of Cardiovascular Risk Factors in the Study Population

Approximately 25% of the included subjects (345 patients) did not have a prior history of hypertension (no previous physician-diagnosed hypertension). Despite this, their blood pressure measurements indicated they could be classified as having at least grade I hypertension. Additionally, a substantial 41.59% (596 patients) of those without a history of dyslipidemia (no previous physician-diagnosed dyslipidemia) had LDLc levels higher than 100 mg/dL.

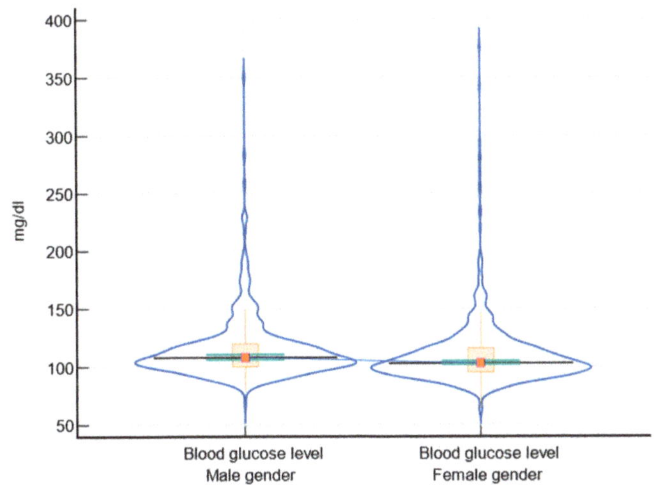

Figure 4. Graphical representation of blood glucose levels between male and female participants, including notched box-and-whisker and violin plot representations (notched box-and-whisker, as well as horizontal lines, markers, connecting lines, and error bars, indicate 95% confidence intervals for medians).

Table 6 displays the classification of the included patients according to the risk factors (BMI > 30 kg/m^2, smoker, SBP $\geq$ 140 mmHg, DBP $\geq$ 90 mmHg, fasting glucose $\geq$ 126 mg/dL, and LDLc $\geq$ 130 mg/dL) they are related to. Figure 5 presents the distribution of these categories.

Table 6. The classification of the included subjects, according to the risk factors they are related to.

Classification	Number of Subjects	Percentage
Subjects without risk factors	218	15.21%
Subjects with 1 risk factor	435	30.35%
Subjects with 2 risk factors	305	21.28%
Subjects with 3 risk factors	268	18.70%
Subjects with 4 risk factors	150	10.46%
Subjects with 5 risk factors	53	3.69%
Subjects with 6 risk factors	4	0.27%

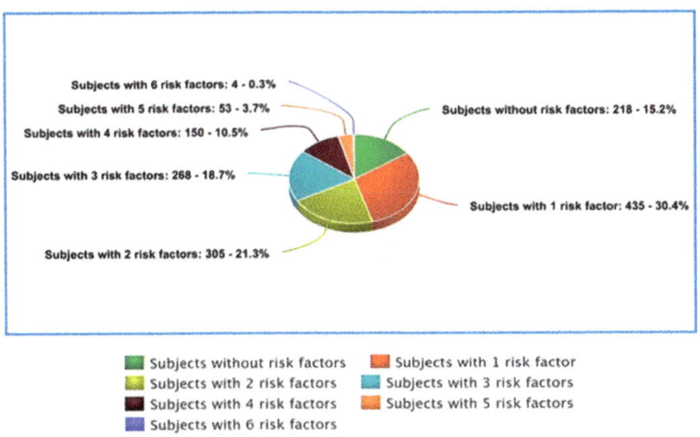

Figure 5. Pie chart graphical representation of included subjects.

3.6. Relative Risk (RR) and Odds Ratio (OR) for Various Outcomes Based on Associated Risk Factors

Individuals with a family history of diabetes (HCA of diabetes) are at a much higher risk of developing diabetes themselves. A higher body mass index (BMI) is strongly linked to elevated blood glucose levels, with the risk increasing as BMI rises. Elevated systolic and diastolic blood pressure levels are also significantly associated with higher blood glucose levels, indicating a strong interplay between hypertension and glucose regulation. Although the presence of a family history of cardiovascular disease (HCA of cardiovascular conditions) slightly increases the risk of coronary disease, this association was not statistically significant. The associations between CVRFs and disease outcomes are presented in Table 7.

Table 7. Associations between cardiovascular risk factors and disease outcomes: relative risk and odds ratios.

Outcome	Group	RR (p-Value)	OR (p-Value)
Diabetes	HCA (diabetes)	3.5 (<0.001)	4.19 (<0.001)
Blood glucose level ≥ 126 mg/dL	BMI ≥ 25 kg/m^2	3.2 (<0.001)	3.76 (<0.001)
Blood glucose level ≥ 126 mg/dL	BMI ≥ 30 kg/m^2	2.26 (<0.001)	2.68 (<0.001)
SBP ≥ 140 mmHg	Blood glucose level ≥ 126 mg/dL	1.66 (<0.001)	2.48 (<0.001)
SBP ≥ 160 mmHg	Blood glucose level ≥ 126 mg/dL	2.56 (<0.001)	3.12 (<0.001)
SBP ≥ 180 mmHg	Blood glucose level ≥ 126 mg/dL	2.54 (<0.001)	2.68 (0.001)
DBP ≥ 90 mmHg	Blood glucose level ≥ 126 mg/dL	1.37 (<0.001)	1.81 (<0.001)
DBP ≥ 100 mmHg	Blood glucose level ≥ 126 mg/dL	1.61 (<0.001)	1.82 (0.001)
DBP ≥ 110 mmHg	Blood glucose level ≥ 126 mg/dL	1.69 (0.066)	1.75 (0.068)
PPA (coronary disease)	HCA (Cardiovascular)	1.71 (0.144)	1.76 (0.148)

4. Discussion

4.1. Cardiovascular Risk Factors among Socioeconomically Disadvantaged Populations in Western Romania: A Comparative Analysis with National and International Studies

This study highlighted a significant prevalence of cardiovascular risk factors among the socioeconomically disadvantaged population in West Romania. PPA conditions such as arterial hypertension (35.58%), dyslipidemia (21.28%), and diabetes (7.39%) were notably prevalent. These findings are consistent with numerous studies that emphasize the disproportionate burden of CVRFs in low-socioeconomic-status populations. For example, a study conducted by Barnett et al. found that individuals in lower SES brackets have a higher prevalence of risk factors such as hypertension, diabetes, and smoking compared to higher SES groups. This is attributed to limited access to healthcare, unhealthy lifestyle choices, and greater psychosocial stress [23]. Furthermore, Kanjilal et al. highlighted that low SES is strongly associated with higher incidences of hypertension and dyslipidemia, paralleling the findings in this West Romania study [24].

The analysis showed significant differences in the median ages of subjects with and without CVRFs. For example, individuals with diabetes had a median age of 65 years, compared to 51 years for those without diabetes. Similarly, those with coronary disease and arterial hypertension also had higher median ages. These findings are similar to others that demonstrated that SES-related disparities significantly impact the onset and progression of CVD. Higher-SES individuals tend to have better access to preventive measures and treatment options, delaying the onset of CVD. Disadvantaged neighborhoods exhibited higher CVD prevalence and poorer health outcomes, emphasizing the role of social determinants in health [25–27].

Our data showed a distribution of BMI classifications among a group of individuals, with the majority falling into the overweight category (33.77%), followed by normal weight (27.63%), obese (21.21%), morbidly obese (15.07%), and underweight (2.30%). This distribution highlights the prevalence of higher BMI categories within the group, which is a common trend observed in various populations globally. Comparing these results with similar studies, a study using the UK Biobank cohort identified similar trends, with a significant portion of the population classified as overweight or obese. This study also highlighted the complexity of obesity, considering various factors like societal influences, individual psychology, and physical activity. Such findings underscore the multifaceted nature of obesity and the need for comprehensive strategies to address it [28,29]. Furthermore, they highlight the ongoing global challenge of obesity and the need for comprehensive approaches to address it. Understanding these trends and their implications can help in developing targeted interventions to improve health outcomes [30,31].

For the HCA of diabetes, the BMI of subjects with diabetes (29.62) was significantly higher than that of those without (27.74), with a p-value of 0.011. This finding aligns with the existing literature, which suggests higher BMI is a risk factor for developing diabetes, particularly in individuals with a family history of the condition [32].

In the case of the cardiovascular HCA, the difference in BMI between subjects with cardiovascular conditions (28.30) and those without (28) was not statistically significant (p-value 0.847). This suggests that while BMI is an important factor, other hereditary factors might play a more critical role in cardiovascular health [33,34]. This suggests that while BMI is a factor, other elements such as genetic predisposition, lifestyle, and other comorbidities play a crucial role in cardiovascular health. Similar findings were reported in a study in the *Journal of the American College of Cardiology*, which emphasized the multifactorial nature of cardiovascular disease [1,35].

Regarding the PPAs of diabetes, coronary disease, arterial hypertension, and dyslipidemia, the BMI of subjects with these conditions was significantly higher than that of those without. This strong association underscores the impact of personal health history on these diseases' risk, consistent with the finding that higher BMI is a significant risk factor for diabetes, coronary disease, arterial hypertension, and dyslipidemia [36,37].

The active smoking rate of 31.71% is notably high. This is consistent with other research indicating a higher smoking prevalence in socioeconomically disadvantaged populations compared to the general population. Nationally, the smoking rate tends to be lower, often around 14–15% in many developed countries [38]. Furthermore, the percentage of ex-smokers (9.79%) is relatively low. This suggests potential barriers to quitting smoking within this population, such as limited access to smoking cessation programs, lack of healthcare support, and higher levels of stress and mental health issues, which are known to affect smoking cessation efforts. Studies consistently show higher smoking rates among socioeconomically disadvantaged groups. For example, research published in the USA indicated that smoking prevalence in the lowest income brackets can be as high as 30–35%, aligning with the 31.71% observed in our data [39,40].

Regarding smoker status, the BMI of smokers (27.66) was slightly lower than that of non-smokers (28), with a p-value of 0.031. This finding is intriguing and aligns with the hypothesis that smoking may suppress appetite and increase metabolism, leading to lower body weight. Furthermore, this small but significant difference is consistent with findings in the *American Journal of Public Health*, which suggest that smokers tend to have a lower BMI but higher risks of other health issues [41,42].

Regarding the BMI of the subjects, the analyzed data highlighted significant differences in cardiovascular risk factors between males and females. Firstly, males have a higher median BMI compared to females, with a statistically significant difference (p = 0.021). This aligns with studies showing that males in disadvantaged populations often have higher BMI due to lifestyle factors and limited access to healthy food options [3]. Both systolic and diastolic blood pressures were higher in males, with highly significant p-values (<0.0001 and 0.001, respectively). These findings are similar to those of the SEPHAR study, which included people from the same geographic area [43,44]. High blood pressure is more prevalent in socioeconomically disadvantaged areas, often due to stress, poor diet, and lack of healthcare access, contributing to increased cardiovascular risk [2,36,45]. Also, males had higher blood glucose levels than females, with a significant p-value (<0.0001). This is consistent with findings that disadvantaged populations have higher rates of diabetes and poor glycemic control due to limited healthcare access [17,46].

It is important to note that the occurrence of diabetes, based on their medical records, was 7.39%. However, 16.41% of individuals had a fasting glucose level exceeding 126 mg/dL. In contrast, the PREDATORR study, conducted from 2012 to 2014, found a diabetes prevalence of 11.6% among the adult Romanian population [46]. A deep analysis of these data showed that impaired glucose regulation (prediabetes, known and unknown diabetes) was found in 28.1% of the study population in the PREDATORR study, compared to 68.11% of our study population with fasting glucose levels higher than 100 mg/dL [46]. The early diagnosis of diabetes is crucial in preventing or delaying the progression of the disease and the onset of complications, such as cardiovascular diseases, neuropathy, and nephropathy, which significantly impact patient outcomes and healthcare resources [47–49].

Total cholesterol levels were slightly higher in females, but the difference was not statistically significant (p = 0.062). HDL levels were significantly higher in females (<0.0001), while LDL levels showed no significant difference (p = 0.562). Disadvantaged populations often have poor lipid profiles due to dietary habits and lack of preventive care [11]. However, regardless of fasting triglyceride levels, males had increased levels. Elevated triglycerides are common in socioeconomically disadvantaged groups, linked to diet and metabolic syndrome [11,50].

The results of this study align with existing research on cardiovascular risk factors in socioeconomically disadvantaged populations, highlighting significant associations between these risk factors and health outcomes. The strong relationship between diabetes and a family history of the disease (HCA) underscores the genetic predisposition in these populations, as supported by studies like those by Sirdah et al. and Wang et al. [51,52]. Furthermore, the significant increase in the risk for elevated blood glucose levels in individuals with higher BMI ($\geq$25 kg/m^2 and $\geq$30 kg/m^2) is consistent with findings from Wondmkun's research, which noted a strong link between obesity and impaired glucose regulation in low-income populations [53]. The progressive increase in the risk of hypertension with elevated blood glucose levels also mirrors the Framingham Heart Study's findings, which highlighted the connection between hyperglycemia and hypertension in at-risk populations [54,55]. Additionally, the observed, albeit not statistically significant, association between coronary disease and a family history of cardiovascular disease suggests a hereditary component that may be influenced by lifestyle and environmental factors, as noted in the INTERHEART study [56,57]. Overall, these findings emphasize the compounded cardiovascular risks faced by disadvantaged populations, reinforcing the need for targeted public health interventions that address both genetic predispositions and socioeconomic factors.

4.2. Comparative Analysis of Cardiovascular Risk Factors in Socioeconomically Disadvantaged Populations: Insights from Recent Romanian Studies

Our study's findings align with and expand upon those in the attached article by Simionescu et al., which examined CVD risk factors and mortality in Romania. Both studies highlight the significant burden of CVDs, particularly among socioeconomically disadvantaged populations, with our research identifying a high prevalence of arterial hypertension, dyslipidemia, and diabetes, which mirrors Simionescu et al.'s emphasis on hypertension as a leading risk factor. While Simionescu et al. discuss the persistent high mortality rates despite increased healthcare infrastructure, our study adds depth by examining the significant correlations between BMI, smoking, and cardiovascular risk factors, reinforcing the complex interplay of lifestyle factors and CVD risk. Both studies underscore the need for enhanced healthcare access and targeted public health policies to address these risk factors, particularly in disadvantaged communities, presenting a compelling case for prioritizing cardiovascular health in Romania's public health strategy [9].

The findings of our study, which highlighted a significant prevalence of CVRFs such as arterial hypertension, dyslipidemia, and diabetes among a socioeconomically disadvantaged population in West Romania, align closely with the results of several key studies in Romania, including those by Simionescu et al., Rosu et al., Weiss et al., and Cinteza et al. (CARDIO-Zone study) [9,58–60]. Both our study and the CARDIO-Zone study reveal high rates of hypertension and diabetes, although our study found even higher rates of undiagnosed cases, particularly of hypertension and dyslipidemia, suggesting gaps in healthcare access and preventive care. Additionally, while the CARDIO-Zone study emphasized regional differences in CVRF prevalence, our research adds to this by examining the complex interplay of BMI, smoking, and CVRFs, further reinforcing the role of lifestyle and socioeconomic factors in cardiovascular health [60]. Moreover, the prevalence of obesity and smoking in our study mirrors that observed in broader Romanian studies, indicating consistent patterns across different populations and regions. Overall, these findings collectively underscore the urgent need for targeted public health interventions and improved healthcare accessibility to mitigate the burden of cardiovascular diseases in Romania, particularly among disadvantaged communities.

All of these findings align with broader research indicating that socioeconomically disadvantaged populations face higher cardiovascular risks due to a combination of biological, behavioral, and psychosocial factors [4,61]. Furthermore, the data from the current study and the PREDATORR and SEPHAR studies collectively indicate high rates of hypertension and metabolic disorders among the Romanian population, particularly in socioeconomically disadvantaged groups. The high prevalence of active smokers in the current study (31.71%) exacerbates these health conditions, highlighting the need for targeted interventions [8,43,44,46].

4.3. Strategies to Reduce Cardiovascular Risk in Socioeconomically Disadvantaged Populations: Addressing Health Equity through Targeted Interventions and Policy Initiatives within the Romanian Population

Efforts to achieve health equity should address the structural, institutional, and environmental barriers faced by marginalized communities. By considering SDOHs, we can inform CVD care, ensure equitable healthcare resource distribution, and reduce observed disparities [3]. To reduce the high prevalence of CVRFs in socioeconomically disadvantaged populations, several targeted interventions could be implemented, focusing on both systemic and community-level strategies [9]. First, increasing access to healthcare is crucial, particularly in underserved areas, through the expansion of community health centers and mobile clinics. These facilities can provide essential services such as regular health screenings, early diagnosis, and the management of conditions like hypertension, diabetes, and dyslipidemia, which are often undiagnosed in these populations. Second, public health campaigns tailored to the specific needs and circumstances of disadvantaged communities could raise awareness about the importance of healthy lifestyles, including diet, physical activity, and smoking cessation. These campaigns should be culturally sensitive and involve community leaders to enhance their effectiveness. Third, implementing policies that address social determinants of health, such as improving access to affordable healthy food options and creating safe spaces for physical activity, is essential. For example, incentivizing grocery stores to stock fresh produce in food deserts or developing urban green spaces can significantly impact community health. Fourth, integrating mental health support into cardiovascular care is important, as chronic stress related to socioeconomic disadvantage contributes to the risk of CVD. Providing mental health services within primary care settings could help mitigate these effects. Lastly, policy-level interventions, such as implementing taxes on sugary drinks and tobacco products, alongside subsidies for healthy food options, could further encourage healthier behaviors. Collectively, these strategies could substantially reduce the burden of CVRFs in socioeconomically disadvantaged populations, leading to improved health outcomes and reduced healthcare disparities [9,62–65].

4.4. Limitations

This study employed a retrospective observational design, which inherently limits the ability to establish causal relationships between socioeconomic factors and CVD outcomes. Observational studies can show associations but not causation, and the findings may be influenced by unmeasured confounding variables. Moreover, factors such as diet, physical activity, alcohol consumption and lifestyle behaviors were not taken into account.

This study was conducted within a specific geographical area (West Romania) and may not be representative of other regions or populations. Furthermore, some analyses within this study were cross-sectional, examining data at a single point in time. This approach does not account for changes in socioeconomic status or health behaviors over time, which can significantly influence cardiovascular health outcomes.

4.5. Future Directions

Future directions should include the integration of digital health technologies and personalized medicine into socioeconomically disadvantaged populations. For example, the use of mobile health (mHealth) applications and telemedicine can play a crucial role in improving access to care in underserved areas. These technologies can facilitate the remote monitoring of cardiovascular risk factors such as blood pressure and glucose levels, enabling timely interventions and continuous patient engagement [66,67]. Additionally, implementing community-based participatory research can empower these populations by involving them in the design and implementation of health interventions, ensuring that the strategies are culturally relevant and more likely to be effective [68]. Another innovative approach could involve the use of genetic screening and precision medicine to identify individuals at higher risk due to hereditary factors, allowing for more targeted and personalized prevention and treatment plans [52,53]. These strategies collectively represent a more holistic and tailored approach to reducing the burden of cardiovascular risk factors in socioeconomically disadvantaged populations [1,30,31].

5. Conclusions

In conclusion, socioeconomically disadvantaged populations exhibit a significantly higher prevalence of cardiovascular risk factors such as diabetes, impaired glucose regulation, hypertension, and dyslipidemia compared to their previously known status. These disparities are likely due to limited access to healthcare, unhealthy lifestyle choices, and greater psychosocial stress, which compound the risk of developing chronic conditions. Therefore, enhanced attention and targeted public health interventions are essential to address these health inequities. Prioritizing preventive care, early diagnosis, and accessible treatment options for these communities is crucial in reducing the burden of cardiovascular diseases and improving overall health outcomes.

Author Contributions: Conceptualization, A.D. and E.R.S.; methodology, A.D. and G.M.V.; software, S.S.; validation, G.M.V., S.S. and S.R.S.; formal analysis, E.R.S.; investigation, A.D.; resources, A.D.; data curation, S.R.S.; writing—original draft preparation, A.D., S.S. and E.R.S.; writing—review and editing, A.D., S.S., S.R.S. and E.R.S.; visualization, G.M.V.; supervision, A.D. and E.R.S.; project administration, A.D. and E.R.S.; funding acquisition, A.D., G.M.V. and S.S. All authors have read and agreed to the published version of the manuscript.

Funding: This project was financed by the European Social Fund through the Operational Programme Human Capital (POCU) and by the Timișoara Local Action Group, with the main aim of improving the health and quality of life of vulnerable people. Project title: Detection of cardiovascular problems and awareness of the population regarding medical problems; SMIS code: 149707. The APC was funded by "Victor Babes" University of Medicine and Pharmacy Timisoara.

Institutional Review Board Statement: This study was conducted in accordance with the Declaration of Helsinki and approved by Ethics Committee of "Neoclinic Concept" Clinique (approval number 1/2024).

Informed Consent Statement: Informed consent was obtained from all subjects involved in this study. Written informed consent was obtained from the patients to publish this paper.

Data Availability Statement: The information is contained within this article in its entirety. For additional information, please feel free to inquire with either the original author or the corresponding author. Public access to the data is restricted as a result of the patient privacy standards that regulate the handling of clinical data.

Acknowledgments: We would like to acknowledge "Victor Babes" University of Medicine and Pharmacy Timisoara for their support in covering the costs of publication for this research paper. We express our gratitude to C.A. Dehelean and Research Center for Pharmaco-Toxicological Evaluations from 'Victor Babes' University of Medicine and Pharmacy Timisoara for their valuable support and encouragement.

Conflicts of Interest: The authors declare no conflicts of interest. The funders had no role in the design of this study; in the collection, analyses, or interpretation of data; in the writing of the manuscript; or in the decision to publish the results.

Abbreviations

CVD	cardiovascular disease
SDOHs	social determinants of health
SES	socioeconomic status
CVRFs	cardiovascular risk factors
EU	European Union
EU-SILC	European Union Statistics on Income and Living Conditions
SMD	severe material deprivation rate
IQR	interquartile range
HCA	hereditary–collateral antecedents
PPA	personal pathologic antecedents
BMI	body mass index
SBP	systolic blood pressure
DBP	diastolic blood pressure
HDL	High-Density Lipoprotein
LDLc	Low-Density Lipoprotein Cholesterol
ATP III	Adult Treatment Panel III
HbA1c	Hemoglobin A1c

References

1. Vaduganathan, M.; Mensah, G.A.; Turco, J.V.; Fuster, V.; Roth, G.A. The Global Burden of Cardiovascular Diseases and Risk: A compass for future health. *J. Am. Coll. Cardiol.* **2022**, *80*, 2361–2371. [CrossRef]
2. Chaturvedi, A.; Zhu, A.; Gadela, N.V.; Prabhakaran, D.; Jafar, T.H. Social Determinants of Health and Disparities in Hypertension and Cardiovascular Diseases. *Hypertension* **2024**, *81*, 387–399. [CrossRef] [PubMed]
3. Fu, Y.; Yu, G.; Maulana, N.; Thomson, K. Interventions to tackle health inequalities in cardiovascular risks for socioeconomically disadvantaged populations: A rapid review. *Br. Med. Bull.* **2023**, *148*, 22–41. [CrossRef] [PubMed]
4. Schultz, W.M.; Kelli, H.M.; Lisko, J.C.; Varghese, T.; Shen, J.; Sandesara, P.; Quyyumi, A.A.; Taylor, H.A.; Gulati, M.; Harold, J.G.; et al. Socioeconomic Status and Cardiovascular Outcomes. *Circulation* **2018**, *137*, 2166–2178. [CrossRef] [PubMed]
5. Over 1 in 5 at Risk of Poverty or Social Exclusion. Available online: https://ec.europa.eu/eurostat/web/products-eurostat-news/-/ddn-20220915-1 (accessed on 24 August 2024).
6. Sebastian, E. Analiză Salvați Copiii. Harta sărăciei coincide cu harta rezultatelor slabe la Evaluarea Națională. Editia de Dimineata 2023. Available online: https://editiadedimineata.ro/analiza-salvati-copiii-harta-saraciei-coincide-cu-harta-rezultatelor-slabe-la-evaluarea-nationala/ (accessed on 24 August 2024).
7. INSSE—Baze de Date Statistice—TEMPO-Online Serii de Timp. Available online: http://statistici.insse.ro/tempoins/index.jsp?page=tempo3&ind=POP105A (accessed on 24 August 2024).
8. Dorobantu, M.; Bădilă, E.; Ghiorghe, S.; O Darabont, R.; Olteanu, M.; Flondor, P. Total cardiovascular risk estimation in Romania. *Data from the SEPHAR study.* **2008**, *46*, 29–37.
9. Simionescu, M.; Bilan, S.; Gavurova, B.; Bordea, E.-N. Health Policies in Romania to Reduce the Mortality Caused by Cardiovascular Diseases. *Int. J. Environ. Res. Public Health* **2019**, *16*, 3080. [CrossRef]
10. Dumitrescu, A.; Doros, G.; Lazureanu, V.E.; Septimiu-Radu, S.; Bratosin, F.; Rosca, O.; Patel, H.; Porosnicu, T.M.; Vitcu, G.M.; Mirea, A.; et al. Post-Severe-COVID-19 Cardiopulmonary Rehabilitation: A Comprehensive Study on Patient Features and Recovery Dynamics in Correlation with Workout Intensity. *J. Clin. Med.* **2023**, *12*, 4390. [CrossRef]
11. Kang, S.Y.; Jeon, T.H.; Yum, K.-S.; Sunwoo, S.; Shin, H.-Y.; Kim, D.H.; Kim, K.; Yoon, J.L.; Choi, J.-K.; Kim, Y.S. Relationship between Dietary Habits and Control of Lipid Profiles in Patients with Dyslipidemia Using Pravastatin. *Nutrients* **2021**, *13*, 3784. [CrossRef]
12. Hahn, R.A. What is a Social Determinant of Health? Back to Basics. *J. Public Health Res.* **2021**, *10*. [CrossRef]
13. Gazibar, M.; Giuglea, L. Inequalities in Romania. World Vision Romania, 2019. Available online: https://www.sdgwatcheurope.org/wp-content/uploads/2019/06/13.1.a-factsheets-RO.pdf (accessed on 24 August 2024).

14. Fina, S.; Heider, B.; Raţ, C. Unequal Romania: Regional Socio-Economic Disparities in Romania. Foundation for European Progressive Studies. 2021. Available online: https://feps-europe.eu/wp-content/uploads/downloads/publications/210622%20unequal%20romania%20en.pdf (accessed on 24 August 2024).
15. Mitrică, B.; Şerban, P.; Mocanu, I.; Grigorescu, I.; Damian, N.; Dumitraşcu, M. Social Development and Regional Disparities in the Rural Areas of Romania: Focus on the Social Disadvantaged Areas. *Soc. Indic. Res.* **2020**, *152*, 67–89. [CrossRef]
16. Ghenciu, L.A.; Haţegan, O.A.; Bolintineanu, S.L.; Dănilă, A.-I.; Iacob, R.; Stoicescu, E.R.; Lupu, M.A.; Olariu, T.R. Human Ocular Toxoplasmosis in Romania: History, Epidemiology, and Public Health: A Narrative Review. *Microorganisms* **2024**, *12*, 1541. [CrossRef] [PubMed]
17. Hassen, H.Y.; Bowyer, M.; Gibson, L.; Abrams, S.; Bastiaens, H. Level of cardiovascular disease knowledge, risk perception and intention towards healthy lifestyle and socioeconomic disparities among adults in vulnerable communities of Belgium and England. *BMC Public Health* **2022**, *22*, 197. [CrossRef] [PubMed]
18. Glossary: At Risk of Poverty or Social Exclusion (AROPE). Available online: https://ec.europa.eu/eurostat/statistics-explained/index.php?title=Glossary:At_risk_of_poverty_or_social_exclusion_(AROPE) (accessed on 24 August 2024).
19. Mancia, G.; Kreutz, R.; Brunström, M.; Burnier, M.; Grassi, G.; Januszewicz, A.; Muiesan, M.L.; Tsioufis, K.; Agabiti-Rosei, E.; Algharably, E.A.E.; et al. 2023 ESH Guidelines for the management of arterial hypertension The Task Force for the management of arterial hypertension of the European Society of Hypertension. *J. Hypertens.* **2023**, *41*, 1874–2071. [CrossRef]
20. American Diabetes Association. 6. Glycemic Targets: Standards of Medical Care in Diabetes—2021. *Diabetes Care* **2021**, *44*, S73–S84. [CrossRef]
21. Eckel, R.H.; Cornier, M.-A. Update on the NCEP ATP-III emerging cardiometabolic risk factors. *BMC Med.* **2014**, *12*, 115. [CrossRef]
22. Expert Panel on Detection, Evaluation, and Treatment of High Blood Cholesterol in Adults. Executive Summary of The Third Report of The National Cholesterol Education Program (NCEP) Expert Panel on Detection, Evaluation, And Treatment of High Blood Cholesterol In Adults (Adult Treatment Panel III). *JAMA* **2001**, *285*, 2486–2497. [CrossRef]
23. Barnett, K.; Mercer, S.W.; Norbury, M.; Watt, G.; Wyke, S.; Guthrie, B. Epidemiology of multimorbidity and implications for health care, research, and medical education: A cross-sectional study. *Lancet* **2012**, *380*, 37–43. [CrossRef] [PubMed]
24. Kanjilal, S.; Gregg, E.W.; Cheng, Y.J.; Zhang, P.; Nelson, D.E.; Mensah, G.; Beckles, G.L.A. Socioeconomic Status and Trends in Disparities in 4 Major Risk Factors for Cardiovascular Disease Among US Adults, 1971–2002. *Arch. Intern. Med.* **2006**, *166*, 2348–2355. [CrossRef]
25. Murray, C.J.L.; Vos, T.; Lozano, R.; Naghavi, M.; Flaxman, A.D.; Michaud, C.; Ezzati, M.; Shibuya, K.; Salomon, J.A.; Abdalla, S.; et al. Disability-adjusted life years (DALYs) for 291 diseases and injuries in 21 regions, 1990–2010: A systematic analysis for the Global Burden of Disease Study 2010. *Lancet* **2012**, *380*, 2197–2223. [CrossRef]
26. Diez Roux, A.V.; Mair, C. Neighborhoods and health. *Ann. N. Y. Acad. Sci.* **2010**, *1186*, 125–145. [CrossRef]
27. Diez Roux, A.V.; Merkin, S.S.; Arnett, D.K.; Chambless, L.; Massing, M.; Nieto, F.J.; Sorlie, P.; Szklo, M.; Tyroler, H.A.; Watson, R.L. Neighborhood of Residence and Incidence of Coronary Heart Disease. *N. Engl. J. Med.* **2001**, *345*, 99–106. [CrossRef] [PubMed]
28. Clark, S.; Lomax, N.; Birkin, M.; Morris, M. A foresight whole systems obesity classification for the English UK biobank cohort. *BMC Public Health* **2022**, *22*, 349. [CrossRef]
29. Zapata, J.K.; Azcona-Sanjulian, M.C.; Catalán, V.; Ramírez, B.; Silva, C.; Rodríguez, A.; Escalada, J.; Frühbeck, G.; Gómez-Ambrosi, J. BMI-based obesity classification misses children and adolescents with raised cardiometabolic risk due to increased adiposity. *Cardiovasc. Diabetol.* **2023**, *22*, 240. [CrossRef] [PubMed]
30. Ong, K.L.; Stafford, L.K.; McLaughlin, S.A.; Boyko, E.J.; Vollset, S.E.; Smith, A.E.; Dalton, B.E.; Duprey, J.; Cruz, J.A.; Hagins, H.; et al. Global, regional, and national burden of diabetes from 1990 to 2021, with projections of prevalence to 2050: A systematic analysis for the Global Burden of Disease Study 2021. *Lancet* **2023**, *402*, 203–234. [CrossRef] [PubMed]
31. Liu, J.; Ren, Z.-H.; Qiang, H.; Wu, J.; Shen, M.; Zhang, L.; Lyu, J. Trends in the incidence of diabetes mellitus: Results from the Global Burden of Disease Study 2017 and implications for diabetes mellitus prevention. *BMC Public Health* **2020**, *20*, 1415. [CrossRef]
32. Ramezankhani, A.; Habibi-Moeini, A.S.; Zadeh, S.S.T.; Azizi, F.; Hadaegh, F. Effect of family history of diabetes and obesity status on lifetime risk of type 2 diabetes in the Iranian population. *J. Glob. Health* **2022**, *12*, 04068. [CrossRef]
33. Loos, R.J.F.; Yeo, G.S.H. The genetics of obesity: From discovery to biology. *Nat. Rev. Genet.* **2022**, *23*, 120–133. [CrossRef]
34. Mahmoud, R.; Kimonis, V.; Butler, M.G. Genetics of Obesity in Humans: A Clinical Review. *Int. J. Mol. Sci.* **2022**, *23*, 11005. [CrossRef]
35. Rogobete, A.F.; Bedreag, O.H.; Popovici, S.E.; Sas, A.M.; Stan, A.T.; Stoicescu, E.R.; Sandesc, D. Detection of Myocardial Injury Using miRNAs Expression as Genetic Biomarkers in Acute Cardiac Care. *J. Cardiovasc. Emergencies* **2016**, *2*, 169–172. [CrossRef]
36. Held, C.; Hadziosmanovic, N.; Aylward, P.E.; Hagström, E.; Hochman, J.S.; Stewart, R.A.H.; White, H.D.; Wallentin, L. Body Mass Index and Association With Cardiovascular Outcomes in Patients With Stable Coronary Heart Disease—A STABILITY Substudy. *J. Am. Heart Assoc.* **2022**, *11*, e023667. [CrossRef]
37. Peters, S.A.E.; Huxley, R.R.; Woodward, M. Diabetes as risk factor for incident coronary heart disease in women compared with men: A systematic review and meta-analysis of 64 cohorts including 858,507 individuals and 28,203 coronary events. *Diabetologia* **2014**, *57*, 1542–1551. [CrossRef] [PubMed]
38. Flor, L.S.; Reitsma, M.B.; Gupta, V.; Ng, M.; Gakidou, E. The effects of tobacco control policies on global smoking prevalence. *Nat. Med.* **2021**, *27*, 239–243. [CrossRef] [PubMed]
39. Keeler, C.; Max, W.; Yao, T.; Wang, Y.; Zhang, X.; Sung, H.-Y. Smoking Behavior in Low- and High-Income Adults Immediately Following California Proposition 56 Tobacco Tax Increase. *Am. J. Public Health* **2020**, *110*, 868–870. [CrossRef]

40. Meza, R.; Cao, P.; Jeon, J.; Warner, K.E.; Levy, D.T. Trends in US Adult Smoking Prevalence, 2011 to 2022. *JAMA Health Forum* **2023**, *4*, e234213. [CrossRef] [PubMed]
41. Chao, A.M.; Wadden, T.A.; Ashare, R.L.; Loughead, J.; Schmidt, H.D. Tobacco Smoking, Eating Behaviors, and Body Weight: A Review. *Curr. Addict. Rep.* **2019**, *6*, 191–199. [CrossRef]
42. E Taylor, A.; Richmond, R.C.; Palviainen, T.; Loukola, A.; E Wootton, R.; Kaprio, J.; Relton, C.L.; Smith, G.D.; Munafò, M.R. The effect of body mass index on smoking behaviour and nicotine metabolism: A Mendelian randomization study. *Hum. Mol. Genet.* **2018**, *28*, 1322–1330. [CrossRef]
43. Dorobantu, M.; Darabont, R.O.; Badila, E.; Ghiorghe, S. Prevalence, Awareness, Treatment, and Control of Hypertension in Romania: Results of the SEPHAR Study. *Int. J. Hypertens.* **2010**, *2010*, 970694. [CrossRef]
44. Dorobantu, M.; Tautu, O.-F.; Dimulescu, D.; Sinescu, C.; Gusbeth-Tatomir, P.; Arsenescu-Georgescu, C.; Mitu, F.; Lighezan, D.; Pop, C.; Babes, K.; et al. Perspectives on hypertension's prevalence, treatment and control in a high cardiovascular risk East European country. *J. Hypertens.* **2018**, *36*, 690–700. [CrossRef]
45. Veisani, Y.; Jenabi, E.; Nematollahi, S.; Delpisheh, A.; Khazaei, S. The role of socio-economic inequality in the prevalence of hypertension in adults. *J. Cardiovasc. Thorac. Res.* **2019**, *11*, 116–120. [CrossRef]
46. Mota, M.; Popa, S.G.; Mota, E.; Mitrea, A.; Catrinoiu, D.; Cheta, D.M.; Guja, C.; Hancu, N.; Ionescu-Tirgoviste, C.; Lichiardopol, R.; et al. Prevalence of diabetes mellitus and prediabetes in the adult Romanian population: PREDATORR study. *J. Diabetes* **2015**, *8*, 336–344. [CrossRef]
47. Rosu, L.M.; Prodan-Bărbulescu, C.; Maghiari, A.L.; Bernad, E.S.; Bernad, R.L.; Iacob, R.; Stoicescu, E.R.; Borozan, F.; Ghenciu, L.A. Current Trends in Diagnosis and Treatment Approach of Diabetic Retinopathy during Pregnancy: A Narrative Review. *Diagnostics* **2024**, *14*, 369. [CrossRef] [PubMed]
48. Dănilă, A.-I.; Ghenciu, L.A.; Stoicescu, E.R.; Bolintineanu, S.L.; Iacob, R.; Săndesc, M.-A.; Faur, A.C. Aldose Reductase as a Key Target in the Prevention and Treatment of Diabetic Retinopathy: A Comprehensive Review. *Biomedicines* **2024**, *12*, 747. [CrossRef] [PubMed]
49. Ghenciu, L.A.; Hațegan, O.A.; Bolintineanu, S.L.; Dănilă, A.-I.; Faur, A.C.; Prodan-Bărbulescu, C.; Stoicescu, E.R.; Iacob, R.; Șișu, A.M. Immune-Mediated Ocular Surface Disease in Diabetes Mellitus—Clinical Perspectives and Treatment: A Narrative Review. *Biomedicines* **2024**, *12*, 1303. [CrossRef]
50. Rygiel, K. Hypertriglyceridemia—Common Causes, Prevention and treatment Strategies. *Curr. Cardiol. Rev.* **2018**, *14*, 67–76. [CrossRef] [PubMed]
51. Sirdah, M.M.; Reading, N.S. Genetic predisposition in type 2 diabetes: A promising approach toward a personalized management of diabetes. *Clin. Genet.* **2020**, *98*, 525–547. [CrossRef]
52. Wang, K.; Kavousi, M.; Voortman, T.; Ikram, M.A.; Ghanbari, M.; Ahmadizar, F. Cardiovascular health, genetic predisposition, and lifetime risk of type 2 diabetes. *Eur. J. Prev. Cardiol.* **2021**, *28*, 1850–1857. [CrossRef]
53. Wondmkun, Y.T. Obesity, Insulin Resistance, and Type 2 Diabetes: Associations and Therapeutic Implications. *Diabetes Metab. Syndr. Obes. Targets Ther.* **2020**, *ume 13*, 3611–3616. [CrossRef]
54. Mahmood, S.S.; Levy, D.; Vasan, R.S.; Wang, T.J. The Framingham Heart Study and the epidemiology of cardiovascular disease: A historical perspective. *Lancet* **2014**, *383*, 999–1008. [CrossRef]
55. Tsao, C.W.; Vasan, R.S. Cohort Profile: The Framingham Heart Study (FHS): Overview of milestones in cardiovascular epidemiology. *Leuk. Res.* **2015**, *44*, 1800–1813. [CrossRef]
56. Macleod, J.; Smith, G.D.; Metcalfe, C.; Hart, C. INTERHEART. *Lancet* **2005**, *365*, 118–119. [CrossRef]
57. Yusuf, S.; Hawken, S.; Ôunpuu, S.; Dans, T.; Avezum, A.; Lanas, F.; McQueen, M.; Budaj, A.; Pais, P.; Varigos, J.; et al. Effect of potentially modifiable risk factors associated with myocardial infarction in 52 countries (the INTERHEART study): Case-control study. *Lancet* **2004**, *364*, 937–952. [CrossRef]
58. Rosu, M. Cardiovascular Risk Assessment in the Adult (Aged 40–79 Years) Romanian Population. *Acta Endocrinol. (Buchar.)* **2018**, *14*, 227–234. [CrossRef]
59. Weiss, E.; Japie, C.; Balahura, A.M.; Bartos, D.; Badila, E. Cardiovascular risk factors in a Roma sample population from Romania. *Rom. J. Intern. Med.* **2018**, *56*, 193–202. [CrossRef]
60. Cinteza, M.; Pana, B.; Cochino, E.; Florescu, M.; Margulescu, A.; Florian, A.; Vinereanu, D.; Iliescu, C. Prevalence and Control of Cardiovascular Risk Factors in Romania Cardio-Zone National Study. *Maedica.* **2007**, *2*, 278–288. Available online: https://www.maedica.ro/articles/2007/2007_Vol2(5)_No4/2007_Vol2(5)_No4_pg277-288.pdf (accessed on 24 August 2024).
61. Lindley, K.J.; Aggarwal, N.R.; Briller, J.E.; Davis, M.B.; Douglass, P.; Epps, K.C.; Fleg, J.L.; Hayes, S.; Itchhaporia, D.; Mahmoud, Z.; et al. Socioeconomic Determinants of Health and Cardiovascular Outcomes in Women: *JACC* Review Topic of the Week. *J. Am. Coll. Cardiol.* **2021**, *78*, 1919–1929. [CrossRef] [PubMed]
62. Ghenciu, L.A.; Hațegan, O.A.; Stoicescu, E.R.; Iacob, R.; Șișu, A.M. Emerging Therapeutic Approaches and Genetic Insights in Stargardt Disease: A Comprehensive Review. *Int. J. Mol. Sci.* **2024**, *25*, 8859. [CrossRef] [PubMed]
63. Graves, B.A. Focused Community-based Research for Eliminating CVD Risk Disparities in a Rural Underserved Population. *Online J. Rural. Nurs. Health Care* **2012**, *12*, 67–77. [CrossRef]
64. Hwang, W.J.; Kang, S.J. Interventions to Reduce the Risk of Cardiovascular Disease among Workers: A Systematic Review and Meta-Analysis. *Int. J. Environ. Res. Public Health* **2020**, *17*, 2267. [CrossRef]

65. Ndejjo, R.; Hassen, H.Y.; Wanyenze, R.K.; Musoke, D.; Nuwaha, F.; Abrams, S.; Bastiaens, H.; Musinguzi, G. Community-Based Interventions for Cardiovascular Disease Prevention in Low-and Middle-Income Countries: A Systematic Review. *Public Health Rev.* **2021**, *42*. [CrossRef]
66. Cruz-Ramos, N.A.; Alor-Hernández, G.; Colombo-Mendoza, L.O.; Sánchez-Cervantes, J.L.; Rodríguez-Mazahua, L.; Guarneros-Nolasco, L.R. mHealth Apps for Self-Management of Cardiovascular Diseases: A Scoping Review. *Healthcare* **2022**, *10*, 322. [CrossRef]
67. Wellmann, N.; Marc, M.S.; Stoicescu, E.R.; Pescaru, C.C.; Trusculescu, A.A.; Martis, F.G.; Ciortea, I.; Crisan, A.F.; Balica, M.A.; Velescu, D.R.; et al. Enhancing Adult Asthma Management: A Review on the Utility of Remote Home Spirometry and Mobile Applications. *J. Pers. Med.* **2024**, *14*, 852. [CrossRef] [PubMed]
68. Haynes, N.; Kaur, A.; Swain, J.; Joseph, J.J.; Brewer, L.C. Community-Based Participatory Research to Improve Cardiovascular Health Among US Racial and Ethnic Minority Groups. *Curr. Epidemiol. Rep.* **2022**, *9*, 212–221. [CrossRef] [PubMed]

biomedicines

MDPI

Article

Clinical and Metabolic Particularities of a Roma Population with Diabetes—Considering Ethnic Disparities in Approaching Healthcare Management

Andrada Cosoreanu [1], Emilia Rusu [1,*], Florin Rusu [2], Silviu Stanciu [2], Ioana Ungureanu [3], Marius Donici [3], Alexandra Visinescu [1], Georgiana Enache [4] and Gabriela Radulian [1]

1 Department of Diabetes, Nutrition and Metabolic Diseases, "Carol Davila" University of Medicine and Pharmacy, 050474 Bucharest, Romania; andrada.cosoreanu@drd.umfcd.ro (A.C.); alexandra-mihaela.visinescu@drd.umfcd.ro (A.V.); gabriela.radulian@umfcd.ro (G.R.)

2 "Doctor Carol Davila" Central Military University Emergency Hospital, 010825 Bucharest, Romania; florinrusumd@yahoo.com (F.R.); silviu.stanciu@umfcd.ro (S.S.)

3 "Nicolae Malaxa" Clinica Hospital, 022441 Bucharest, Romania; ioana.ungureanu97@yahoo.com (I.U.); mdonici@yahoo.com (M.D.)

4 "Pompei Samarian" Emergency Hospital, 910071 Calarasi, Romania; georgianamd@yahoo.com

* Correspondence: emilia.rusu@umfcd.ro; Tel.: +40-742959946

Abstract: The Roma population is Europe's largest ethnic minority, yet data on the prevalence of non-communicable diseases remain scarce in medical literature. This study aimed to compare the clinical and metabolic particularities of a Roma population with diabetes with a group of non-Roma. We conducted an observational, transversal study and evaluated 808 adult patients with diabetes mellitus, from a tertiary diabetes care hospital. The prevalence of metabolic syndrome was high among both groups, 94.3% in the Roma patients and 89.1% in the non-Roma. A slightly higher mean value of the triglyceride–glucose (TyG) index was observed among the Roma group (10.07 ± 0.71 versus 9.71 ± 0.82). Among the non-Roma, variables that were significantly associated with the TyG index were glycated hemoglobin (HbA1c), total cholesterol (TC), high density lipoprotein–cholesterol (HDL-c), and low-density lipoprotein-cholesterol (LDL-c), while among the Roma, HbA1c and HDL-c were correlated with this index. There were no differences concerning myocardial infarction; however, the number of patients with a history of stroke was 2.1 times higher in the Roma group compared to the non-Roma group. The prevalence of cardiovascular risk factors, cardiovascular disease, and microvascular complications among the study's Roma population are quite significant, underscoring the importance of ethnic disparities in approaching healthcare management strategies.

Keywords: clinical characteristics; metabolic particularities; anthropometric assessment; Roma population

1. Introduction

The Roma population constitutes one of the largest ethnic minorities in Europe, estimated at 10–12 million. In countries with significant Roma populations (Southern, Central, and Eastern Europe), collecting statistical data on health and its determinants based on ethnic status remains challenging [1].

While the connection between extremely adverse socio-economic conditions and the poor health status among Roma is quite clear, the discrepancies noted in comparisons between the Roma population and the general population do not seem to be entirely explained by their inferior socio-economic status. Recent research into the genetic basis of the high risk of various non-communicable diseases among Roma additionally supports the fact that their health status is influenced by a mix of different health-related factors [1].

Studies have highlighted the elevated prevalence of both communicable and non-communicable diseases among the Roma population. Their health and living standards in Central and Eastern Europe are reported to be lower compared to the general population. Studies suggest a higher incidence of diseases like diabetes, coronary heart disease, and obesity within this minority group. Social determinants such as poverty, limited healthcare access, inadequate nutrition, and cultural traditions play significant roles in these disparities. Additionally, due to frequent consanguineous marriages within the Roma community, there is a heightened risk of genetically inherited illnesses emerging among them [1,2]. Therefore, research also indicates a reduced life expectancy among Roma compared to the majority population, their population pyramid typically showing a higher proportion of younger individuals and a lower concentration of elderly individuals, suggesting a predominantly progressive demographic trend [3].

Moreover, an important marker in understanding metabolic health disparities is the triglyceride–glucose (TyG) index, which correlates with an increased risk of developing metabolic syndrome, insulin resistance, and cardiovascular events. The TyG index has proven to be an useful marker for early identification of and intervention in metabolic health issues [4].

For many years, the Roma population has been notably overlooked in health policy and research, with only recent developments beginning to address this issue. In response to emerging data concerning the health disparities faced by the Roma, the European Commission and other international entities have advocated the necessity of measures to narrow the health gap between the Roma and the broader population [1].

Therefore, the aim of this study was to compare the clinical and metabolic profiles of Roma and non-Roma patients with diabetes in a tertiary care center in Bucharest, Romania. Specifically, we assessed the prevalence of metabolic syndrome, obesity, hypertension, dyslipidemia, cardiovascular disease, and health-related behaviors (smoking and alcohol consumption), along with anthropometric and paraclinical measurements in both groups.

2. Materials and Methods

2.1. Study Design and Setting

We conducted an observational, transversal study in October 2022 and March 2024. We evaluated 808 adult patients with diabetes mellitus, aged between 18 and 89 years old who were attending a tertiary hospital providing diabetes care, "Nicolae Malaxa" Clinical Hospital in Bucharest, Romania. The study was accomplished following the Strengthening the Reporting of Observational Studies in Epidemiology (STROBE) guidelines for observational studies [5]. All data were collected in adherence to the hospital's standard protocols for managing patients with diabetes. The study was approved by the Ethics Committee for Clinical Studies of the "Nicolae Malaxa" Clinical Hospital, with the approval number 75/2022. All participants involved in the study granted their informed consent for the collection of data and the subsequent utilization of medical information for research objectives.

2.2. Study Population

The study consisted of adult patients diagnosed with type 1 (T1DM) or type 2 diabetes mellitus (T2DM) who underwent consultations at the hospital's inpatient department throughout the study's duration, agreed to participate, and signed an informed consent form. On the contrary, an age lower than 18 years, the absence of diabetes, pregnancy, and rejection of signing the informed consent form represented exclusion criteria.

2.3. Data Collection

The data were obtained from the medical records of the patients hospitalized during the study period. Data collection was comprehensive and included multiple aspects of the patients' medical and personal history, including family history of diabetes, duration of diabetes, personal medical history of obesity, hypertension, heart failure, myocardial infarction, stable angina, stroke, hepatic steatosis, dyslipidemia, metabolic syndrome, lower limb amputations, history of behaviors related to health (smoking and alcohol consumption), presence of microvascular diabetes-related complications (chronic kidney disease, peripheral neuropathy, orthostatic hypotension, retinopathy), socio-economic and demographic factors (age, gender, place of residence), clinical measurements (anthropometric indicators), and paraclinical assessment.

The places of residence were sorted according to urban and rural areas.

Regarding the health-related behaviors, for smoking assessment, patients were classified as smokers (active or former smokers) and non-smokers, depending on their self-evaluation responses, while for alcohol consumption evaluation, based on the participants' self-assessment of their drinking habits, they were categorized as drinkers or non-drinkers.

2.4. Clinical Measurements

The following anthropometric indicators were assessed for each participant, including height (cm), weight (kg), waist circumference (cm), hip circumference (cm), and body mass index (kg/m^2). WC and HC were determined using a measuring tape, following the standard procedures.

2.5. Paraclinical Assessment

The laboratory parameters analyzed were fasting plasmatic glycemia (FPG), glycated hemoglobin (HbA1c) level, serum creatinine, estimated glomerular filtration rate (eGFR), urinary albumin to creatinine ratio (UACR), uric acid, serum urea, aspartate aminotransferase (AST), alanine aminotransferase (ALT), gamma-glutamyl transferase (GGT), total cholesterol (TC), high-density lipoprotein–cholesterol (HDL-c), low-density lipoprotein–cholesterol (LDL-c), triglycerides (TG), and triglyceride–glucose (TyG) index, a surrogate indicator for the evaluation of insulin resistance.

HbA1c level was determined using the validated high-performance liquid chromatography (HPLC) method [6]; the device used to determine it was produced by BIO-RAD. The batch number for HbA1c was 64573120. The other parameters were determined using spectrophotometry [7] incorporated into Mindray devices. The batch number for biochemistry was 2023071301.

eGFR was assessed using the 2021 Chronic Kidney Disease Epidemiology Collaboration (CKD-EPI) formula [8].

UACR was obtained using spot urine samples, calculated by dividing the total urinary albumin value in milligrams by the creatinine concentration in grams.

LDL-c levels were derived either through calculation using a formula—TC minus HDL-c minus TG/5—if TG levels were below 400 mg/dL, or through direct laboratory measurement if TG levels exceeded 400 mg/dL [9].

TyG was calculated using the following formula: ln [TG (mg/dL) × FPG (mg/dL)/2] [10]. While there are no universally established cutoff values for the TyG index, according to various research studies, we divided it into quartiles by the 25th, the 50th, and the 75th percentiles and treated categorized variables as follows: quartile 1: $\leq$9.36, quartile 2: 9.37–9.91, quartile 3: 9.92–10.45, and quartile 4: $\geq$10.46.

2.6. Definitions

Diabetes mellitus was defined according to the ADA (American Diabetes Association) guideline criteria [11].

Resting blood pressure was measured using the auscultatory method with the patient in a seated position. Hypertension was characterized by systolic blood pressure (SBP) exceeding 140 mmHg and diastolic blood pressure (DBP) surpassing 90 mmHg, according to the AHA (American Heart Association) guidelines [12], as well as current use of blood pressure-lowering medication or a documented medical history of physician-diagnosed hypertension.

To classify the nutritional status according to BMI (body mass index), we used the definition of the World Health Organization (WHO): underweight was defined by a BMI < 18.5 kg/ m^2, normal weight by a BMI between 18.5 and 24.9 kg/m^2, overweight as a BMI between 25 and 29.9 kg m^2, and obesity by a BMI over 30 kg/m^2 [13].

The diagnosis of hepatic steatosis was made either through imaging techniques, such as an abdominal ultrasound performed during the hospitalization, or a medically recorded history of it.

Dyslipidemia was diagnosed by laboratory tests of the lipid profile according to present guidelines or current use of lipid-lowering medication [9].

Metabolic syndrome was diagnosed using the harmonized definition, with any three of the following criteria: waist circumference >94 cm for males and >80 cm for females, a raised level of triglycerides (TG) $\geq$ 150 mg/dL, or specific treatment for this lipid abnormality; a reduced level of high-density lipoprotein cholesterol (HDL-c) < 40 mg/dL in men, <50 mg/dL in women, or specific treatment for this lipid abnormality; increased blood pressure, systolic $\geq$ 130 or diastolic $\geq$ 85 mmHg, or treatment of previously diagnosed hypertension; and previously diagnosed type 2 diabetes mellitus [14].

The diagnosis of chronic kidney disease was established based on the Kidney Disease Improving Global Outcomes (KDIGO) criteria using the estimated glomerular filtration rate and albuminuria [15].

Eye fundus examination, part of the ophthalmological evaluation, was employed to evaluate diabetic retinopathy following the protocol outlined in The Early Treatment for Diabetic Retinopathy Study [16].

The ankle–brachial index test was conducted to evaluate peripheral arterial disease; the test outcome was determined by the ankle-to-brachial blood pressure ratio, and a value below 0.9 was indicative of the diagnosis [11].

2.7. Study Outcome

The primary endpoint was to assess the clinical and metabolic particularities of a sample Roma population in comparison with a corresponding group of non-Roma patients.

2.8. Statistical Analysis

The IBM SPSS 19th version was used for performing the statistical analysis. The normally distributed continuous variables were presented as mean $\pm$ SD (standard deviation) and non-normal variables were reported as median $\pm$ IQR (interquartile range), while the categorical variables were presented as absolute counts and percentages. Normality tests which were employed included the Kolmogorov–Smirnov test with a Lilliefors correction for significance and the Shapiro–Wilk statistic [17,18]. For quantitative variables, analysis of variance (ANOVA) was used for comparisons among groups, while for categorical variables, the χ^2 test was used. For non-normally distributed variables, we applied the Kruskal–Wallis test. Linear regression analysis was performed to identify factors associated with the TyG index. Statistical significance was set at a 95% confidence interval.

3. Results

3.1. General Characteristics of the Patients

The general characteristics of the patients are summarized in Table 1. The study included 458 Roma patients and 350 Caucasian participants, of which the majority were men (54.6% and 51.5%, respectively). In both groups, most of the patients included had T2DM, reaching 95.1% the Caucasian group and 87.8% among the Roma patients. However, more Roma patients had T1DM (12.2% versus 4.9%). More than half of the participants from both groups did not have a family history of diabetes.

Regarding the place of residence, irrespective of their ethnicity, most of the patients lived in urban areas (65.1% of the Caucasian patients and 52.2% of the Roma patients).

Table 1. General characteristics of the patients.

Variables		Non-Roma Patients (n = 350)	Roma Patients (n = 458)	p-Value
Gender	Men	54.6% (n = 191)	51.5% (n = 236)	0.391
	Women	45.4% (n = 159)	48.5% (n = 222)	
Place of residence	Urban area	65.1% (n = 228)	52.2% (n = 239)	0.0001
	Rural area	34.9% (n = 122)	47.8% (n = 219)	
Type of diabetes	T1DM	4.9% (n = 17)	12.2% (n = 56)	0.0001
	T2DM	95.1% (n = 333)	87.8% (n = 402)	
Family history of diabetes	Yes	47.1% (n = 165)	45.4% (n = 208)	0.625
Smoking (former or active smokers)	Yes	26.3% (n = 92)	50.4% (n = 231)	0.0001
Alcohol consumption	Yes	25.1% (n = 88)	26.9% (n = 123)	0.583

A large proportion of Caucasian patients were non-smokers (73.7%) compared to the corresponding group, where the majority of the Roma were smokers (both former or active smokers, 50.4%). Alcohol consumption accounted for 26.9% in the Roma group, while in the Caucasian group, slightly fewer patients (25.1%) were alcohol users (Table 1).

3.2. *Prevalence of Comorbidities*

Regarding the associated diseases, a significant percentage of the Caucasian patients had hypertension (81.1%), approximately 15% more than in the Roma group (67.7%). There were slight differences regarding dyslipidemia, with 78.5% among the non-Roma and 76.7% among the Roma. Apart from this, a predominance of obesity was noticed, with more than half of the patients in both groups categorized as obese (62.2% in the Roma group and 50.3% in the Caucasian group). The prevalence of metabolic syndrome was significantly high among both groups, reaching 94.3% in the Roma patients and 89.1% in the non-Roma (p = 0.008) (Figure 1). Hepatic steatosis was present in 55.3% of the Caucasian participants and 48.5% in the Roma subjects (Figure 1).

Analyzing the prevalence of cardiovascular disease, there were no differences concerning personal history of myocardial infarction, which approximately 12% of the patients from each group had; however, the number of patients with a history of stroke was 2.1 times higher in the Roma group compared to non-Roma participants (42 versus 20 patients, p = 0.067). The prevalence of stable angina and heart failure was significantly lower in the Caucasian group (p = 0.0001). Peripheral artery disease was significantly more frequent in the Caucasian group compared to the Roma (21.7% versus 9.6%). A modest percentage of patients suffered from lower limb amputations, with no differences observed between the two groups (Figure 1).

Detailed data regarding the number of patients with these associated diseases are provided in Supplementary Table S1.

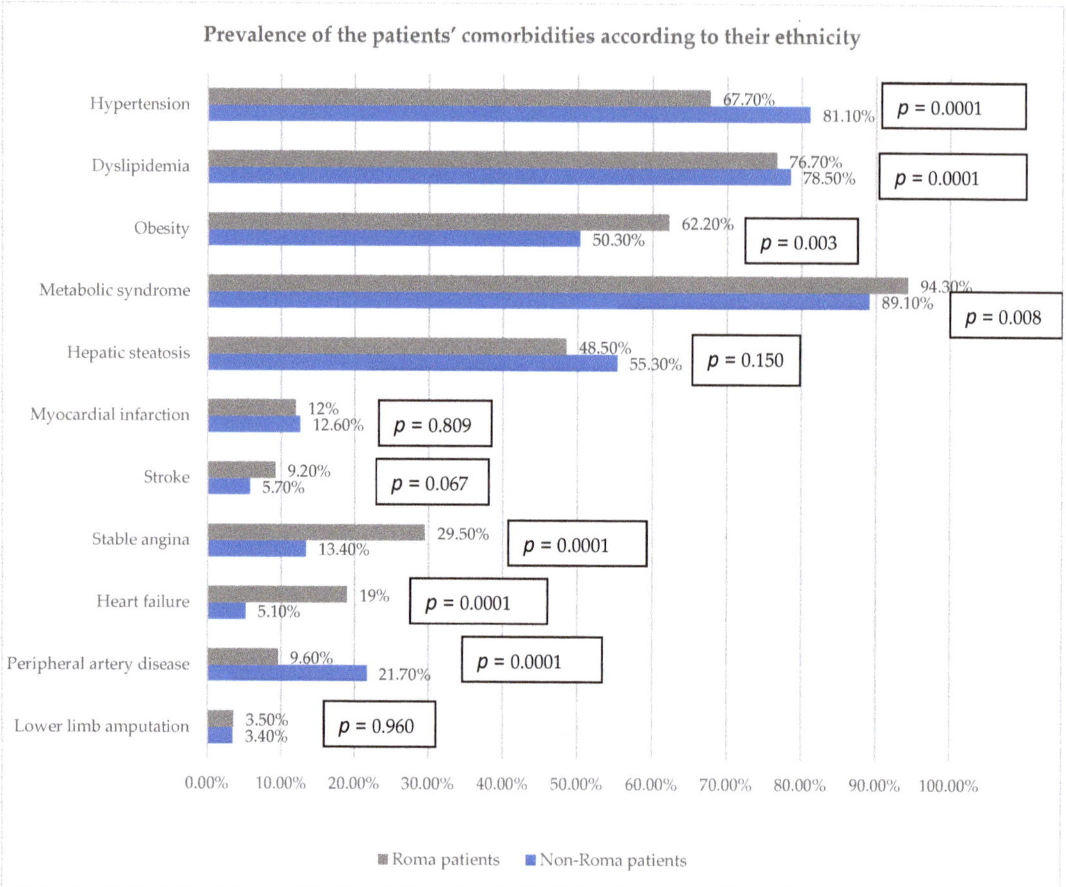

Figure 1. Prevalence of the patients' comorbidities according to their ethnicity.

3.3. *Prevalence of Diabetic Complications*

The most prevalent microvascular complication was peripheral polyneuropathy, exceeding 70% in both groups (Figure 2). In the Roma population, chronic kidney disease was present in 22.1% of the patients, while in the Caucasian group, nearly 35% were associated with this complication. Apart from this, almost a third of the participants from both groups were associated with diabetic retinopathy, a slightly higher percentage being observed among the Caucasian patients (38.3% versus 33.25%). Orthostatic hypotension was more prevalent in the Roma population compared to the corresponding group, accounting for 14.6% (Figure 2).

Comprehensive information on the number of patients with these associated conditions can be found in Supplementary Table S2.

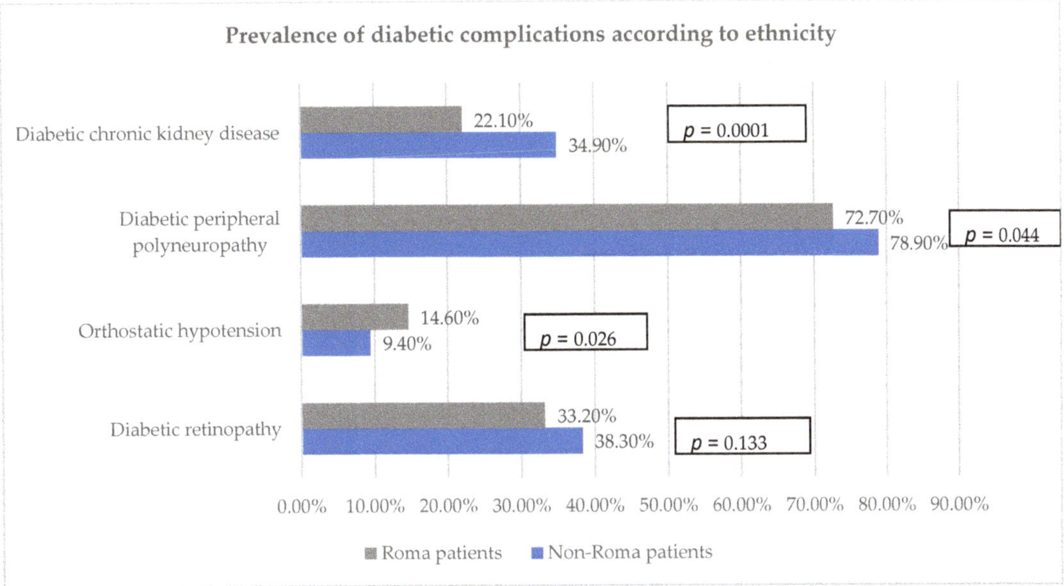

Figure 2. Prevalence of diabetic complications according to ethnicity.

3.4. Clinical and Paraclinical Assessments

Comparing the Roma population with the Caucasian group, the mean age was lower in the Roma group (55.62 ± 11.55 versus 62.06 ± 10.6 years); moreover, the median duration of diabetes was significantly lower (6.00 versus 11.00 years, p-value = 0.0001) (Table 2).

Analyzing the anthropometric measurements, the average height of the Caucasian patients was slightly higher compared to the opposite group (166.83 ± 9.68 cm versus 164.54 ± 9.27 cm), but the average weight, waist circumference, and hip circumference, however, were higher among the Roma patients (87.51 ± 20.12 kg versus 84.81 ± 17.82 kg, 110 ± 15.87 cm versus 103.73 ± 14.70 cm, and 108.61 ± 14.40 cm versus 104.82 ± 14.02 cm, respectively). Concerning the mean BMI, the same trend was observed (32.28 ± 7.03 kg/m^2 versus 30.41 ± 5.06 kg/m^2).

Regarding the paraclinical assessments, the Roma patients had a slightly higher mean HbA1c level compared to the non-Roma group (9.91 ± 2.45% versus 9.07 ± 2.09%); apart from this, the mean values of the lipid profile were also significantly higher in this ethnic group, with the exception of the mean value of HDL-c, which was higher among the Caucasian patients. Concerning the insulin resistance measured by the TyG index, a slightly higher mean value was observed among the Roma group (10.07 ± 0.71 versus 9.71 ± 0.82). The mean values of the renal profile parameters (creatinine level and uric acid level, respectively) were higher among the Roma patients, but there were no differences regarding the mean urea level. However, the median value of the eGFR level was lower among the Roma patients (80.00 ± 41.00 mL/min/1.73 m^2 versus 83.00 ± 45.00 mL/min/1.73 m^2), but the median value of the urinary albumin to creatinine ratio was quite similar (25.00 ± 31.28 mg/g versus 25.13 ± 104.27 mg/g, respectively). The mean values of the hepatic enzymes were higher among the Roma population compared to the corresponding group (Table 2).

The differences between patients with T1DM and T2DM cand be found in Supplementary Table S3.

Table 2. Mean values of the analyzed parameters according to ethnicity.

Parameters	Non-Roma Patients (n = 350)	Roma Patients (n = 458)	Total (n = 808)	p-Value
	Mean ± SD	Mean ± SD	Mean ± SD	
Age (years)	62.06 ± 10.6	55.62 ± 11.55	58.41 ± 11.59	0.0001
Duration of diabetes (years)	11.00 ± 8.18 *	6.00 ± 6.89 *	9.00 ± 7.77 *	0.0001
Height (cm)	166.83 ± 9.68	164.54 ± 9.27	165.67 ± 9.54	0.001
Weight (kg)	84.81 ± 17.82	87.51 ± 20.12	86.19 ± 19.06	0.059
WC (cm)	103.73 ± 14.70	110.00 ± 15.87	107.08 ± 15.64	0.0001
HC (cm)	104.82 ± 14.02	108.61 ± 14.40	107.20 ± 14.36	0.011
BMI (kg/m^2)	30.41 ± 5.60	32.28 ± 7.03	31.36 ± 6.43	0.0001
HbA1c (%)	9.07 ± 2.09	9.91 ± 2.45	9.53 ± 2.33	0.0001
FPG (mg/dL)	226.35 ± 87.96	232.00 ± 117.42 *	243.59 ± 106.46	0.0001
TC (mg/dL)	192.66 ± 65.29	217.12 ± 63.41	205.67 ± 65.40	0.0001
HDL-c (mg/dL)	49.40 ± 14.09	45.57 ± 9.91	47.38 ± 12.20	0.0001
TG (mg/dL)	192.06 ± 138.62	234.39 ± 123.45	214.54 ± 132.39	0.0001
LDL-c (mg/dL)	103.64 ± 48.67	123.11 ± 52.59	113.79 ± 51.64	0.0001
TyG index	9.71 ± 0.82	10.07 ± 0.71	9.90 ± 0.78	0.36
Creatinine (mg/dL)	0.96 ± 0.37	1.04 ± 0.43	1.00 ± 0.40	0.010
eGFR (mL/min/1.73 m^2)	83.00 ± 45.00 *	80.00 ± 41.00 *	83.00 ± 41.00 *	0.255
Urea (mg/dL)	44.56 ± 20.08	44.34 ± 18.49	44.43 ± 19.16	0.904
Uric acid (mg/dL)	5.99 ± 1.98	6.16 ± 2.36	6.06 ± 2.15	0.578
UACR (mg/g)	25.13 ± 104.27 *	25.00 ± 31.28 *	24.14 ± 65.7 *	0.003
AST (UI/L)	20.00 ± 22.66 *	23.00 ± 25.88 *	22.00 ± 13.18 *	0.086
ALT (UI/L)	24.00 ± 27.31 *	29.00 ± 28.75 *	27.00 ± 23.00 *	0.002
GGT (UI/L)	33.35 ± 102.97 *	44.00 ± 47.58 *	42.00 ± 38.00 *	0.081

Abbreviations: WC (cm)—waist circumference, HC (cm)—hip circumference, BMI (kg/m^2)—body mass index, HbA1c (%)—glycated hemoglobin, FPG (mg/dL)—fasting plasmatic glycemia, TC (mg/dL)—total cholesterol, HDL-c (mg/dL)—high-density lipoprotein–cholesterol, LDL-c (mg/dL)—low-density lipoprotein–cholesterol, TG (mg/dL)—triglycerides, TyG index—triglyceride–glucose index, eGFR (mL/min/1.73 m^2)—estimated glomerular filtration rate, UACR (mg/g)—urinary albumin to creatinine ratio, AST (UI/L)—aspartate aminotransferase, ALT (UI/L)—alanine aminotransferase, GGT (UI/L)—gamma-glutamyl transferase. The data are represented as mean ± SD (standard deviation) and median ± IQR (marked with "*", IQR—interquartile range). The statistical significance was considered at a p-value < 0.05.

3.5. Evaluation of the Insulin Resistance among the Study Groups

Regarding the insulin resistance analyzed using the TyG index, our results revealed that a greater percentage of the patients from the Caucasian group belonged to the first quartile (34%), while most of the Roma patients belonged to the second one (36.9%). Among the fourth quartile, there were significantly more Roma patients than non-Roma patients (24.5% versus 18.6%, $p < 0.001$) (Figure 3).

Details about the number of patients belonging to each quartile are available in Supplementary Table S4.

Concerning the differences between patients with T1DM and T2DM, extended data can be found in Supplementary Table S5.

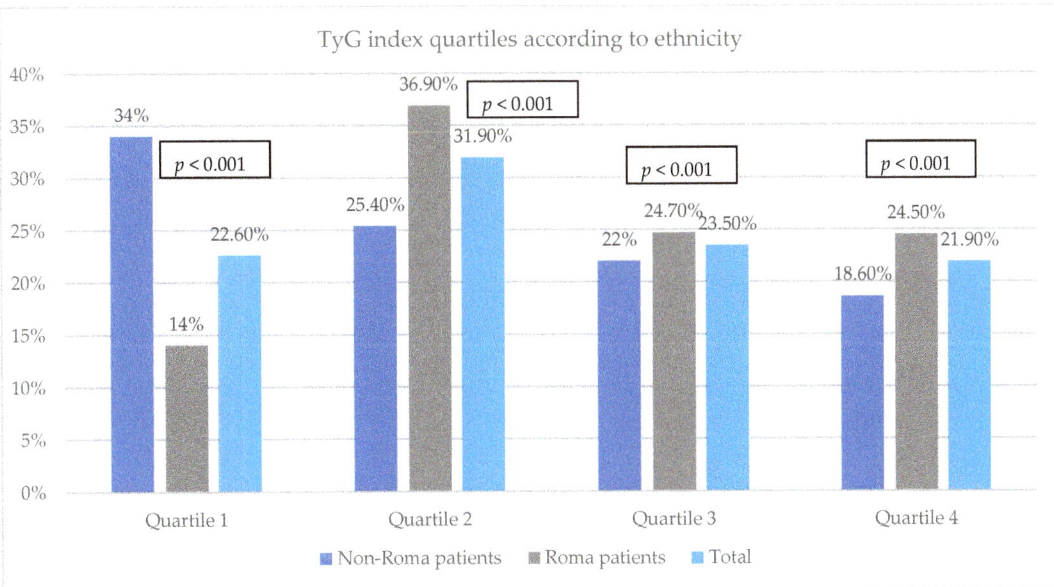

Figure 3. TyG index quartiles according to ethnicity.

Among patients from the fourth quartile of the TyG index, the mean age of the non-Roma subjects was significantly higher compared to the Roma (62.05 ± 11.67 versus 55.26 ± 11.73, $p < 0.001$); however, the average value of the HbA1c was more elevated among the Roma group (11.66 ± 2.05 versus 9.55 ± 2.36, $p < 0.001$). Regarding the anthropometric measurements, the mean values of weight, WC, and HC were higher in the Roma group compared to the non-Roma group. Concerning the renal profiles, the mean values of the creatinine, eGFR, urea, and uric acid were higher among the Roma, but conversely, the median value of the UACR was more elevated in the Caucasian group of patients. Analyzing the hepatic laboratory tests, the median value of the ALT was higher among the Roma, but with a GGT level which was more elevated among the non-Roma (Table 3).

Table 3. Characteristics of the patients from the fourth quartile of the TyG index according to ethnicity.

Parameters	Forth Quartile of the TyG index		*p*-Value
	Non-Roma Patients (*n* = 65)	**Roma Patients (*n*= 112)**	
Age (years)	62.05 ± 11.67	55.26 ± 11.73	<0.001
Duration of diabetes (years)	12.00 ± 4.50 *	6.00 ± 9.30 *	<0.001
Height (cm)	167.03 ± 9.27	164.88 ± 8.27	0.123
Weight (kg)	85.55 ± 17.83	90.64 ± 20.30	0.102
WC (cm)	104.44 ± 15.26	112.65 ± 15.48	0.006
HC (cm)	106.74 ± 8.82	109.07 ± 13.49	0.422
BMI (kg/m^2)	31.33 ± 4.23	31.83 ± 6.98	0.159
HbA1c (%)	9.55 ± 2.36	11.66 ± 2.05	<0.001
FPG (mg/dL)	255.50 ± 100.50 *	337.50 ± 108.50 *	0.010

Table 3. *Cont.*

Parameters	Forth Quartile of the TyG index		p-Value
	Non-Roma Patients (n = 65)	Roma Patients (n= 112)	
TC (mg/dL)	244.28 ± 93.54	247.82 ± 70.12	0.775
HDL-c (mg/dl)	45.44 ± 13.72	42.52 ± 9.71	0.103
TG (mg/dL)	401.25 ± 178.75	363.50 ± 125.93	0.102
LDL-c (mg/dL)	104.35 ± 40.20	127.42 ± 32.80	0.006
Creatinine (mg/dL)	1.02 ± 0.43	1.09 ± 0.43	0.661
eGFR (mL/min/1.73 m^2)	76.63 ± 29.26	78.16 ± 24.09	0.716
Urea (mg/dL)	42.26 ± 17.36	49.56 ± 19.82	0.500
Uric acid (mg/dL)	5.90 ± 2.13	6.80 ± 2.80	0.363
UACR (mg/g)	45.80 ± 150.08 *	36.00 ± 60.20 *	0.047
AST (UI/L)	40.88 ± 20.00	23.00 ± 15.5 *	0.320
ALT (UI/L)	27.83 ± 20.09 *	31.00 ± 26.25 *	0.904
GGT (UI/L)	94.13 ± 95.00 *	44.00 ± 27.00 *	0.076

Abbreviations: WC (cm)—waist circumference, HC (cm)—hip circumference, BMI (kg/m^2)—body mass index, HbA1c (%)—glycated hemoglobin, FPG (mg/dL)—fasting plasmatic glycemia, TC (mg/dL)—total cholesterol, HDL-c (mg/dL)—high-density lipoprotein–cholesterol, LDL-c (mg/dL)—low-density lipoprotein–cholesterol, TG (mg/dL)—triglycerides, TyG index—triglyceride–glucose index, eGFR (mL/min/1.73m^2)—estimated glomerular filtration rate, UACR (mg/g) —urinary albumin to creatinine ratio, AST (UI/L)—aspartate aminotransferase, ALT (UI/L)—alanine aminotransferase, GGT (UI/L)—gamma-glutamyl transferase. The data are represented as mean ± SD (standard deviation) and median ± IQR (marked with "*", IQR- interquartile range). The statistical significance was considered at a p-value < 0.05.

3.6. Factors Associated with TyG Index

To evaluate the factors associated with the TyG index, we used univariate analysis (Pearson correlation). The statistical analysis is presented in Supplementary Table S6.

In non-Roma participants, TyG was positively correlated with weight, HbA1c level, TC, LDL-c, and UACR, while among the Roma group, univariate analysis revealed a positive association between TyG index and HbA1c level, TC, LDL-c, creatinine level, and UACR, as well as a negative association with HDL-c. Multiple linear regression was conducted to estimate the independent correlation of the TyG index with the aforementioned parameters. Variables that were significantly associated with the TyG index among the non-Roma were HbA1c level, TC, HDL-c, and LDL-c (Table 4). In multivariate analysis, variables that were correlated with TyG index among the Roma participants were the HbA1c level and HDL-c (Table 4).

Table 4. Factors associated with TyG index according to ethnicity.

Variables	B	SE	p-Value	95% CI	
				Lower	Upper
Non-Roma patients					
Weight (kg)	−0.001	0.002	0.706	7.215	8.420
HbA1c (%)	0.148	0.018	<0.001	0.112	0.183
TC (mg/dL)	0.015	0.001	<0.001	0.012	0.017
HDL-c (mg/dL)	−0.022	0.003	<0.001	0.028	−0.015
LDL-c (mg/dL)	−0.012	0.002	<0.001	−0.015	−0.009
ALT (UI/L)	0.0007	0.001	0.945	−0.002	0.002

Table 4. *Cont.*

Variables	B	SE	*p*-Value	95% CI	
				Lower	Upper
UACR (mg/g)	0.0001	0.0001	0.059	0.0001	0.0001
Roma patients					
HbA1c (%)	0.150	0.027	<0.001	0.096	0.204
TC (mg/dL)	0.004	0.003	0.232	−0.002	0.009
HDL-c (mg/dL)	−0.017	0.008	0.030	−0.032	−0.002
LDL-c (mg/dL)	0.0001	0.004	0.911	−0.008	0.007
Creatinine (mg/dL)	−0.071	0.170	0.678	−0.411	0.269
UACR (mg/g)	0.001	0.001	0.344	−0.001	0.002

Abbreviations: HbA1c (%)—glycated hemoglobin, TC (mg/dL)—total cholesterol, HDL-c (mg/dL)—high-density lipoprotein–cholesterol, LDL-c (mg/dL)—low-density lipoprotein–cholesterol, ALT (UI/L)—alanine aminotransferase, UACR (mg/g)—urinary albumin to creatinine ratio, B—standard beta coefficient, SE—standard error, CI—confidence interval. The statistical significance was considered at a p-value < 0.05.

4. Discussion

The data that we used are from a Romanian sample of adults among whom T2DM was predominant. We analyzed the clinical and metabolic particularities of a Roma population compared to a corresponding group of non-Roma, including the prevalence of cardiovascular risk factors, cardiovascular disease, health-related behaviors, and anthropometric and paraclinical measurements.

Although T2DM was predominant, interestingly, there were approximately twice as many Roma patients with T1DM compared to non-Roma patients (12.2% versus 4.9%). There is limited specific research on the prevalence of T1DM in the Roma population compared to the general population; therefore, the exact reasons for this higher prevalence could be multifactorial and complex. Further research focusing on the interplay between genetic, environmental, and social factors is needed to fully understand these disparities [19].

Regarding the prevalence of cardiovascular risk factors, the most frequent factors identified in our study were hypertension, obesity, dyslipidemia, smoking, and alcohol consumption. Our findings are comparable with the results from a paper by Enache et al. that analyzed a group of Roma patients from Călărași County, Romania. The prevalence of obesity in our study was likewise higher among the Roma patients; however, greater rates were observed, with approximately 60% in the Roma group and 50% in the Caucasian group versus 45.2% and 43.9%, respectively. Hypertension and dyslipidemia were also significantly prevalent among both groups, but the rates were correspondingly higher among the Caucasian participants [20]. Nevertheless, data from another study that compared Roma patients from Călărași County with the general population showed higher percentages regarding the prevalence of obesity, but even so, the rates were lower than in the results in our paper, with obesity being present in 43.2% of the non-Roma and 43.3% of the Roma. What should be mentioned is that diabetes (known and newly diagnosed) was present in only 10% and 13.6% of the Roma patients, respectively [21].

Weiss et al. implied a prevalence of 33% of obesity, 33.62% of hypertension, 26.92% of dyslipidemia, and 42.55% of smoking among the analyzed Roma patients, suggesting lower rates compared to our study; nonetheless, only 15.13% of the patients had diabetes mellitus [22].

In the Predatorr study, a representative study in Romania that included more than 2500 patients aged between 20 and 79 years old, the prevalence of obesity was 56.4% in patients with known diabetes and 52.3% in patients with unknown diabetes. Similar rates were observed only among the non-Roma, the prevalence of obesity among the Roma being higher; however, the prevalence of hypertension was around 64% in patients with both known or unknown diabetes, and similar rates were observed only among the Roma. Concerning smoking status, the prevalence was around 50% in patients with both known and unknown diabetes. Our paper identified the same rate among the Roma, and a lower rate was observed among the non-Roma [23].

In analyzing our results in comparison with those from a Roma population in Serbia, among whom the prevalence of previously diagnosed diabetes was 5.9% and newly diagnosed T2DM was 5.2%, we found that only a third of the patients presented a family history of diabetes; our findings, however, suggest a higher percentage of patients with a positive family history of diabetes (45.4%) [24].

In Slovakia, a sample from the Roma population had a BMI above 25 kg/m^2 (55.8% of the Roma men and 53.4% of the Roma women, respectively), while a significant proportion of them had a BMI higher than 30 kg/m^2 (28.8% of the Roma men and 26.2% of the Roma women, respectively), with a higher mean waist circumference in women than in men [25]. In our study, we analyzed the Roma in comparison with a corresponding group of non-Roma and identified a higher mean BMI value among them (32.28 kg/m^2 versus 30.4 kg/m^2), as well as higher mean waist and hip circumferences (110.00 cm versus 103.73 cm, and 108.61 cm versus 104.82 cm, respectively). It would be intriguing to investigate potential disparities between genders.

In Hungary, data from a sample of Roma people implied that, regarding the anthropometric parameters, they had a lower mean height and weight, but with no differences regarding the average BMI compared to the general population; in our study, only the average weight was higher among the Roma group compared to the non-Roma, and concerning the mean BMI, there were also slight differences between the two groups [1].

Although the high frequency of communicable diseases among the Roma is firmly highlighted by the current medical literature, data regarding the prevalence of non-communicable diseases, including cardiovascular disease, are still modest. The prevalence of heart disease among the adult Roma population is considered to be around 10% [26]. However, it remains the main cause of premature mortality among this ethnic group, according to a paper from Slovakia [27]. Our study revealed corresponding results: 12% of the Roma participants were associated with myocardial infarction and 9.2% had a history of stroke. Nonetheless, higher rates were observed concerning stable angina and heart failure, with 29.5% of the Roma patients and 19% of them, respectively.

Regarding the prevalence of metabolic syndrome among the Roma, our study revealed a significant percentage of 94.3%, slightly higher compared to the non-Roma (89.1%). Data from the medical literature, however, identified a prevalence of 36.38% among the Roma individuals in Hungary and 29.28% in Slovakia [1,23,28].

Piko et al. analyzed the changes in the prevalence of metabolic syndrome and its components between 2011 and 2018 among a Hungarian sample of the Roma population and identified an increase in the prevalence of central obesity, hypertension, and metabolic syndrome in 2018, as well as an increased TG level. However, in 2018, a reduction in previously diagnosed diabetes mellitus or raised FPG, as well as a reduced HDL-c level, were observed [29]. The increased prevalence of metabolic syndrome among Roma patients is likely due to a combination of genetic predisposition, socio-economic challenges, lifestyle factors, and limited access to healthcare. Tackling these disparities necessitates a comprehensive strategy that involves enhancing healthcare access, encouraging healthier lifestyles, and implementing targeted interventions for this vulnerable population [29–31].

Adany et al. analyzed the TyG index among a sample Roma population from Hungary and identified that there were no differences in comparison with a corresponding group from the general Hungarian population (an average value of 4.88 was found in both groups) [32]. In our study, however, a higher mean value of the TyG index was found among the Roma group (10.07 ± 0.71 versus 9.71 ± 0.82). Among the general population, the TyG index has been positively associated with TC, LDL-c, very-low-density lipoprotein–cholesterol (VLDL-c), uric acid, AST, and ALT [33]. Accordingly, in our study, among the non-Roma group, TyG was positively correlated with TC, HDL-c, and LDL-c.

The TyG index has been associated with various components of metabolic syndrome, including obesity, dyslipidemia, hypertension, and hyperglycemia [4]. Accordingly, in our study, we observed high mean values of TyG index among both groups, as well as high prevalences of obesity, dyslipidemia, hypertension, and metabolic syndrome.

Concerning the paraclinical examination, a study from Bulgaria revealed higher mean values of the total cholesterol, triglycerides, and LDL-c among a Roma population compared to a non-Roma group, but a higher average HDL-c level among the latter [34]. These results are in concordance with our findings.

Regarding the prevalence of diabetic microvascular complications among the Roma population, data from the medical literature are scarce. Of the general population with T2DM, chronic kidney disease is considered to affect 25% of the patients, retinopathy is considered to be present in 21% of the patients, and approximately more than 50% of the patients have polyneuropathy [35]. Our study revealed corresponding data regarding the prevalence of chronic kidney disease among the Roma, but with higher rates observed with reference to peripheral neuropathy and retinopathy. A paper by Weiss et al. identified that retinopathy affected 12.5% of the Roma diabetic patients [22].

Regarding the prevalence of amputations, a recent study from Romania suggested that 51.2% of the total number of non-traumatic amputations were in patients with diabetes [36]. Other papers indicated a prevalence of 3.6% in the general Romanian population, while a comparison between non-Roma and Roma patients implied a higher prevalence among the former group (7.5% versus 2.3%) [37,38]. Our study identified a percentage of around 3.5% among both groups.

Overall, considering all results, our study revealed that there are no major differences between the two groups of patients with diabetes mellitus. Apart from this, the results align with those in another recent paper published regarding diabetes distress [39]. These findings are in agreement with the genetic study of Nardos et al., which suggested that genetic predispositions are similar between the Roma and the general population [40]. However, minor differences in clinical and paraclinical assessments and complications in our study could likely be more attributable to disparities in social and living conditions rather than genetic differences, which further emphasizes the importance of addressing social inequalities to improve diabetes management and outcomes in the Roma population. The European Commission and Romanian government have implemented policies to improve Roma health, education, and social services, such as the National Roma Integration Strategy and the EU Framework for National Roma Integration Strategies. While progress has been made, gaps remain in terms of effectively reaching the Roma population. Healthcare providers can bridge the gap by offering culturally competent care and advocating for policy changes. Understanding the Roma's socio-economic and cultural context is essential for improving patient outcomes and reducing health disparities [41].

5. Limitations of the Study

In addressing the constraints of our research, participant recruitment was confined to a single tertiary care hospital amid the COVID-19 pandemic, which may not be representative of the general Roma and non-Roma populations with diabetes, although the sample size is reasonable. Moreover, our study relied on self-reported data for health behaviors like smoking and alcohol consumption, which can be inaccurate due to social desirability bias (people under-reporting unhealthy behaviors).

Apart from this, our study did not collect specific data on healthcare management strategies, such as the frequency of primary healthcare utilization or participation in health education programs among the Roma population. Future studies should aim to include these variables to provide a more comprehensive understanding of healthcare management strategies and their impact on health outcomes within this population. By incorporating these aspects, we can better understand the disparities in healthcare access and outcomes between Roma and non-Roma patients and develop targeted interventions to address these gaps.

While our findings align with larger studies comparing the general population to ethnic minorities, there is a scarcity of data on Roma patients. Consequently, we acknowledge the imperative for additional research in this area, with a more in-depth analysis to identify the specific genetic and environmental factors contributing to the higher cardiovascular risk in the Roma population. Considering conducting a longitudinal study to investigate cause-and-effect relationships between observed factors and health outcomes by partnering with community leaders and healthcare professionals from the Roma community could contribute significantly to improving cardiovascular health outcomes and reducing ethnic disparities in healthcare for the Roma population.

6. Conclusions

Taking the above into consideration, the prevalence of cardiovascular risk factors, cardiovascular disease, and microvascular complications among the study Roma population is quite significant, underscoring the importance of considering ethnic disparities in approaching healthcare management strategies. Regarding the anthropometric and paraclinical assessments, our data demonstrated different characteristics of the Roma in comparison to a corresponding group of non-Roma, highlighting the importance of tailoring healthcare interventions to the specific needs and cultural context of this ethnic minority. Further research is warranted to explore the underlying factors contributing to these differences as well as potential genetic or environmental factors, and to develop targeted interventions in high-risk populations.

Supplementary Materials: The following supporting information can be downloaded at: https://www.mdpi.com/article/10.3390/biomedicines12071422/s1, Table S1. Prevalence of the patients' comorbidities according to their ethnicity; Table S2. Prevalence of diabetic complications according to ethnicity; Table S3. Mean values of the analysed parameters according to ethnicity and type of diabetes; Table S4. TyG index quartiles according to ethnicity; Table S5. TyG index quartiles according to ethnicity and type of diabetes; Table S6. Univariate analysis between TyG index and different variables according to ethnicity.

Author Contributions: Conceptualization, A.C. and E.R.; methodology, A.C., E.R. and G.R.; software, E.R.; validation, A.C., E.R., G.E. and G.R.; formal analysis, A.C. and E.R.; investigation, F.R.; resources, A.C., I.U., M.D. and A.V.; data curation, G.E.; writing—original draft preparation, A.C., E.R. and S.S.; writing—review and editing, A.C. and E.R.; visualization, S.S.; supervision, E.R. and G.R.; project administration, A.C.; funding acquisition, A.C. and E.R. All authors have read and agreed to the published version of the manuscript.

Funding: This research was funded by the University of Medicine and Pharmacy Carol Davila, through the institutional program "Publish not Perish".

Institutional Review Board Statement: The study was conducted in accordance with the Declaration of Helsinki, and approved by the Ethics Committee of "Nicolae Malaxa" Clinical Hospital, Bucharest, Romania (approval number 75 on 5 September 2022).

Informed Consent Statement: Informed consent was obtained from all subjects involved in the study.

Data Availability Statement: The data presented in this study are available upon request from the corresponding author. The data are not publicly available due to the hospital's privacy policy.

Conflicts of Interest: The authors declare no conflicts of interest.

References

1. Kósa, Z.; Moravcsik-Kornyicki, Á.; Diószegi, J.; Roberts, B.; Szabó, Z.; Sándor, J.; Ádány, R. Prevalence of metabolic syndrome among Roma: A comparative health examination survey in Hungary. *Eur. J. Public Health* **2015**, *25*, 299–304. [CrossRef]
2. Kanapeckiene, V.; Valinteliene, R.; Berzanskyte, A.; Kevalas, R.; Supranowicz, P. Health of Roma children in Vilnius and Ventspils. *Medicina* **2009**, *45*, 153–161. [CrossRef]
3. Nunes, M.A.; Kučerová, K.; Lukáč, O.; Kvapil, M.; Brož, J. Prevalence of diabetes mellitus among Roma populations—A systematic review. *Int. J. Environ. Res. Public Health* **2018**, *15*, 2607. [CrossRef] [PubMed]

4. Simental-Mendía, L.E.; Rodríguez-Morán, M.; Guerrero-Romero, F. The product of fasting glucose and triglycerides as surrogate for identifying insulin resistance in apparently healthy subjects. *Metab. Syndr. Relat. Disord.* **2008**, *6*, 299–304. [CrossRef]
5. Cuschieri, S. The STROBE guidelines. *Saudi J. Anaesth.* **2019**, *13*, S31–S34. [CrossRef]
6. Thomas, D.; Seeman, T.; Potter, A.; Hu, P.; Crimmins, E.; Herningtyas, E.H.; Sumantri, C.; Frankenberg, E. HPLC-based measurement of glycated hemoglobin using dried blood spots collected under adverse field conditions. *Biodemography Soc. Biol.* **2018**, *64*, 43–62. [CrossRef] [PubMed]
7. Spectrophotometry | NIST. Available online: https://www.nist.gov/programs-projects/spectrophotometry (accessed on 14 June 2024).
8. Chen, R.Y.; Shi, J. Evaluation of the CKD-EPI 2021 creatinine equation using laboratory data: Considerations for practice changes among clinical laboratories in British Columbia, Canada. *Clin. Biochem.* **2024**, *123*, 110686. [CrossRef] [PubMed]
9. Mach, F.; Baigent, C.; Catapano, A.L.; Koskinas, K.C.; Casula, M.; Badimon, L.; Chapman, M.J.; De Backer, G.G.; Delgado, V.; Ference, B.A.; et al. 2019 ESC/EAS guidelines for the management of dyslipidaemias: Lipid modification to reduce cardiovascular risk. *Eur. Heart J.* **2019**, *41*, 111–188. [CrossRef]
10. Selvi, N.M.K.; Nandhini, S.; Sakthivadivel, V.; Lokesh, S.; Srinivasan, A.R.; Sumathi, S. Association of triglyceride- glucose index (TyG index) with HbA1c and insulin resistance in type 2 diabetes mellitus. *Maedica* **2021**, *16*, 375–381.
11. American Diabetes Association Professional Practice Committee. Standards of care in diabetes-2024. *Diabetes Care* **2024**, *47*, S5–S10. [CrossRef]
12. Unger, T.; Borghi, C.; Charchar, F.; Khan, N.A.; Poulter, N.R.; Prabhakaran, D.; Ramirez, A.; Schlaich, M.; Stergiou, G.S.; Tomaszewski, M.; et al. 2020 International Society of Hypertension Global Hypertension Practice Guidelines. *Hypertension* **2020**, *75*, 1334–1357. [CrossRef]
13. Body Mass Index (BMI). Available online: https://www.who.int/data/gho/data/themes/topics/topic-details/GHO/body-mass-index (accessed on 2 April 2024).
14. Alberti, K.G.; Eckel, R.H.; Grundy, S.M.; Zimmet, P.Z.; Cleeman, J.I.; Donato, K.A.; Fruchart, J.C.; James, W.P.T.; Loria, C.M.; Smith, S.C., Jr. Harmonizing the metabolic syndrome: A joint interim statement of the International Diabetes Federation Task Force on Epidemiology and Prevention; National Heart, Lung, and Blood Institute; American Heart Association; World Heart Federation; International Atherosclerosis Society; and International Association for the Study of Obesity. *Circulation* **2009**, *120*, 1640–1645. [PubMed]
15. Stevens, P.E.; Ahmed, S.B.; Carrero, J.J.; Foster, B.; Francis, A.; Hall, R.K.; Herrington, W.G.; Hill, G.; Inker, L.A.; Kazancıoğlu, R.; et al. KDIGO 2024 Clinical practice guideline for the evaluation and management of chronic kidney disease. *Kidney Int.* **2024**, *105*, S117–S314.
16. Relhan, N.; Flynn, H.W. The early treatment diabetic retinopathy study historical review and relevance to today's management of diabetic macular edema. *Curr. Opin. Ophthalmol.* **2017**, *28*, 205–212. [CrossRef] [PubMed]
17. Massey, F.J. The Kolmogorov-Smirnov Test for Goodness of Fit. *J. Am. Stat. Assoc.* **1951**, *46*, 68–78. [CrossRef]
18. Shapiro, S.S.; Wilk, M.B. An Analysis of Variance Test for Normality (Complete Samples). *Biometrika* **1965**, *52*, 591. [CrossRef]
19. Kolarčik, P.; Geckova, A.M.; Orosova, O.; van Dijk, J.P.; Reijneveld, S.A. Predictors of health-endangering behaviour among Roma and non-Roma adolescents in Slovakia by gender. *J. Epidemiol. Community Health* **2010**, *64*, 1043–1048. [CrossRef] [PubMed]
20. Enache, G.; Rusu, E.; Ilinca, A.; Rusu, F.; Costache, A.; Jinga, M.; Pănuş, C.; Radulian, G. Prevalence of overweight and obesity in a Roma population from Southern Romania—Calarasi county. *Acta Endocrinol.* **2018**, *14*, 122–130. [CrossRef] [PubMed]
21. Rusu, E.; Enache, G.; Rusu, F.; Cosoreanu, A.; Cîrstea, C.; Baleanu, M.; Radulian, G. 1466-P: Prevalence of glucose intolerance in the Roma population from a rural area in the south part of Romania: Călărași county. *Diabetes* **2020**, *69* (Suppl. S1), 1466-P. [CrossRef]
22. Weiss, E.; Japie, C.; Balahura, A.M.; Bartos, D.; Badila, E. Cardiovascular risk factors in a Roma sample population from Romania. *Rom. J. Intern. Med.* **2018**, *56*, 193–202. [CrossRef]
23. Mota, M.; Popa, S.G.; Mota, E.; Mitrea, A.; Catrinoiu, D.; Cheta, D.M.; Guja, C.; Hancu, N.; Ionescu-Tirgoviste, C.; Lichiardopol, R.; et al. Prevalence of diabetes mellitus and prediabetes in the adult Romanian population: PREDATORR study. *J. Diabetes.* **2016**, *8*, 336–344. [CrossRef] [PubMed]
24. Beljić Zivković, T.; Marjanović, M.; Prgomelja, S.; Soldatovic, I.; Koprivica, B.; Acković, D.; Zivković, R. Screening for diabetes among Roma people living in Serbia. *Croat. Med. J.* **2010**, *51*, 144. [CrossRef] [PubMed]
25. Fedacko, J.; Pella, D.; Jarcuska, P.; Siegfried, L.; Janicko, M.; Veselíny, E.; Pella, J.; Sabol, F.; Jarcuska, P.; Mareková, M.; et al. Prevalence of cardiovascular risk factors in relation to metabolic syndrome in the Roma population compared with the non-Roma population in the eastern part of Slovakia. *Cent. Eur. J. Public Health* **2014**, *22*, S69–S74. [CrossRef] [PubMed]
26. Health and the Roma Community, Analysis of the Situation in Europe. Available online: www.gitanos.org (accessed on 16 April 2024).
27. Ginter, E.; Krajcovicova-Kudlackova, M.; Kacala, O.; Kovacic, V.; Valachovicova, M. Health status of Romanies (Gypsies) in the Slovak Republic and in the neighbouring countries. *Bratisl. Lek. Listy* **2001**, *102*, 479–484. [PubMed]
28. Fedacko, J.; Pella, D.; Jarcuska, P. Clinical and biochemical determinants of metabolic syndrome among Roma and non-Roma subjects in the eastern part of Slovakia. *Cent. Eur. J. Public Health* **2014**, *22*, S75–S80. [CrossRef] [PubMed]

29. Piko, P.; Dioszegi, J.; Kosa, Z.; Sandor, J.; Moizs, M.; Adany, R. Changes in the prevalence of metabolic syndrome, its components, and relevant preventive medication between 2011 and 2018 in the northeast hungarian roma population. *J. Pers. Med.* **2021**, *11*, 595. [CrossRef] [PubMed]
30. Cook, B.; Wayne, G.F.; Valentine, A.; Lessios, A.; Yeh, E. Revisiting the evidence on health and health care disparities among the Roma: A systematic review 2003–2012. *Int. J. Public Health.* **2013**, *58*, 885–911. [CrossRef] [PubMed]
31. Piko, P.; Werissa, N.A.; Adany, R. Genetic susceptibility to insulin resistance and its association with estimated longevity in the Hungarian general and Roma populations. *Biomedicines* **2022**, *10*, 1703. [CrossRef] [PubMed]
32. Ádány, R.; Pikó, P.; Fiatal, S.; Kósa, Z.; Sándor, J.; Bíró, É.; Kósa, K.; Paragh, G.; Bácsné Bába, É.; Veres-Balajti, I.; et al. Prevalence of insulin resistance in the Hungarian general and Roma populations as defined by using Data generated in a complex health (Interview and Examination) Survey. *Int. J. Environ. Res. Public Health* **2020**, *17*, 4833. [CrossRef]
33. Araújo, S.P.; Juvanhol, L.L.; Bressan, J.; Hermsdorff, H.H.M. Triglyceride glucose index: A new biomarker in predicting cardiovascular risk. *Prev. Med. Rep.* **2022**, *29*, 101941. [CrossRef]
34. Delcheva, G.; Stankova, T.; Stefanova, K.; Bivolarska, A. Assessment of health status and cardiovascular risk factors in a Roma population sample from South Bulgaria. *Cent. Eur. J. Public Health* **2023**, *31*, 115–119. [CrossRef]
35. Faselis, C.; Katsimardou, A.; Imprialos, K.; Deligkaris, P.; Kallistratos, M.; Dimitriadis, K. Microvascular complications of type 2 diabetes mellitus. *Curr. Vasc. Pharmacol.* **2020**, *18*, 117–124. [CrossRef]
36. Rusu, E.; Coman, H.; Coșoreanu, A.; Militaru, A.M.; Popescu-Vâlceanu, H.C.; Teodoru, I.; Mihai, D.A.; Elian, V.; Gavan, N.A.; Radulian, G. Incidence of Lower extremity amputation in Romania: A nationwide 5-year cohort study, 2015–2019. *Medicina* **2023**, *59*, 1199. [CrossRef]
37. Ghid de Management al Diabetului Zaharat. 2021. Available online: https://societate-diabet.ro/wp-content/uploads/2021/07/Ghidul-SRDNBM-2021.pdf (accessed on 16 April 2024).
38. Coşoreanu, A.; Rusu, E.; Baleanu, M.; Marinescu, M.; Iordache, S.; Vlad, A.M.; Rusu, F.; Enache, G.; Radulian, G. Prevalence of limb amputations in a Roma population compared to Caucasians, in patients with diabetes mellitus. *Rom. J. Orthop. Surg. Traumatol.* **2020**, *3*, 41–48. [CrossRef]
39. Cosoreanu, A.; Rusu, E.; Mihai, D.A.; Rusu, F.; Pantea, I.; Paunica, I.; Ungureanu, I.; Radulian, G. Diabetes distress among the Roma population from a tertiary care center in Romania. *Cureus* **2024**, *16*, e60348. [CrossRef] [PubMed]
40. Werissa, N.A.; Piko, P.; Fiatal, S.; Kosa, Z.; Sandor, J.; Adany, R. SNP-based genetic risk score modeling suggests no increased genetic susceptibility of the Roma population to type 2 diabetes mellitus. *Genes* **2019**, *10*, 942. [CrossRef] [PubMed]
41. EU Roma Strategic Framework for Equality, Inclusion and Participation for 2020–2030 Justice and Consumers. Available online: https://commission.europa.eu/publications/new-eu-roma-strategic-framework-equality-inclusion-and-participation-full-package_en (accessed on 14 June 2024).

biomedicines

MDPI

Article

Age-Related Glucose Intolerance Is Associated with Impaired Insulin Secretion in Community-Dwelling Japanese Adults: The Kumamoto Koshi Study

Kazuki Fukuda [1,†], Masaki Haneda [2,†], Naoto Kubota [1,2], Eiichi Araki [1,2,3,4] and Kazuya Yamagata [1,5,*]

1 Center for Metabolic Regulation of Healthy Aging (CMHA), Faculty of Life Sciences, Kumamoto University, Kumamoto 860-8556, Japan; fudakazuki@kumamoto-u.ac.jp (K.F.); nkubota0511@kumamoto-u.ac.jp (N.K.); earaki@gpo.kumamoto-u.ac.jp (E.A.)
2 Department of Metabolic Medicine, Faculty of Life Sciences, Kumamoto University, Kumamoto 860-8556, Japan; msk_asp72@yahoo.co.jp
3 Research Center for Health and Sports Sciences, Kumamoto Health Science University, Kumamoto 861-5598, Japan
4 Diabetes Center, Kikuchi Medical Association Hospital, Kumamoto 861-1306, Japan
5 Department of Medical Biochemistry, Faculty of Life Sciences, Kumamoto University, Kumamoto 860-8556, Japan
* Correspondence: k-yamaga@kumamoto-u.ac.jp; Tel.: +81-96-373-5068; Fax: +81-96-364-6940
† These authors contributed equally to this work.

Abstract: Background/Objectives: Glucose tolerance progressively declines with age. However, the effects of aging on insulin secretion and insulin sensitivity in Japanese subjects are unclear. **Methods**: We conducted an oral glucose tolerance test (OGTT) in residents aged between 22 and 85 years in Koshi City, Kumamoto Prefecture, Japan, to clarify the characteristics of insulin secretion and insulin sensitivity in older adults. Participants were recruited using a flyer, and the OGTT was performed after an overnight fast (12–16 h) between 8:00 and 10:30 am. **Results**: HOMA-IR and the Matsuda index are indices of insulin action. No correlation of age with HOMA-IR or the Matsuda index was found, whereas HOMA-β, the insulinogenic index, and the disposition index, all indices of insulin secretion, were negatively correlated with age in all participants and in individuals with normal glucose tolerance. Multiple regression analysis showed that age was an explanatory factor for insulin secretion. **Conclusions**: Impaired insulin secretion may contribute to age related glucose intolerance in Japanese individuals.

Keywords: age; elderly; insulin secretion; insulin sensitivity

1. Introduction

Glucose tolerance progressively declines with age [1,2]. Older people are more glucose intolerant than young individuals, and the total diabetes prevalence exceeds 20% in every age group between 65 and 95 years worldwide [3]. Insulin resistance and impaired insulin secretion are the major underlying mechanisms of hyperglycemia in type 2 diabetes. The effects of aging on insulin action and insulin secretion have been studied in detail, but the results are controversial. Regarding insulin action, many studies indicate that insulin resistance develops with age [4–6], but some studies did not find such an association [7–9]. The effect of aging on insulin secretion is also unclear. Previous studies have been inconsistent, reporting that aging increases [6,10], decreases [4,7,11–13], or does not change [5,14,15] insulin secretion. This variability may be due to confounding factors associated with aging, such as obesity and insulin resistance [1].

Ethnic differences in insulin sensitivity and insulin secretion are widely recognized, and Japanese people are characterized by higher insulin sensitivity and lower insulin secretion [16–18]. Controversial results have also been reported on the effect of aging on insulin sensitivity and insulin secretion in Japanese people. One study reported that both the homeostasis model assessment of insulin resistance (HOMA-IR), an index of insulin resistance; and the homeostasis model assessment of β-cell function (HOMA-β), a marker of β-cell function; declined with age [19], suggesting that insulin secretion decreases with age while insulin sensitivity increases. On the other hand, another study showed an age-dependent deterioration of insulin sensitivity using the Matsuda index, but no age-dependent change in the insulinogenic index, a marker of glucose-stimulated early insulin secretion, in Japanese subjects after the age of 65 [20]. Insulin secretion in an oral glucose tolerance test (OGTT) was also comparable between middle-aged and elderly Japanese individuals [21]. Therefore, the effect of aging on insulin sensitivity and insulin secretion in Japanese people remains unclear.

Characterizing insulin secretion and insulin action in older people would be useful for developing appropriate strategies for the prevention and treatment of type 2 diabetes. Accordingly, in the present study, we conducted OGTT in residents aged between 22 and 85 years in Koshi City, Kumamoto Prefecture, Japan, to assess the prevalence of diabetes and impaired glucose tolerance (IGT) and to clarify the characteristics of insulin secretion and insulin sensitivity in older individuals.

2. Materials and Methods

2.1. Study Design and Participants

Koshi City is a rural area in Kumamoto Prefecture, Japan. A flyer was distributed to all households (approximately 20,000 households) in Koshi City, informing them that a glucose tolerance test would be performed on the residents and inviting them to participate in the study. The following were excluded from the study on the basis of self-reported information: people being treated for diabetes; people with fasting blood glucose of 126 mg/dl or more or HbA1c of 6.5% or more on physical examination; and people who had undergone gastric resection. From August 2020 to August 2021, a total of 160 residents aged 22 to 85 years agreed to participate in the study and underwent an OGTT. This study was conducted in accordance with the Declaration of Helsinki. The study protocol was approved by the ethics committees of the Kumamoto University Graduate School of Medicine (No. 2602, 8 November 2022). Both written informed consent and opt-out informed consent were obtained from all participants.

2.2. Anthropometrics and Biochemical Measurements

A 75-g OGTT was carried out after an overnight fast (12–16 h) between 8:00 and 10:30 am. Blood samples were collected at 0, 30, 60, and 120 min. Based on plasma glucose levels, participants were categorized as having normal glucose tolerance (NGT; fasting plasma glucose [FPG] < 110 mg/dL and 2-h plasma glucose [2hPG] < 140 mg/dL), isolated impaired fasting glucose (IFG; FPG = 110–125 mg/dL and 2hPG < 140 mg/dL), IGT (FPG < 126 mg/dL and 2hPG = 140–199 mg/dL), and diabetes mellitus (FPG $\geq$ 126 mg/dL and/or 2hPG $\geq$ 200 mg/dL) according to World Health Organization criteria. Plasma glucose levels were measured by hexokinase enzymatic analysis, HbA1c levels were measured by high-performance liquid chromatography, and serum insulin levels were measured by chemiluminescent enzyme-linked immunosorbent assay. These measurements were conducted by BML, Inc. (Kumamoto, Japan).

Calf circumference, grip strength, and body composition were also measured by a qualified physician (K.F.) in the 88 individuals who agreed to participate. Calf circumference and grip strength were measured bilaterally, and the larger value was used for analysis. Skeletal muscle mass and body fat mass were measured by bioelectrical impedance analysis (BIA, InBody® 270, Inbody Japan Co. Ltd., Tokyo, Japan). The skeletal muscle index was calculated as skeletal muscle mass/(height)^2. Percent body fat was calculated as (body fat mass/body weight) × 100.

2.3. Calculation of Indices of Insulin Secretion and Insulin Sensitivity

HOMA-IR, an index of insulin resistance, was calculated as fasting serum insulin (μU/mL) × FPG (mg/dL)/405 [22]. The Matsuda index was calculated as {10,000/square root of (FPG [mg/dL] × fasting insulin [μU/mL] × mean glucose [mg/dL] × mean insulin during OGTT [μU/mL])} [23]. HOMA-β was calculated as (fasting insulin [μU/mL] × 360)/(FPG [mg/dL] − 63) [22]. The insulinogenic index was calculated as (insulin at 30 min − insulin at 0 min)/(glucose at 30 min − glucose at 0 min) [24]. The disposition index was calculated as the Matsuda index × (AUC-insulin/AUC-glucose), as previously reported [25].

2.4. Statistical Analysis

Data are presented as the mean ± standard deviation (SD). To approximate a normal distribution, HOMA-IR, Matsuda index, HOMA-β, insulinogenic index, and disposition index values were logarithmically transformed before statistical analysis. Differences in means were tested using an unpaired two-tailed Student's *t*-test or one-way analysis of variance (ANOVA) with Tukey's post hoc test. Frequencies were compared using the chi-square test. Pearson's correlation coefficient analysis was performed to assess the relationship between two variables. Multivariate stepwise regression analysis was performed to explore the relationship of the indices of insulin secretion and insulin sensitivity with age, sex, body mass index (BMI), percent body fat, skeletal muscle index, calf circumference, and grip strength. A value of $p < 0.05$ was considered to be statistically significant. All statistical analyses were performed using Prism version 10 (GraphPad Software, Boston, MA, USA).

3. Results

3.1. Diabetes and Prediabetes Prevalence by Age Group

Participants were divided into four groups—group 1, 20–39 years; group 2, 40–59 years; group 3, 60–74 years; group 4, 75 years or older—according to age. The characteristics of each group are shown in Table 1. BMI was comparable among the four groups, while FPG was significantly higher in the two groups aged 60 years or older than in the two groups aged under 60 years.

Figure 1A shows the plasma glucose levels during the 75-g OGTT. The area under the curve (AUC) of plasma glucose during the OGTT (AUC-glucose) was significantly higher in the groups aged 60 years or older than in the groups aged under 60 years (Figure 1B), indicating that the older individuals were more glucose intolerant. Consistently, HbA1c was positively correlated with age (Figure 1C). The proportion of individuals with NGT decreased with age. On the other hand, the prevalence of newly diagnosed diabetes increased with age (0%, 2.0%, 15.5%, and 21.4% for groups 1–4, respectively). The prevalence of IGT also markedly increased with age (4.0%, 16.3%, 25.9%, and 42.9% for groups 1–4, respectively), whereas the prevalence of isolated IFG did not increase with age (Table 1 and Figure 1D). The prevalence of IGT tended to be higher in women than in men in younger age groups (aged 20–59 years) (Figure 1E,F), but the difference was not significant.

Table 1. Characteristics of the individuals in the different age groups.

Groups	Group 1 (20–39)	Group 2 (40–59)	Group 3 (60–74)	Group 4 (75–)	p
n (M, F)	25 (11, 14)	49 (26, 23)	58 (31, 27)	28 (14, 14)	
Age (years)	32.6 ± 4.4	49.1 ± 6.2	67.6 ± 3.9	78.4 ± 3.4	
NGT, n (%)	24 (96.0)	40 (81.6)	33 (56.9)	9 (32.1)	
IFG, n (%)	0 (0)	0 (0)	1 (1.7)	1 (3.6)	
IGT, n (%)	1 (4.0)	8 (16.3)	15(25.9)	12(42.9)	
DM, n (%)	0 (0)	1 (2.0)	9 (15.5)	6 (21.4)	
BMI (kg/m^2)	23.7 ± 4.8	22.2 ± 2.8	23.0 ± 3.3	22.9 ± 2.7	0.343
FPG (mg/dL)	88.6 ± 5.7	91.4 ± 8.5	99.4 ± 10.3 ***, †††	98.3 ± 12.2 **, †	<0.001
HbA1c (%)	5.43 ± 0.24	5.45 ± 0.32	5.76 ± 0.33 ***, †††	5.79 ± 0.37 ***, †††	<0.001
F-IRI (μU/mL)	6.62 ± 6.5	4.83 ± 2.3	5.29 ± 3.2	5.39 ± 3.1	0.259
HOMA-IR (μU/mL·mg/dL)	1.48 ± 1.53	1.11 ± 0.58	1.32 ± 0.84	1.35 ± 0.88	0.483
Matsuda Index ((mg/dL·μU/mL)$^{-1}$)	7.25 ± 3.7	7.65 ± 3.6	6.84 ± 3.4	6.40 ± 3.4	0.403
HOMA-β (μU/mL/mg/dL)	90.6 ± 72	64.0 ± 29	54.2 ± 34 ***	58.9 ± 38 *	0.002
Insulinogenic Index (μU/mL/mg/dL)	1.05 ± 0.9	0.82 ± 0.7	0.59 ± 0.5 *	0.58 ± 0.7 *	0.006
Disposition Index ((mg/dL)$^{-2}$)	2.40 ± 0.9	2.20 ± 0.8	1.64 ± 0.6 ***, †††	1.58 ± 0.7 ***, ††	<0.001
Body Fat Mass (kg) §	21.1 ± 12.4	14.8 ± 5.7 *	14.0 ± 3.9 **	13.0 ± 5.5 **	0.006
Body Fat Percentage (%) §	29.5 ± 11.0	25.5 ± 7.9	24.9 ± 6.1	23.3 ± 7.4	0.181
Skeletal Muscle Mass (kg) §	25.8 ± 5.9	23.6 ± 4.5	23.2 ± 5.0	22.4 ± 4.4	0.276
Skeletal Muscle Index (kg/m^2) §	7.21 ± 1.3	6.65 ± 0.9	6.58 ± 1.0	6.49 ± 1.0	0.206
Calf Circumference (cm) §	37.7 ± 4.7	35.3 ± 2.1 *	34.7 ± 2.5 **	33.5 ± 2.4 ***	0.001
Grip Strength (kg) §	33.5 ± 9.9	32.8 ± 9.7	30.5 ± 9.1	26.8 ± 7.3	0.150

Data are shown as the mean ± SD. NGT, normal glucose tolerance; IFG, impaired fasting glucose; IGT, impaired glucose tolerance; DM, diabetes mellitus; BMI, body mass index; FPG, fasting plasma glucose; HbA1c, glycated hemoglobin (hemoglobin A1c); F-IRI, fasting immunoreactive insulin; HOMA-IR, homeostatic model assessment for insulin resistance; HOMA-β, homeostatic model assessment β-cell function. § Data were available for 88 of the participants (group 1, n = 14; group 2, n = 30; group 3, n = 29; and group 4, n = 15). * $p < 0.05$ vs. Group 1, ** $p < 0.01$ vs. Group 1, *** $p < 0.001$ vs. Group 1, † $p < 0.05$ vs. Group 2, †† $p < 0.01$ vs. Group 2, ††† $p < 0.001$ vs. Group 2.

3.2. Relationship Between Age and Indices of Insulin Sensitivity

Increased body weight/adiposity and decreased muscle mass have been suggested to contribute to the reduced insulin sensitivity in older adults [2]. We thus investigated the relationship between aging and various parameters related to fat and muscle mass. No correlation between age and BMI was observed in the participants (Figure 2A). In terms of adiposity, there was a significant negative correlation between age and body fat mass ($r = -0.28$, $p < 0.01$) (Figure 2B). There was a nonsignificant tendency for the percentage of body fat to decrease with age (Figure 2C). Calf circumference ($r = -0.22$, $p < 0.05$) and grip strength ($r = -0.37$, $p < 0.001$) were negatively correlated with age (Figure 2D,E), and similar trends were observed for age with skeletal muscle mass ($r = -0.18$) and the skeletal muscle index ($r = -0.18$) (Figure 2F,G). A previous Japanese study reported a decrease in the HOMA-IR with age [19]. However, no correlation was found between age and indices of insulin action (HOMA-IR and Matsuda index) (Figure 2H,I), indicating that insulin sensitivity did not change with age in the participants.

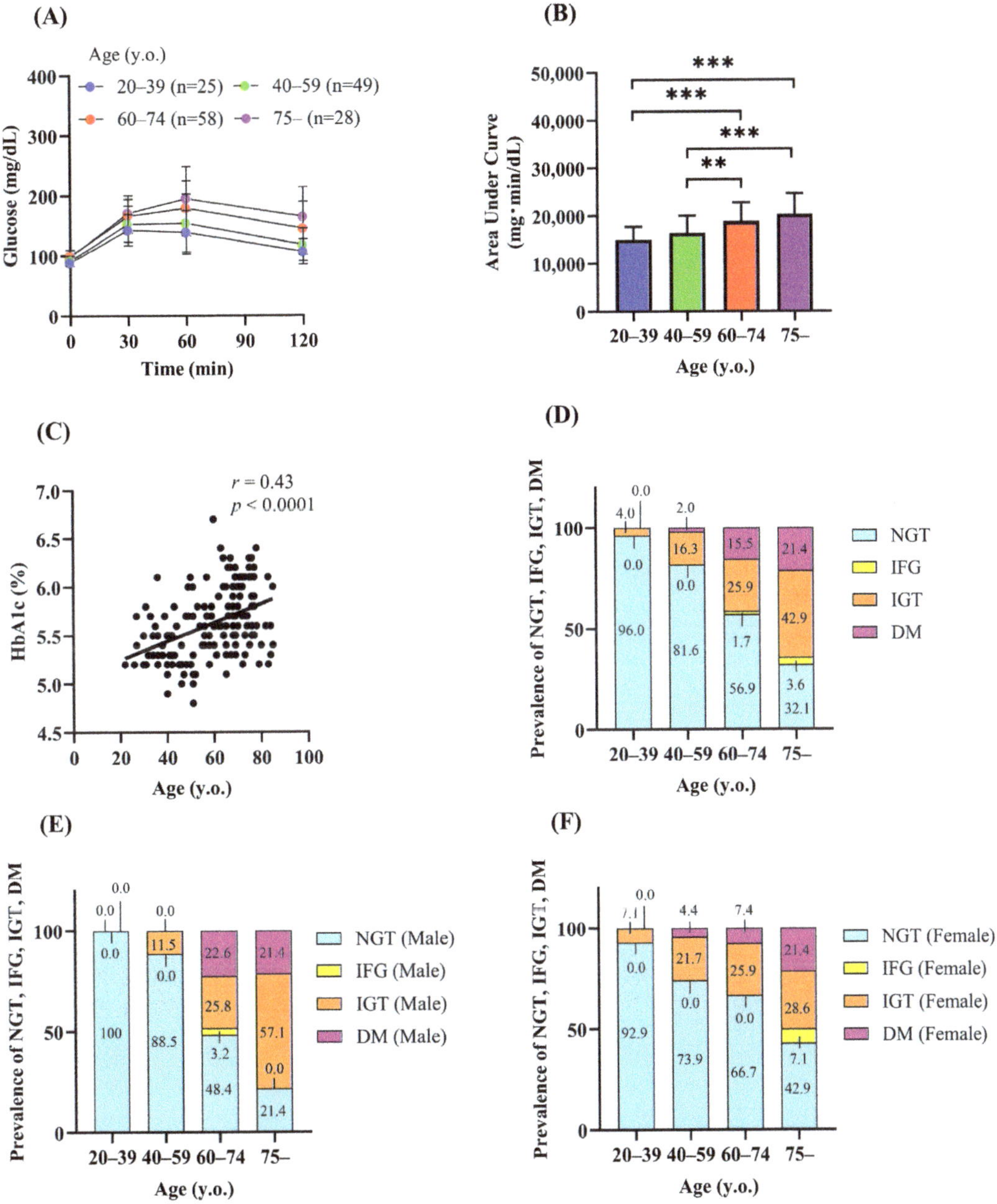

Figure 1. Prevalence of diabetes and impaired glucose tolerance in Koshi City. Plasma glucose (**A**) and the area under the curve of plasma glucose (**B**) during the 75-g OGTT. Correlation between age and HbA1c (**C**). Prevalence of normal glucose tolerance (NGT), impaired fasting glucose (IFG), impaired glucose tolerance (IGT), and diabetes (DM) (**D–F**). Data are shown as the mean ± SD. ** $p < 0.01$, *** $p < 0.001$.

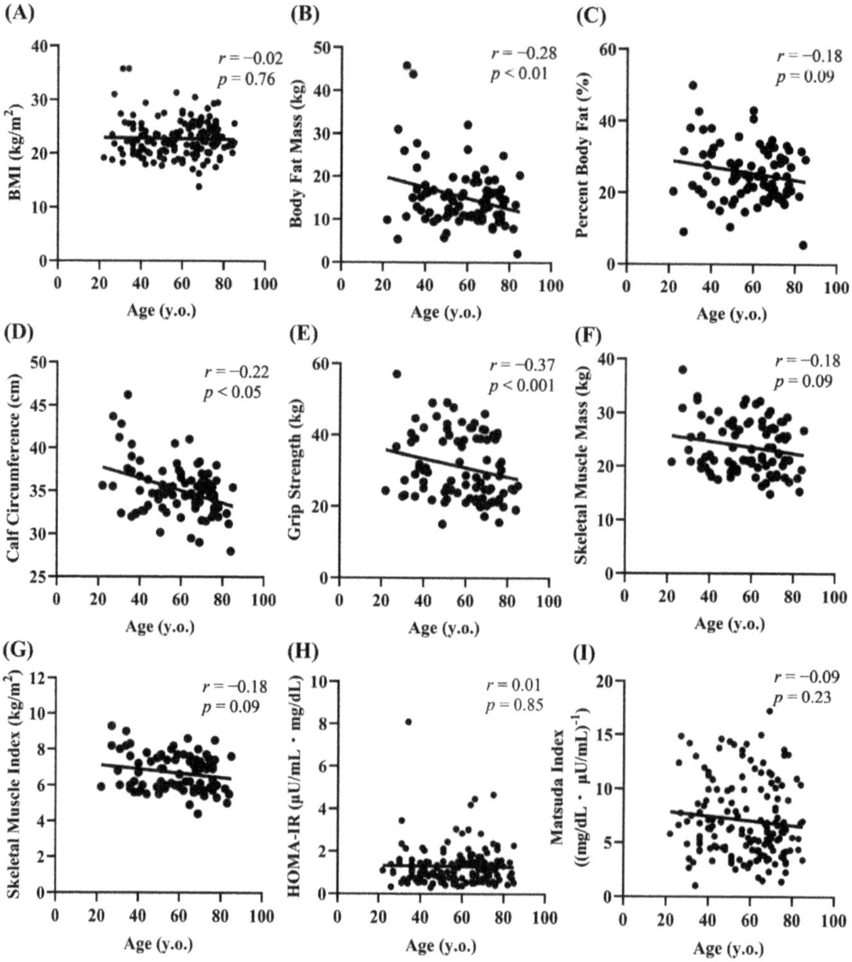

Figure 2. Relationship of age with fat/muscle mass parameters and the insulin sensitivity index. Correlation of age with adiposity (**A–C**), muscle mass (**D–G**), and the insulin sensitivity index (**H**,**I**).

3.3. Relationship Between Age and Indices of Insulin Secretion

We next investigated the relationship between age and the indices of insulin secretion. A significant negative correlation between age and HOMA-β was observed ($r = -0.31$, $p < 0.0001$) (Figure 3A). HOMA-β was significantly lower in groups 2–4 than in group 1 and in group 3 than in group 2 (group 1, 90.6 μU/mL/mg/dL; group 2, 64.0 μU/mL/mg/dL; group 3, 54.2 μU/mL/mg/dL; group 4, 58.9 μU/mL/mg/dL) (Figure 3B). The AUC of plasma insulin during the OGTT did not differ significantly among the age groups (Figure 3C,D). However, the insulinogenic index, a marker of early insulin secretion, declined with age ($r = -0.33$, $p < 0.0001$) and was significantly lower in the groups aged 60 years or older than in age group 1 (Figure 3E,F), suggesting that aging impairs early insulin secretion. The disposition index reflects the ability of β-cells to upregulate insulin secretion in response to a decrease in insulin sensitivity [25], and an age-dependent decline in the disposition index has been reported in Japanese adults between their 20s and 50s [26]. The disposition index was negatively correlated with age ($r = -0.43$, $p < 0.0001$), and the values were also significantly decreased in the groups aged 60 years or older than in the groups aged under 60 years (Figure 3G,H). Although HOMA-β, the insulinogenic index, and the disposition index decreased with age, these indices did not differ between groups 3 (60–74 years) and 4 (75 years or older) (Figure 3B,F,H). These findings may suggest that there is a limit to the decline in insulin secretion with age, or that the rate of the decline is slower in people over the age of 60.

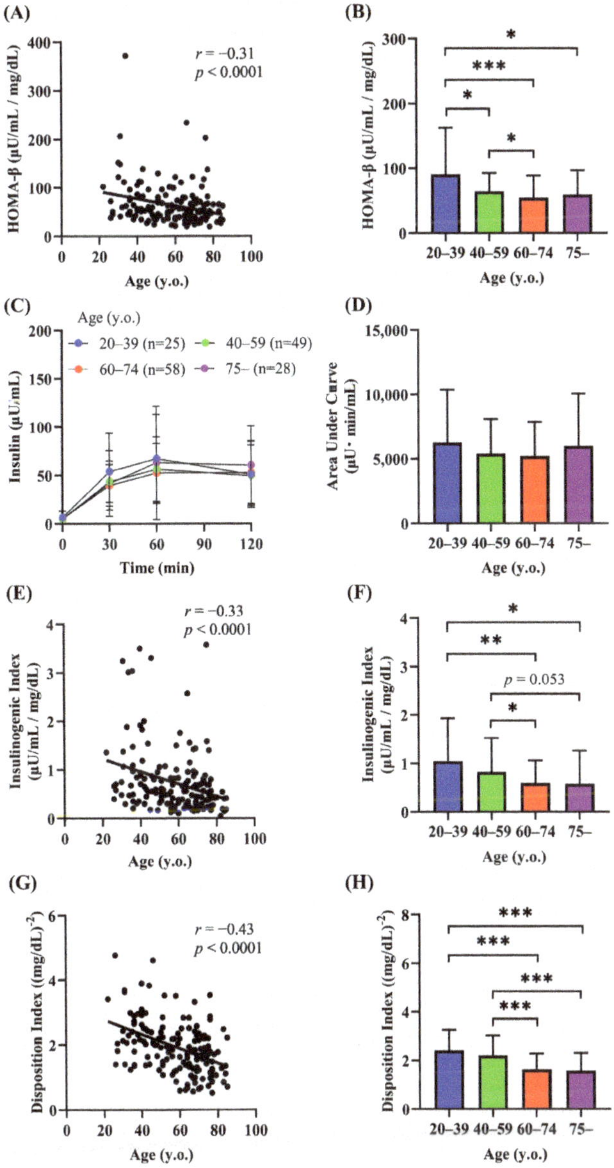

Figure 3. Relationship between age and indices of insulin secretion. Correlation of age with HOMA-β (**A**,**B**), insulin levels during the OGTT (**C**,**D**), insulinogenic index (**E**,**F**), and disposition index (**G**,**H**). Data are shown as the mean ± SD. * $p < 0.05$, ** $p < 0.01$, *** $p < 0.01$.

3.4. Effects of Aging in People with NGT

Insulin secretion is impaired in individuals with IGT and type 2 diabetes [16], and the prevalence of both IGT and diabetes was higher in the older groups (Figure 1D). To rule out the possibility that the lower insulin secretion in the older participants was simply due to the high prevalence of IGT and type 2 diabetes, we examined the effects of aging in people with NGT. A significant positive correlation between age and HbA1c was still observed (Figure 4A). Because HOMA-β, the insulinogenic index, and the disposition index were reduced in the groups aged 60 years or older than in those aged under 60 years, people with NGT (n = 106) were divided into two groups (Table 2): 60 years or older (older group) and under 60 years (younger group). The AUC-glucose was significantly higher in the older group than in the younger group (Figure 4B,C). Consistent with the previous findings, HOMA-β, the insulinogenic index, and the disposition index were negatively correlated with age ($r = -0.27$ to -0.34) (Figure 4D–F). No correlation was found between age and the indices of insulin action (Figure 4G,H).

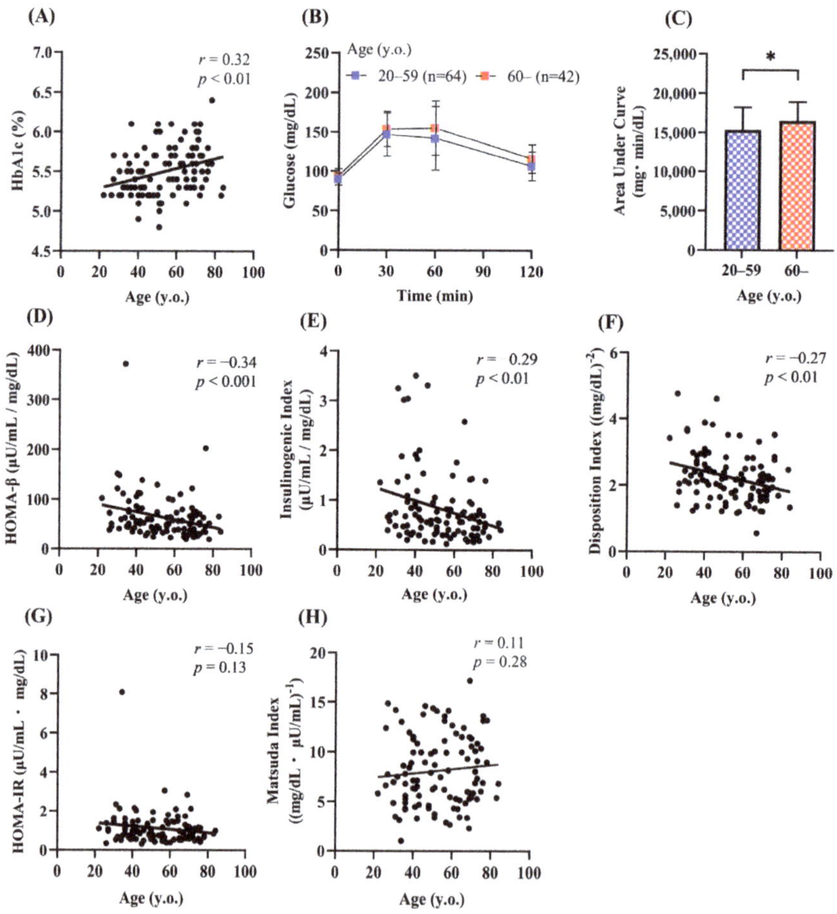

Figure 4. Effects of aging on glucose tolerance, insulin secretion, and insulin sensitivity in people with NGT. Correlation of age with the HbA1c (**A**), HOMA-β (**D**), insulinogenic index (**E**), disposition index (**F**), HOMA-IR (**G**), and Matsuda index (**H**) in the NGT group (n = 106). Plasma glucose (**B**) and the area under the curve of plasma glucose (**C**) during the 75-g OGTT. Data are shown as the mean ± SD. * $p < 0.05$.

Table 2. Characteristics of NGT individuals.

Groups	Younger Group (20–59)	Older Group (60–)	*p*
n (M, F)	64 (34, 30)	42 (18, 24)	
Age (years)	42.6 ± 9.6	70.1 ± 5.5	
BMI (kg/m^2)	22.5 ± 3.5	22.4 ± 3.1	0.919
FPG (mg/dL)	89.9 ± 7.7	94.2 ± 8.7	0.009
HbA1c (%)	5.43 ± 0.29	5.59 ± 0.28	0.006
F-IRI (μU/mL)	5.21 ± 4.3	4.28 ± 2.1	0.194
HOMA-IR (μU/mL·mg/dL)	1.18 ± 1.03	1.00 ± 0.53	0.351
Matsuda Index ((mg/dL·μU/mL)$^{-1}$)	7.97 ± 3.6	8.38 ± 3.5	0.474
HOMA-β (μU/mL/mg/dL)	71.4 ± 50	53.3 ± 33	0.006
Insulinogenic Index (μU/mL/mg/dL)	0.94 ± 0.8	0.65 ± 0.5	0.043
Disposition Index ((mg/dL)$^{-2}$)	2.38 ± 0.8	2.03 ± 0.6	0.023
Body Fat Mass (kg) §	15.6 ± 7.6	13.2 ± 4.4	0.158
Body Fat Percentage (%) §	25.2 ± 8.2	23.2 ± 6.7	0.321
Skeletal Muscle Mass (kg) §	24.6 ± 5.1	23.4 ± 4.7	0.343
Skeletal Muscle Index (kg/m^2) §	6.91 ± 1.0	6.49 ± 1.0	0.117
Calf Circumference (cm) §	36.0 ± 3.3	34.6 ± 2.6	0.077
Grip Strength (kg) §	34.4 ± 9.7	29.4 ± 8.6	0.042

Data are shown as the mean ± SD. BMI, body mass index; FPG, fasting plasma glucose; HbA1c, glycated hemoglobin (hemoglobin A1c); F-IRI, fasting immunoreactive insulin; HOMA-IR, homeostatic model assessment for insulin resistance; HOMA-β, homeostatic model assessment β-cell function. § Data were available for 63 of the participants (younger group, n = 38; older group, n = 25).

Previous studies showed that insulin secretion is associated with adiposity and skeletal muscle mass in Japanese people [27,28]. We next investigated the determinants of insulin secretion in people with NGT. HOMA-β was negatively associated with age (r = −0.34) and positively associated with BMI (r = 0.45), body fat mass (r = 0.36), percent body fat (r = 0.32), and calf circumference (r = 0.32) (Table 3). The insulinogenic index was negatively correlated with age (r = −0.35) and positively correlated with BMI (r = 0.25), body fat mass (r = 0.35), and percent body fat (r = 0.34). The disposition index showed a marginal negative correlation with age (r = −0.24) (Table 3). By multiple regression analysis, age and BMI were shown to be independent determinants of HOMA-β (Table 4). On the other hand, age was the only explanatory factor for the insulinogenic index and disposition index (Table 4).

Table 3. Correlation coefficients of the relationship between indices of insulin secretion and various parameters.

	HOMA-β		Insulinogenic Index		Disposition Index	
	r	*p*	*r*	*p*	*r*	*p*
Age	−0.34	0.007	−0.35	0.004	−0.24	0.058
Sex	−0.17	0.187	−0.09	0.502	−0.21	0.096
BMI	0.45	0.0002	0.25	0.049	−0.23	0.073
Body Fat Mass	0.36	0.004	0.35	0.005	−0.08	0.518
Percent Body Fat	0.32	0.012	0.34	0.006	0.03	0.808
Skeletal Muscle Mass	−0.08	0.527	−0.06	0.656	−0.17	0.182
Skeletal Muscle Index	0.09	0.469	0.001	0.991	−0.23	0.076
Calf Circumference	0.32	0.010	0.15	0.256	−0.20	0.109
Grip Strength	0.03	0.818	0.001	0.992	−0.17	0.190

The Pearson correlation coefficient (r) and each probability value (p) are shown. Statistically significant results ($p < 0.05$) are shown in bold. Individuals with NGT (n = 106) are included in the analysis. Body composition data were available for 63 NGT individuals.

Table 4. Multiple regression analysis for indices of insulin secretion.

	HOMA-β		Insulinogenic Index		Disposition Index	
	Std β	p	Std β	p	Std β	p
Age	−0.064	0.043	−0.053	0.013	−0.028	0.040
Sex	−0.144	0.238	0.049	0.547	−0.015	0.771
BMI	0.144	0.011	0.056	0.134	−0.019	0.423
Percent Body Fat	−0.027	0.483	0.021	0.408	0.007	0.671
Skeletal Muscle Index	−0.064	0.433	−0.055	0.315	0.004	0.905
Calf Circumference	0.012	0.841	−0.018	0.655	−0.012	0.653
Grip Strength	0.041	0.417	0.006	0.855	−0.005	0.819

The standardized regression coefficient (Std β) and each probability value (p) are shown. Statistically significant results ($p < 0.05$) are shown in bold. Individuals with NGT (n = 106) are included in the analysis. Body composition data were available for 63 NGT individuals.

4. Discussion

In the present study, we conducted OGTT in residents aged between 22 and 85 years in Koshi City, Kumamoto Prefecture, Japan, to assess the prevalence of diabetes and IGT. The prevalence of newly diagnosed diabetes was low (1 in 74: 1.4%) in individuals younger than 60 years but increased with age, peaking at 21.4% in the oldest age group (75 years or older). The prevalence of IGT, but not isolated IFG, also increased with age, and the peak prevalence of IGT exceeded 40% at the age of 75 years or older, indicating the importance of performing OGTT to detect glucose intolerance in older people. The high prevalence of type 2 diabetes and IGT in the older participants is consistent with reports from European and Asian countries [29,30].

Many previous studies have reported that insulin resistance increases with age [4–6,20], but we did not observe a worsening of insulin resistance with increasing age. It has been reported that insulin action, as measured by the euglycemic insulin clamp, decreases with age in Europeans, but that the age-related increase in insulin resistance is no longer statistically significant after adjustment for BMI [31]. We also found that BMI, but not age, is an independent determinant of HOMA-IR and the Matsuda index in NGT individuals by multiple regression analysis (Supplementary Table S1). Body fat accumulation is strongly associated with insulin resistance [2], and body fat mass did not increase with age in this study. The fact that BMI/adiposity did not increase with age may be one reason why insulin resistance was not worse in older people in this study. Further studies are needed in this regard.

In addition to obesity, the development of insulin resistance in older adults has been suggested to be associated with the loss of skeletal muscle mass [32,33]. While we observed a marginal correlation between age and the skeletal muscle index, multiple regression analysis did not show that the skeletal muscle index was a significant contributor to HOMA-IR and the Matsuda index in individuals with NGT (Supplementary Table S1). Similarly, no correlation between skeletal muscle mass and the Matsuda index was reported in another Japanese study [20]. These results may suggest that a reduction in skeletal muscle mass has less impact on insulin sensitivity in older people, at least in Japanese individuals with NGT.

Regarding insulin secretion in Japanese subjects, one study reported that HOMA-β declined with age [19], suggesting that insulin secretion decreases with age. On the other hand, another study showed no age-related change in the insulinogenic index in Japanese subjects after the age of 65 [20]. Insulin secretion in an OGTT was also comparable between middle-aged and older Japanese subjects [21]. Therefore, the effect of aging on insulin secretion in Japanese is controversial. In the present study, we found a significant negative correlation of age with HOMA-β, the insulinogenic index, and the disposition index in all participants and in those with NGT. In addition, age was shown to be the only independent determinant of these insulin secretion indices in a multiple regression analysis. Our results suggest that an age-related decline in insulin secretion plays an important role in the development of glucose intolerance in older Japanese adults. Chronic inflammation is a hallmark of aging, and the circulating levels of inflammatory cytokines and biomarkers (such as CRP) increase with age [34]. Because inflammation-related cytokines/adipokines such as IL-6, TNFα, and adiponectin have been reported to regulate insulin secretion [35–37], measuring these molecules would provide additional information on the age-related impairment of insulin secretion. The accumulation of senescent β-cells, another hallmark of aging, may also explain, at least in part, the age-related insulin secretion defect [38]. Senolysis (removal of senescent β-cells) has been reported to improve insulin secretion in mice [39].

In this study, the highest prevalence of type 2 diabetes and IGT was seen in the group aged over 75 years. However, we did not find a significant difference in insulin secretion between the groups aged 65–74 years and 75 years or older. The reasons why the highest frequency of glucose intolerance was observed in the group aged 75 years or older are unclear. Normal insulin secretion is pulsatile, but abnormalities in insulin pulsatility have been reported in older adults [1,2]. Further studies are needed to clarify the reasons for the high prevalence of glucose intolerance in the very old group.

There are several limitations to this study. First, because of the cross-sectional design, it is inappropriate to assess the cause–effect relationship and to extrapolate the age-related decline in insulin secretion for each individual. Second, we found the age-related decline in insulin secretion in Japanese subjects, but the number of participants was relatively small. Third, insulin secretion is affected by oxidative stress, endoplasmic reticulum stress, inflammation, and hypoxia [40]. However, we did not measure parameters related to these stresses. Fourth, we cannot exclude the possibility of selection bias in the study. We enrolled only non-diabetic individuals on the basis of self-reported information. It is therefore possible that people with increased insulin resistance were already diagnosed with diabetes and therefore excluded from the study. Finally, we did not assess the lifestyle of the participants, such as their dietary habits and physical activity.

5. Conclusions

In conclusion, this study showed that the age-related high prevalence of diabetes and IGT is associated with impaired insulin secretion rather than insulin resistance in Japanese individuals. Further studies are necessary to understand why insulin secretion declines with age in order to develop new strategies for the prevention and treatment of type 2 diabetes.

Supplementary Materials: The following supporting information can be downloaded at: https://www.mdpi.com/article/10.3390/biomedicines13020380/s1, Supplementary Table S1: Multiple regression analysis for indices of insulin resistance.

Author Contributions: Conceptualization, K.F., M.H. and K.Y.; methodology, K.F., M.H. and K.Y.; software, M.H.; validation, K.F., M.H. and K.Y.; formal analysis, K.F. and M.H.; investigation, K.F., M.H., N.K., E.A. and K.Y.; resources, K.F. and M.H.; data curation, K.F., M.H. and K.Y.; writing—original draft preparation, K.Y.; writing—review and editing, N.K. and E.A.; visualization, K.F. and M.H.; supervision, N.K. and E.A.; project administration, K.F. and K.Y.; funding acquisition, E.A. and K.Y. All authors have read and agreed to the published version of the manuscript.

Funding: This work was supported by a Grant-in-Aid for Scientific Research (B) (22H03129), a Grant-in-Aid for Challenging Research (Exploratory) (23K18302), a grant from Takeda Science Foundation, and a grant from Manpei Suzuki Diabetes Foundation.

Institutional Review Board Statement: The study was conducted in accordance with the Declaration of Helsinki. This study was approved by the ethics committees of the Kumamoto University Graduate School of Medicine (No. 2602, 8 November 2022).

Informed Consent Statement: Written informed consent and opt-out informed consent were obtained from all participants.

Data Availability Statement: The data that support the findings of this study is available on request to the corresponding author. The data are not publicly available due to privacy or ethical restrictions.

Acknowledgments: The authors thank Miyagawa K., Kiyohara Y., Koga K., Sato M., the staff at Kikuchi Yojyoen, and the staff at Koshi Town Hall who contributed to data collection. We also thank Tsuyama T., Takeshita M., Sakaguchi M., Igata M., and Matsumura T. (Kumamoto University) for their helpful discussion.

Conflicts of Interest: The authors declare no conflicts of interest.

References

1. Chang, A.M.; Holter, J.B. Aging and insulin secretion. *Am. J. Physiol. Endocrinol. Metab.* **2003**, *284*, E7–E12. [CrossRef]
2. Scheen, A.J. Diabetes mellitus in the elderly: Insulin resistance and/or impaired insulin secretion? *Diabetes Metab.* **2005**, *31*, 5S27–5S34. [CrossRef]
3. GBD 2021 Diabetes Collaborators. Global, regional, and national burden of diabetes from 1990 to 2021, with projections of prevalence to 2050: A systematic analysis for the Global Burden of Disease Study 2021. *Lancet* **2023**, *402*, 203–234. [CrossRef]
4. Chen, M.; Bergman, R.N.; Pacini, G.; Porte, D., Jr. Pathogenesis of age-related glucose intolerance in man: Insulin resistance and decreased b-cell function. *J. Clin. Endocrinol. Metab.* **1985**, *60*, 13–20. [CrossRef]
5. DeFronzo, R.A. Glucose intolerance and aging: Evidence for tissue insensitivity to insulin. *Diabetes* **1979**, *28*, 1095–1101. [CrossRef]
6. Coon, P.J.; Rogus, E.M.; Drinkwater, D.; Muller, D.C.; Goldberg, A.P. Role of body fat distribution in the decline in insulin sensitivity and glucose tolerance with age. *J. Clin. Endocrinol. Metab.* **1992**, *75*, 1125–1132.
7. Ahren, B.; Pacini, G. Age-related reduction in glucose elimination is accompanied by reduced glucose effectiveness and increased hepatic insulin extraction in man. *J. Clin. Endocrinol. Metab.* **1998**, *83*, 3350–3356. [CrossRef]
8. Boden, G.; Chen, X.; DeSantis, R.A.; Kendrick, Z. Effects of age and body fat on insulin resistance in healthy men. *Diabetes Care* **1993**, *16*, 728–733. [CrossRef]
9. Xiao, J.; Weng, J.; Ji, L.; Jia, W.; Lu, J.; Shan, Z.; Liu, J.; Tian, H.; Ji, Q.; Yang, Z.; et al. Worse pancreatic β-cell function and better insulin sensitivity in older Chinese without diabetes. *J. Gerontol. A Biol. Sci. Med. Sci.* **2014**, *69*, 463–470. [CrossRef]
10. Guminer, B.; Polonsky, K.S.; Beltz, W.F.; Wallace, P.; Brechtel, G.; Fink, R.I. Effects of aging on insulin secretion. *Diabetes* **1989**, *38*, 1549–1556. [CrossRef]
11. Basu, R.; Breda, E.; Oberg, A.L.; Powell, C.C.; Man, C.D.; Basu, A.; Vittone, J.L.; Klee, G.G.; Arora, P.; Jensen, M.D.; et al. Mechanisms of the age-associated deterioration in glucose tolerance. *Diabetes* **2003**, *52*, 1738–1748. [CrossRef]
12. Chang, A.M.; Smith, M.J.; Galecki, A.T.; Bloem, C.J.; Halter, J.B. Impaired β-cell function in human aging: Response to nicotinic acid-induced insulin resistance. *J. Clin. Endocrinol. Metab.* **2006**, *91*, 3303–3309. [CrossRef]
13. Ihm, S.H.; Matsumoto, I.; Sawada, T.; Nakano, M.; Zhang, H.; Ansite, J.D.; Sutherland, D.E.R.; Hering, B.L. Effect of donor age on function of isolated human islets. *Diabetes* **2006**, *55*, 1361–1368. [CrossRef]
14. Broughton, D.L.; James, O.W.; Alberti, K.G.; Taylor, R. Peripheral and hepatic insulin sensitivity in healthy elderly human subjects. *Eur. J. Clin. Invest.* **1991**, *21*, 13–21. [CrossRef]
15. Elahi, D.; Muller, D.C.; McAloon-Dyke, M.; Tobin, J.D.; Andres, R. The effect of age on insulin response and glucose utilization during four hyperglycemic plateaus. *Exp. Gerontol.* **1993**, *28*, 393–409. [CrossRef]
16. Yabe, D.; Seino, Y.; Fukushima, M.; Sino, S. β cell dysfunction versus insulin resistance in the pathogenesis of type 2 diabetes in east Asians. *Curr. Diab Rep.* **2015**, *15*, 36. [CrossRef]
17. Kodama, K.; Tojjar, D.; Yamada, S.; Toda, K.; Patel, C.J.; Butte, A.J. Ethnic differences in the relationship between insulin sensitivity and insulin response. *Diabetes Care* **2013**, *36*, 1789–1796. [CrossRef]
18. Møller, J.B.; Pedersen, M.; Tanaka, H.; Ohsugi, M.; Overgaard, R.V.; Lynge, J.; Almind, K.; Vasconcelos, N.M.; Poulsen, P.; Keller, C.; et al. Body composition is the main determinant for the difference in type 2 diabetes pathophysiology between Japanese and Caucasians. *Diabetes Care* **2014**, *37*, 796–804. [CrossRef]
19. Hirose, H.; Takayama, M.; Iwano, Y.; Kawabe, H. Effects of aging on visceral and subcutaneous fat areas and on homeostasis model assessment of insulin resistance and insulin secretion capacity in a comprehensive health checkup. *J. Atheroscler. Thromb.* **2016**, *23*, 207–215. [CrossRef]

20. Naito, H.; Kaga, H.; Someya, Y.; Tabata, H.; Kakehi, S.; Tajima, T.; Ito, N.; Yamasaki, N.; Sato, M.; Kadowaki, S.; et al. Fat accumulation and elevated free fatty acid are associated with age-related glucose intolerance: Bunkyo health study. *J. Endocrine Society* **2024**, *8*, bvad164. [CrossRef]
21. Shimizu, M.; Kawazu, S.; Tomono, S.; Ohno, T.; Utsugi, T.; Kato, N.; Ishi, C.; Ito, Y.; Murata, K. Age-related alteration of pancreatic β-cell function. *Diabetes Care* **1996**, *19*, 8–11. [CrossRef]
22. Matthews, D.R.; Hosker, J.P.; Rudenski, A.S.; Naylor, B.A.; Treacher, D.F.; Turner, R.C. Homeostasis model assessment: Insulin resistance and β-cell function from fasting plasma glucose and insulin concentrations in man. *Diabetologia* **1985**, *28*, 412–419. [CrossRef]
23. Matsuda, M.; DeFronzo, R.A. Insulin sensitivity indices obtained from oral glucose tolerance testing: Comparison with the euglycemic insulin clamp. *Diabetes Care* **1999**, *22*, 1462–1470. [CrossRef]
24. Gastaldelli, A.; Ferrannini, E.; Miyazaki, Y.; Matsuda, M.; DeFronzo, R.A.; San Antonio metabolism study. Beta-cell dysfunction and glucose intolerance: Results from the San Antonio metabolism (SAM) study. *Diabetologia* **2004**, *47*, 31–39. [CrossRef]
25. Retnakaran, R.; Shen, S.; Hanley, A.J.; Vuksan, V.; Hamilton, J.K.; Zinman, B. Hyperbolic relationship between insulin secretion and sensitivity on oral glucose tolerance test. *Obesity* **2008**, *16*, 1901–1907. [CrossRef]
26. Komada, H.; Sakaguchi, K.; Takeda, K.; Hirota, Y.; Hashimoto, N.; Okuno, Y.; Seino, S.; Ogawa, W. Age-dependent decline in β-cell function assessed by an oral glucose tolerance test-based disposition index. *J. Diabetes Investig.* **2011**, *2*, 293–296. [CrossRef]
27. Fukuda-Akita, E.; Okita, K.; Okauchi, Y.; Ryo, M.; Nakamura, T.; Funahashi, T.; Iwahashi, H.; Shimomura, I.; Miyagawa, J.; Yamagata, K. Impaired early insulin secretion in Japanese type 2 diabetes with metabolic syndrome. *Diabetes Res. Clin. Pract.* **2008**, *79*, 482–489. [CrossRef]
28. Sakai, S.; Tanimoto, K.; Imbe, A.; Inaba, Y.; Shishikura, K.; Tanimoto, Y.; Ushiroyama, T.; Terasaki, J.; Hanafusa, T. Decreased β-cell function is associated with reduced skeletal muscle mass in Japanese subjects without diabetes. *PLoS ONE* **2016**, *11*, e0162603. [CrossRef]
29. DECODE Study Group. Age- and sex-specific prevalence of diabetes and impaired glucose regulation in 13 European cohorts. *Diabetes Care* **2003**, *26*, 61–69. [CrossRef]
30. The DECODA Study Group. Age- and sex-specific prevalence of diabetes and impaired glucose regulation in 11 Asian cohorts. *Diabetes Care* **2003**, *26*, 1770–1780. [CrossRef]
31. Ferrannini, E.; Vichi, S.; Beck-Nielsen, H.; Laakso, M.; Paolisso, G.; Smith, U. Insulin action and age. European Group for the Study of Insulin Resistance (EGIR). *Diabetes* **1996**, *45*, 947–953. [CrossRef] [PubMed]
32. Lee, S.W.; Youm, Y.; Lee, W.J.; Choi, W.; Chu, S.H.; Park, Y.R.; Kim, H.C. Addendicular skeletal muscle mass and insulin resistance in an elderly Korean population: The Korean social life, health and aging project-health examination cohort. *Diabetes Metab. J.* **2015**, *39*, 37–45. [CrossRef] [PubMed]
33. Barzilay, J.I.; Cotsonis, G.A.; Walston, J.; Schwartz, A.V.; Satterfield, S.; Miljkovic, I.; Harris, T.B.; Health ABC Study. Insulin resistance is associated with decreased quadriceps muscle strength in nondiabetic adults aged >70 years. *Diabetes Care* **2009**, *32*, 736–738. [CrossRef]
34. López-Otín, C.; Blasco, M.A.; Partridge, L.; Serrano, M.; Kroemer, G. Hallmarks of aging: An expanding universe. *Cell* **2023**, *186*, 243–278. [CrossRef]
35. Suzuki, T.; Imai, J.; Yamada, T.; Ishigaki, Y.; Kaneko, K.; Uno, K.; Hasegawa, Y.; Ishihara, H.; Oka, Y.; Katagiri, H. Interleukin-6 enhances glucose-stimulated insulin secretion from pancreatic beta-cells: Potential involvement of the PLC-IP3-dependent pathway. *Diabetes* **2011**, *60*, 537–547. [CrossRef] [PubMed]
36. Zhang, S.; Kim, K.H. TNF-α inhibits glucose-induced insulin secretion in a pancreatic β-cell line (INS-1). *FEBS Lett.* **1995**, *377*, 237–239. [CrossRef]
37. Okamoto, M.; Ohara-Imaizumi, M.; Kubota, N.; Hashimoto, S.; Eto, K.; Kanno, T.; Kubota, T.; Wakui, M.; Nagai, R.; Noda, M. Adiponectin induces insulin secretion in vitro and in vivo at a low glucose concentration. *Diabetologia* **2008**, *51*, 827–835. [CrossRef] [PubMed]
38. Aguayo-Mazzucato, C. Functional changes in beta cells during ageing and senescence. *Diabetologia* **2020**, *63*, 2022–2029. [CrossRef] [PubMed]
39. Aguayo-Mazzucato, C.; Andle, J.; Lee, T.B., Jr.; Midha, A.; Talemal, L.; Chipashvili, V.; Hollister-Lock, J.; van Deursen, J.; Weir, G.; Bonner-Weir, S. Acceleration of β Cell Aging Determines Diabetes and Senolysis Improves Disease Outcomes. *Cell Metab.* **2019**, *30*, 129–142. [CrossRef]
40. Yamagata, K.; Tsuyama, T.; Sato, Y. Roles of beta-cell hypoxia in the progression of type 2 diabetes. *Int. J. Mol. Sci.* **2024**, *25*, 4186. [CrossRef]

biomedicines

MDPI

Article

The Influence of COVID-19 in Glycemic Control: Predictive Value of Inflammation and Metabolic Parameters

Minodora Andor [1,2], Dana Emilia Man [3,4,*], Daciana Carmen Nistor [5,6], Valentina Buda [7] and Simona Dragan [3,4]

1 Discipline of Medical Semiotics II, Department V—Internal Medicine—1, "Victor Babes" University of Medicine and Pharmacy, 300041 Timisoara, Romania; andor.minodora@umft.ro
2 Multidisciplinary Heart Research Centre, "Victor Babes" University of Medicine and Pharmacy, 300041 Timisoara, Romania
3 Department VI—Cardiology, University Clinic of Internal Medicine and Ambulatory Care, Prevention and Cardiovascular Recovery, "Victor Babes" University of Medicine and Pharmacy, 300041 Timisoara, Romania; simona.dragan@umft.ro
4 Research Centre of Timisoara Institute of Cardiovascular Diseases, "Victor Babes" University of Medicine and Pharmacy, 300041 Timisoara, Romania
5 Department of Functional Sciences, Physiology, Center of Immuno-Physiology and Biotechnologies (CIFBIOTEH), "Victor Babes" University of Medicine and Pharmacy, 300041 Timisoara, Romania; daciana_nistor@umft.ro
6 Centre for Gene and Cellular Therapies in Cancer, 300723 Timisoara, Romania
7 Department I, Faculty of Pharmacy, University Clinic of Clinical Pharmacy, Communication in Pharmacy, Pharmaceutical Care, "Victor Babes" University of Medicine and Pharmacy, 300041 Timisoara, Romania; buda.valentina@umft.ro
* Correspondence: man.dana@umft.ro

Abstract: Background/Objectives: Predicting post-COVID-19 diabetes is crucial for enhancing patient care and public health. This study investigates the role of metabolic factors in predicting the glycemic outcomes in patients recovering from moderate to severe COVID-19. Methods: We conducted a retrospective analysis of 135 patients without pre-existing diabetes, selected from a cohort of 1980 individuals hospitalized between January 2020 and December 2022. Metabolic parameters, including blood glucose, Homeostasis Model Assessment of Insulin Resistance (HOMA-IR), Triglyceride/Glucose (TyG) index, and high-sensitivity C-reactive protein (hs-CRP), were assessed at discharge and followed up after 4 months (T4) and 12 months (T12). Results: Statistical analysis revealed significant correlations of initial glycemia, HOMA-IR, and hs-CRP with the subsequent glycemic levels at T4 and T12. Multiple regression analysis confirmed that initial glycemia, HOMA-IR, and hs-CRP were strong predictors of elevated glycemia, while the TyG index did not show a significant predictive value. Conventional diabetes risk factors, including body mass index (BMI) and lipid profiles, showed low predictive power for post-COVID-19 glycemia. Conclusions: This research highlights the critical role of metabolic and inflammatory pathways in managing glycemic control in COVID-19 patients. Markers like blood glucose, HOMA-IR, and hs-CRP are significant predictors of blood glucose levels, while the TyG index appears less helpful in this context. Early, targeted interventions based on these markers can improve patient outcomes and reduce the risk of post-COVID-19 complications like diabetes.

Keywords: post-COVID-19 diabetes; glycemic outcomes; metabolic factors; HOMA-IR; hs-CRP; TyG index; insulin resistance; predictive analysis; COVID-19 recovery

1. Introduction

Predicting the development of diabetes (DM) after COVID-19 is not just valuable but also essential for optimizing patient care, reducing the burden of diabetes-related complications, and improving overall public health outcomes. It allows for proactive management, personalized healthcare, and better resource allocation, ultimately leading to a more effective and efficient healthcare delivery. After the COVID-19 pandemic, numerous studies have demonstrated changes in the metabolic profile, with an increase in the incidence of diabetes. Previous studies indicated that DM is associated with an increased risk of severe COVID-19, acute respiratory distress syndrome (ARDS), and in-hospital mortality [1–3]. People with persistent long COVID symptoms can experience pulmonary and extrapulmonary manifestations, including the occurrence of DM. More intriguingly, a recent meta-analysis reported that newly diagnosed DM is frequently seen in patients with COVID-19 [4]. The world has expressed concern about a two-way relationship between these two conditions [5,6]. A follow-up of children with COVID-19 has identified that the incidence of newly diagnosed type 1 DM has increased [7]. Individuals with DM are at greater risk of severe outcomes if they contract COVID-19. This includes increased rates of hospitalization, need for intensive care, and mortality [8].

Additionally, DM can impair the immune response, making it harder for the body to fight off infections, including COVID-19. This can lead to more severe disease progression [9]. Chronic hyperglycemia is associated with increased inflammation, which can exacerbate the inflammatory response seen in severe COVID-19 cases [10]. Some patients who contract COVID-19 have been observed to develop DM even though the classical risk factors for DM are not present. This could be due to the virus's direct damage to pancreatic beta cells, stress-induced hyperglycemia, or the use of certain medications (e.g., steroids) [11]. Moreover, patients with pre-existing DM may experience severe complications like diabetic ketoacidosis and a hyperosmolar hyperglycemic state when presenting with COVID-19. These conditions often require significantly higher doses of insulin and more intensive medical management [12].

Predicting the development of DM after a COVID-19 infection can be highly useful for several reasons. Identifying individuals at risk of developing post-COVID-19 DM can enable early interventions, such as lifestyle modifications (diet and exercise) and pharmacologic therapy, to prevent or delay the onset of DM. By monitoring individuals identified as at-risk for early signs of hyperglycemia, healthcare professionals can be vigilant and attentive, allowing for timely medical intervention and management. Prediction models can help healthcare providers create personalized treatment plans that address both the acute effects of COVID-19 and the potential for developing DM [13].

Healthcare systems can allocate resources more effectively by identifying patients who may require more intensive follow-up and management. The early detection and management of DM can prevent or reduce the risk of complications such as cardiovascular disease, neuropathy, nephropathy, and retinopathy, which are commonly associated with uncontrolled DM.

Predicting the development of DM can provide valuable data for public health officials to understand the long-term impacts of COVID-19 on population health.

Purpose of the Study

Experimental observations and data from the literature suggest that blood glucose values, or even the onset of DM, are influenced by both metabolic factors and comorbidities [14–16]. In our study, we aimed to investigate these hypotheses by examining the influence of metabolic factors (blood glucose values, HOMA-IR, TyG index) during the acute phase of COVID-19 infection in a group of patients who were subsequently followed up at 4 months and 12 months. Additionally, we considered the comorbidities present before the COVID-19 infection that could contribute to the onset of DM or at least influence elevated glycemic levels.

To make an effective prediction, we used clinical and biological data from a cohort admitted with moderate and severe forms of COVID-19 at the Cardiological Rehabilitation Clinic in Timisoara, Romania.

2. Materials and Methods

A retrospective study was performed on a cohort of patients hospitalized between January 2020 and December 2022 at the Cardiovascular Rehabilitation Center of the Institute of Cardiovascular Diseases, Timisoara, Romania. The inclusion/exclusion criteria are presented in Figure 1.

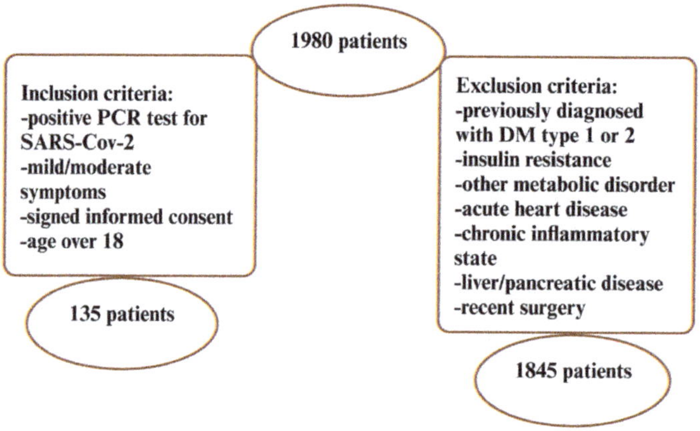

Figure 1. Inclusion/exclusion criteria (created with BioRender.com). Abbreviations: PCR—polymerase chain reaction; SARS-CoV-2—severe acute respiratory syndrome coronavirus 2; DM—diabetes mellitus.

2.1. Clinical Variables and Laboratory Parameters

Demographic data and epidemiological factors such as gender, age, body mass index, smoking status, hypertension status, or other previous cardiovascular comorbidities, along with clinical and laboratory data, were analyzed. This included an evaluation of cardiovascular risk factors, as well as a review of personal pathological history and comorbidities. Inflammatory marker analysis and the biochemical function test Basic Metabolic Panel (BMP), including the determination of glucose, calcium, electrolytes (Sodium, Potassium, Chloride, Bicarbonate, Blood Urea Nitrogen (BUN) and Creatinine), Estimated Glomerular Filtration Rate (eGFR), Alanine Aminotransferase (ALT) and Aspartate Aminotransferase (AST), Alkaline Phosphatase (ALP), bilirubin, albumin, complete blood count, were carried out. Hemoglobin A1c (HbA1c), insulin levels, HOMA-IR, and TyG index were also analyzed. Fasting serum samples were collected at specific intervals, stored at −80 °C, and tested for proinsulin, HbA1c, and basal blood glucose. Additionally, during the arginine stimulation test and at 4 and 12 months (T0, T4, T12), they were analyzed for insulin, C-peptide, and glucagon. Insulin secretion was measured using an intravenous arginine stimulation test, with blood samples taken at baseline and 2, 5, 10, and 30 min after a 5 g arginine injection. The Acute Insulin Response to Glucose (AIRglucose) was calculated, and beta cell function and insulin resistance were assessed using the insulin-to-proinsulin ratio, HOMA-IR, and TyG index.

Insulin resistance was calculated using the HOMA-IR formula and the Triglyceride/Glucose (TyG) index equation.

$$\text{HOMA-IR} = \text{fasting insulin } [(\mu U/mL) \times \text{fasting glucose } (mg/dL)]/405 \quad (1)$$

$$\text{TyG} = \text{Ln } [\text{TG } (mg/dL) \times \text{fasting glucose } (mg/dL)/2] \quad (2)$$

2.2. Statistical Analysis

Our data were stored in an Excel spreadsheet. To assess the influence of metabolic parameters on the prediction of glycemic values post-COVID-19, we performed multiple linear regressions with the dependent variable being glycemia at the 4-month (Glyc-T4) control and at the 12-month (Glyc-T12) control. The significance level for the correlation coefficient in both simple and multiple linear regression was set at $p = 0.05$. The independent variables were the following metabolic parameters determined during hospitalization for an acute episode of COVID-19, just before discharge when the acute episode was considered cured: blood glucose, Triglyceride/Glucose index (TyG), Homeostasis Model Assessment for Insulin Resistance (HOMA-IR), and high-sensitivity C-reactive protein (hs-CRP).

Since comorbidities prior to COVID-19 infection could have an impact on elevated blood glucose values, another multiple linear regression was performed with the same dependent variables (Glyc-T4 and Glyc-T12) but a different set of independent variables: blood glucose at discharge from the acute episode of COVID-19, body mass index (BMI), waist/hip ratio (W/H), and the lipid profile consisting of the values of total cholesterol (TC), triglyceride (TG), LDL-cholesterol (LDLc), and HDL-cholesterol (HDLc).

2.3. Ethics Approval and Patient-Informed Consent

Written informed consent was obtained from all patients for routine admission to our tertiary university hospital for future research and study purposes. Before commencing the study, ethics approval was obtained from the Ethics Committee for Scientific Research of the Cardiovascular Institute of Timisoara (ref. nr. 2193/25 March 2024). The study was carried out following the Declaration of Helsinki.

3. Results

The data were processed, leading to the following descriptive statistics results. The blood glucose values are shown in Table 1. The average blood glucose values at T4 and T12 increased compared to the initial average value. The application of the paired t-test showed that these increases were statistically significant (Table 1).

Table 1. Differences between Glyc-T0 and Glyc-T4 and Glyc-T0 and Glyc-T12.

	Glyc-T0	**Glyc-T4**	**Glyc-T12**
Mean	104.8 ± 33.7	116.2 ± 34.45	119.3 ± 33.1
Pearson correlation with Glyc-T0		0.865	0.770
$P(T \leq t)$ two-tail		9.25×10^{-12}	1.12×10^{-11}

Glyc-T0—initial glycemia; Glyc-T4—glycemia at the 4-month control; Glyc-T12—glycemia at the 12-month control.

As a first analysis, we examined the pairwise correlations between multiple measurements at discharge and glycemia at T4 and T12. We observed that glycemia at T4 and T12 correlated with initial glycemia, HOMA-IR, and hs-CRP, measured at discharge after the acute episode of COVID-19, with correlation coefficients greater than 0.3 (see Table 2).

Table 2. Pairwise correlation between the studied parameters.

	Glyc-T12	**Glyc-T4**	**Glyc-T0**	**TyG**	**HOMA-IR**	**hs-CRP T0**	**W/H**	**BMI**	**TC**	**TG**	**HDLc**	**LDLc**
Glyc-T12	1											
Glyc-T4	**0.949**	1										
Glyc-T0	**0.770**	**0.865**	1									
TyG	**0.418**	**0.430**	**0.444**	1								
HOMA-IR	**0.617**	**0.581**	**0.340**	0.170	1							
hs-CRP T0	**0.539**	**0.493**	0.227	0.220	**0.638**	1						
W/H	0.100	0.057	0.001	−0.063	0.030	0.041	1					
BMI	0.150	0.108	0.066	−0.016	0.089	−0.003	0.294	1				
TC	−0.145	−0.143	−0.111	0.217	−0.092	−0.077	0.007	−0.067	1			
TG	0.015	−0.012	−0.044	**0.828**	−0.040	0.073	−0.114	−0.076	**0.376**	1		
HDLc	−0.120	−0.117	0.015	−0.407	−0.119	−0.195	−0.094	0.019	0.186	−0.362	1	
LDLc	−0.135	−0.121	−0.090	0.028	−0.075	−0.084	0.130	−0.016	**0.790**	0.108	0.016	1

Glyc-T12—glycemia at the 12-month control; Glyc-T4—glycemia at the 4-month control; Glyc-T0—initial glycemia; TyG—Triglyceride/Glucose index; HOMA-IR—Homeostasis Model Assessment for Insulin Resistance; hs-CRP T0—high-sensitivity C-reactive protein at T0; W/H—waist/hip ratio; BMI—body mass index; TC—total cholesterol; TG—triglyceride; HDLc—HDL-cholesterol; LDLc—LDL-cholesterol. Bold values highlight important findings.

We used multiple regression analysis to build a better predictive model of long-term glycemia. We performed multiple regressions predicting glycemia at T4 and T12 with the following independent variables: glycemia at T0, TyG, HOMA-IR, hs-CRP, W/H, BMI, TC, TG, LDLc, and HDLc.

The R value for the T4 prediction was 0.933, while for the T12 prediction, it was 0.886. For the T4 prediction, we observed that three coefficients were significantly predictive: glycemia at T0, HOMA-IR, and hs-CRP. For T12, we observed the same three coefficients being significantly predictive: Glyc-T0, HOMA-IR, and hs-CRP (Table 3).

Table 3. Multiple regression—prediction of glycemia dependence on all factors at T4 and T12.

	Glyc-T4		**Glyc-T12**	
R	**0.933**		**0.886**	
	Coefficients	***p*-Value**	**Coefficients**	***p*-Value**
Intercept	29.79	0.673	−51.60	0.557
Glyc-T0	0.792	$\mathbf{3.72 \times 10^{-21}}$	0.580	$\mathbf{5.04 \times 10^{-10}}$
TyG	−5.828	0.720	10.01	0.621
HOMA-IR	1.659	$\mathbf{2.05 \times 10^{-5}}$	2.026	$\mathbf{2.77 \times 10^{-5}}$
hs-CRP T0	0.293	$\mathbf{4.14 \times 10^{-5}}$	0.338	**0.00013**
W/H	18.11	0.368	38.84	0.121
BMI	0.157	0.319	0.305	0.121
TC	0.022	0.651	0.0053	0.932
TG	0.0075	0.835	−0.0076	0.865
HDLc	−0.214	0.069	−0.071	0.623
LDLc	−0.038	0.426	−0.042	0.474

Glyc-T4—glycemia at the 4-month control; Glyc-T12—glycemia at the 12-month control; Glyc-T0—initial glycemia; TyG—Triglyceride/Glucose index; HOMA-IR—Homeostasis Model Assessment for Insulin Resistance; hs-CRP T0—high-sensitivity C-reactive protein at T0; W/H—waist/hip ratio; BMI—body mass index; TC—total cholesterol; TG—triglyceride; HDLc—HDL-cholesterol; LDLc—LDL-cholesterol. Bold values highlight important findings.

In a follow-up multiple regression analysis, we examined the dependence of blood glucose at T4 on blood glucose at T0, TyG, HOMA-IR, and hs-CRP. Applying multiple linear correlation analysis led to the results presented in Table 4. A strong multiple correlation was observed. We noted that the parameters of blood glucose at T0, HOMA-IR, and hs-CRP provided strongly significant contributions (all $p < 0.001$), while the contribution of TyG appeared to be insignificant ($p > 0.05$). Similarly, we examined the dependence of the T12 glucose values on the same parameters and observed a very strong multiple correlation. Consistent with the findings from the T4 glucose analysis, the contributions of blood glucose at T0, HOMA-IR, and hs-CRP were significant, while the TyG contribution remained insignificant ($p > 0.05$) (Table 4).

Table 4. Multiple linear regression allowing for the estimation of Glyc-T4 and Glyc-T12 dependence on metabolic factors—selected by prediction significance.

	Glyc-T4		**Glyc-T12**	
R	**0.929**		**0.876**	
	Coefficients	***p*-Value**	**Coefficients**	***p*-Value**
Intercept	17.99	6.17×10^{-6}	33.56	1.19×10^{-10}
Glyc-T0	0.767	$\mathbf{9.53 \times 10^{-46}}$	0.618	$\mathbf{4.82 \times 10^{-28}}$
HOMA	1.713	$\mathbf{8.82 \times 10^{-6}}$	2.082	$\mathbf{1.61 \times 10^{-5}}$
hs-CRP T0	0.313	$\mathbf{8.63 \times 10^{-6}}$	0.362	$\mathbf{3.76 \times 10^{-5}}$

Glyc-T4—glycemia at the 4-month control; Glyc-T12—glycemia at the 12-month control; Glyc-T0—initial glycemia; HOMA—Homeostasis Model Assessment; hs-CRP T0—high-sensitivity C-reactive protein at T0. Bold values highlight important findings.

Even though TyG has been reported [17,18] as a reliable surrogate marker of insulin resistance and an independent predictor of DM, our results do not provide evidence for its significance in predicting the evolution of glycemia. If TyG is eliminated from the above table, after recalculations, the results are those in Table 5.

Table 5. Multiple linear correlation allowing for the estimation of Glyc-T4 and Glyc-T12 dependence on conventional diabetes risk factors.

	Glyc-T4		**Glyc-T12**	
R	**0.204**		**0.244**	
	Coefficients	***p*-Value**	**Coefficients**	***p*-Value**
Intercept	114.6	0.048	85.72	0.120
W/H	16.27	0.762	39.45	0.443
BMI	0.444	0.293	0.572	0.155
TC	−0.027	0.837	−0.024	0.846
TG	−0.006	0.883	0.0074	0.848
HDLc	−0.295	0.316	−0.245	0.382
LDLc	−0.066	0.603	−0.082	0.496

Glyc-T4—glycemia at the 4-month control; Glyc-T12—glycemia at the 12-month control; W/H—waist/hip ratio; BMI—body mass index; TC—total cholesterol; TG—triglyceride; HDLc—HDL-cholesterol; LDLc—LDL-cholesterol.

Hence, we could write the resulting relations for the predicted values pred_Glyc-T4 (Figure 2) and pred_Glyc-T12:

$$\text{Pred\_Glyc-T4} = 17.99 + 0.767 \times \text{Glyc-T0} + 1.713 \times \text{HOMA} + 0.313 \times \text{hs-CRP-T0} \quad (3)$$

$$\text{Pred\_Glyc-T12} = 33.56 + 0.618 \times \text{Glyc-T0} + 2.082 \times \text{HOMA} + 0.362 \times \text{hs-CRP-T0} \quad (4)$$

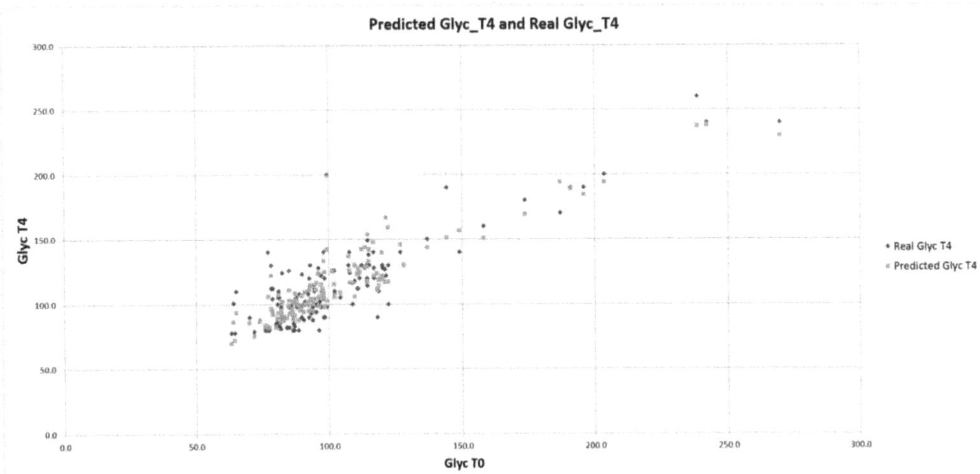

Figure 2. Predicted Glyc-T4 calculated with Equation (3). Glyc-T4—glycemia at the 4-month control; Glyc-T0—initial glycemia.

A similar plot was used to predict Glyc-T12. A second track mentioned in the study's hypothesis is the dependence of blood glucose variations on conventional DM risk factors prior to the COVID-19 infection, which could impact changes in blood glucose values. These comorbidities are reflected by W/H, BMI, and lipid profile. Applying multiple linear correlation analyses for T4 blood glucose showed a low correlation coefficient. Similarly, for blood glucose at T12, a low correlation coefficient was found (Table 5). As shown in the tables, none of the coefficients had a statistically significant contribution.

4. Discussion

Research shows an increased likelihood of developing DM after COVID-19, especially in the first six months post-infection and in patients with more severe illness [19–22]. The probability of DM onset appears to increase with the intensity of the infection, with critically ill patients at the highest risk [23–25]. According to Xie et al. [21], certain groups, such as elderly individuals, Black patients, and those with conditions like cardiovascular disease, obesity, or hypertension, face a heightened risk of post-COVID-19 diabetes.

Our findings indicated that the blood sugar levels recorded at admission were strong indicators of future glycemic issues, highlighting the need for early blood sugar monitoring in patients hospitalized with COVID-19. Additionally, insulin resistance, measured using HOMA-IR, was a reliable predictor of elevated blood glucose, suggesting that individuals with higher resistance at the onset of illness are more prone to developing hyperglycemia. While the hyperinsulinemic–euglycemic clamp remains the gold standard for evaluating insulin sensitivity, HOMA-IR is widely used for its practicality [26–28]. Furthermore, hs-CRP, a marker of inflammation, was identified as a significant predictor of blood sugar imbalances in our study, reflecting the role of inflammation in the metabolic issues seen during COVID-19.

While Geetha et al. [29] have found no correlation between other inflammatory markers like ferritin, lactate dehydrogenase (LDH), and D-dimer with new-onset hyperglycemia, our data point to the importance of inflammation in glycemic control during the infection. Elevated hs-CRP levels indicate that the immune response triggered by the virus can interfere with normal glucose metabolism, worsening the condition in patients with COVID-19. Despite previous studies suggesting that the TyG index helps predict type 2 DM, it did not show predictive value for higher blood sugar in our cohort of COVID-19 patients. Park et al. [30] reported that both TyG and HOMA-IR were linked to an increased risk of DM, with TyG often being more accurate for early detection. However, our study found that markers like HOMA-IR and hs-CRP were more effective in predicting glycemic disturbances in COVID-19. Frailty has been associated with an increased risk of hospitalization in diabetic patients, and the combined effects of the SARS-CoV-2 pandemic and type 2 DM have been shown to contribute significantly to frailty. In this context, a study compared clinical and laboratory indices of frail and non-frail diabetic patients during the COVID-19 pandemic, as defined by the Edmonton Frail Scale scores. The results revealed significant differences between the frail and the non-frail groups in terms of blood urea, serum creatinine, eGFR, plasma albumin, TC, TG, HbA1c, mean platelet volume (MPV), and monocyte/lymphocyte ratio (MLR). These findings suggest that frailty in diabetic patients during COVID-19 can be linked to specific metabolic and inflammatory markers, whose determination is essential for managing both DM and frailty in this population [31].

Our research highlights the critical need for early blood sugar monitoring and using indicators such as HOMA-IR and hs-CRP to assess patients at risk of developing glycemic complications during COVID-19. Although the TyG index is valuable in other contexts, it appears less effective in predicting hyperglycemia during COVID-19 than markers like HOMA-IR and inflammation levels. This approach can help healthcare providers better identify at-risk patients and intervene promptly to manage blood sugar and improve the recovery outcomes.

5. Conclusions

This research highlights the complex interplay between metabolic and inflammatory pathways in COVID-19 and underscores the potential benefits of early and targeted interventions. In addition to blood glucose at T0, HOMA-IR and hs-CRP significantly contribute to predicting blood glucose at T4 and T12; however, the TyG index does not have additional predictive power compared to these factors.

The study emphasizes the need for a multifaceted approach to managing COVID-19 patients, where understanding and monitoring the glycemic control play a central role. Tailoring interventions based on markers like blood glucose levels, HOMA-IR, and hs-CRP could lead to better outcomes. The findings also suggest that not all commonly used markers (like the TyG index) are universally applicable, highlighting the importance of context-specific research.

Additionally, the inflammatory marker hs-CRP was found to predict worse glycemic control in COVID-19 patients, reflecting how inflammation interacts with metabolic processes. On the other hand, markers like the TyG index, though beneficial in non-COVID-19 populations for predicting insulin resistance, do not hold the same predictive power in the context of COVID-19. This underscores the importance of context-specific research and intervention strategies.

In summary, COVID-19 exacerbates metabolic and inflammatory disturbances, making early and targeted interventions essential to managing glycemic control and mitigating the risk of complications like DM in post-COVID-19 recovery.

These findings underscore the intricate relationship between metabolic factors, inflammation, and glycemic control, particularly post-COVID-19 recovery. Monitoring and managing these parameters can provide valuable insights for predicting and mitigating the risk of DM onset and managing the blood glucose levels in post-COVID-19 patients. By leveraging this knowledge, healthcare providers can develop more effective, personalized treatment plans to improve patient outcomes.

Author Contributions: Conceptualization, M.A.; methodology, D.E.M.; software, D.C.N.; validation, S.D.; formal analysis, D.C.N.; investigation, D.E.M.; resources, S.D.; data curation, D.E.M.; writing—original draft preparation, M.A.; writing—review and editing, V.B. and S.D.; project administration, M.A. All authors have read and agreed to the published version of the manuscript.

Funding: We would like to acknowledge "Victor Babes" University of Medicine and Pharmacy of Timisoara, Romania for their support in covering the costs of publication for this research paper.

Institutional Review Board Statement: Ethics approval was obtained from the Ethics Committee for Scientific Research of the Cardiovascular Institute of Timisoara (ref. nr. 2193/25 March 2024). The study was conducted in accordance with the Declaration of Helsinki.

Informed Consent Statement: Written informed consent was obtained from all patients as part of the routine admission to our tertiary university hospital for future research and study purposes, before commencing the study.

Data Availability Statement: The data presented in this study are available on reasonable request from the corresponding author.

Conflicts of Interest: The authors declare no conflicts of interest.

Abbreviations

AIRglucose	Acute insulin response to glucose
ALP	Alkaline phosphatase
ALT	Alanine aminotransferase
ARDS	Acute respiratory distress syndrome
AST	Aspartate aminotransferase
BMI	Body mass index
BMP	Basic metabolic panel
BUN	Blood urea nitrogen
COVID-19	Coronavirus disease
DM	Diabetes mellitus
eGFR	Estimated glomerular filtration rate
Glyc-T0	Initial glycemia
Glyc-T4	Glycemia at the 4-month control
Glyc-T12	Glycemia at the 12-month control

HbA1c	Glycated hemoglobin
HDLc	HDL-cholesterol
HOMA-IR	Homeostasis Model Assessment of Insulin Resistance
hs-CRP	High-sensitivity C-reactive protein
LDH	Lactate dehydrogenase
LDLc	LDL-cholesterol
MLR	Monocyte/lymphocyte ratio
MPV	Mean platelet volume
PCR	Polymerase chain reaction
SARS-Cov-2	Severe acute respiratory syndrome coronavirus 2
TC	Total cholesterol
TG	Triglyceride
TyG	Triglyceride/Glucose
W/H	Waist/hip ratio

References

1. Huang, I.; Lim, M.A.; Pranata, R. Diabetes mellitus is associated with increased mortality and severity of disease in COVID-19 pneumonia—A systematic review, meta-analysis, and meta-regression. *Diabetes Metab. Syndr.* **2020**, *14*, 395–403. [CrossRef] [PubMed]
2. Kumar, A.; Arora, A.; Sharma, P.; Anikhindi, S.A.; Bansal, N.; Singla, V.; Khare, S.; Srivastava, A. Is diabetes mellitus associated with mortality and severity of COVID-19? A meta-analysis. *Diabetes Metab. Syndr.* **2020**, *14*, 535–545. [CrossRef] [PubMed]
3. Guo, L.; Shi, Z.; Zhang, Y.; Wang, C.; Do Vale Moreira, N.C.; Zuo, H.; Hussain, A. Comorbid diabetes and the risk of disease severity or death among 8807 COVID-19 patients in China: A meta-analysis. *Diabetes Res. Clin. Pract.* **2020**, *166*, 108346. [CrossRef]
4. Khunti, K.; Valabhji, J.; Misra, S. Diabetes and the COVID-19 pandemic. *Diabetologia.* **2023**, *66*, 255–266. [CrossRef]
5. Sathish, T.; Kapoor, N.; Cao, Y.; Tapp, R.J.; Zimmet, P. Proportion of newly diagnosed diabetes in COVID-19 patients: A systematic review and meta-analysis. *Diabetes Obes. Metab.* **2021**, *23*, 870–874. [CrossRef] [PubMed]
6. Sathish, T.; Tapp, R.J.; Cooper, M.E.; Zimmet, P. Potential metabolic and inflammatory pathways between COVID-19 and new-onset diabetes. *Diabetes Metab.* **2021**, *47*, 101204. [CrossRef]
7. Bornstein, S.R.; Rubino, F.; Khunti, K.; Mingrone, G.; Hopkins, D.; Birkenfeld, A.L.; Boehm, B.; Amiel, S.; Holt, R.I.; Skyler, J.S.; et al. Practical recommendations for the management of diabetes in patients with COVID-19. *Lancet. Diabetes Endocrinol.* **2020**, *8*, 546–550. [CrossRef]
8. Rahmati, M.; Keshvari, M.; Mirnasuri, S.; Yon, D.K.; Lee, S.W.; Il Shin, J.; Smith, L. The global impact of COVID-19 pandemic on the incidence of pediatric new-onset type 1 diabetes and ketoacidosis: A systematic review and meta-analysis. *J. Med. Virol.* **2022**, *94*, 5112–5127. [CrossRef] [PubMed]
9. Riddle, M.C.; Buse, J.B.; Franks, P.W.; Knowler, W.C.; Ratner, R.E.; Selvin, E.; Wexler, D.J.; Kahn, S.E. COVID-19 in People With Diabetes: Urgently Needed Lessons From Early Reports. *Diabetes Care* **2020**, *43*, 1378–1381. [CrossRef]
10. Norouzi, M.; Norouzi, S.; Ruggiero, A.; Khan, M.S.; Myers, S.; Kavanagh, K.; Vemuri, R. Type-2 Diabetes as a Risk Factor for Severe COVID-19 Infection. *Microorganisms* **2021**, *9*, 1211. [CrossRef]
11. Vasbinder, A.; Anderson, E.; Shadid, H.; Berlin, H.; Pan, M.; Azam, T.U.; Khaleel, I.; Padalia, K.; Meloche, C.; O'Hayer, P.; et al. ISIC Study Group, Inflammation, Hyperglycemia, and Adverse Outcomes in Individuals with Diabetes Mellitus Hospitalized for COVID-19. *Diabetes Care* **2022**, *45*, 692–700. [CrossRef] [PubMed]
12. Sabri, S.; Bourron, O.; Phan, F.; Nguyen, L.S. Interactions between diabetes and COVID-19: A narrative review. *World J. Diabetes* **2021**, *12*, 1674–1692. [CrossRef] [PubMed]
13. Zahedi, M.; Kordrostami, S.; Kalantarhormozi, M.; Bagheri, M. A Review of Hyperglycemia in COVID-19. *Cureus* **2023**, *15*, e37487. [CrossRef] [PubMed]
14. Santos, A.; Magro, D.O.; Evangelista-Poderoso, R.; Saad, M.J.A. Diabetes, obesity, and insulin resistance in COVID-19: Molecular interrelationship and therapeutic implications. *Diabetol. Metab. Syndr.* **2023**, *13*, 23. [CrossRef]
15. Ren, H.; Yang, Y.; Wang, F.; Yan, Y.; Shi, X.; Dong, K.; Yu, X.; Zhang, S. Association of the insulin resistance marker TyG index with the severity and mortality of COVID-19. *Cardiovasc. Diabetol.* **2020**, *19*, 58. [CrossRef]
16. Chee, Y.J.; Ng, S.J.H.; Yeoh, E. Diabetic ketoacidosis precipitated by Covid-19 in a patient with newly diagnosed diabetes mellitus. *Diabetes Res. Clin. Pract.* **2020**, *164*, 108166. [CrossRef]
17. Fadini, G.P.; Morieri, M.L.; Longato, E.; Avogaro, A. Prevalence and impact of diabetes among people infected with SARS-CoV-2. *J. Endocrinol. Investig.* **2020**, *43*, 867–869. [CrossRef]
18. Alizargar, J.; Bai, C.H.; Hsieh, N.C.; Wu, S.V. Use of the triglyceride-glucose index (TyG) in cardiovascular disease patients. *Cardiovasc. Diabetol.* **2020**, *19*, 8. [CrossRef] [PubMed]
19. Park, H.M.; Lee, H.S.; Lee, Y.J.; Lee, J.H. The triglyceride-glucose index is a more powerful surrogate marker for predicting the prevalence and incidence of type 2 diabetes mellitus than the homeostatic model assessment of insulin resistance. *Diabetes Res. Clin. Pract.* **2021**, *180*, 109042. [CrossRef]

20. Kim, S.H.; Arora, I.; Hsia, D.S.; Knowler, W.C.; LeBlanc, E.; Mylonakis, E.; Pratley, R.; Pittas, A.G. New-Onset Diabetes After COVID-19. *J. Clin. Endocrinol. Metab.* **2023**, *108*, e1164–e1174. [CrossRef]
21. Xie, Y.; Al-Aly, Z. Risks and burdens of incident diabetes in long COVID: A cohort study. *Lancet. Diabetes Endocrinol.* **2022**, *10*, 311–321. [CrossRef] [PubMed]
22. Estiri, H.; Strasser, Z.H.; A Brat, G.; Semenov, Y.R.; Patel, C.J.; Murphy, S.N. Evolving Phenotypes of non-hospitalized Patients that Indicate Long COVID. *BMC Med.* **2021**, *19*, 249. [CrossRef] [PubMed]
23. Daugherty, S.E.; Guo, Y.; Heath, K.; Dasmariñas, M.C.; Jubilo, K.G.; Samranvedhya, J.; Lipsitch, M.; Cohen, K. Risk of clinical sequelae after the acute phase of SARS-CoV-2 infection: Retrospective cohort study. *BMJ* **2021**, *373*, n1098. [CrossRef]
24. Birabaharan, M.; Kaelber, D.C.; Pettus, J.H.; Smith, D.M. Risk of new-onset type 2 diabetes in 600 055 people after COVID-19: A cohort study. *Diabetes Obes. Metab.* **2022**, *24*, 1176–1179. [CrossRef]
25. Zhang, J.; Shu, T.; Zhu, R.; Yang, F.; Zhang, B.; Lai, X. The Long-Term Effect of COVID-19 Disease Severity on Risk of Diabetes Incidence and the Near 1-Year Follow-Up Outcomes among Postdischarge Patients in Wuhan. *J. Clin. Med.* **2022**, *11*, 3094. [CrossRef]
26. Turner, R.C.; Holman, R.R.; Matthews, D.; Hockaday, T.D.; Peto, J. Insulin deficiency and insulin resistance interaction in diabetes: Estimation of their relative contribution by feedback analysis from basal plasma insulin and glucose concentrations. *Metab. Clin. Exp.* **1979**, *28*, 1086–1096. [CrossRef]
27. Matthews, D.R.; Hosker, J.P.; Rudenski, A.S.; Naylor, B.A.; Treacher, D.F.; Turner, R.C. Homeostasis model assessment: Insulin resistance and beta-cell function from fasting plasma glucose and insulin concentrations in man. *Diabetologia* **1985**, *28*, 412–419. [CrossRef] [PubMed]
28. Shashaj, B.; Luciano, R.; Contoli, B.; Morino, G.S.; Spreghini, M.R.; Rustico, C.; Sforza, R.W.; Dallapiccola, B.; Manco, M. Reference ranges of HOMA-IR in normal-weight and obese young Caucasians. *Acta Diabetol.* **2016**, *53*, 251–260. [CrossRef]
29. Geetha, H.S.; Singh, G.; Sekar, A.; Gogtay, M.; Singh, Y.; Abraham, G.M.; Trivedi, N. Hyperglycemia in COVID-19 infection without diabetes mellitus: Association with inflammatory markers. *World J. Clin. Cases* **2023**, *11*, 1287–1298. [CrossRef]
30. Park, B.; Lee, H.S.; Lee, Y.J. Triglyceride glucose (TyG) index as a predictor of incident type 2 diabetes among nonobese adults: A 12-year longitudinal study of the Korean Genome and Epidemiology Study cohort. *Transl. Res. J. Lab. Clin. Med.* **2021**, *228*, 42–51. [CrossRef]
31. Tel, B.M.A.; Bilgin, S.; Kurtkulagi, O.; Kahveci, G.; Duman, T.T.; Sagdic, T.; Aktas, G. Frailty in Diabetic Subjects during COVID-19 and Its Association with HbA1c, Mean Platelet Volume and Monocyte/Lymphocyte Ratio. *Clin. Diabetol.* **2022**, *11*, 119–126. [CrossRef]

MDPI AG
Grosspeteranlage 5
4052 Basel
Switzerland
Tel.: +41 61 683 77 34

Biomedicines Editorial Office
E-mail: biomedicines@mdpi.com
www.mdpi.com/journal/biomedicines

www.ingramcontent.com/pod-product-compliance
Lightning Source LLC
Chambersburg PA
CBHW061812210926
51850CB00006B/677
9783725850952